PHYSICAL AGENTS

A Comprehensive Text for Physical Therapists

PHYSICAL AGENTS

A Comprehensive Text for Physical Therapists

Bernadette Hecox, PT, MA
Associate Professor in Clinical Physical Therapy, Retired
Program in Physical Therapy
Columbia University
New York, New York

Tsega Andemicael Mehreteab, PT, MS
Clinical Associate Professor
Department of Physical Therapy
School of Education
New York University
New York, New York

Joseph Weisberg, PT, PhD
Dean
Barry Z. Levine School of Health Sciences
Touro College
Dix Hills, New York

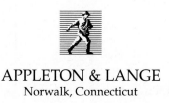

APPLETON & LANGE
Norwalk, Connecticut

Copyright © 1994 by Appleton & Lange
Simon & Schuster Business and Professional Group

94 95 96 97 98 / 10 9 8 7 6 5 4 3 2

Prentice Hall International (UK) Limited, *London*
Prentice Hall of Australia Pty. Limited, *Sydney*
Prentice Hall Canada, Inc., *Toronto*
Prentice Hall Hispanoamericana, S.A., *Mexico*
Prentice Hall of India Private Limited, *New Delhi*
Prentice Hall of Japan, Inc., *Tokyo*
Simon & Schuster Asia Pte., Ltd., *Singapore*
Editora Prentice Hall do Brasil Ltda., *Rio de Janeiro*
Prentice Hall, *Englewood Cliffs, New Jersey*

Library of Congress Cataloging-in-Publication Data

Hecox, Bernadette.
    Physical agents : a comprehensive text for physical therapists /
Bernadette Hecox, Joseph Weisberg, Tsega Andemicael Mehreteab.
        p.   cm.
    ISBN 0–8385–8040–8
    1. Physical therapy.   I. Weisberg, Joseph.   II. Andemicael
Mehreteab, Tsega.   III. Title.
    [DNLM: 1. Physical Therapy—methods. WB 460 H449p 1993]
RM700.H43 1993
615.8′2—dc20
DNLM/DLC
for Library of Congress   93–4700
                                                            CIP

Acquisitions Editor: Cheryl Mehalik
Production Editor: Sondra Greenfield
Designer: Michael J. Kelly
Cover Designer: Kathy Hornyak

PRINTED IN THE UNITED STATES OF AMERICA

ISBN 0-8385-8040-8
9 780838 580400
90000

This book is dedicated to the memory of our friend, coauthor and colleague, Diana Fond. Diana's contribution to this book is interwoven in each page. She was a team member of the Physical Agents Review Committee (PARC) since its inception. She contributed not only her knowledge of the subject matter but also her ability to keep us organized and on track. Her thoughtfulness, encouragement, and warm sense of humor helped us to finish this multiyear project.

Diana was a wonderful person, educator and clinician whose desire for excellence in the physical therapy profession we will always remember. Her untimely death is a loss to the profession. We miss her; we love her.

CONTENTS

FOREWORD

All those who contributed to this book have been physical agents instructors in schools of physical therapy in the New York City area. Five such schools are situated within a subway ride of one another. Several years ago, the instructors from these five schools began meeting to discuss problems and share ideas about the physical agents used in physical therapy.

We soon discovered that we shared similar problems and decided to organize as a group to work toward solving some of them. We called ourselves the Physical Agents Review Committee (PARC). As a result of a questionnaire sent to all schools of physical therapy in the United States, we discovered that our problems were similar to those of other instructors. This book evolved from our work as members of the committee.

One major problem that confronted all of us was the difficulty of finding reading material for our students that not only contained the appropriate content but also was written in an educationally sound manner. In many cases, we were forced to consult books and journals published for members of other disciplines such as anatomy, physiology, and physics to obtain pertinent background information. In many cases, these sources were extremely difficult to read. Thus, we decided to write a book that contained the information we all agreed was essential and appropriate for our own work and would be useful for others as well.

Bernadette Hecox
Associate Professor in Clinical Physical Therapy (retired)
Columbia University

PREFACE

This text includes all the modalities that are commonly discussed in entry-level physical agents courses. It covers the topics and has the depth of information that we, the authors, consider to be appropriate for such a course. We believe the book can serve the needs of those who teach students about physical agents, entry-level students in physical therapy and in assistant physical therapy programs, and clinicians who use the modalities or plan to conduct research projects in this area.

We have chosen to cover many and varied physical agents in this text. As all physical therapists know, physical agents can be beneficial to patients as treatments in themselves or as adjuncts to other techniques such as massage, joint mobilization, or therapeutic exercise within a total treatment program. We have based our choice of agents on the guidelines of the American Physical Therapy Association, which state that the practice of physical therapy

> includes but is not limited to the use of physical agents: heat, cold, water, air, sound, compression, electricity, and electromagnetic radiation [along with] other physical measures . . . [to] detect, assess, prevent, correct, alleviate, and limit physical disability, bodily malfunction and pain from injury, disuse, and any other bodily and mental conditions.

Thus, we cover numerous physical agents, including heat, cold, light, water, ultrasound, electrotherapy of all types, and special techniques such as traction. In our opinion, it is essential for students and clinicians to understand the use of these physical agents fully to fulfill their responsibilities.

The book discusses the physics, biophysics, anatomy, and physiology required to explain how each physical agent affects the human body. It also provides guidelines for the application of these modalities and describes recent changes in their application resulting from the advent of newer equipment or from experimental data that validate or invalidate specific treatment theories and techniques. We have found that the techniques outlined in the book, although satisfactory, are by no means the only ways to administer treatment.

The book is divided into six sections. Section I reviews basic information on how the human body responds to the various modalities. Section II presents all the thermal agents that are commonly used in physical therapy. Section III discusses the hydrotherapy modalities that are generally used today and briefly describes modalities that are popular in other countries but are used less frequently in the United States. Section IV covers the uses of therapeutic electricity and electrophysiologic testing procedures. Section V discusses other physical agents such as ultraviolet light and traction. The final section, Section VI, contains two chapters: the first chapter contains clinical problems for review; the second offers suggestions for laboratory experiments.

We have attempted to write the book using a simple and clear format. Information that is appropriate for entry-level students has been carefully selected, and the content is presented in a practical manner. To help the student follow the content better, we have repeated some information in several chapters or referred to other chapters where background information can be found.

Finally, we have included information that supplements or clarifies the text of the chapter. For example, some chapters contain problem-solving questions that pertain directly to the practice of physical therapy. We expect that a two-semester course is necessary to cover the contents of the book thoroughly. However, instructors can easily modify or select topics they wish to cover in a one-semester course for physical therapy students or in a program for physical therapy assistants.

Bernadette Hecox
Tsega Andemicael Mehreteab
Joseph Weisberg

CONTRIBUTORS

Mary Jane Day, PT, MS
Assistant Professor in Clinical Physical Therapy
Program in Physical Therapy
Columbia University
New York, New York

Diana Fond, PT, MA
Instructor
Department of Physical Therapy
School of Education
New York University
New York, New York

Lynn Geisel, PT, BS
Research and Program Coordinator
Department of Rehabilitation Medicine
Rusk Institute
New York University Medical Center
New York, New York

Bernadette Hecox, PT, MA
Associate Professor in Clinical Physical Therapy (retired)
Program in Physical Therapy
Columbia University; New York, New York

Andrew L. McDonough, PT, MS
Clinical Associate Professor and Director
Department of Physical Therapy
School of Education
New York University
New York, New York

Tsega Andemicael Mehreteab, PT, MS
Clinical Associate Professor
Department of Physical Therapy
School of Education
New York University
New York, New York

Arthur Nelson, Jr., PT, PhD
Professor
Department of Physical Therapy
School of Education
New York University
New York, New York

Dina Fine Rhodes, PT, MA
Former Assistant Director
EMG Biofeedback Department
International Center for the Disabled
New York, New York

Ronald W. Sweitzer, PT, MS
Director
Pleasantville Physical Therapy & Sports Care PC
Lecturer
Program in Physical Therapy
Hunter College
New York, New York

Joseph Weisberg, PT, PhD
Dean
Barry Z. Levine School of Health Sciences
Touro College
Dix Hills, New York

ACKNOWLEDGMENTS

This book could not have been completed without the understanding and support of our many friends and colleagues. We especially want to thank our students, whose inquisitiveness challenged and inspired us to write this book.

My deepest thanks to the many students who commented on my original class handouts or shared the references from their master's thesis with me, to the faculty and staff of the physical therapy and occupational therapy programs at Columbia University for the countless ways they helped, to Dr Dan Lemons and Dr Shu Chien for their input and reviewing of the Thermal and Circulatory Physiology sections, to Douglas Westfeld and Kate Harrigan for being both photographers and models, to Harriet Ayers for making midnight hours at the word processor pleasant, and to all my family members and friends for enabling me to sustain a sense of humor.

Bernadette Hecox

I would like to acknowledge my husband, Ammanuel, for his tireless support throughout the development of this text and for his invaluable assistance in designing my computer-generated diagrams. Special thanks also to my students for their constant feedback throughout this endeavor and to my sons, Hagos and Berhe, for their understanding and patience.

Tsega Andemicael Mebreteab

I wish to thank my wife, Rina, and my children, Arel, Yaron, Orah, and Yael, for their support and understanding. Special thanks to Les Schonbrun for his thorough review and suggestions and to my administrative staff for their assistance in typing my manuscript.

Joseph Weisberg

SECTION 1

APPROACHING
PHYSICAL AGENTS

Everyone who responsibly includes physical agents as part of a treatment program must have an understanding of related physical, biological and psychological information. Prerequisite courses required for any students entering physical therapy programs include general courses containing this information.

This section includes a few topics selected from these general courses that are especially meaningful to clinicians who include physical agents in their treatment programs. Each chapter reviews information on one topic focusing on factors related to physical therapy treatments in general and to physical agents in particular.

The topic of Chapter One is The Skin. Biological factors pertaining to the skin and its accessory organs, and the wound healing processes are reviewed. Skin conditions which are commonly observed when applying physical agents are described. The final part of the chapter applies some of this information directly to physical therapy procedures.

Chapter Two is a brief review of peripheral vascular and lymphatic circulations. Emphasis is on the role these systems play in controlling the temperature of local body tissues and general body temperature, and on the mechanisms which control the flow of blood and lymphatics through the body. The last part of the chapter gives examples of how this information can be applied when considering physical therapy procedures.

Chapter Three discusses *edema,* a condition frequently seen in patients receiving physical agents treatments. It includes information about the causes and various types of edema, and considerations concerning physical therapy intervention.

Chapter Four discusses *pain/spasms,* both the physical and psychological components. These signs and symptoms are perhaps seen more than any others in physical therapy. Former pain theories are reviewed briefly to help the reader relate to the theories presently being considered, which are discussed in more detail. Information concerning the conditions called "spasms" is given as well as the relationship between pain and spasms.

Chapter Five reviews the *electro-magnetic spectrum* and electro-magnetic theories. Frequencies, wave lengths and depth of penetration into the body must be considered for many physical agents, especially the radiation therapies and Short Wave Diathermy. The basic laws of radiated energy included in this chapter will be referred to in future chapters, especially the Infrared, Ultraviolet and Microwave chapters.

The intention of including these background information chapters is to avoid redundancy in future chapters. The many chapters which would otherwise need to include this information may only summarize and refer the reader to the chapter in this section that contains more detailed information.

1

Skin

Andrew L. McDonough, PT, MS

S kin is the largest organ of the body, representing approximately two square meters of surface area in the mature adult.[1] Skin consists of layers of tissue, through which underlying structures can be treated with various modalities. This chapter describes the structural and functional aspects of the skin and related structures and discusses some common skin conditions and diseases that physical therapists should be aware of when treating patients with physical agents. Knowledge of the structure and function of the skin and the effect of physical agents on the skin will help the therapist determine the efficacy of various modalities. It also will permit the modification of treatment regimens if changes are observed in the condition of the skin.

STRUCTURE AND FUNCTION

The basic structure of the skin includes a thin layer of epithelial cells overlying a mesh of connective tissue (Fig. 1–1). The average thickness of the skin is 1 to 2 mm; however, its thickness can range from 0.5 mm in the eyelids to as much as 5 mm in the interscapular region.[2] Thicker skin (eg, bunions) may develop over areas that are subjected to excessive mechanical stresses. Accessory organs (eg, hair follicles, sweat glands, receptors) are supported and protected by the enveloping skin.

Skin has a variety of interrelated physiological and mechanical functions: protection, sensation, and regulation.

Protection. The skin protects against infection by acting as an important intermediary between the environment and other organs. In addition, it retains or excludes fluid, primarily water, by a layer of waterproof keratin, a waxlike substance located in the most superficial layer of the epidermis. The barrier function of the

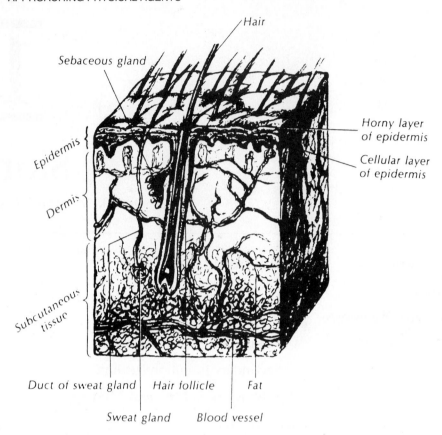

Figure 1–1. Diagrammatic section of the skin showing the epidermis, dermis, subcutaneous tissue, and structures that it envelops (eg, hair follicles, sweat glands, neuroreceptors, and blood vessels). (*Reproduced, with permission from Bates B.* A Guide to Physical Examination and History Taking, *4th ed. Philadelphia, Pa: JB Lippincott. 1987:134.*)

skin can be appreciated when some or all of the skin is lost through burn injury. In such instances, water lost to the outside environment may lead to significant, sometimes life-threatening, alterations in concentrations of electrolytes.[3]

Sensation. Sensory function can be attributed to the skin because it serves as the interface between the outside environment and the afferent nervous system. Several types of receptors that react to physical stimuli are embedded in the skin. Because these receptors signal the patient regarding physical agents applied to the surface, they are important factors in determining the tolerance of such modalities.

Regulation. The skin regulates body temperature and fluid balance by working in conjunction with the circulatory system. When heat must be conserved, the skin insulates the body with an underlying layer of fat. When excess heat must be removed to avoid a potentially catastrophic rise in core temperature, sweat glands are activated to liberate heat.

GENERAL APPEARANCE

The general appearance of the skin yields important information about its health and the function of underlying organs. For example, increased amounts of hair suggest a disturbance of sex hormones.[4] Thick coarse hair situated over the spine may indicate the failure of the vertebral column to close during development, as in spina bifida.[5]

Many pathologies can cause atrophy of the skin (loss of substance). The most common cause of skin atrophy is the occlusion of small arteries. The degree of atrophy depends on the amount of oxygen deprivation relative to the oxygen requirements of the tissue. Sweat glands, hair follicles, and neurons cannot tolerate a low concentration of oxygen and will atrophy first. Fibroblasts, the primary cells of connective tissue, can tolerate relatively low concentrations of oxygen and will be affected the least. Oxygen deprivation causes skin to be shiny, dry, and hairless. This type of skin is easily damaged and heals extremely slowly. These manifestations are often seen in the lower limbs of patients with diabetes and related peripheral vascular diseases.[6]

The color and texture of the skin suggests metabolic or mechanical disorders such as the following:

- *Jaundiced* (yellow) skin is often associated with liver or gallbladder disease, whereas bronze skin may be symptomatic of glandular disorders.[2]
- *Cyanosis* (bluish color) is associated with diminished or absent circulation or decreased concentrations of oxygen in the blood, whereas the blackened, apparently charred, skin associated with gangrenous lesions indicates a total absence of blood supply.
- *Erythema* (reddened skin) secondary to dilation and congestion of superficial vessels may be a response to a heightened emotional state (eg, blushing) or to thermal injury (eg, mild sunburn).
- *Mottled erythema* refers to harmful reactions to infrared radiation. White patches interspersed with vivid red blotches warn that a burn is likely to occur.[7] The mottling is the result of a vasomotor response manifested by dilation of capillaries in the dermis.
- *Erythema ab Igne* is a persistent erythema and pigmentation produced by long-term exposure to excessive nonburning heat. This type of erythema begins as a mottling caused by local hemostasis and becomes a meshlike erythema that leaves pinkish-rose or dark purplish-brown patches.[8]
- *Blisters*, vesicles of fluid that collect between the layers of skin, or smaller vesicles called *blebs*, may indicate damage caused by burns. For example, blistering of the skin, among other factors, distinguishes first- from second-degree burns. Blisters also may suggest increased mechanical stress: for example, when skin rubs against poorly fitting shoes.
- *Decubitus ulcers* (sores) indicate compression or shear stress to skin over bony prominences resulting from prolonged periods of immobilization, especially when cutaneous sensation is impaired or absent.
- *Wheals*, or hives, are localized pruritic (itchy) skin eruptions caused by a histamine reaction that is usually brought on by allergic responses to certain foods, insect bites, or inhaled substances such as pollen or mold spores. Minor irritations such as those caused by severe heat, intense itching, or rough massage may produce temporary local wheals.
- *Rashes* may be associated with primary disease of the skin or may be caused by local or systemic allergic or autoimmune responses. For example, the peculiar "butterfly" rash over the bridge of the nose caused by deposits of antibodies (immunoglobulins and other compounds) is common in systemic lupus erythematosus.[9]

Conversely, certain localized patches such as freckles, birthmarks, and "age spots" are usually physiologically inconsequential.[10]

GROSS AND MICROSCOPIC STRUCTURE

The skin consists of two layers: a multicellular epidermis and a dense, irregular, underlying layer of connective tissue called the dermis or corium (Fig. 1–1). The *epidermis* is derived from ectoderm and may include two or as many as five strata of cells, the thickness of which vary over different body areas.[11] Different modalities have their primary effect on different strata: for example, the primary effect of ultraviolet light occurs in the two deepest layers of epidermis, whereas resistance to electrical current occurs primarily in the most superficial layers.

Epidermis

Most of the cells that make up the epidermis are of the epithelial type. *Melanocytes* represent a second cell type and are found principally in the deepest two layers of the epidermis (stratum malpighi) and produce melanin, a pigment that imparts a tannish to blackish color to the skin. A third, less numerous cell type is the *Langerhans cell.*[3] This irregularly shaped cell with an indented nuclei is probably a form of macrophage (phagocyte) and thus is a component of the immune system.

The following five layers of cells may be present in the epidermis (listed in order from deepest to most superficial): basale, spinosum, granulosum, lucidum, and corneum (Figs. 1–1 and 1–2). The two deepest layers, basal and spinosum, col-

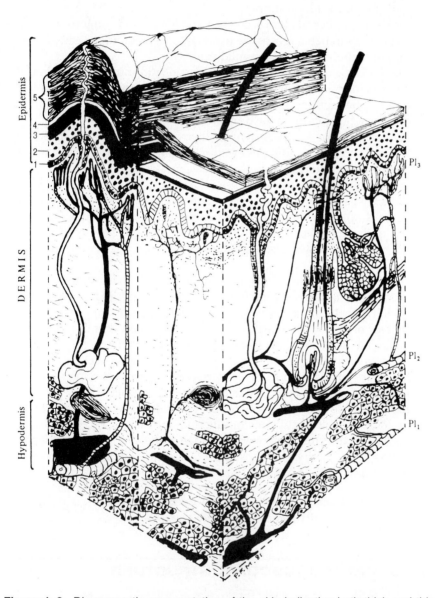

Figure 1–2. Diagrammatic representation of the skin indicating both thick and thin skin (not to scale). Five layers of cells in the epidermis: 1 = basale; 2 = spinosum; 3 = granulosum; 4 = lucidum; 5 = corneum. Pl_{1-3} = levels of the three plexuses of blood vessels. (*Reproduced, with permission from Millington PF, Wilkinson R. Skin. New York: Cambridge University Press. 1983: frontispiece*).

lectively known as the *stratum malpighi,* have well-developed nuclei and are the most viable layers. The remaining, more superficial layers show progressively less cellular vitality. This is especially true of the most superficial layer, the stratum corneum.

Stratum malpighi. The deepest layer of the stratum malpighi, the *stratum basale,* also called the stratum germinativum, is a single layer of high cuboidal to low columnar cells that are anchored to a basement membrane (Figs. 1–2 and 1–3). The nuclei of these cells tend to be oval and eccentrically located in the cytoplasm, usually close to the basement membrane. The mitotic figures often seen in this layer indicate a reproductively active stratum. In addition to a well-defined nucleus, a large number of ribosomes are found, indicating an active capacity to synthesize protein. The basal cells abut one another and are connected to their neighbors by a series of interdigitating cytoplasmic processes.

The overlying layer of the stratum malpighi, the *stratum spinosum,* is several cell layers thick and consists of cells that vary in shape from cuboidal to columnar in the lower regions to polygonal to squamous in more superficial layers (Fig. 1–3). These cells are bound together by cytoplasmic processes that appear, under high magnification, as "spines" (spinosum), suggesting a layer of spiny or prickle cells.[4]

Superficial layers. The deepest of the three more superficial layers of the epidermis, the *stratum granulosum,* is usually two to five cell-layers thick. These cells begin to take on a more elongated and flattened appearance (Fig. 1–3). The fact that fewer interdigitating processes are found in this layer than in the other two layers suggests reduced intercellular communication and, accordingly, less cellular vitality. Some dead cells also are found in this layer. Keratohyalin granules, produced in this stratum, ascend to the stratum corneum (keratinization) and exclude or retain water.[2]

The optically clear layer called *stratum lucidum* is typically three to five cell layers thick (Fig. 1–2). These cells lack nuclei and the cell borders are poorly defined. The cytoplasm has a semifluid consistency and contains eleidin, a compound believed to be a transformation product of keratohyalin.[2]

The most superficial layer of cells, the *stratum corneum,* is a translucent stratum that consists of many layers of dead cells that are periodically sloughed. Also known as the stratum disjunctivum, the cytoplasm in this layer of cells is replaced by "soft keratin," a product of the keratinization process that transforms epithelial cells into hardened scales and gives skin its characteristic waterproofing properties.[2] Subsequent hardening of and reduction of fluid in this layer, especially in "thick" skin, increases resistance to electrical currents.[12,13] Finally, this configuration of scales excludes foreign bodies that might lead to infection.

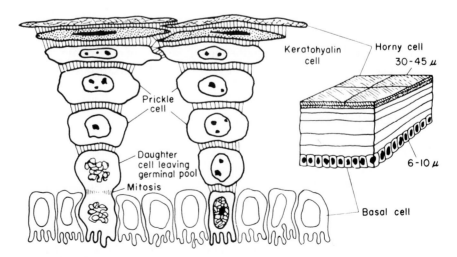

Figure 1–3. Diagrammatic section of the skin illustrating stratum spinosum "prickle cells." (*Adapted from Pinkus. In Handbuch der Haut- und Geschlech-tskrankheiten, Ergänzungswerk, 1, 2, 1965. Courtesy of Springer-Verlag.*)

Dermis

The dermis or corium is derived from mesoderm and is composed of two layers of irregular connective tissue called papillary and reticular layers. No clear demarcating line is noted between these layers. Dermis is usually 0.5 to 5 mm thick (Fig. 1–2).[4]

The uppermost layer, the *papillary layer*, which is usually thinner than the reticular layer, anchors the dermis to the overlying epidermis. It is essentially a layer of loose connective tissue composed primarily of collagen and some elastic fibers. Accessory skin organs are supported and maintained by this layer and by the underlying reticular layer.

The *reticular layer*, as its name suggests, is a meshwork (reticulum) of denser connective tissue composed of coarse collagen fibers and some elastic and reticular fibers. Some deep accessory organs such as hair follicles are found in this layer, and the muscles that control facial expression are inserted here.

Lines of tension created by movement of underlying joints tend to orient the collagen of the dermis parallel with these lines. This preferential orientation of collagen establishes a "grain" to the skin called Langer's lines. Surgical incisions made parallel with Langer's lines result in a cleanly cut wound that heals with minimal scarring. Incisions made transversely across Langer's lines result in gaping wounds with ragged edges that heal more slowly and result in thick, sometimes hypertrophic, scar formation; keloids—raised scars often seen in black skin—are such scars. Thick scars tend to concentrate wave energy that, if sufficiently intense, can cause burns.

THIN VERSUS THICK SKIN

In areas where the skin is subjected to substantial mechanical stress, it is strengthened and referred to as "thick" skin. Specific sites of thick skin include the soles and palms, the pads of the fingers and toes, and parts of the external genitalia.[2] The remainder of the body is covered with "thin" skin. (see Fig. 1–2)

Thick skin can be distinguished from thin skin in several ways. First, the epidermis of thick skin has five well-developed cell layers. The stratum corneum is usually well fortified with as many as 50 layers of keratinized cells. In thin skin, situated in less mechanically stressed areas (eg, the dorsal surface of the hand), one or more cell layers is absent. The stratum malpighi is always intact; however, the thickness of the stratum spinosum may be reduced. Second, the dermis of thick skin, in section, appears to be corrugated. A downward protrusion of the epidermis toward the dermis is called an epidermal (rete) peg, whereas an upward extension of the papillary layer toward the epidermis is called a dermal papilla. This arrangement of layers serves to strengthen thick skin in a manner that is similar to the way that corrugated cardboard is stronger than a flat piece of cardboard (Fig. 1–4).

ACCESSORY ORGANS

Hair follicles. During the third month of fetal development, a downward projection of epidermis invaginates the dermis. The space created by this action gives rise to a hair follicle (Fig. 1–5). In the deepest part of that cavity, a cluster of germinal matrix cells consolidates and gives rise to a hair.[4] Epithelial cells in the upper part of the follicle contribute to an external root sheath that connects with the surface of the skin. These cells nearest the surface are keratinized. Matrix cells also generate a tubular internal root sheath composed of soft keratin that extends part way up the follicle (Fig. 1–5).

Sebaceous glands. Associated with the hair follicles are *sebaceous glands*, oil-producing glands that drain into the upper part of the follicle or, occasionally, directly onto the skin surface (Fig. 1–5). *Sebum,* a fatty secretory product, is produced by the disintegration of cells lining the gland. This process is known as the holocrine

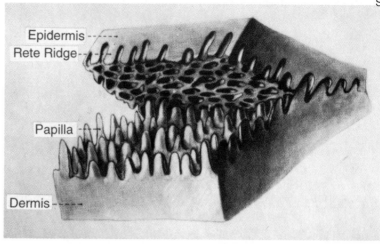

Figure 1–4. Vertical section of the skin showing the epidermal pegs and dermal papillae. (*Reproduced with permission from Copenhauer WM, Kelly DE, Wood RI. 8th ed.* Bailey's Textbook of Histology *Baltimore, Md: Williams & Wilkins. 1978:424.*)

mode of secretion.[2] Sebum coats and lubricates the hair shaft and the area adjacent to it as the shaft emerges from the skin. This protective coating prevents excess evaporation of water from the stratum corneum and probably acts to conserve heat. Prolonged exposure to water can reduce the amount of sebum on the skin.

Sebum is expressed from the gland onto the hair by contraction of the arrector pili muscle (Fig. 1–5). This bundle of smooth muscle fibers is attached to a sheath of connective tissue investing the hair shaft. After looping around the sebaceous gland, the arrector pili muscle inserts into the papillary layer of the dermis. When the muscle contracts, the gland is squeezed and its contents are expressed onto the hair shaft.[2] Excessive production of sebum, especially during puberty, leads to localized pockets of oil that are deposited on the skin. Subsequent bacterial infection may lead to acne. Male hormones (in adolescent males and females) apparently lead to a rapid turnover of glandular cells and overproduction of sebum.

Concurrent with its action on the sebaceous gland, the arrector pili muscle pulls the hair shaft into an erect or semierect position. Known as "gooseflesh" or "goosepimples," this action represents an attempt to trap a thin layer of air against the skin to prevent loss of heat to the outside environment. Because hair is sparsely distributed over the human body, this mechanism is relatively ineffective. Arrector pili muscles are not associated with the hairs of the beard or pubic regions; they also are not found in the eyelids, eyebrows, or eyelashes.

Sweat glands (see Fig. 1–1). Humans have two types of sweat glands: apocrine and eccrine. The apocrine glands are situated primarily in the axillary and genital regions. The eccrine (merocrine) glands are distributed throughout the body; large concentrations are found in the skin of the soles and palms.

Both the duct and the secretory parts of apocrine glands lie coiled in the dermis. Larger glands often extend deep into the hypodermis, subcutaneous connective tissue deep to the skin, also known as superficial fascia.[14] The lumen is lined with a layer of cuboidal or low columnar cells that continuously secrete small amounts of sweat into the hair follicle and, occasionally, directly onto the surface of the skin. Apocrine sweat glands, which are innervated by the autonomic nervous system, are activated primarily by emotional or painful stimuli.[2] At first, the sweat produced is odorless, but it is quickly contaminated and degraded by bacteria, causing its characteristic odor.

Eccrine sweat glands, excluding those found in the palms and soles, are activated by increased heat and are part of a thermoregulatory mechanism. The eccrine glands found in the palms and soles are activated primarily by changes in emotional state (eg, nervousness) rather than by the thermoregulatory apparatus. The secretory part of the gland is situated in the subcutaneous tissue space immediately below the dermis. A tortuous duct courses through both layers of the skin,

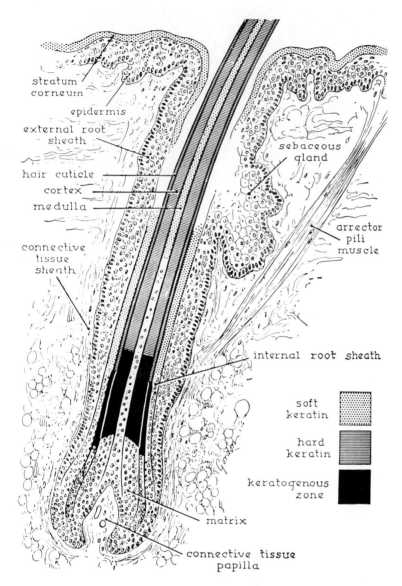

Figure 1–5. Diagram of a hair in a hair follicle showing adjacent structures. (*Reproduced with permission from Ham AW, Cormack DH, eds.* Histology, *8th ed. Philadelphia, Pa: JB Lippincott: 1979:630. Based on Leblond C: Ann NY Acad Sci. 1951;53:464.*)

delivering sweat directly to the surface. Eccrine glands are innervated by the sympathetic division of the autonomic nervous system, and most are linked to and controlled by the hypothalamus.[4] Electrical stimulation is used to treat excessively active sweat glands.

VASCULAR SUPPLY

The epidermis is an avascular layer of cells that relies on diffusion of fluids for sustenance.[11] Unlike the epidermis, the dermis (especially the papillary layer) has an extensive vascular supply. Arteries supplying this region extend from the hypodermis and reach upward toward and through the reticular layer. At this level, an arterial network that gives rise to capillary beds in the papillary layer is established. These capillaries are especially numerous near the stratum basale of the epidermis (Fig. 1–2).

The papillary layer of the dermis is drained by lymphatic capillaries lined with a single layer of endothelial cells. At the junction of these cells are fibrils that anchor the capillary to enveloping connective tissue and are tensed when excess fluid accumulates in the intercellular spaces. Tension on the fibrils forces the cellular junctions to open, permitting fluid to enter the lymphatic capillary. Accumulated fluid moves through progressively larger vessels that accompany veins in the hypodermis. These larger lymphatics become afferent ducts flowing toward lymph nodes that filter the collected fluid. Lymph is eventually collected by the thoracic duct, which ultimately joins the left brachycephalic vein.

TANNING AND COLORATION

Skin color results from a combination of factors, including the relative abundance of melanocytes and the presence of blood. Melanocytes produce *melanin* (brown or black granules) in the stratum malpighi. Blood is found in networks of vessels in the reticular layer and deeper aspects of the papillary layer of the dermis (Fig. 1–1).

Skin tanning is a protective mechanism against exposure to ultraviolet (UV) radiation, which stimulates the production of melanin in deeper strata. Melanin appears to ascend into the more superficial zones, causing a darkening of the skin. This tanning partially blocks penetration of UV radiation, thus reducing injury secondary to sunburn or other damaging effects of UV radiation.

Caucasian skin has relatively small concentrations of melanin in the deeper recesses of the stratum malpighi. Interspersed blood vessels impart a pinkish tinge to the skin. Darker skin contains more melanin, which is distributed more homogeneously throughout the epidermis. Increased concentrations of carotene account for the yellow tones characteristic of some Asians. *Albinism* refers to skin that is unable to produce melanin and therefore is unable to block the harmful effect of UV radiation.

NEURAL RECEPTORS

Because skin supports and maintains various types of *receptors,* it can be considered to be an integral part of the afferent (sensory) nervous system. Receptors in the epidermis, the dermis, and the hypodermis report various sensations. *Nociceptors* transmit sensations of pain, *thermoreceptors* are sensitive to changes in temperature, and *mechanoreceptors* report sensations of pressure, touch, vibration, or two-point discrimination (Fig. 1–6).[15] Although classification schemes for receptors differ, two general categories can be distinguished and are based in part on the status of encapsulation: free nerve endings, which are unencapsulated and unmyelinated as they approach the surface of the skin, and encapsulated (corpuscular) receptors, which have both myelinated and unmyelinated fibers (eg, Meissner's corpuscles, which are mechanoreceptors).[15] Table 1–1 summarizes the main receptors associated with the skin and indicates their sites and probable functions.

HEALING OF WOUNDS

Two types of wound healing can be distinguished. Simple incisions, which involve only minor loss of tissue and have edges that are close together, heal by "primary intention." Surgical incisions typically heal in this manner. Large gaping wounds, which are characterized by substantial removal or loss of tissue and widely separated ragged edges, heal by "secondary intention." The primary difference between the two types of wound healing is the type of wound created, not the ongoing physiologic processes, which are essentially the same.

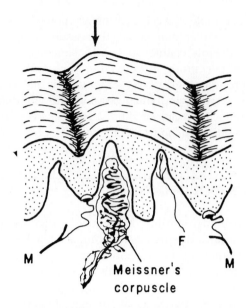

Figure 1–6. Neural receptors in the skin. (*Reproduced, with permission from Carpenter MB, Sutin J.* Human Neuroanatomy. *Baltimore, Md: Williams & Wilkins: 1983;162.*) (*Modified with permission from* Advances in Biology of Skin. (*Montagna W, ed. 1965:*) *Pergamon Press.*)

Primary Intention Healing

Immediately after injury or incision, blood fills the space between the apposed edges of the wound, forming a small clot. An acute inflammatory response ensues, the end stage of which represents the beginning of a reparative process. Twenty-four to 36 hours after the injury, epithelial cells from the cut edges of the adjacent epidermis migrate into the small cavity between the dermis and the previously formed clot to form a continuous sheet.[16] During the next 24 hours, epidermal cells migrate and invade the space where connective tissue will develop to complete the healing process. Next, rapid infiltration by capillary buds from the hypodermis and deposition of macrophages clear the area of debris. Vascularization of the wound facilitates the deposition of collagen fibers, which ultimately fill and repair the defect. The newly established tissue is strengthened through apparent bonding of adjacent collagen fibers. Eventually (within 6 to 12 months), the pinkish color imparted by vascularized tissue fades as vessels disintegrate and are reabsorbed. Over time, the

TABLE 1–1. NEURAL RECEPTORS OF THE SKIN

Receptor	Encapsulated?	Type*	Function	Location†	Distribution (approx.)
Free nerve ending	No	T,M,N	Pain Temperature	Ep, Dr	Entire body‡
Merkel's discs	No	M	Touch	Ep, Dr	Palms, soles§ Fingers (volar aspects)
Meissner's corpuscles	Yes	M	Touch 2-pt. Discrimination	Dr‖	Palms, soles§, fingers, toes (volar aspects), lips, eyelids, volar forearm, external genitalia
Pacinian corpuscles	Yes	M	Pressure Vibration	Hd	Hands, feet, penis, nipple
Golgi-Mazzoni corpuscles	Yes	M	Pressure Vibration	Hd	Fingers, tendons
Ruffini organs	No	M	Proprioception	Dr?, HD¶	Entire body, tendons, ligaments, joint capsules, deep fascia

*T = thermoreceptor, M = mechanoreceptor, N = nociceptor.
†Ep = epidermis, Dr = dermis, Hd = hypodermis.
‡Nonglabrous (hair-covered) surfaces.
§Glabrous (without hair) surfaces.
‖Near epidermis.
¶More prevalent in visceral structures.

size of the scar decreases, in part because of remodeling forces generated by mechanical stresses created by muscular contractions and motion of the joints.

Secondary Intention Healing

Healing by secondary intention initially involves an inflammatory period, followed by an ensuing reparative phase. First, a large clot fills the defect, consolidating and splinting the wound to cushion and protect it from further injury. Epidermal cells adjacent to the wound are then stimulated to migrate into the wound cavity between the clot above and the viable tissue below. Fibrolytic enzymes are apparently secreted by epidermal cells to break down necrotic tissue.[16] Debris is removed from the wound by an influx of phagocytes brought by capillaries that infiltrate the base of the wound from the hypodermis. The initial appearance of these cells as red dots or "granules" marks the emergence of granulation tissue. Although granulation tissue also forms in wound healing by primary intention, considerably more is laid down in open wounds and thus quantitatively distinguishes secondary from primary intention healing. With the onset of granulation, the epidermis continues to migrate, ultimately covering the granulation tissue and establishing a line of demarcation between the scab and the new tissue below. Eventually, the scab is sloughed at this line. Through regenerative processes (mitosis), the epidermis gradually thickens and begins to organize into a multilayered covering. Because the new epidermis is typically thinner than the original tissue it replaced, it is less able to withstand mechanical stress, thus providing the possibility for reinjury.

The resultant scar, a consolidation of dense randomly oriented collagen, is thicker and less compliant than the original tissue. Large thick scars may become moderately or severely distorted. Skin contractures may develop and may restrict underlying structures, especially joints. Excessive collagen accumulates in a scar, especially after a burn, and may lead to the formation of hypertrophic scar tissue. The collagen of these raised nodular areas is initially deposited in an unorganized manner, which results in a cosmetically unsightly mass that may limit movement of the skin, joints, or both.

Large scars, including keloids, are typically devoid of melanocytes and accessory skin organs, including hair follicles, sebaceous glands, and sweat glands. Cutaneous receptors also may be absent. The loss of melanin makes these tissues sensitive to exposure to UV radiation, which tends to be concentrated in the scar. Similarly, other forms of energy (eg, electricity) conducted over or through a scar may be concentrated and cause thermal damage to adjacent tissues.[13] Subsequent damage also may result secondary to lack of sensation in the affected area. Because patients may be unaware of excessive accumulation of energy that can lead to burns in a denervated area, they must limit their exposure to sunlight until scar formation can be reduced, cutaneous innervation regenerates, or both. Conversely, some physical agents, which will be discussed in later chapters, may hasten wound healing and reduce or prevent adhesions and excessive scarring.

APPLICATION TO PHYSICAL THERAPY

For clinicians, habitual observations of the appearance of their patients' skin is vital. This chapter has discussed skin conditions that are signs of health and others that are signs of local or systemic physical problems. When considering the use of physical agents, observing the condition of the patient's skin and understanding how the condition of the skin affects the results of treatment with various physical agents are especially important. Pretreatment observations may suggest that a particular physical agent is indicated, should be used cautiously, or should not be used at all. Generally applied principles can be drawn from the information provided in this chapter. The following examples illustrate how some skin conditions might affect treatments with physical agents.

BREAKS IN THE SKIN. Breaks in the skin may cause changes in the concentrations of electrolytes in body fluids or invite infections or cross contamination, including possible susceptibility to the human immunodeficiency virus (HIV). Such breaks may indicate that sterile techniques are necessary, especially **if hydro-therapy** is indicated. Areas with no skin (eg, a decubitus ulcer) have markedly less electrical resistance. Thus, when electrical modalities are used, current should be applied carefully over such areas because far less voltage is needed than is required over intact skin.

ROUGH OR THICK SKIN. Because the electrical resistance of rough or thick skin is greatly increased, such skin should be abraded. This will reduce the voltage needed to permit the flow of an electrical current.

THICK SCARS. Because energy tends to concentrate in scarred areas, diathermy and infrared, UV, microwave, and other radiation therapies should be used cautiously over these areas. If the areas are covered and protected, the treatment can be given to areas around rather than over the scar.

SENSORY RECEPTORS. Intact sensory receptors and nerves may contribute to the relief of symptoms and enable the patient to report whether the treatment dosage is intense enough to cause pain or tissue damage. If the sensory receptors are not intact, most thermal and electrical modalities should be used cautiously or not at all because the patient cannot report the intensity of the dosage.

GLANDS. Sebaceous glands lubricate the skin. Excessive use of water or radiation modalities tend to reduce the amount of sebum available and cause dryness. However, if the goal is to diminish the activity of the gland—for example, when treating acne—hydrotherapy or radiation may be useful. Overactive sweat glands can be treated with various unidirectional (galvanic) electrical modalities, which may retard sweating.

COLOR. Because bluish-black color of the skin indicates severe circulatory problems, heat therapies in that area are generally contraindicated. Sometimes, however, mild heat, if used cautiously, can be applied in an attempt to achieve a slight increase in blood flow to the area. Electrical stimulation that produces muscle contractions, thereby increasing blood flow, also is used.

The patient's skin color must be carefully noted before and after treatments. When using UV radiation, both the potentially beneficial and potentially harmful effects are related to the color of the skin being irradiated. The skin color of both the patient and the treating clinician must be considered. Therapists or patients with albinism should not be exposed to UV radiation.

After treatment, the condition of the patient's skin should again be noted. Therapists should be able to recognize and distinguish between normal, expectable changes and changes that indicate an overdose of treatment or abnormal reactions to treatment.

■   KEY TERMS

skin	stratum lucidum
jaundice	stratum corneum
cyanosis	**dermis (corium)**
erythema	papillary layer
blisters	reticular layer
blebs	**keloids**
wheals	**sebaceous glands**
hives	**sebum**
epidermis	**melanin**
stratum malpighi	**receptors**
stratum basal	nociceptors
stratum spinosum	thermoreceptors
stratum granulosum	mechanoreceptors

REFERENCES

1. Lockhart RD, Hamilton GF, Fyfe FW: *Anatomy of the Human Body.* Philadelphia, Pa: JB Lippincott; 1972.
2. Kelly DE, Wood RL, Enders, AC: *Bailey's Textbook of Histology.* 18th ed. Baltimore, Md: Williams & Wilkins; 1984.
3. Ham AW: Experimental study of histopathology of burns with particular reference to sites of fluid loss in burns of different depths. *Ann Surg.* 120:689, 1944.
4. Ham AW, Cormack DH: *Histology.* 8th ed. Philadelphia, Pa: JB Lippincott; 1979.
5. Salter RB: *Textbook of Disorders and Injuries of the Musculoskeletal System.* Baltimore, Md: Williams & Wilkins; 1983.
6. Burnside JW: *Physical Diagnosis.* 16th ed. Baltimore, Md: Williams & Wilkins; 1981.
7. Griffin J: *Physical Agents for Physical Therapists.* Springfield, Ill: Charles C Thomas; 1978.
8. Andrews G, Domonkas A: *Diseases of the Skin.* 5th ed. Philadelphia, Pa: WB Saunders; 1963.
9. Rodman GP, Schumacher R: *Primer on the Rheumatic Diseases.* 8th ed. Atlanta, Ga: Arthritis Foundation; 1983.
10. Robbins SL, Angell M, Kumer V: *Basic Pathology.* 3rd ed. Philadelphia, Pa: WB Saunders; 1981.
11. Gray H, Goss CM, eds: *Gray's Anatomy of the Human Body.* 29th ed. Philadelphia, Pa: Lea & Febiger; 1976.
12. Schriber WJ: *A Manual of Electrotherapy.* 4th ed. Philadelphia, Pa: Lea & Febiger; 1975.
13. Wolf SL, ed: *Electrotherapy.* New York: Churchill Livingstone; 1981.
14. Montagna W, Parakkal PF: *The Structure and Function of Skin.* 3rd ed. New York: Academic Press; 1974.
15. Carpenter MB, Sutin J: *Human Neuroanatomy.* 8th ed. Baltimore, Md: William & Wilkins; 1983.
16. Walter JB: *An Introduction to the Principles of Disease.* 2nd ed. Philadelphia, Pa: WB Saunders; 1982.

2

Peripheral Circulatory Systems

Bernadette Hecox, PT, MA

Many physical agents can affect the vascular or lymphatic systems of the peripheral circulation or both. Depending on the agent and the patient's status, the agents may be beneficial or harmful. This chapter reviews these systems as they apply to the use of the physical agents discussed in later chapters. It focuses on the circulation to skin, muscle, and bone.

PERIPHERAL VASCULAR SYSTEM

Blood leaves the heart through the arterial system and flows through arteries that continually branch and diminish in size. Eventually, the blood flows to the arterioles, the smallest arteries, and then to the capillary beds. At the capillary region, O_2 and other nutrients are dispersed to the tissues and CO_2 and other wastes enter the blood stream. This deoxygenated blood returns to the heart through the venous system:* first through the venules, the smallest veins; then from smaller to larger veins; and eventually joins the great veins, which carry the blood back to the heart. The blood flow continues through the pulmonary system to the lungs, where the wastes are exchanged for nutrients, then returns to the heart to repeat the cycle.

Control of Blood Flow

Control of blood flow is largely related to the circumference of the *lumen,* or hollow center, of blood vessels. The circumference can actively change through *vasoconstriction* and *vasodilation.* Narrowing or widening of the lumen can be the result

---

*Although venous blood is often called "deoxygenated" blood, this term is a misnomer in the purest sense because venous blood still contains O_2, but less of it than does arterial blood. For example, partial pressure of O_2 in arterial blood can be 95 mm Hg; in venous blood, it can be 40 mm Hg.[1]

of central nervous system control, local reactions, humoral control, or all of these mechanisms. The exact involvement of each is, as yet, not completely known.

Control by the central nervous system. The sympathetic branch of the autonomic system carries both vasoconstricting and vasodilating fibers. Chemical transmitters are released from the nerve endings at target areas. The adrenergic nerves release norepinephrine, which acts directly on the receptors of smooth muscle within the vessels to cause vasoconstriction. Normal vascular motor tone represents a continuous mild vasoconstriction. Cholinergic nerves release acetylcholine (ACh), which causes vessels to dilate. The specific action of ACh is not known: ACh may act to diminish the release of norepinephrine, thereby inhibiting constriction, or it may produce dilation directly.

Control by local reactions. Vasoactive agents released in local tissues, including histamine, bradykinin, and some of the prostaglandins, may act to dilate vessels or to affect the endothelial cells of the vessels directly. This activity of endothelial cells may leave gaps between cells, thereby increasing the permeability of the cell membrane. Histamine is released whenever tissues are damaged or are subjected to a noxious stimulus. Formation of bradykinin results from activation of precursor enzymes and may be related to the activity of sweat glands.

Humoral control. The humoral control of vasomotor tone refers to the effect of all the substances mentioned above as well as the effect of many other ions: These ions not only act locally but also travel in the blood stream. The concentration of ions in the blood stream affects vasomotor activity.[2,3]

Thermal Regulatory Function

The peripheral vascular system serves to regulate the temperature of both local tissues and the body. Two of the ways it accomplishes this are by transferring **heat** to and from vessels, other tissues, and the environment and by transferring **blood** through the peripheral circulatory systems and between the peripheral and other circulatory systems.

Heat Transfer

The peripheral vascular system is one major means by which loss and gain of body heat are controlled. Heat is transported by the circulating blood, and heat exchange occurs between blood and other tissues and/or the environment. The location and arrangement of the vessels also affects the distribution of body heat. Blood returns to the heart through both deep and superficial veins. The superficial veins located in the superficial fascia travel various courses before joining major veins. For example, the saphenous veins in the legs remain superficial until they join the deep femoral veins at the groin, and the cephalic veins in the arms are superficial until they join the axillary veins. In general, deep veins run parallel to the arteries (Fig. 2–1). The arrangement of two or more veins parallel to an artery is referred to as *venae comitantes*.[4] To some extent, this parallel position influences both core and tissue temperatures.

The blood leaving the heart is at approximately core temperature. Depending on the temperature of tissues, the environment, or both in the cutaneous capillary region, the incoming arterial blood may be warmer or cooler than the venous blood that is flowing in the opposite direction in veins adjacent to the arteries. For example, in a cold environment, blood leaving the capillaries, venous blood will be cooler than arterial blood. Until the temperature of the parallel veins and arteries is in equilibrium, some heat will transfer to the arteries or veins carrying the cooler blood, thus contributing to the maintenance of a constant core temperature.

This conductive transfer of heat (not blood) is termed *countercurrent exchange* (CCE). In hotter environmental conditions, more venous blood appears to be directed through superficial veins; in colder environmental conditions, it appears to be directed through the deep-lying venae comitas.[5] Fig. 2–2 illustrates the CCE that might occur in the arm (1) if the room temperature is 50° F (10° C), with more blood

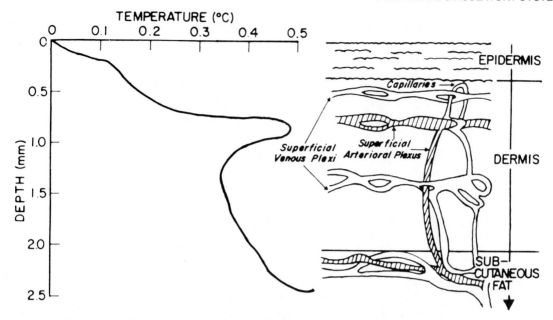

Figure 2–1. Diagrammatic rendering of the skin and subcutaneous circulation. On reaching the subcutaneous layer, the arteries and veins follow a similar course. (*Reproduced with permission from Carlson D, Loren D, and Hsieh, Arnold CL. Temperature and Humidity. In Slonim, NB ed.* Environmental Physiology. *St. Louis, Missouri: CV Mosby, 1974:70*).

flowing through the deeper veins, and (2) if the room temperature is 86° F (30° C), with more blood flowing through the superficial veins.

Heat transfer by conduction also occurs between the blood vessels and the tissues through which they pass. Usually, the deeper the tissues, the higher their temperature. Although the heat exchange with either adjacent vessels or other tissues is a factor in maintaining a constant core temperature, the exchange is limited because of the rapid velocity at which blood flows through any area. Heat exchange is especially limited in areas where the temperature gradient between either the adjacent vessels or other tissues is low.

Shunting Mechanisms

When the demand for blood to a particular area of the body is greater than the amount usually provided—eg, when the temperature of the tissues in that area is dangerously increased or decreased—the mechanism of *shunting* can occur. In general, shunting refers to the temporary closing or reduction of blood flow to one area of the body so that more blood can flow to another area that is in danger of being damaged. Three shunt mechanisms can be activated by thermal agents, fevers, or environmental conditions: anteriovenous (A-V) shunts, shunts from deeper systems to the cutaneous circulation, and shunts to and from different branches of the peripheral circulation. *A-V shunts (arteriovenous anastomosis)* involve specific vessels through which blood flows only under extreme hot or cold conditions. These shunts are described later in this chapter. The shunting of blood to the cutaneous circulation while reducing the flow to deeper circulatory systems brings more blood to the surface for cooling when the internal temperature is elevated. The shunting of blood to and from different branches of the peripheral circulation occurs, which is discussed more in Chapter 9.[6,7] In extremely hot weather, half of the total cardiac output is shunted from elsewhere to the skin.

Of interest to physical therapists is the evidence that branches to the superficial and deeper muscles are not derived from the same vessels. Vessels passing through superficial muscles are mainly the superficial capillaries and their terminal arterioles and venules, whereas the circulation to the underlying deep muscles is completely independent of the cutaneous circulation.[8] Thus, shunting does not occur between superficial and underlying muscles in a local area. Blood flow to

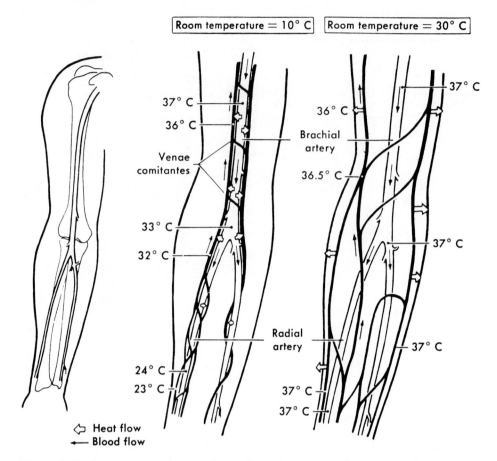

| Room temperature = 10° C | Room temperature = 30° C |

Heat flow
Blood flow

Figure 2–2. Countercurrent heat exchange in the human arm. Intravascular temperatures show that patterns of venous blood flow in the arm adjust to counteract thermal environmental stress. In the cold (10° C), venous blood flow is mainly through the deep venae comitantes, which receive heat from blood flowing out in the arteries and thereby minimize loss of body heat. In a warm environment (30° C), venous blood flow is mainly in superficial veins that, being close to the surface, increase the loss of body heat. Note the various courses of the veins situated in the superficial fascia and the parallel courses of the deep arteries and veins. (*Reproduced with permission from Frisancho AR.* Human Adaptation. *St. Louis, Missouri: CV Mosby Co, 1979:17*).

deep muscles appears to be directly related to their metabolic demands. An extremely low percentage of total blood flows through muscles at rest, but the percentage can increase 15- to 25-fold with exercise.[3]

Determinants of Arterial and Capillary Flow

Arterial Flow

The blood pressure and the amount of blood flow to the capillaries are determined by cardiac stroke volume and peripheral resistance. Factors controlling peripheral resistance include the size and pliability of arterial vessels and the integrity of the smooth muscles in these vessels. When the smooth muscles within the arteries and arterioles contract, the vessels constrict, which increases the peripheral resistance to blood flow, thus increasing the blood pressure. When these muscles relax, the vessels dilate, allowing more profuse flow and decreasing the blood pressure. When tissue metabolism increases, the vessels supplying those tissues dilate, thus increasing the amount of blood flow to the area necessary to meet its metabolic demands. Neural problems affecting the sympathetic nervous system or peripheral vascular diseases may alter the normal processes of constriction and dilation. For example, arteriosclerosis, which narrows the lumen of the arteries and renders them less pliable, prevents normal flow to the capillaries.

Capillary Flow

Capillaries, the vessels that connect the arterioles and venules, are composed of a single layer of endothelial cells surrounded by a more or less continuous basement membrane.[9] Metabolically, the endothelium is highly active and can synthesize or break down many chemical substances.[10] Variations in capillary structure are categorized according to the type of organs in which they are situated (ie, somatic or visceral) or by their histological appearance.[9] Because capillaries are microscopic in size, averaging 5 μm in diameter, blood cells must adapt in shape to pass through them.[10] One square inch of tissue may have as many as 1.5 million capillaries.[11] The diameter of each capillary is extremely small; however, if all the capillaries in one area were combined, their total area, taken in cross-section, would be far greater than the cross-section of the large arteries and veins for which they are connecting channels.

The capillary membrane is semipermeable, allowing the O_2 and nutrients in arterial blood to be transported through this membrane to the interstitial fluid and hence to body cells. CO_2 and wastes are transported in the opposite direction and return to the heart through venous and lymphatic vessels.

The transport of blood gases such as O_2 and CO_2 across capillary membranes occurs by diffusion. Water and small solutes such as glucose and amino acids pass through intercellular clefts between endothelial cells. Proteins, which are large water solutes, are transported either through wider clefts or by vesicles that enable them to move across the endothelium.[12] Fluids are transported via filtration caused by hydrostatic and osmotic pressure (see Chapter 3.)

Precisely how transport occurs across the membrane is under investigation.[12] Although the structural basis determines the permeability of capillaries,[13] vasoactive substances, including bradykinin, histamine, and the prostaglandins, are believed to participate, either directly or by interaction, in altering the permeability of the capillary membrane.[12]

There is general agreement that transcapillary transport increases as the temperature increases. But how much is the result of the decreased viscosity of blood that occurs with a rise in temperature, alterations in the geometry of the transcapillary pathway, or other mechanisms has not been fully explained.[10,14]

Atrioventricular Shunts

A-V shunts (arteriovenous anastomosis) are anatomical channels that connect arterioles directly with venule vessels. The function of these shunts is to protect cutaneous tissues from damage caused by excessive heat or cold and possibly to prevent extremely high core temperatures.[15] When the temperature of peripheral tissue is within the normal range, these shunts are closed; however, they open when the temperature of tissues is high or low enough to endanger them. When shunts are open, a large amount of blood flows through them, increasing local blood flow. These shunts are coiled channels with thick musculature that is under the control of the sympathetic nervous system. This central control activates the shunts when the tissue temperature increases to approximately 104° F (40° C),[11] reducing the sympathetic vasoconstrictor tone[16] thus increasing cutaneous blood flow and enhancing heat loss.

The shunting activity caused by cold appears to be a strictly local response, with no need for central input. Evidence indicates that, at specific cold temperatures, various neurotransmitters that control vasoconstriction and dilation are released and that these neurotransmitters may control the activity of the shunts.[16] Some authors have theorized that an "axon reflex" (see Chapter 9) may activate these shunts.[17] When shunts open as a result of tissue cooling, blood continues to flow through the area by bypassing the capillaries, thus rewarming the skin of the tissues. Although shunts are found throughout the skin, they are richly concentrated in the areas most susceptible to damage by cold: the fingers, toes, nail beds, face, lips, and ears.

Determinants of Venous Flow

In addition to its function of controlling both local tissue and core temperatures, the peripheral venous system is responsible for transporting deoxygenated blood and much of the metabolic waste away from local tissues. Removal of metabolic wastes can reduce pain and muscle spasms caused by excessive accumulation of acid in muscles or other tissues. The return of blood to the heart is controlled by (1) the blood pressure gradient, (2) the integrity of the valves and muscles of the veins, (3) "muscle pumps," and (4) the volume of flow.

Blood pressure gradient. The amount of pressure and the *pressure gradient* are crucial determinants of venous flow. Fluid always flows in the direction from higher to lower pressure. If no pressure gradient is present, no blood flows. The gradual decrease in blood pressure that occurs along the path of the vessels after blood leaves the heart dictates the direction of flow. Venous pressure, which is lower than arterial pressure, gradually declines to just a few mm Hg before entering the right atrium of the heart. Thus, blood accumulates in the veins. Obviously, the pressure-gradient factor alone cannot maintain a sufficient flow of blood to the heart. The other three factors mentioned above help increase the rate of venous return.

Integrity of the veins. Although muscles in the walls of veins are not as numerous as they are in arterial vessels, they do contract and relax to assist the pumping of blood through the veins. As blood passes through the veins, with each stroke, the pressure increases as the muscles contract and decreases when the muscles relax. During each stroke, the increase in pressure forces bicuspid valves in the veins to open; between strokes as muscles relax; the valves close. The "one-way" valve mechanism prevents a backflow of blood between strokes. However, distended or varicose veins limit adequate closing of the valves, which makes the valves less effective and flow of blood toward the heart more difficult.

Muscle pumps. Rhythmical contractions of skeletal muscle also help pump and maintain venous flow. Venous flow in the legs is assisted by the tricep surae muscles in particular and in the trunk primarily by the abdominal muscles. Actions of the muscles in the trunk are often called the abdominal and respiratory pumps. When these muscles are less active, as occurs in prolonged bed rest, fluids that are usually returned by veins and lymph vessels may accumulate in the distal extremities. To prevent this accumulation of fluid, **the legs of nonambulatory patients** should be positioned frequently at horizontal or elevated levels, and external pressures such as elastic bandages or stockings should be applied.

Volume of flow. Normally, two-thirds of the peripheral blood supply is on the venous side. Whenever a higher-than-normal percentage of blood remains on the venous side, the volume of blood returning to the heart is decreased. A reduction in cardiac filling ultimately results in less than normal cardiac output.

Any conditions that retard venous return to the heart create a condition called *venous pooling.* Wherever venous pooling occurs, more deoxygenated blood remains in tissues. This stagnant blood may cause local stasis ulcers, or other stasis dermatological conditions.

Venous pooling also can be caused by systemic problems such as congestive heart failure (CHF). If the heart is unable to pump enough blood through the pulmonary system, as is the case in CHF, blood may be dammed up on the venous side. The venous pressure gradient may reverse, becoming higher in veins near the heart than in those near the capillaries. Pooling of venous blood in the extremities would then indicate that excessive fluid already exists in the region of the lungs and heart. In such systemic conditions, the use of any physical agents that may force fluid back to the thoracic region is contraindicated.

LYMPHATIC SYSTEM

The lymphatic system begins in the capillary area. Lymph channels have openings that can expand enough to permit proteins as well as other large molecules to pass from the interstitium into the lymphatic system. The interstitial fluid, including large molecules, that passes through these channels is termed *lymph.*

Like veins, lymphatic channels contain valves; thus, the lymph can move in only one direction. Much like venous flow, any pressure from contraction of the walls of the lymphatic channels themselves or from outside pressure such as muscle contractions, will squeeze these channels and cause the lymph to move toward the heart. The lymph flowing through the channels from the upper right quadrant of the body empties into the right lymphatic duct. The rest of the body's channels drain into the thoracic duct. Ultimately, the lymph ducts join the great veins near the heart, where the lymph mixes with the venous blood returning to the heart.[9]

Lymph nodes are situated along the route of the lymphatic vessels and are arranged in clusters at various locations throughout the body. Much, but not all, of the lymph passes through and temporarily accumulates in these nodes. When the nodes must be surgically removed, some of the lymph flowing toward the great veins may be blocked.

The lymphatic process, as presented here, is based on the most commonly accepted theory. However, mounting evidence indicates that lymphatic return to venous blood may take place by somewhat different pathways (see Chapter 3).[12] As newer information is acquired, additional insights regarding all aspects of care of peripheral circulatory problems may be available.

An understanding of the physiological activities of all body systems and how physical agents affect them is the basis for determining the indications, contraindications, and cautious use of physical agents in patient treatments. For this reason, this overview of the peripheral circulatory systems relevant to physical agent treatments has been included in this text.

APPLICATION TO PHYSICAL THERAPY

The peripheral circulatory systems must function properly to supply the body tissues with oxygen and other nutrients; remove excess fluids, CO_2, and metabolic wastes; and help maintain a constant body temperature. Malfunctioning of some parts of these systems often occurs.

Because humans are bipedal, gravity is a powerful force in reducing blood flow from distal segments of the extremities—especially from the lower limbs—back to the heart. With increasing age or certain life-styles, the risk of some type of peripheral vascular disease is relatively high.

Peripheral vascular disease (PVD) is a general name for any problems involving the peripheral circulatory systems. These problems range from mild to severe to even life threatening. Peripheral vascular disease includes problems related to the arterial, venous or lymphatic circulations (The lymphatic dysfunctions are discussed in Chapter 3.)

Arterial Dysfunctions

Factors preventing normal arterial function include the following: (1) cardiac problems, which *prevent* sufficient cardiac stroke volume, (2) dysfunction of the sympathetic nerves, which control constriction and dilation of the smooth muscles within the vessels or deficiencies in the arterial vessels, and (3) *arteriolosclerosis,* a thickening of the walls of the arterioles, which causes a loss of pliability that reduces the ability of the vessel to constrict and dilate. In turn, this decreases the flow of oxygenated blood.

Clinical Signs and Symptoms

The skin may be paler or cooler than normal. The pulse may be weak. The radial pulse in the upper extremities and the dorsal pulse or posterior tibial pulses in the lower extremities can be palpated to determine whether the pulse is weak. Leg cramps are a common complaint.

Physical Therapy Treatments

Extremities can be alternately elevated and lowered to allow gravity to help the flow of blood through the arterial vessels. In addition, brief periods of walking should be encouraged, and patients with severe arterial dysfunction should stand for very brief periods throughout the day.

Whenever there is a lack of oxygenated blood flow, physical agents must be used cautiously. The affected extremity should be kept warm, but intense heat modalities should be avoided because they increase tissue metabolism. To prevent tissue damage, the circulation must meet metabolic demands for oxygen. Although intermittent pneumatic compression pumps are sometimes used, the specific recommended dosages must be followed carefully.

Details of treatment for arteriole insufficiency are beyond the scope of this chapter. However, clinicians are advised to become knowledgeable in this area before performing any aggressive therapies.

Venous Dysfunctions

The common venous dysfunctions are varicose veins, local stasis ulcers, and venous phlebitis and thrombosis.

Varicose Veins

This condition refers to veins that are distended and often twisted. Whenever excessive amounts of blood are pooled in the veins for a prolonged period, the increase in venous pressure can cause the vessels to become permanently enlarged. This prevents the valves from closing. As a result, these valves become incompetent. Because gravitational forces tend to draw fluids downward, varicose veins often occur in the lower extremities, where varicosities can develop in superficial or deep veins.

Superficial varicosities are visible and can be diagnosed easily, but the diagnosis of varicosities of deeper veins requires specific testing. Skin in the involved area may be bluer or paler than normal because of the accumulation of deoxygenated blood. Patients commonly complain of pressure or pain in the affected extremity.

Local Stasis Ulcers

Local stasis ulcers are caused by the lack of oxygen and decreased clearing of CO_2 and metabolites from a local area. They develop as the duration and severity of varicosities increases.

Clinical Signs and Symptoms

In the early stages, patients may complain of tenderness in the area, and rashes can be observed. If untreated, the condition can eventually progress to open (superficial) ulcers.

Venous Phlebitis and Thrombosis

Venous phlebitis is an inflammation within the vein. Venous thrombosis involves formation of a crusty clot on the inside wall of the vein that usually occurs as consequence of the phlebitis. Whenever these conditions exist, there is the danger of the clot detaching from the wall. A dislodged clot is called an embolism, which may travel through the blood stream and lodge elsewhere in the veins or in the lungs or heart. The result may be local necrosis, a heart attack, or death.

Clinical Signs and Symptoms

Areas of phlebitis are usually warm, pink, swollen, and tender. A superficial thrombosis can be palpated. Although therapists sometimes test for deep vein thrombosis by applying deep pressure to an area to elicit pain, this test is not conclusive. Positive results serve as a warning that the patient should be seen by a cardiovascular specialist. **Negative tests do not confirm the absence of a deep thrombus.** Whenever a thrombus is suspected, a cardiovascular specialist should be notified.

Physical Therapy Procedures

Before any treatments are initiated, the patient must be thoroughly tested to determine the type and severity of the vascular problem. For less severe venous problems, the following therapeutic procedures are usually indicated to prevent more serious problems:

- Patients with problems in the lower extremities should be encouraged to walk, run, rise on their toes, and so forth to maximize muscle contractions. Static standing should be discouraged because it may increase venous pooling.
- The involved extremity should be elevated at least to a horizontal position whenever possible.
- Gentle massage can be given to move the stagnant blood and relieve the pressure. If a thrombus is suspected, however, **massage is contraindicated.**
- Intermittent pneumatic compression treatments are commonly given, often followed by exercises with the involved extremities elevated to a near vertical position to take advantage of the gravitational force. At the end of the treatment, an elasticized garment or ace bandage is applied immediately while the extremity is in an elevated position.
- Electrical stimulation as well as active exercises are recommended for the intermittent pumping action of the muscles in the extremity.
- If extremities are cold only mild local heat should be used.
- With any peripheral vascular disease, patients should be advised against wearing tight bands such as garters, which may interfere with circulation.

The clinical considerations presented in this chapter are by no means complete. They represent a sample that we hope will help the student understand the relationship between the anatomy and physiology of the peripheral circulation and the reasons why physical agents may or may not be indicated for patients with peripheral circulatory problems.

■ KEY TERMS

lumen
vasoconstriction
vasodilation
venae comitantes
countercurrent exchange (CCE)
shunting
AV shunts
capillaries
pressure gradient

muscle pumps
venous pooling
lymph
peripheral vascular disease
  arteriosclerosis
  varicose veins
  local stasis ulcers
  venous phlebitis and thrombosis

REFERENCES

1. Selkurt E, ed: *Basic Physiology for the Health Sciences.* 2nd ed. Boston: Little Brown; 1982:344.
2. Roddie IC, Shepherd JT, Abboud FM, eds. Circulation to skin and adipose tissue. In: *Handbook of Physiology,* 2nd ed. Bethesda, MD: American Physiological Society; 1984:285–317.
3. Guyton A: *Human Physiology and Mechanisms of Diseases.* 4th ed. Philadelphia, PA: WB Saunders; 1987:135–137, 183.
4. *Stedman's Medical Dictionary.* 25th ed. Baltimore, MD: Williams & Wilkins; 1990.
5. Leithead C, Lind A: *Heat Stress and Heat Disorders.* Philadelphia, PA: FA Davis, 1964:10.
6. Rowell L: Human cardiovascular adjustments to exercise and thermal stress. *Physiol Rev.* 1974; 54:75–159.

7. Rowell L, Marx H, Bruce R, et al: Reductions in cardiac output, central blood volume, and stroke volume with thermal stress in normal men during exercise. *Clin Invest.* 1966; 45:1801–1816.

8. Weinbaum S, Jiji LM, Lemons D: Theory and experiment for the effect of vascular microstructure on surface heat transfer. *Biomech Eng.* 1984; 106:337.

9. Carola R, Harley J, Noback C: *Human Anatomy & Physiology,* New York: McGraw-Hill; 1990.

10. Noring S: Dynamics of blood flow. *P & S J* (Columbia University College of Physicians & Surgeons). Fall 1983:4–13.

11. Lockhart R, Hamilton G, Fyfe F: *Anatomy of the Human Body.* Philadelphia PA: JB Lippincott; 1965: *Vascular System.* 586; 583.

12. Baez S, Knobel E, eds. Microcirculation. In: *Ann Rev Physiol.* Palo Alto, CA: Ann Rev Inc. 1977; 39:394, 400–407.

13. Mellander S, Hall VE, eds. Systemic circulation: local control. In: *Ann Rev Physiol.* Palo Alto, CA: Ann Rev Inc. 1970: 32:313–344.

14. Wolf M, Watson P: Effects of temperature on transcapillary water movement in isolated cat hindlimb. *Am J Physiol.* 249(4):H792–H798.

15. Hales J, Iriki M, Tsuchiijak K, et al: Thermally-induced cutaneous sympathetic activity related to blood flow through capillaries and arteriovenous anastomoses. *Pflug Arch.* 1978; 375:17–24.

16. Lehmann J, ed. Heat. In: *Therapeutic Heat and Cold.* 3rd ed. Baltimore, MD: Williams & Wilkins; 1982:418. Chap 10. Lehmann & DeLatteur: Therapeutic Heat 464–562.

17. Shepherd J, Vanhoutte P: Cold vasoconstriction and cold vasodilation in Vanhoutte P, Leusen I, eds: *Vasodilation.* New York: Raven Press; 1981:263–271.

3

Edema

Bernadette Hecox, PT, MA

Physiologic Factors

   Factors Regulating Exchange of Fluids

   Factors That Disrupt Normal Fluid Exchange

Clinical Aspects

Acute and Chronic Edema

Amount of Swelling

Consistency of the Fluid

Site and Size of the Edematous Area

Application to Physical Therapy

Edema is a condition in which the amount of fluid within interstitial spaces is greater than normal. This excessive intercellular fluid can be localized to one area of the body such as a hand or an ankle, or it can be more general, involving an entire extremity or the entire body. *Effusion* refers specifically to an excess of fluid in a cavity: for example, the pleural space or excessive synovial fluid in a joint. *Lymphedema* is the accumulation of interstitial fluid caused by an obstruction in lymph channels that prevents reabsorption of proteins from the interstitium.

When the swelling caused by excess fluid increases pressure on the sensory nerves, it causes pain. When such pressure blocks blood flow to tissues, it can cause necrosis. Excessive fluid, either intra-articular effusion or extra-articular edema, that crowds a joint decreases the range of motion and function of those joints. If edema is allowed to persist, osteoporosis of bone caused by lack of use or infections such as low-grade cellulitis may occur. Edema and slow venous flow predisposes the patient to thrombosis or pulmonary embolisms.[1,2] Chronic lymphedema predisposes tissues to bacterial infection.[3] Thus, edema should not be regarded lightly; it should be treated aggressively and as soon as possible.

Many physical agents can be useful for either preventing edema or hastening its resolution. However, because some agents have the potential to increase edema, physical agents are contraindicated for some edematous conditions. The following information should help guide clinicians who must decide whether and how to use physical agents with patients with edema or with conditions that may cause edema to develop.

PHYSIOLOGIC FACTORS

Approximately 60% of body weight is water.[4,5] The water within the body cells is called intracellular fluid and all that is outside the cells is called extracellular fluid. Extracellular fluids include the fluids within the blood vessels, called plasma, and the fluids in the interstitial spaces, called interstitial fluid. Normally, the interstitial fluid accounts for approximately 16% of an adult's body weight.[6]

Many authorities explain that the content of the interstitial fluid exists in both a "free fluid" and a tissue "gel" state and that, in healthy individuals, most interstitial fluid is in the gel state. Any large concentration in the free fluid state is edema. Theoretically, the gel serves several purposes. The gel matrix contains negatively charged mucopolysaccharides, which attract and hold positively charged sodium ions (Na+). Because sodium is an osmotic substance, its concentration in the gel enhances the passage of water across the capillary membrane, through osmosis, into the gel. The gel also acts as a "filler" holding cells apart and enabling the interstitial fluid to remain relatively immobilized and thus localized. If all the interstitial fluid was free fluid that is none was in the gel state—gravity would pull all the fluid to lower regions of the body. For example, when a person was standing with arms at sides, all the fluid would shift to the distal parts of the arms and legs. Such pooling of interstitial fluid is observed with edema, which is an excess of "free fluid."

Because of a pressure gradient between the interstitial space and blood, fluid is constantly being exchanged across the capillary membrane between the interstitial space and plasma. The capillary membrane is semipermeable. A delicate balance between the gradients of the forces drawing fluids in each direction maintains a normal amount of fluid in the interstitium. Guyton[6] stated that the interstitial pressure is normally negative—ie, less than the atmospheric pressure—and that "the *physical* cause of edema is positive pressure in the interstitial spaces." He noted that if edema is prolonged (hours to years), tissues will stretch accordingly, causing the pressure in the spaces to become even more positive and thus encouraging more edema. This theory lends support to the importance of preventing or hastening the reduction of edema.

Because physical therapists must understand how the delicate balance between the concentrations of fluids in blood and the interstitium is maintained and what can disturb that balance so that edema develops, a review of the related physiology is presented here.

In 1896 Starling[7] presented a theory explaining how fluids are normally transported between blood and interstitium. He explained that the two-way exchange of fluid between capillaries and interstitium occurred at the capillary membrane because of hydrostatic and osmotic pressure gradients. If all factors were normal, the net effect of the gradients would result in a normal amount of interstitial fluid, thus no edema. This theory is referred to as "Starling's hypothesis of the capillaries." Basically, that hypothesis still stands, and "although hydrolic and osmotic pressure differs across different barriers, Starling's equation has universal applicability."[7] In the 20th century, however, many authors have presented new evidence that contributes to our current understanding. A brief discussion of the factors that regulate the exchange of fluids between blood and interstitium follows. The reader may find it helpful to refer to Figs. 3–1, 3–2, and 3–3, which illustrate these transactions. One must bear in mind that capillaries may be only 0.5 mm long[8] and that the figures are not drawn to scale; they are presented only to clarify the fluid exchange concepts that will be discussed.

Factors Regulating Exchange of Fluids

Hydrostatic Pressure

Hydrostatic pressure always causes fluids moving through a semipermeable membrane to flow from the higher pressure side to the lower pressure side of the membrane. In this case, the plasma pressure is higher than the interstitial fluid pressure at the capillary membrane. In a "model" capillary, one can estimate that the blood plasma pressure at the arteriole end of a capillary is 25 mm Hg and 10 mm Hg at the venule end. This pressure within the capillary forces fluids out of the capillary into the interstitium. Fig. 3–1 illustrates the differences in processes at either end.

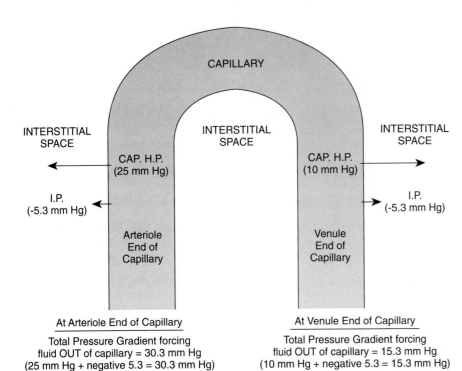

INTERSTITIAL SPACE

INTERSTITIAL SPACE

INTERSTITIAL SPACE

CAPILLARY

CAP. H.P.
(25 mm Hg)

CAP. H.P.
(10 mm Hg)

I.P.
(-5.3 mm Hg)

I.P.
(-5.3 mm Hg)

Arteriole
End of
Capillary

Venule
End of
Capillary

At Arteriole End of Capillary

Total Pressure Gradient forcing
fluid OUT of capillary = 30.3 mm Hg
(25 mm Hg + negative 5.3 = 30.3 mm Hg)

At Venule End of Capillary

Total Pressure Gradient forcing
fluid OUT of capillary = 15.3 mm Hg
(10 mm Hg + negative 5.3 = 15.3 mm Hg)

Figure 3–1. Effect of hydrostatic pressure on fluid exchange between a capillary and the interstitial space. The model illustrates the difference in the total pressure gradient forcing fluid *out* of the capillary at its arteriole and venule ends. Although the negative interstitial pressure (IP) is constant, the hydrostatic pressure (CAP H.P.) of the capillary is greater at the arteriole end than at the venule end.

Interstitial Pressure

As stated earlier, the interstitial pressure is normally negative, averaging approximately –5.3 mm Hg. Negative pressure acts as a suction; thus, negativity on the interstitial side of the membrane also favors transport out of capillary into the interstitial space. So far, we have shown two forces that cause fluids to flow out of capillaries: (1) the capillary pressure (25 mm Hg at the arteriole end and 10 mm Hg at the venule end) and (2) interstitial pressure, which is negative (5.3 mm Hg). When the effects of these two forces are combined, a pressure gradient of 30.3 mm Hg at the arteriole end forces fluids out of the capillary (capillary pressure of 25 mm Hg and negative interstitial pressure of 5.3 mm Hg), whereas the pressure gradient at the venule end of the capillary is only 15.3 mm Hg, which forces fluids out (capillary pressure of 10 mm Hg and negative interstitial pressure of 5.3 mm Hg). Thus, the total gradients differ at the two ends—the pressure forcing fluid out of the capillary is 15 mm Hg greater at the arteriole end (see Fig. 3–1).

Osmotic Pressure

Next, osmotic pressure must be considered. *Osmotic pressure* is the pressure that causes fluids to pass from areas of lower concentration to areas of higher concentration of an osmotic substance. Both protein and sodium ions are examples of osmotic substances. The major osmotic pressure at the capillary membrane is caused by a concentration of plasma protein (primarily albumin) at the membrane. Because protein molecules are large, most are unable to pass from the plasma through the membranes to the interstitium. Thus, they accumulate in the capillary at the membrane, creating osmotic pressure of approximately 19 mm Hg and drawing fluids into the capillaries. Osmotic pressure resulting from a concentration of protein is called *oncotic pressure* (OP) or *colloid osmotic pressure* (COP). The plasma colloid osmotic pressure (PCOP) is augmented approximately 50% by the so-called "Donnan effect," which explains that because protein molecules are negative, they attract a large number of positive ions, mainly sodium ions. Because sodium is also an osmotic substance, the concentration of osmotically active sodium molecules increases wherever the proteins accumulate. This effect increases the total PCOP by 9 mm Hg, making the total PCOP 28 mm Hg, which tends to force fluids into the capillaries.

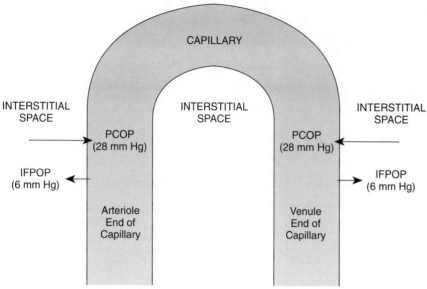

NET Colloid Osmotic Pressure (COP) = 22 mm Hg forcing fluids INTO Capillary
PCOP (28 mm Hg) — IFPOP (6 mm Hg) = 22 mm Hg

Figure 3–2. Effect of osmotic forces on fluid exchange between the capillary and the interstitial space. The net colloid osmotic pressure (COP) is the same at both ends of the capillary. PCOP = plasma colloid osmotic pressure, IFCOP = interstitial fluid colloid osmotic pressure.

Although most proteins do not pass through the membrane, a small percentage do pass to the interstitial fluid, creating an opposing osmotic pressure on the interstitial side of the membrane. This pressure is an *interstitial fluid colloid osmotic pressure* (IFCOP) of 6 mm Hg, which tends to draw fluids in the opposite direction of the PCOP: that is, into the interstitial space. The sum of these osmotic forces (PCOP-28 mm Hg into capillaries minus IFCOP 6 mm Hg out of capillaries) leaves a net osmotic force of 22 mm Hg, which draws fluids into the capillaries (see Fig. 3–2).

Direction and Amount of Pressure Gradient

Finally, the direction and amount of the pressure gradient at the arterial and venule ends of the capillaries can be determined. At the arterial end, if the net osmotic pressure forcing fluids into capillaries (22 mm Hg) is subtracted from the net hy-

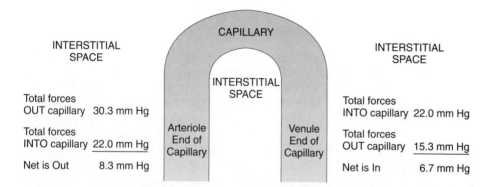

Figure 3–3. Difference in net pressure at the arteriole and venule ends of the capillary that effects exchange of fluid between the capillary and the interstitium. Total pressure forcing fluids *out* of the capillary = Cap. hydrostatic pressure and the negative interstitial pressure. Total pressure forcing fluids *into* the capillary = plasma colloid osmotic pressure (PCOP) minus interstitial fluid colloid osmotic pressure (IFCOP). The net pressure at the arteriole end is 8.3 mg Hg, which forces fluids *out* of the capillary. The net pressure at the venule end is 6.7 mm Hg, which forces fluids *into* the capillary. Thus, in this model, the 1.6 mm Hg difference in pressure tends to force fluid *out* of the capillary into the interstitial space.

drostatic force out (30.3 mm Hg), the remainder is 8.3 mm Hg, which forces fluids out of capillaries (see Fig. 3–3).

The numbers change, however, at the venule end of the capillary. Here, the net force out are only 15.3 mm Hg because the capillary hydrostatic pressure at the venule end is only 10 mm Hg. Subtracting the outward force from the net osmotic force drawing fluids into the capillaries (22 mm Hg), the remainder is 6.7 mm Hg, which draws fluids back into the capillaries. Comparing the net at each end (8.3 mm Hg out at the arteriole end and 6.7 mm Hg in at the venule end), one sees a difference of 1.6 mm Hg, which tends to force fluids out of the capillaries (see Fig. 3–3).

This small, overall resultant effect of forcing fluid out indicates that a small percentage of fluid will not be reabsorbed into the blood stream. This interstitial residue is primarily albumin protein. Under normal circumstances, this residue does not cause edema because the proteins will be taken into the lymphatic system (see Chapter 2).

Factors That Disrupt Normal Fluid Exchange

From the previous discussion, we see that the delicate balance that maintains normal volume of interstitial fluid depends on (1) the permeability of the capillary membrane, (2) the hydrostatic pressure of the capillary, (3) negative interstitial pressure, (4) the PCOP, (5) the IFCOP, and (6) an intact lymphatic system. Changes in any of these factors that can disrupt the delicate balance are discussed below.

Capillary permeability. The permeability of capillaries appears to increase when vasoactive substances such as histamine or bradykinin are released in the tissues, when tissue temperatures increase or when they decrease excessively. The inflammatory process activates vasoactive substances and also increases the temperature of tissues. Capillary permeability may be the factor that causes the edema observed with tissue irritation or trauma or with the application of thermal modalities.

Capillary hydrostatic pressure. The hydrostatic pressure of capillaries increases whenever arterial flow to the capillary region increases or when some condition prevents the free return of blood flow through the veins. Increased arterial flow can occur when metabolic activity is increased: for example, with exercise or increased tissue temperature. Capillary hydrostatic pressure also increases with any pooling of blood in veins. Pooling occurs when veins are distended (eg, varicose veins) or when systemic problems create an excessive amount of fluids in the central body (eg, renal problems or congestive heart failure). This excessive fluid forces blood to back up in veins.

Any pressure on veins (eg, a fetus pressing down on the femoral veins of a pregnant woman) can block the flow. Even straps on leg braces or elastic tops on socks, if narrow and tight, can create strong pressure on leg tissues and block venous return. Standing erect for long periods when one is not using muscle pumps causes pooling in the lower extremities, especially in a hot environment.

Injury to tissue. More fluid flows to the interstitium after injury to tissue, including burns because the physical disruption of the capillaries allows more protein to escape to the interstitium. This reduces the gradient between the PCOP and the IFCOPs, thus reducing the osmotic force that draws fluids back into the capillaries. Similarly, any conditions that increase the amount of an osmotic substance (eg, protein or sodium) in the interstitium will destroy the balanced osmotic pressure gradient. An imbalance in salt-regulatory hormones exemplifies this situation.

Obstruction in the lymphatic system. Finally, obstructions within the lymphatic system prevent the uptake of lymphatic substances. Surgical removal of lymph nodes (eg, with a radical mastectomy) or a systemic condition (eg, elephantiasis) can cause lymphedema. Table 3–1 outlines the common causes of edema and indicates which factor controlling the delicate pressure balance was disturbed.

Although edema ultimately results from disturbances of the delicate balance of capillary membrane pressures, the cause of the disturbances may be many and

**TABLE 3–1. FACTORS ALTERING NORMAL EXCHANGE OF FLUID
AT CAPILLARY MEMBRANES**

Physiological Factor Change	Cause	Result
Increased capillary membrane permeability	Inflammatory process Temperature change Release of histamine, kinines, or other vasoactive chemicals	Increased flow out of the capillary (edema)
Increased capillary hydrostatic pressure	Arterial dilatation (increased flow to capillary) Venous obstruction (reduced flow from capillary) Systemic problem: ie, congestive heart failure (blood backflow to capillary) Renal problems causing fluid retention	Increased flow out of the capillary (edema)
Reduced plasma COP*	Reduced plasma protein caused by hypoproteinemia with severe burns or physical disruption of capillaries (eg, trauma)	Reduced flow into the capillary from the interstitium (edema)
Increased interstitial COP*	Increased protein in interstitium Excessive extracellular sodium (eg, imbalance in salt regulating hormones)	Increased flow out of the capillary (edema)
Lymphatic obstructions	Systemic diseases (eg, elephantitis-filariasis) Lymphatic resection (after cancer)	Lymphedema

*COP = colloid osmotic pressure.

complex, as illustrated by the shoulder-hand-finger syndrome of the hemiplegic patient. The pain, joint limitations, and swelling that are part of this syndrome interfere with therapeutic exercise and the patient's functional recovery. Impairment of venous and lymphatic circulation and immobilization of the involved extremity and therefore less muscle-pumping activity, are primarily responsible for these problems. Cailliet[1] pointed out, however, that since the syndrome is seen in patients with and without sympathetic nerve involvement, the motor and sensory deficits of the central nervous system are initially responsible for the syndrome.

The subject of edema can be studied in many ways. This physiologic overview is limited to factors most pertinent for a text about physical agents. More complete information can be found in current physiology texts.[9,10,11] Staub and Taylor's text[3] is recommended for in-depth information about both current physiologic theories and therapeutic considerations. The need for more study is stressed because researchers in this field do not always agree and no one conclusive hypothesis accounts for all the facts concerning edema. For example, the generally accepted role of the lymphatic system is now questioned.[12] The information provided in this chapter is based on theories commonly accepted at this time.

CLINICAL ASPECTS

When describing edema, clinicians must consider (1) whether it is acute or chronic, (2) the amount of swelling that has occurred, (3) the consistency of the fluid, and (4) the site and size of the edematous area.

Acute and Chronic Edema

Acute edema, as the term implies, refers to a swelling that has occurred recently and rapidly: for example, the sudden swelling that occurs immediately after an injury such as an ankle sprain. *Chronic edema* refers to a swelling that persists for some time: that is, a swelling related to a trauma or injury that remains beyond the time expected for normal healing or a swelling that develops gradually because of systemic problems or other factors that disturb the normal physiologic mechanisms maintaining the balance between the fluids in the capillaries and the interstitial spaces.

Amount of Swelling

The "free fluid" in the interstitium may increase as much as 30% above normal before it is noticeable. But whenever free fluid is increased to the extent that the interstitial fluid pressure changes from negative to positive, marked edema occurs.[6] The extent of edema in a body part can be ranked on a continuum from 1+ (barely detectable) to 4+ (swelling of the area to 1.5 or 2 times its normal size).

Consistency of the Fluid

The consistency of the fluid is the basis for the following classifications of edema: "transudate" versus "exudate" and "pitting" versus "nonpitting." *Transudate edema* is the mild edema that is part of the inflammatory process. The fluid, primarily water and dissolved electrolytes, is clear. *Exudate edema* involves the fluid that occurs with a more extreme stage of inflammation. It may appear as a milky or pus-type fluid because of an increased protein content, primarily leukocytes.[13]

Edema is classified as pitting if a depression (pit) appears when the examiner presses a finger into the swollen tissues and the pit remains for a few seconds after the finger is removed, then gradually recedes. The fluid moves away from the pressure site, then slowly returns, because the substance was indeed "fluid" and could move freely. Massive pitting edema is seen in cases of extreme neglect in treating the condition.[2]

Edema is classified as nonpitting if the fluid does not move with the finger pressure: ie, no pitting is observed. This occurs when the interstitial fluid is coagulated or the tissue cells are swollen from disease, trauma, or inadequate nourishment. Longstanding nonpitting edema may progress to a state in which the skin is golden brown in color. This condition is often called "brawny" edema. Eventually, fibrous tissue deposits may form,[14] a condition referred to as "fibrosis" edema.

Site and Size of the Edematous Area

The site of edema must be noted because, if it is near a nerve plexus or major blood vessel, the resultant pressure can block nerve conduction or blood flow and lead to further complications. If it is within a joint, the function of that joint may be decreased. One also should note the size of the area because a localized edema that spreads may indicate that the condition is becoming worse. If the edema is generalized—ie, observed throughout the body or in more than one extremity—it may indicate a systemic problem such as heart failure or renal disease.[15] Generalized edema is also called anasarca or dropsy.

APPLICATION TO PHYSICAL THERAPY

Edema can interfere with any treatments the therapist may be giving, such as mobilization or therapeutic exercise. The pain and discomfort caused by the extra pressure on nerves can set up a vicious pain cycle. Additional fluid at joints can reduce range of motion, leading to decreased function of those joints. The position of the joint that decreases the fluid pressure is one of flexion; thus, people with edematous joints tend to avoid full extension, which in turn encourages shortening of flexor muscles, tendons, and joints structures. A wisely selected physical modality or combination of modalities and appropriate dosages may improve an edematous condition and be extremely helpful before other procedures are initiated.

Physical Therapy Interventions used to prevent or treat edema include the following:

- Application of *mild* superficial heat or cold to reduce pain or spasms.
- Immediate application of cold to prevent or reduce immediate posttrauma swelling. The cold may cause temporary local vasoconstriction and thus decrease the flow of arterial blood to the capillary region and also may reduce the inflammatory reactions. This may prevent an increase in capillary hydrostatic pressure and in capillary permeability.
- Application of compression bandages or garments to block fluid accumulation in the interstitium.
- Instructions to patients regarding positioning: for example, keep edematous extremities elevated to at least a horizontal position whenever possible and avoid static flexed-joint positions as much as possible. Fluid has less opportunity to accumulate at joints if the joint is in extension or close-pack position.
- Application of external pressure via massage to move the fluids through the vessels. Foldi[16] recommended that the massage begin at the "root"—the trunk region just proximal to the swollen extremity—to prevent blockage of fluid flow as the extremity is massaged. Then, one can massage distally to move fluids back toward the trunk.[16]
- Application of intermittent compression pumps to produce external pressure to vessels that simulates the on-off pressure of muscle contractions.
- Use of ultrasound to deter formation of fibrotic tissue.
- Use of active exercise or electrical stimulation of muscles to increase muscle pumping action and thus encourage venous and lymphatic return of fluids.

The first four modalities may be useful to prevent edema in cases of acute trauma: for example, immediately after a strain or sprain. However, controversy exists regarding the use of either heat or cold.[16,17] (This subject is discussed in Section II of this text.)

Treatment of **chronic problems** requires an aggressive and prolonged approach. In such cases, additional modalities such as massage, ultrasound, intermittent positive pressure pumps, electrical stimulation of muscles, or all of these may be recommended.

When generalized edema exists, the therapist must give careful consideration to the use of physical agents. If the condition is extensive, physical agents may be ineffective. With some systemic problems, they may be useful, although incapable of helping the primary problem. For example, if swelling is sufficient to prevent joint movement and thus functioning of an extremity, even a temporary reduction of the swelling may allow some joint movement and thus some muscle contraction and active movement of the part. This activity, in turn, decreases the edema and improves the function.

When the therapist uses these modalities in such cases, he or she must be in consultation with the primary physician because, in some systemic problems (eg, renal problems or congestive heart failure), a modality that reduces edema locally is **contraindicated.** In such cases, the body is attempting to deal with excessive fluid that impinges on heart, lungs, and other organs in the trunk by sending more of the fluid to the extremities. Therefore, forcing the fluid back to the central body would be dangerous.

Before applying any physical agents, whether to treat edema or some unrelated problem, the therapist must check the patient's chart, obtain the patient's history, and understand any edema-related physical problems the patient may have to rule out contraindications. In succeeding chapters as each physical agent is addressed, indication and contraindications for their use are given. Many are related to how a particular agent may effect edema. The information presented in this chapter should enable the physical therapist to understand why an agent should or should not be used for various conditions.

■ KEY TERMS

effusion

Lymphedema

Starling's hypothesis of the capillaries

osmotic pressure

oncotic pressure (OP)

colloid osmotic pressure (COP)

Donnan effect

plasma colloid osmotic pressure (PCOP)

interstitial fluid colloid osmotic pressure (IFCOP)

acute edema

chronic edema

transudate edema

exudate edema

REFERENCES

1. Cailliet R: *The Shoulder in Hemiplegia*. Philadelphia, PA: FA Davis; 1980.
2. Fishman A, Wyngaarden J, Smith L, eds: Heart failure. In: *Cecil's Textbook of Medicine*. 17th ed. Philadelphia, PA: WB Saunders; 1985.
3. Staub N, Taylor A, eds: *Edema*. New York: Raven Press; 1984.
4. Carola R, Harley J, Noback C: *Anatomy and Physiology*. New York: McGraw-Hill; 1990.
5. Anthony C, Thiboneau G. Fluid and electrolyte balance. In: *Textbook of Anatomy and Physiology*. 11th ed. St. Louis, MO: CV Mosby; 1983:569.
6. Guyton A: *Textbook of Medical Physiology*. 6th ed. Philadelphia, PA: WB Saunders; 1981: 376.
7. Witte CL, ed. The introduction to classics in lymphology. In: *Lymphology*, 1984;17(4):124.
8. Lockhart R, Hamilton G, Fyfe F: *Anatomy of the Human Body*. Philadelphia, PA: JB Lippincott; 1965:580.
9. Boyd W, Sheldon H: *Introduction to the Study of Disease*. 8th ed. Philadelphia, PA: Lea & Febiger; 1980.
10. Berne R, Levy M: *Cardiovascular Physiology*. 4th ed. St. Louis, MO: CV Mosby; 1981: chaps 6 and 7.
11. Guyton A: *Human Physiology and Mechanism of Disease*. 4th ed. Philadelphia, PA: WB Saunders; 1987.
12. Baez S, Knobile E, eds. Microcirculation. In: *Ann Rev Physiol*. Palo Alto, CA: Ann Rev Inc. 1977, vol 39, 391–415.
13. Reed B. Zarrou, Michlovitz S: Inflammation and repair and the use of thermal agents. In: *Thermal Agents in Rehabilitation*. Philadelphia, PA: FA Davis; 1990, 5–7.
14. Abramson D, Miller D: *Vascular Problems in Musculoskeletal Disorders*. New York: Springer-Verlag; 1981.
15. *Dorland's Illustrated Medical Dictionary*. 27th ed. Philadelphia, PA: WB Saunders; 1988.
16. Foldi E: Lymphedema. In: Staub, N., Taylor, A., eds. *Edema*. New York: Raven Press; 1984:657–677.
17. Marek J, Jezdensky S, Ochonsky P: Effects of local cold and heat therapy in traumatic oedema of the rat hind paw. *Acta Universitatis Palackiane Olomucensis*. 1973;65–66:203–226.

4

Pain

Joseph Weisberg, PT, PhD

P ain is the major complaint of most patients. Finding ways to minimize the devastating effects of pain—psychological,[1] socioeconomic,[2] and physiological[3]—is a major challenge for those who care for people suffering from pain. To deal with the problem effectively, one must understand that pain is a multidimensional phenomenon: ie, the experience of pain is modulated by a wide range of factors such as the sensitivity of the particular tissue involved, the person's mental state, the attitudes of the culture toward pain, and the person's previous experience of pain. Patients who suffer from chronic or acute pain are often extremely irritable and depressed. Consequently, the physical therapist must be aware of its psychological as well as neurophysiological aspects.

THEORIES

One of the oldest theories of pain was postulated by Aristotle, who believed that pain was a reaction to excessive stimulation. This stimulation was said to be carried by the blood to the heart, where it was perceived as an unpleasant experience. It should be noted that Aristotle was cognizant of the psychological aspects of pain.[4]

Specificity Theory

Acceptance of the concept that pain is a sensory modality led to the development of neurophysiologic theories of pain. In 1894 Von Frey proposed a doctrine of specific nerve energies—the specificity theory of pain. This doctrine implied that each sensory modality was subserved by morphologically specific nerve endings: that is, pain by free nerve endings, light touch by Merkel's corpuscles, flutter (vibration) by Meissner's corpuscles, and pressure touch by pacinian corpuscles. Von Frey's theory grew out of Muller's concept, which stated that the quality of the

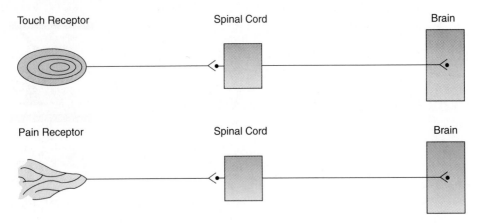

Figure 4–1. A diagram representing the concept of the specificity theory of pain.

sensation depended on the properties of the nerve[5] and from the evidence gained by microscopic investigation, especially the identification of specific receptors in the skin. According to Von Frey's theory, pain is a specific sensation that is triggered when specific receptors in the skin are stimulated. This stimulation travels along specific pathways in the spinal cord to reach specific projection areas in the brain: namely, the pain center, where the stimulus is appreciated (Fig. 4–1). The anatomical evidence for this theory was that similar stimulation of a different type of receptor produced different sensations and that a different stimulus to the same type of receptor produced the same sensation. The objections to this theory are many; the most obvious is the fact that a wide spectrum of sensations can be transmitted from tissue served by one type of nerve ending. For example, free nerve endings can transmit the sensation of pain, touch, or pressure.

Pattern Theory

The realization that pain and other sensations were not simple stimulus-response phenomena led Goldschneider (1896) to develop the pattern theory. This theory suggested that the pattern of stimulation (its intensity and frequency) of nerve endings determined whether the brain would interpret the stimuli as pain (Fig. 4–2). The theory implied that a group of nerve endings and their associated nerve fibers formed a "pain spot." Such spots are the primary areas for initiation of a train of impulses in the pain pathways.[4] The stimulation of these spots results in the perception of pain when the proper "pain" centers in the brain are activated. Actually, the conscious perception of various nuances of pain are probably expres-

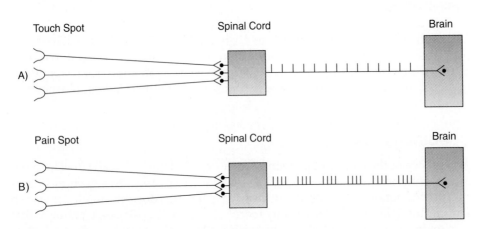

Figure 4–2. A diagram representing the concept of differentiation between pain and touch according to the pattern theory of pain.

sions of the stimulation of different combinations of nerve endings and the resulting complex interactions in the "pain centers" in the brain.[6]

In 1943 Livingston expanded on the pattern theory to explain how pain could occur long after an initial injury. Subsequently, Weddell and Sinclair (1947) suggested that the size of the nerve fiber as well as the frequency and intensity of the stimulus were the determinants of the sensation and perception of pain. This theory was challenged by the fact that receptor specialization does exist to a great extent.

Both the specificity and pattern theories were probably valid to a certain degree; however, both were criticized for overemphasizing the sensation of pain and underemphasizing the perception of pain.[7] Although the functional role of all known nociceptors and their corresponding afferent fibers has been established, no detectable structural differences of general pain receptors, (free nerve endings), explain the functional differences. Moreover, the unimodal nociceptor responds to only one type of noxious stimulus, whereas the polymodal nociceptor might respond equally to mechanical, thermal, or chemical stimuli. In addition, it has been determined that different nerve fibers mediate different sensations. Large myelinated (A-alpha) fibers transmit messages perceived as vibrations, and small myelinated (A-delta) fibers transmit messages perceived as sharp, prickling, dermatomic pain; proprioception; and temperature. The unmyelinated (C) fibers transmit burning sclerodermic pain, a poorly localized deep aching. Pain mediated by A-delta fibers is more severe but of short duration, whereas the pain mediated by C-fibers is dull and continuous. Although dull, the effects of this continuous pain accumulates and is subjectively viewed as more disabling.

Gate Theory

In 1965 Melzack and Wall proposed the *gate theory* of pain,[8] which they subsequently revised in 1978 (see Fig. 4–3). They originally postulated that interneurons in the substantia gelatinosa in the dorsal horn of the spinal cord acted as a gate to modulate sensory input. These cells project to second order neurons of pain or temperature pathways located in lamina V called transmission cells. Melzack and Wall postulated that this was where modulation of peripheral stimuli occurred through the activity of interneurons. The gate was considered to be related to the different amounts of input from large and small fibers to the system. For example, the input of large A fibers could be viewed as exciting the inhibitory interneuron in

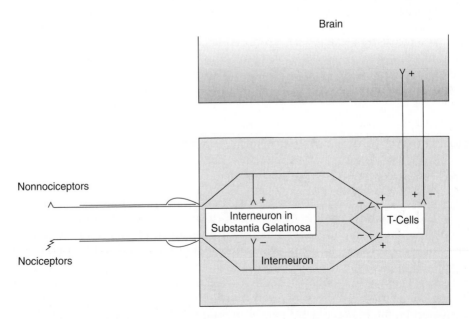

Figure 4–3. A diagram representing Melzack and Wall's revised gate theory of pain.

the substantia gelatinosa. This A fiber input, which reduced the excitation level of the transmission cells, might result in "closing the gate" at that level, thus decreasing the number of ascending nociceptive stimuli. In turn, the small C fibers could be regarded as stimulators of the excitatory interneurons, thereby tending to "open the gate." The gate could be "opened" or "closed" further by descending excitatory or inhibitory pathways from the brain, thus decreasing or increasing the firing of transmission cells. This original theory was criticized for its simplicity and the fact that it does not explain pain mediated by A fibers. Nonetheless, it did spark renewed interest in pain control that led to the development of transcutaneous electrical nerve stimulation (or TENS), which is currently an effective and widely used modality for the relief of chronic and acute pain.

Melzack and Wall revised their theory, incorporating a more complex neural mechanism in the dorsal horn. In this revision, they hypothesized that the control at the gate was the result of the activities of nociceptive and non-nociceptive neurons rather than the activities of large- and small-diameter afferent fibers (see Fig. 3).[9] The gate theory offered an explanation for a clinical prediction: namely, that direct stimulation of sensory fibers by transcutaneous electrical stimulation diminishes the pain. However, the gate control theory remains just a theory. No solid anatomical evidence is available to support the existence of this mechanism.

Biochemical Theories

Over the past 50 years, biochemical theories of pain have emerged that involve pain-producing substances, pain-mediating substances, and pain chemoreceptors such as endogenous opioids and the opiate receptors located on the membrane of certain neurons in the brain. *Endorphins* and *enkephalins* modify sensory input and function as "natural" narcotics. They are found in high concentrations in the periaqueductal gray area and the thalamus, in structures associated with the limbic system, and in the substantia gelatinosa, where they can affect the transmission of pain. The neurotransmitter of the C fibers released into the substantia gelatinosa is a peptide called substance P, which excites neurons in the dorsal horn. This excitation is of long duration but of gradual onset.[10] The release of substance P can be blocked by morphine and results in analgesia. Substance P may be significant in the transmission of pain; endorphins and enkephalins, when released, inhibit the transmission of this substance.[11]

Other chemical substances have been associated with pain. For example, an imbalance of dopaminergic and serotoninergic substances influences the neurotransmission of pain.[11] Acetylcholine, histamine, bradykinin, prostaglandin, capaicin, and potassium ions also have been implicated, and the injection of bradykinin into the viscera actually has produced lasting pain. A good example of pain that is most likely to be produced by these substances is angina pectoralis. During a heart attack, bradykinin and prostaglandin are released, probably because of the ischemia in the muscle, which causes the sensitization of the nociceptor.[12]

ANATOMIC AND PHYSIOLOGIC ASPECTS

Nociceptive Receptor System

The *nociceptive receptor system* consists of two varieties. The first type is the free nerve ending found mostly in the cornea of the eye, the teeth, tendons, and ligaments. The second type is a continuous tridimensional plexus of unmyelinated nerve fibers that weave in all directions throughout the tissue and around blood vessels (except for blood vessels in the central nervous system, CNS).[13] Mechanical distortion, changes in the chemical composition of tissue fluid, or thermal changes may stimulate these receptors. The person suffering from pain elicited by mechanical distortion might describe the pain as pressure pain, stabbing pain, or prickling pain, whereas pain caused by a thermal or chemical agent is usually described as a burning pain. When the pain receptors around blood vessels are activated, the pain is usually described as a throbbing pain.

Most nociceptors are innervated by unmyelinated afferent fibers (C-fibers) with small diameters or by finely myelinated (A-delta) fibers. The C-fibers in the skin can be stimulated by mechanical irritation, which is likely to cause a prickling pain (see Table 4–1).[14]

Certain pain sensations are associated with certain pathologies. Trauma to muscle or nerve cells usually causes a deep "boring" pain; spasm causes intermittent recurrent pain; cramps cause deep pressure pain that is initially sharp, then achy; inflammation (myositis, tendinitis) produces a deep ache; and ischemia in the muscle causes deep intermittent pain. Rodbard[12] suggested that every time a muscle contracts, toxic catabolites are released, then cleared by the circulation. When more catabolites are produced than can be cleared by the circulation (whether because of poor circulation or excessive muscle contraction), they accumulate and irritate the nociceptor, causing pain.

The sympathetic nerves themselves do not mediate sensation. However, because pain-mediating fibers travel with the sympathetic nerves, interruption of the sympathetic nerves (sympathectomy) also cuts these pain fibers, thus obliterating the pain (visceral or neuropathic). Sympathectomy to an extremity may have an additional beneficial effect of decreasing pain by increasing the blood supply to the extremity.[15]

Some pain receptors have high thresholds; others have low thresholds. The stronger the stimulus, the larger the recruitment of stimulated receptors, thus the stronger the sensation. However, because the pain threshold is different in young and old (older people have higher thresholds) and in men and women (men have higher thresholds),[16] different individuals perceive pain differently. Thus, a person's reaction to the stimuli cannot be accurately predicted.[17] For example, the pain threshold of thermal pain receptors is said to be 45° C;[8] for some people, however, exposure to a stimulus of 42° C would be perceived as pain, whereas others would find that exposure to a stimulus of 45° C is relatively comfortable.

The action potentials carried by the primary afferent neurons via the A delta and C fibers produce neural activity that is conveyed via two basic pathways to the higher centers in the brain. The A delta and C fibers terminate in the dorsal horn of the spinal cord where some neural processing occurs. Each pathway transmits somewhat different types of pain sensations.

Pathway I

The axons of some transmission cells (see Fig. 4–3) of the dorsal horn cross over (decussate) and ascend as the lateral spinothalamic tract (or pathway) and terminate in the thalamus. Some collateral fibers of this tract terminate in the brain stem. Other neurons of the thalamus associated with this pathway terminate in the postcentral gyrus (somatosensory cortex) of the cerebral cortex. This pathway transmits information perceived as sharp, discriminative, and relatively localized sensations of pain.

TABLE 4–1. CHARACTERISTICS OF TYPE A AND C PAIN FIBERS

Fiber Type	Location	Distribution in a Given Area	Myelinated?	Conduction Velocity	Receptors	Perceived Pain Sensation
A	Skin and mucous membranes	Several spots within 1 sq cm; half as much as C fibers	Yes	Fast: 5–30 m/s	Mechanical, thermal, and chemical	Pricking, localized, sharp, stabbing; short duration, usually of sudden onset
C	Throughout the body except for nervous tissue in the brain	Spotty; twice as much as A fibers	No	Slow; 0.5–2 m/s	Mechanical, thermal, and chemical	Persistent, diffuse, throbbing, burning, itching, aching; often after the initial sharp pain

Pathway II

The axons of other transmission cells ascend in the same tract and terminate in the brainstem (reticular formation) and the midbrain tectum, including the periventricular gray matter. From these regions, neurons have axons that terminate in some thalamic nuclei and in some structures of the limbic system. Axons of neurons of the thalamus project to the structures of the limbic system, basal ganglia, and cerebral cortex. This pathway, known as the spinoreticulothalamic pathway, conveys information perceived as diffuse, poorly localized somatic and visceral pain.

TYPES OF PAIN

The three types of pain are acute, chronic, and referred. *Acute pain* may last from seconds to days and is usually a result of potential or actual tissue damage. *Chronic pain* lasts for many months or years, and its mechanism is poorly understood. *Referred pain* is pain that is perceived to be in areas other than where the nociceptors were stimulated (eg, pain in the shoulder that is referred from the gallbladder). At times, this phenomenon may be associated with the fact that both areas—the area where the pain is perceived and the area where the nociceptors were irritated—are innervated by nerves traveling through a common root: for example, on the same dermatome (see Table 4–2).

In essence, the perception of pain begins with the stimulation of certain receptors. Acute pain is believed to be an alarm that triggers activities to protect the body from noxious stimuli. The actual perception of the sensation occurs in the higher centers of the brain. A good example of this is a person with amputation who feels pain in the absent limb (the phantom limb phenomenon). The pain sensation occurs because the area in the brain associated with the amputated limb is stimulated.

The perception of pain and the reaction to pain is based on a complex of anatomical, physiological, chemical, and psychological factors, many of which are still

TABLE 4–2. THE CHARACTERISTICS OF THE DIFFERENT TYPES OF PAIN

Type of Pain	Onset	Duration	Pain Sensation	Cause	Associated Condition	Medication	Prognosis	Type of Nerve Fiber
Acute	Sudden, recent	Short: seconds-days	Sharp, localized	Tissue damage often easy to localize and diagnose	Usually none	Usually effective	Usually good	A C
Chronic	Slow, gradual	Long: months-years	Dull, diffuse	Prolonged nerve compression or pain spasm cycles poorly understood; often difficult to localize and diagnose	Poor posture, depression, hopelessness, drug abuse	Usually ineffective	Usually poor	Mostly C
Referred*	Dependent on primary cause	Dependent on primary cause	Dependent on primary cause	Irritation in area other than where pain is experienced.				

*Referred pain is poorly understood and difficult to diagnose.

poorly understood. In totality, pain can be defined as an unpleasant sensory and emotional experience that is associated with actual or potential tissue damage or is simply the result of an unpleasant emotional state.[18] Because pain is a perceptual experience, it should be viewed only as a symptom, not as a root cause. The clinician must realize that stimulation of pain receptors will not always evoke the experience of pain and that the number of nerve fibers and the frequency of discharge of the fibers carrying the nociceptive impulses will not always be directly related to the intensity of the pain.

ASSESSMENT

Assessing pain is not a simple task. Because pain is subjective, it is basically an unmeasurable experience. However, ways have been developed to measure pain for both clinical and experimental purposes. Three mechanical devices can help to quantify the intensity of the pain: the pressure threshold meter, the tissue compliance meter, and the thermograph.

The *pressure threshold meter* measures the patient's pressure-pain threshold. This device is easy to operate. First, identify the most sensitive spot. Second, apply the rubber disk at the end of the device to the skin surface over that spot. Third, gradually increase the pressure on the spot until the patient indicates that he or she is experiencing pain or discomfort. The pressure indicator registers the amount of pressure required to elicit the pain (see Fig. 4–4).[19]

The *tissue compliance meter* measures the softness or firmness of tissue. The de-

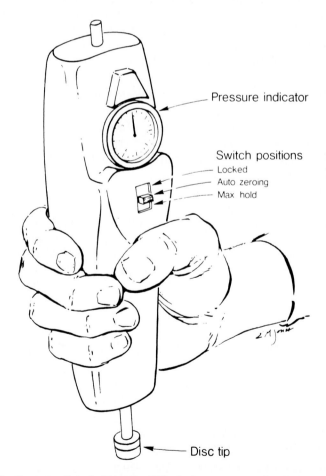

Figure 4–4. Pressure threshold meter. This device measures the amount of pressure needed to elicit pain. (*Reproduced with permission from* Current Therapy in Psychiatry. *AP Ruskin, ed. 1984:127 WB Saunders.*)

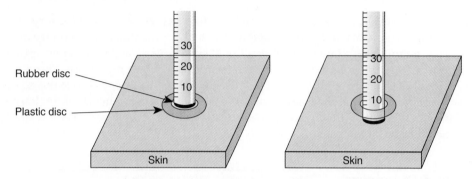

Rubber disc
Plastic disc
Skin
Skin

Figure 4–5. Tissue compliance meter. This meter measures the firmness of tissue. The degree of firmness can be correlated with the severity of pain.

gree of firmness can be correlated with the severity of pain. This device also measures tolerance to compression. The apparatus consists of a rubber disk with a surface area of 1 sq cm that is surrounded by a flat plastic disk (see Fig. 4–5). As the disk is pressed against the tender tissue, the rubber tip compresses the tissue while the plastic disk stays on the surface. The depth of the compressed tissue is recorded by an electronic transducer on a graph.[19]

Thermography is a method of measuring surface temperature. In many conditions, pain is associated with temperature changes. For example, inflammation increases the surface temperature, whereas spasm and vasoconstriction reduce the surface temperature. Therefore, thermography can be used to document inflammation, spasm, or both related to pain and discomfort. One type of thermographic device uses scanning mirrors that reflect infrared radiation onto an infrared electronic transducer. The infrared pattern is then displayed on a cathode ray tube and photographed. The second type of device is a contact thermograph that uses a flexible sheet coated with liquid crystals (Flexitherm system). Seven temperatures are represented by seven colors, and the sensitivity from one temperature to the next is usually a difference of 1° C. Thermography must be done in a draft-free room maintained at 65° F, and it should be repeated after 15–20 minutes to validate the findings. Because of constant variations in surface temperature, the findings are considered to be positive only when they display a difference of more than 1° C and when the area of change is more than 25% of the part tested.[19]

One simple way to assess pain clinically is with self-rating pain scales. The smaller the scale, the less sensitive and the more reliable the measurement. A scale containing four or five categories is sufficient (see Fig. 4–6).

Assessing the source of pain is more complex. Asking the patient to describe the pain may help to identify its source. For example, throbbing pain may indicate that a blood vessel is involved, burning pain may indicate chemical irritation within the tissue, and stabbing pain may indicate mechanical irritation.

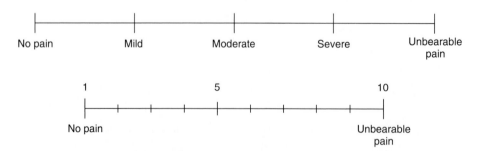

No pain   Mild   Moderate   Severe   Unbearable pain

1   5   10

No pain   Unbearable pain

Figure 4–6. Pain scale. One simple way to make a clinical assessment of pain is to use a self-rated pain scale such as this. The smaller the scale, the less sensitive and more reliable the measurement.

Pain questionnaires were developed to evaluate pain intensity more thoroughly. One popular instrument is the McGill Pain Questionnaire, which qualifies the pain as the patient subjectively describes it. This instrument uses three parameters: the pain-rating index, the number of words the patient uses to describe the pain, and the patient's rating of the intensity of the current pain on a five-point scale (1 to 5).[20] To complete the clinical assessment, however, the therapist also must pay attention to the patient's occupation, psychological state, and educational and sociological background.

MUSCLE SPASM (MUSCLE HOLDING STATE)

Muscle spasm is one cause of pain that is often treated with physical modalities. The literature is unclear about the meaning of the term muscle spasm. Even medical dictionaries lack a clear definition of what the term means. For example, *Stedman's Medical Dictionary* defines spasm as "an involuntary muscle contraction; if painful, referred to as a cramp. . . . Increased muscular tension and shortness which can't be released voluntarily and which prevent lengthening of the muscle involved."[21] Moreover, the term does not represent a specific pathology or a specific dysfunction. Therefore, the authors suggest that the term "muscle holding state," which describes the continuous contracted state of muscles, should be used.

There are three different types of muscle-holding states: *involuntary muscle holding, voluntary muscle holding,* and *chemical muscle holding.*[22] The interrelationship between the three different types of muscle holding and dysfunction is illustrated in Fig. 4–7. The pain associated with the spasm is probably caused by stimulation of mechanosensitive or chemosensitive pain receptors or both.[23]

The term muscle spasm is often used to describe a pathophysiological state of muscles. The spasm is a symptom of a pathological condition, not of the pathology itself. Some authorities combine spasm with the term cramp, contracture, or both.[21,24] Others differentiate between the terms simply by stating that the cramp is painful.[21] EMG recordings of muscle cramps show irregular high-frequency, high-voltage, profuse bursts of motor unit potential, whereas the EMG recordings of muscle contracture (spasm) show little or no electrical activity in the muscle affected by the contraction.[25] Physiologically, the state of contraction is sustained when there is enough calcium present in the sarcomere to uncover binding sites between the actin and myosin fibers. Therefore, an agent or a condition that promotes release of calcium or inhibits its reaccumulation will cause a muscle to go into spasm.[26]

Spasticity also describes a pathophysiological state of muscles. This term is not interchangeable with the terms spasm, cramp, and contracture. Spasticity is associated with upper motor neuron lesions; the spastic muscle is hypersensitive to stretching: that is, it will contract strongly even with a small sudden stretch.[27]

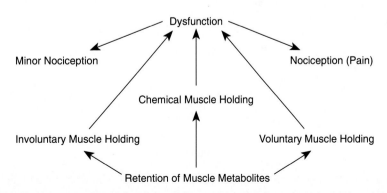

Figure 4–7. The interrelationship between the three different types of muscle holding and dysfunction. (Adapted from Paris SV).

Muscle spasm can have a variety of causes, including an orthopedic disorder or the sequela of a peripheral nervous system disorder. In the case of orthopedic disorders, the muscle spasm is secondary to and develops as a result of pain; it does not cause the pain. On the other hand, a neurogenic spasm can be painful.[28] A postural spasm is one that arises from an imbalance of the postural mechanism caused by overstimulation of or inhibition within the peripheral nervous system in patients with an intact CNS. This type of spasm tends to lead to a fixed muscular contracture and, ultimately, to atrophy.[29]

An incidental spasm occurs as a result of a noxious stimulus that produces a momentary reaction. The minor derangements of reflex control produced by a muscle spasm may result in a remarkable aberration in the rhythm of body movements. Incidental muscle spasm is also referred to as a protective spasm.[30] Some authors object to the term protective primarily because, at times, such a spasm may be destructive, especially if left untreated. For example, a spasm that develops around an infected joint to prevent movement and further deterioration can be viewed as a protective spasm, whereas the severe spasm that may accompany fractures and cause displacement of the bones can only be viewed as a destructive spasm.[30,31]

A muscle spasm also may develop as a response to an abnormality in the physiologic environment of the muscle. For example, a deficiency of muscle phosphorylase or phosphofructokinase or an increase in the concentration of calcium or iodacetate within the myofibril increases the likelihood of a muscle cramp.[27] Consequently, muscle spasm is a dominant response to many pathological states whether those states are local, systemic, or even psychological.

Muscle spasm is identified primarily by palpation and is characterized by the symptoms of local pain and tenderness, restriction of motion, and, when severe enough, impaired activities of daily living. Symptoms associated with spasms are part of a vicious cycle. The cycle begins with a specific pathology (trauma or stress) that causes pain, inflammation, dysfunction, muscle spasm, or all of these. The spasm then may cause local ischemia (increasing the concentration of metabolites), which leads to more pain, inflammation, or both, which in turn results in more spasm (see Fig. 4–8).[31]

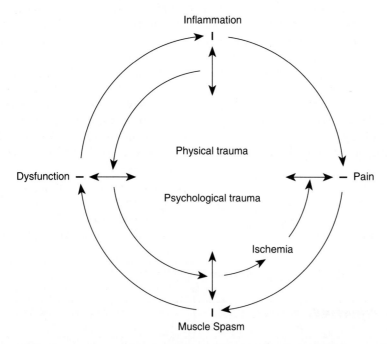

Figure 4–8. Pain cycle showing the interrelationship between physical and psychological trauma and signs and symptoms. The outer cycle shows the cause and effect relationship in a clockwise direction. The inner cycle shows other cause and effect relationships in a counterclockwise direction (pain, muscle spasm, ischemia, more pain).

Because muscle spasm is a symptom, one must identify the cause and the mechanism by which it developed to treat it effectively. The cause of muscle spasm is not always obvious. The muscle may be susceptible because of its physiological condition. On the other hand, a spasm can be triggered by irritation of any of the following structures: sensory organ or nerve, motor end plate (the most pain-sensitive site in muscle), motor nerve, or the CNS. Whatever the cause of the spasm, one can reasonably assume that, during the early stage, the structure of a muscle in a holding state is essentially the same as that of a contracted muscle.[32]

Although most musculoskeletal spasms are not life-threatening, their impact on quality of life is substantial. Pain associated with spasm is among the most important causes of absenteeism from work.

TREATMENT

Treatment should first be directed at the cause, provided the cause can be identified. Spasm that is widespread throughout the body might be caused by an abnormal physiological state, and its treatment might involve medication, a change in diet, or both. Localized spasm is more likely to be induced mechanically, and its treatment might involve correction of a joint dysfunction, improving the patient's posture, or changing the patient's work habits. Psychological stress contributes to overall tension and spasm in specific vulnerable sites and can be treated by teaching the patient how to use relaxation techniques and, at times, by suggesting psychotherapy.

In some cases, addressing the cause of spasm may not bring the immediate relief necessary for the patient to function. This problem usually arises either during the acute stage, when the pain is disabling, or when the condition has become chronic and the tissue has already undergone some physiological changes. Under these conditions, the clinician will have to incorporate specific modalities into the treatment plan that are directed at the spasm itself. Many treatments are available that can effectively reduce muscle spasm and help restore normal length and function of the muscle. Physicians often use local injections, systemic medications, or both to achieve relief. Physical therapists often use massage, exercise, heat, cold, ultrasound, phonophoresis, electrical stimulation, iontophoresis, and biofeedback to reduce pain and promote relaxation. The specific effects of each physical agent will be discussed in subsequent chapters.

■ KEY TERMS

gate theory	pressure threshold meter
endorphins	tissue compliance meter
enkephalins	thermography
nociceptive receptor system	muscle spasm
Pathway I	involuntary muscle holding
Pathway II	voluntary muscle holding
acute pain	chemical muscle holding
chronic pain	spasticity
referred pain	

REFERENCES

1. Nolan MF: Pain: the experience and its expression. *Clin Mgt, Phys Ther.* 1990;10(1):22–25.
2. French S: Pain: some psychological and sociological aspects. *Physiotherapy.* 1989;75:255–260.
3. Bullingham RES: Physiological mechanism in pain. Smith G, Covino BG, eds. *Acute Pain.* London, UK: Butterworth; 1985:

4. Luce JM, Thompson RL II, Getto CJ, et al: New concepts of chronic pain and their implication. *Hosp Pract.* April 1985:113.

5. Newton RA: Contemporary views on pain and the role played by thermal agents in managing pain symptoms. In: Michlovitz SL, ed. *Thermal Agents in Rehabilitation.* Philadelphia, PA: FA Davis; 1986:20

6. Novack C, Demarest: *The Nervous System: Introduction and Review.* New York: McGraw-Hill; 1986:92

7. Martin J: Receptor physiology and submodality coding in the somatic sensory system. In: Kandel F, Schwartz J, eds. *Principles of Neural Science.* 2nd ed. New York: Elsevier Science Publishers; 1985:294

8. Melzack R, Wall PD: Pain mechanism: a new theory. *Science.* 1965;150:971.

9. Wall PD: The gate control theory of pain mechanism: a reexamination and restatement. *Brain.* 1978;101:1

10. Kahn CH, et al: The role of neurotransmitters in processing pain stimuli. *Hosp Pract.* 1989;24:169–170.

11. Kantor TG: Physiology and treatment of pain and inflammation. *Am J Med.* 1986;80(suppl 3A):118.

12. Rodbard S: Pain associated with muscular activity. *Am Heart J.* 1975;90:84–92.

13. Thompson FF: *The Brain: An Introduction to Neuroscience.* New York: WM Freeman; 1985:141

14. Willis WD, Jr: *The Pain System.* New York: S Karger; 1985:264

15. Gildenberg PL, Bevaul RA: *The Chronic Pain Patient.* New York: S Karger; 1985:138

16. Wolff BB: Perceptions of pain. *Science.* 1980

17. Charman RA: Pain theory and physiotherapy. 1989;75:247–254.

18. Wyke BD: Neurological aspect of pain therapy: a review of some current concepts. In: Swerdlow M, ed. *The Therapy of Pain.* Philadelphia, PA: JB Lippincott; 1981;4

19. Fischer AA: Diagnosis and management of chronic pain in physical therapy and rehabilitation. In: Ruskin AP, ed. *Current Therapy in Psychiatry.* Philadelphia, PA: WB Saunders; 1984:130

20. Melzack R: The McGill Pain Questionnaire: major properties and scoring methods. *Pain.* 1975;1:277–299.

21. *Illustrated Stedman's Medical Dictionary.* 23rd ed. Baltimore, MD: William & Wilkins; 1976:1304.

22. Paris SV: Institute of Graduate Health Sciences. 1982.

23. Gayton AC: *Medical Physiology.* Philadelphia, PA: WB Saunders; 1986:594.

24. O'Donoghue DH: *Treatment of Injuries to Athletes.* 4th ed. Philadelphia, PA: WB Saunders; 1984:86.

25. Layzer RB, Rowland LP: Cramps. *N Engl J Med.* 1971;285:31–38.

26. West JB: *Best and Taylor's Physiological Basis of Medical Practice.* 11th ed. Baltimore, MD: Williams & Wilkins; 1985.

27. Khalili AA: Nerve Blocks. In: Basmajian JV, Kirby LR, eds. *Medical Rehabilitation.* Baltimore, MD: Williams & Wilkins; 1984:95

28. Cyriax J: *Textbook of Orthopedic Medicine.* Vol. 1. *Diagnosis of Soft Tissue Lesions.* 8th ed. Philadelphia, PA: Bailliere Tindall; 1982:7.

29. Capener RN: Orthopedic Aspects of Muscle Spasm.

30. Ritchie AE: Muscle spasm: its role in the natural order of biological activities. pp. 111–112. Proceedings of a symposium on skeletal muscle spasm, pp. 101–105, London, UK: British Medical Association; November 1961.

31. Cailliet R: *Soft Tissue Pain and Disability.* Philadelphia, PA: FA Davis; 1977:33

32. Barer R: Muscle structure in relation to spasm. Proceedings of a symposium on skeletal muscle spasm, p. 53; British Medical Association House, London, UK: November 1961.

5

Electromagnetic Spectrum

Joseph Weisberg, PT, PhD

All substances with temperatures above absolute zero (–273° C) emit radiant energy. The emission and transmission of this energy has been explained by two theories: (1) the quantum theory, and (2) the electromagnetic wave theory.

According to the *quantum theory*, the indivisible unit of radiant energy is the photon, which is the smallest entity of radiant energy produced by either electronic or molecular motion of high velocity or by the kinetic energy released from the collision of molecules. The energy (E) content, or quantum, of each photon is proportional to the frequency of the photons emitted and is determined by the formula

$$E = H \times f,$$

where H is Planck's universal constant and f is the frequency in cycles per second. X-rays, for example, are potentially destructive because of their high frequency and photon energy.

According to the *electromagnetic wave theory*, the energy is transmitted by oscillatory motion in the form of electromagnetic waves. The shorter the wavelength, the higher the frequency of oscillation. As explained by the quantum theory, the higher the wave frequency, the higher the energy content. The frequency of the wave emitted by the different modalities used in physical therapy determines the depth of penetration (see Fig. 5–1). In general, all modalities used by physical therapists have lower photon energy and they serve either to increase or decrease the kinetic or thermal energy of body tissues or to induce a photochemical reaction in the absorbing media.

The electromagnetic spectrum is a representation of various wave energies arranged in the order of their wavelength, frequency, or both (see Fig. 5–2). Wavelength is defined as the distance from the peak of one wave to the identical peak of the next wave and is measured in units ranging from nanometers (10^{-9}m) to meters (see Fig. 5–3). The frequency is defined as the number of oscillations or cycles per second, or Hertz. The spectrum that is commonly used extends from wavelengths of 0.0001 nm or (10^{21} cycles/s), the cosmic ray, to wavelengths of $.5 \times 10^{15}$nm (60 cycles/s), a long wave of electric power that is in clinical use (see Fig. 5–2).

The wave propagates in a straight line, but it can undergo reflection (see Fig. 5–4), refraction (see Fig. 5–5), and absorption by the media it encounters. The amount of reflection, refraction, and absorption that occurs will depend on the type of media and the angle of the rays in relation to those media. Ideally, any radiated material, including body tissues, should be at right angles to the wave for maximum absorption. Different wavelengths have different designations (eg, infrared

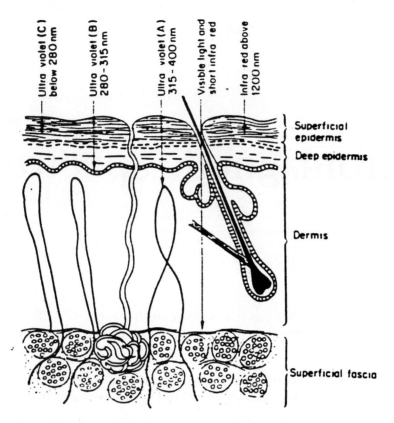

Figure 5–1. Cross-section of the skin showing the extent of penetration of radiation of different frequencies. (*Reproduced with permission from* Electrotherapy and Actinotherapy. *Clayton EB. 1949: Williams & Wilkins.*)

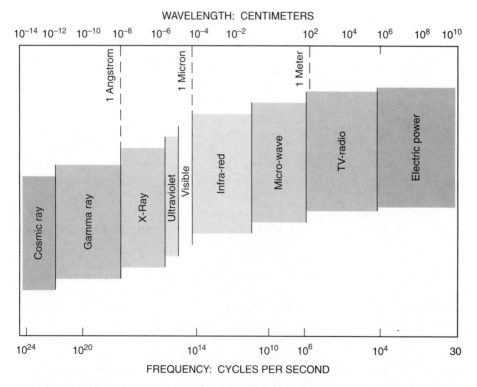

Figure 5–2. Electromagnetic spectrum of radiant energy. (*Reproduced with permission from* Therapeutic Electricity and Ultraviolet Radiation. *Stillwell KG. 3rd ed. 1983: Williams & Wilkins.*)

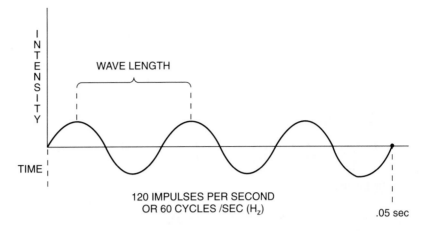

Figure 5–3. Wavelength. Wavelength is the distance from the peak of one wave to the identical peak of the next wave. Frequency is the number of oscillations or cycles per second. Here, the frequency is 60 Hz.

and ultraviolet) and some waves have specific medical uses. Table 5–1, displays the wavelength, the frequency of the wave, its designation, and its medical use.

Electromagnetic waves can travel through a vacuum at the highest speed. As the density of the medium increases, however, the velocity decreases. Sound and ultrasound are not part of the electromagnetic spectrum because they have different physical characteristics: for example, they cannot travel through a vacuum. These waves are discussed in Chapter 13.

Rays of radiant energy such as light can be affected by a medium in four different ways:

TABLE 5–1. THE ELECTROMAGNETIC SPECTRUM

Wavelength (range in nm)*	Frequency The upper limit (cycle/s, or Hz)	Designation	Medical Use
0.0001–0.01	3.0×10^{21}	Cosmic rays	Not known
0.01–0.14	2.14×10^{18}	Gamma rays	Radium therapy
0.14–120	5.9×10^{15}	X-rays	Diagnosis and treatment
180–280	1.03×10^{15}	Short (far) ultraviolet (UVC)	Diagnosis and treatment
280–315	9.0×10^{14}	Long (near) ultraviolet (UVB)	Diagnosis and treatment
280–400	7.5×10^{14}	Long (near) ultraviolet (UVA)	Diagnosis and treatment
400–800	3.75×10^{14}	Visible light: violet, blue, green	Not fully explored (seasonal depression)
632	4.74×10^{14}	Cold laser	Not fully explored (tissue healing, pain)
800–1500	2.0×10^{14}	Short (near) infrared	Superficial heat
1500–15000	2.0×10^{13}	Long (far) infrared	Superficial heat
$1.5 \times 10^4 – 1 \times 10^9$	3.0×10^8	Microwave	Diathermy (deep heat)
$1 \times 10^9 – 3 \times 10^9$	10^8	Radar	Not known
$3 \times 10^9 – 30 \times 10^9$	10^7	Short wave diathermy	Deep heat
$30 \times 10^9 – 300 \times 10^9$	10^6	Long wave diathermy	Deep heat
$300 \times 10^9 – 30 \times 10^{12}$	10^4	Broadcast	Not known
$.5 \times 10^{15}$	60	Electric power	Muscle and nerve stimulation

*Millimicron (nm) is equal to 10 angstrom (Å) or 10^{-7} cm.

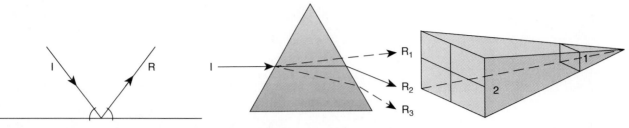

Figure 5–4. Reflection (I = rays of incident, R = rays of reflection). The angle-of-incident ray is equal to the angle of the reflected ray.

Figure 5–5. Refraction through a prism (I = rays of incident, R = rays of refraction).

Figure 5–6. The law of inverse squares. This law states that because of the diversion of the rays, the intensity of the wave varies inversely with the square of the distance between the source of the radiant energy and the tissue absorbing the rays.

1. They can be reflected by the medium (eg, a mirror).
2. They can be absorbed by the medium (eg, one with a dark, nonshiny surface).
3. They can be refracted by the medium (eg, a prism, which refracts the sunlight into its different wavelengths, producing a rainbow effect).
4. They can penetrate through the medium (eg, clear glass).

When energy penetrates or transmits through a medium, some of it is absorbed in the process. Therefore, having 100% of emitted energy available at deeper tissues is impossible. Biological tissue exposed to radiant energy will be affected by that energy. According to the *Grotthuss Draper law*, waves of different wavelengths produce different effects, and the extent of the effect will be determined by the amount of the energy that is absorbed by the tissue.

When radiant energy such as infrared and ultraviolet is used in treatment, the skin is invariably exposed and will reflect some of the rays. The amount of reflection will be related to the patient's complexion (amount of melanin in the skin), the texture of the skin (scaly or smooth), and the oiliness or dryness of the skin. The skin will absorb some of the rays, and the energy from those rays will affect the skin. Some rays have a predominantly photochemical effect, whereas others simply increase the skin temperature.

In addition to the quality of the skin, three laws govern the dosage of radiant energy the tissue receives: the inverse square law, the cosine law, and the Bunsen Roscoe law of reciprocity. The *inverse square law* states that the intensity of the wave varies inversely with the square of the distance between the source of the radiant energy and the absorbing tissue because of the divergence of the rays (see Fig. 5–6). For example, if the distance between the source and the surface decreases from 2 feet to 1 foot, the intensity of the dosage is increased four times, as expressed in the following formula:

$$I = \frac{1}{D^2}, \text{ where I = intensity and D = distance.}$$

To avoid overexposure, the distance must be kept in mind.

The *cosine law* states that maximum absorption of radiant energy occurs when the source is at right angles to the absorbing surface. When the source is not at a right angle to the absorbing surface, the angle formed by the source and the perpendicular to the absorbing surface determines the effect of the energy. The relationship between the angle of the rays and the amount absorbed is expressed by the following formula (see Fig. 5–7).

$$\text{Cos ABC} = \frac{AB}{BC}$$

When the angle is 60°,

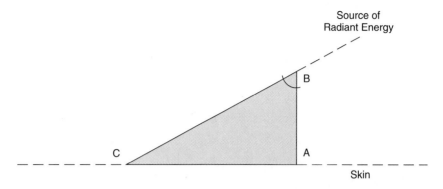

Figure 5–7. The cosine of the angle of incidence. This law states that maximum absorption of radiant energy occurs when the source of the energy (BC) is at a right angle (CAB) to the absorbing surface (AC).

$$\frac{AB}{BC} = \frac{1}{2}$$

Because the cosine of 60° is 0.5, only 50% of the output is available for absorption at that angle of incidence.

The *Bunsen Roscoe law of reciprocity* states that the intensity and duration of the dose of radiant energy are inversely proportional:

$$\text{Energy (E)} = \text{intensity (I)} \times \text{time (T)}$$

The practical meaning of this law is that the intensity and duration of the dose can be manipulated even when one wants the amount of energy delivered to the patient to remain constant. This relationship can be shown by rearranging the above formula in the following way:

$$I = \frac{E}{T} \text{ or } T = \frac{E}{I}$$

The principles and laws just outlined must be considered when planning treatments using electromagnetic waves (ie, when determining dosage and when positioning equipment) if the treatments are to be both effective and safe.

■ **KEY TERMS**

quantum theory
electromagnetic wave theory
electromagnetic spectrum
Grotthuss-Draper law

inverse square law
cosine law
Bunsen Roscoe law of reciprocity

SECTION 2
THERMAL AGENTS

Whether using a sunbath to relax aching muscles or splashing cool water on the temples when overheated, people throughout the ages have treated physical complaints and sought relief from discomfort by applying heat or cold to their bodies in some way. At present, both heat and cold are widely used physical therapy modalities. A thermal modality is sometimes the primary part of a treatment program. Such a program is acceptable when it is likely that the physiological or psychological changes produced of themselves can alleviate the patient's problem (eg, when one applies ice immediately after an injury to stop bleeding or soaks in a hot bath to sooth mental anxiety and tension). More often, however, thermal modalities are used as an adjunct to other physical therapy treatments. For example, before therapeutic exercise—passive range of motion or mobilization procedures—heat or cold can be applied to prepare body tissues or reduce pain. Thus, patients may benefit more from the treatment procedures that are to follow.

Much of our present use of thermal modalities is based on empirical evidence—clinical observations that patients exhibit positive reactions after thermal modalities are applied. Because of research done so far, we have some scientific understanding of how and why these reactions occur. With the passive procedures mentioned above, studies have shown that either heat or cold can be beneficial, but the rationale for using each one differs. For example, some evidence indicates that collagen tissues become more elongated when heated and that cold, by altering the activity of peripheral nerves, allows muscles to relax. Thus, heat might be chosen if scar tissue limits the range of motion and cold might be chosen if the limitation is the result of muscle splinting.

Conclusive evidence is lacking regarding some physiological responses to changes in tissue temperature and, in some instances, controversy exists concerning the therapeutic benefits. Some therapists believe that heat should always be applied before muscle strengthening exercises, whereas others believe that only cold should be used. Although studies can be cited to reinforce either viewpoint, more studies need to be done to determine whether and when one thermal agent is significantly better clinically than the other.

To select and apply thermal modalities rationally, the physical therapist should know why and how each modality is used. Chapter 6 defines and discusses terms that are commonly used to differentiate the various thermal modalities and the dosages used. Chapters 7, 8, and 9 discuss basic thermal physics and physiology. Chapter 10 compares the effects of heat versus cold, the therapeutic implications of which should help therapists make judgments about the use of specific modalities in specific situations. Chapters 11 through 14 discuss each specific thermal modality. Chapter 15, the final chapter in the section, contains basic information about monitoring signs and symptoms and about ambient conditions to consider when applying thermal modalities to patients.

6

Terminology

Bernadette Hecox, PT, MA

Categories of Thermal Modalities	Dosage Terms and Reactions
Heat Modalities	Dosage Reactions
Cold Modalities	Specific Dosages
Local Versus General Applications	**Key Terms**
Local Versus Systemic Reactions	**Review Questions**

T his chapter defines terms that are often used when discussing thermal modalities. Familiarity with these terms and their meanings can help the physical therapist to understand the content of the chapters in this thermal section and to communicate effectively with other health professionals as well.

CATEGORIES OF THERMAL MODALITIES

Heat Modalities

Heat modalities can be categorized as either superficial or deep. A *superficial heat modality* refers to heat that, when applied at a maximally safe clinical dosage, is only capable of raising the temperature of superficial tissues to a therapeutically significantly level.[1] Although these modalities may increase the skin temperature by 18° F (10° C), the increase in temperature of tissues 1 cm deep will be less than 6° F (3° C) and that of tissues 2 cm deep about 2° F (1.3° C).[1,2]

Superficial heat can be either moist or dry, depending on the source of the heat. If the source is the sun, other sources of infrared radiation, or any modality with little moisture (eg, a heating pad or warm dry air), it is called a *dry heat* modality. If the heat source is water, another fluid, moist air, or a modality containing moisture (eg, a hot pack), it is called *moist heat.*

The term *deep heat modality* implies that a form of energy other than heat is transmitted through the skin and is absorbed in deeper tissues, where it increases the kinetic action of molecules. Thus, forms of energy such as electromagnetic energy (diathermy) and acoustic energy (ultrasound), which can be transmitted to deeper tissues, increase the temperature of those tissues. These modalities produce heat as a result of energy conversion (see Chapter 7).

Cold Modalities

Because all cold modalities are applied to and will cool the surface tissue more than the deeper tissues, no terms differentiate deep from superficial. These modalities are categorized according to the specific modality: for example "apply ice" versus "apply a cold pack." The general term used to describe cold modalities is *cryotherapy*.

LOCAL VERSUS GENERAL APPLICATIONS

Local application refers to the application of a thermal modality to only one area of the body: for example, placing a hot water bottle or ice pack on a painful shoulder. *General application* refers to the application of heat or cold to all or much of the body, as in taking a shower, bath, or staying in a warm room. The terms local and general refer only to the amount of the body being treated, not to the amount of heat absorbed or given off. Naturally, if heat of the same temperature and duration is used in a general and a local application, the general agent will provide more heat input. However, a brief warm shower, although a general application, may provide less heat input than a heating pad, a local agent that is "on" all night. The modalities shown in Fig. 6–1A and B can be clearly described as local or general. However, a modality applied to larger areas of the body (see Fig. 6–1C) requires a more specific description.

LOCAL VERSUS SYSTEMIC REACTIONS

A *local reaction* refers to physiological changes occurring at the site of a local application, including localized sweating with heat, pilo erection (goose bumps) with cold, and changes in local metabolic rate, blood flow, and skin condition with both heat and cold. A *systemic reaction* refers to physiological changes occurring in the various systems of the body. For example, if enough heat is added to or taken from the body (regardless of whether by a prolonged local or general thermal modality), the core temperature may change. The results may include systemic reactions such

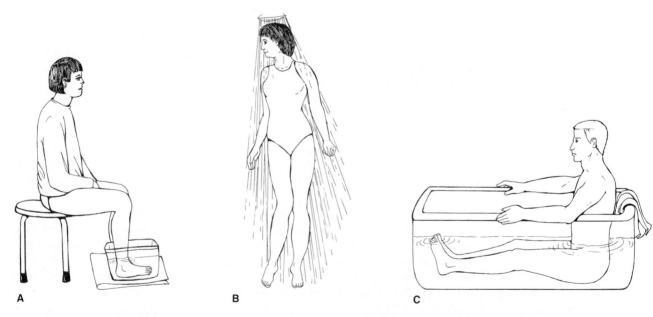

A   **B**   **C**

Figure 6–1. Examples of applications of a thermal modality. The modality is water in this case. **(A)** The immersion of one foot or ankle is a local application. **(B)** A full-body shower is a general application. **(C)** Sitting waist high in water is not considered to be either a local or general application. A more specific description is required.

as generalized sweating or shivering and cardiovascular changes such as increased or decreased pulse rate and blood pressure. With application of a local heat modality, the rate at which the modality is able to increase tissue temperature is an important factor that influences the degree of local containment of the heat and the duration of the treatment. If the HEAT input causes the *tissue temperature* (TT) to rise faster than the local vascular system can convect the heat into the general circulation, the result is a greater local heating effect. Conversely, if a modality requires 10 min to increase the TT above 107° F (42° C) and the goal of the therapist is to have a significant *tissue temperature rise* (TTR) lasting 15 min, a 25-min treatment is required. The usual 20-min treatment would not be long enough.[3] These physiological responses are mentioned here because they affect the dosage given. Such responses will be discussed in more detail in later chapters of this section.

DOSAGE TERMS AND REACTIONS

For safe and effective use, thermal modalities should be applied in appropriate doses. The dosage will vary with each modality and with each patient's needs. *General dosage* terms can be used to describe the effect that the modality has on the patient, whereas specific dosage terms describe precise treatment factors.

Heat or cold treatments are often described in the following general terms: mild, moderate, and vigorous. One can say "mild heat may be helpful" or "vigorous heat is indicated." These general terms relate to the degree to which the reactions to the dosage occurs or they describe the desired effect.

Dosage Reactions

Thermal modalities can produce changes in tissue temperature, and changes in firing of thermal sensory neurons. Either can result in local or systemic reactions or both.

Changes in Tissue Temperature

With a *mild dose* of heat or cold, the desired effect is no more than a slight change in the TT in the area where the modality is applied. Benefits are probably related to the sensation of warmth or coolness. A *moderate dose* is expected to increase the TT to approximately 102°–106° F (39°–41° C), with only a slight increase in blood flow. With a *vigorous dose*, the goal is a TTR to approximately 107°–113° F (42°–45° C). In this range, one can anticipate maximum beneficial physiological effects without tissue damage.

A temperature in deeper tissues of 109°–113° F (43°–45° C) is required to increase blood flow significantly in those tissues.[3,4] Thus, the term *significant heating* implies that tissues should be heated to that range to achieve a marked increase in blood flow.

In general, if the patient's vascular status is good, it is considered safe to heat tissues up to approximately 113° F (45° C) for 30 min to 50 min, whereas tissue damage occurs at even slightly higher temperatures.[5] However, patients may not tolerate temperatures higher than 109° F (43° C), for at approximately that temperature, one begins to perceive pain, signaling the danger of tissue damage at higher temperatures. With prolonged vigorous heating, the patient's core temperature may rise to well above 100° F (37.8° C).[6]

With cold, a TT near freezing may be tolerable for brief periods. However, as the TT falls to 68° F (20° C) or less, the tissues approach a *critical range*. Although tissues are not frozen in the range between 68°–32° F (20°–0° C), pain is perceived, neural activity gradually diminishes, and protective vascular adjustments are activated.[7] Heating or cooling beyond safe limits may damage tissues, sometimes irreparably.[5,8,9] Table 6–1 notes significant physiological effects that occur at various temperatures.

Changes in Firing of Thermal Sensory Neurons

Thermoreceptors are found in cutaneous tissues throughout the body. Whenever these receptors are subject to any change in temperature, the rate of firing of the thermal sensory neurons changes and the body responds instantaneously to a sensation of heat or cold. Depending on (1) the size of the area subjected to the temper-

TABLE 6–1. EFFECTS OF VARIOUS TEMPERATURES ON TISSUES

Temperatures	Degrees		Effect
	Fahrenheit	Celsius	
Increased temperature*	109.0	43.0	Pain threshold
	113.0	45.0	Severe pain; safety limit for 30 min of heat application.
	118.0	47.8	Blisters appear in 20 min; tissue necrosis occurs in 1 hr.
	126.0	52.0	Blisters appear in 30 sec; tissue necrosis occurs in 1 min.
	149.0	65.0	Tissue necrosis occurs in 1 sec.
Decreased temperature*†‡§‖	73.4	23.0	Activity of peripheral nerves begins to decline markedly.
	68–32	20–0	Critical range.
	50.0	10.0	Redness and swelling in 1 hr.
	48.2	9.0	Velocity of nerve conduction ceases.
	41.0	5.0	Paralysis of peripheral nerves occurs.
	28.6	−1.9	Marked pain or swelling occurs in 4–7 min.
	28.0	−2.2	Skin freezes.

*Krusen F, ed: *Handbook of Physical Medicine and Rehabilitation.* 2nd ed. Philadelphia, PA: WB Saunders; 1971:261–272.
†Burton A, Edhold O: *Man in a Cold Environment.* London, UK: Edward Arnold; 1955:225,227,230.
‡Holdcroft A: *Body Temperature Control.* London, UK: Bailliere-Tindall; 1980:1,12–26.
§Lehmann J, ed: *Therapeutic Heat and Cold.* 3rd ed. Baltimore, MD: Williams & Wilkins; 1982:65,128–129,175,179,212–213.
‖Williamson C, Schultz J: Time-temperature relationships in thermal blister formation. *J Invest. Dermatol.* 1949 12(1):41–47.

ature change, (2) the temperature gradient between the skin and the applied modality, and (3) the rate of heat exchange, autonomic nervous system responses and behavioral responses, sometimes called *thermal shock reactions,* occur.

If the thermal modality applied is approximately the same temperature as the skin (a mild dose) or if the rate of change in skin temperature is gradual, the responses of the autonomic system are usually those associated with comfort: for example, relaxation and analgesia. With a moderate dose, one can expect a more pronounced sensation of heat or cold and a more stimulating reaction. With a vigorous dose, if the temperature gradient and rate of change are sufficient, the result is the "fight or flight" reaction, which includes changes in the activity of the cardiovascular system.[6,7,10] For example, if the skin temperature is 84° F (28.9° C) and a person slowly gets into a 90° F (32.2° C) bath or an 80° F (26.7° C) lake, the body will react only slightly to the temperature change—an experience usually perceived as pleasurable. However, everyone is familiar with the strong reactions that occur when one jumps into an extremely hot bath (105° F, 40.6° C) or an extremely cold lake (68° F, 20° C).

Many factors, including age, individual sensitivity, past experiences related to thermal sensation, and pathological conditions, will affect a person's reactions to thermal shock. Thus, when applying a thermal modality, the therapist must consider the effect of both the temperature gradient and the rate at which the patient experiences the change. For example, when treating a patient in a Hubbard tank, lower the patient into the tank slowly to avoid a thermal shock reaction.

Specific Dosages

The following specific factors must be considered for each thermal modality:

- The intensity of the heat or cold per area of the patient to which it is applied: ie, how much and how fast the modality can affect tissues or systems.

- The duration of each treatment.
- The frequency with which the treatment will be given.

Because variations in techniques alter the intensity and therefore the thermal changes, the techniques recommended when applying the modality also should be known. If, at a given temperature, one hot pack is applied with only two layers of toweling and another is applied with eight layers, the intensity of heat that the patient receives will obviously be much greater with the former. Recommended dosages per technique, based on clinical experience, scientific studies, or both, are those producing changes in TT that are considered to be optimal for safe and therapeutically beneficial treatment.

The factors that dictate the dosage for each thermal modality differ for several reasons. Each modality is composed of different substances with different thermal qualities, and the means by which each transfers heat to the patient also varies. These factors are discussed in subsequent chapters in this section.

Another important consideration is whether the modality is connected to a constant source of heat production such as a heat lamp or a heating pad, which can either maintain or increase its temperature and heat output as long as it is connected to the source of electrical energy. A modality such as a hot pack or a hot water bottle will not maintain its initial heat output for more than a few minutes, whereas a modality that provides constant heat produces a greater TTR, systemic reaction, or both. The latter modalities pose an inherently greater danger of overheating both locally and systemically.

Special attention must be paid to the dosages for deep heat modality treatments because the temperature of deeper tissues may be higher than that of superficial tissues. Thus, skin sensation may not indicate the temperature rise in the deeper tissues where the damage may occur.

To predict the temperature changes in deeper tissues more objectively, the National Council on Radiation & Measurements of the Food and Drug Administration has quantified the amount of high-frequency electromagnetic energy per unit of tissue mass absorbed in the tissues through the use of a unit called the *specific absorption rate* (SAR), which is expressed in watts per kilogram. The therapeutic range of this absorption extends from approximately 50 w/kg to 170 w/kg, and the rate of TTR corresponds somewhat to the SAR. In vascularized tissues, a low SAR (50 w/kg) will generally cause a TTR of 1.4° F (0.8° C)/min and a high SAR (170 w/kg) will cause a TTR of 4.9° F (2.7° C)/min. As with all thermal modalities, the final TT depends on the duration of the treatment and on physiological factors, especially the patient's vascular status.[11–13] However, physiological factors differ for each patient, and, because the skin temperature does not indicate the deep TTR the clinician has no way of determining the exact dosage that each patient should receive.

Although one can use the percentage of power (energy) or SAR level readout on the high-frequency device as a guide, the dosage for deep heat modalities must ultimately be determined by the patient's report of the sensation of heat he or she experiences. Table 6–2 suggests the dosage level, duration and frequency of treatments to be used when deep heat modalities are used for acute, subacute, or chronic conditions. These suggestions are based on the patient's subjective reporting of the warmth experienced and the SAR dosage factors that produce similar sensations of warmth. These factors include the percentage of power output required to produce a specific SAR that can be predicted to cause a specific rate of TTR.

Finally, the fact that care must be used with all thermal modalities cannot be over emphasized. The *specific dosage* must be determined according to each patient's physical status and pathology, which can greatly influence the local and systemic reactions that thermal changes may produce. Recommended dosages for each modality as well as precautions and contraindications based on pathology and physical status are discussed in subsequent chapters.

TABLE 6–2. DOSAGE GUIDE FOR DEEP HEAT TREATMENTS*†‡

Condition Being Treated	Treatment			Heat Sensation Reported by Patient	Percentage Output of Energy from the Device	Specific Absorption Rate (SAR) (w/kg)	Rate of Tissue Temperature Rise (° C/min)
	Dosage Level	Duration of Treatment	Frequency of Treatments				
Acute inflammation	1. Lowest	1–3 min	Daily for 1–2 wks	None; dose is just below any sensation of heat	1/4 maximum output	25–50 w/kg	0.4°–0.8° C/min
Subacute resolving	2. Low	3–5 min	Daily for 1–2 wks	Barely felt	1/2 maximum output	50–75 w/kg	0.8°–1.2° C/min
Inflammatory conditions	3. Medium	5–7 min	Daily for 1–2 wks	Distinct but pleasant heat sensation	3/4 maximum output	75–125 w/kg	1.2°–2° C/min
Usual chronic conditions	4. High	5–7 min	Daily or 2 times/wk for 1 wk to 1 mo	Definite heat sensation, well within tolerance	maximum output	125–170 w/kg	2.0°–2.7° C/min

*Kloth L: Lecture delivered at the APTA Combined Section Meeting. Anaheim, CA: February 1986.
†Michlovitz S: *Thermal Agents in Rehabilitation*. Philadelphia, PA: FA Davis; 1986.
‡Therapeutic shortwave and microwave diathermy. *FDA Bulletin* 85–8237. December 1984.

■ KEY TERMS

superficial heat modality
  dry heat
  moist heat
deep heat modality
cryotherapy
local application
general application
local reaction
systemic reaction
general dosage

mild dose
moderate dose
vigorous dose
specific dosage
tissue temperature (TT)
tissue temperature rise (TTR)
significant heating
critical range
thermal shock reaction
specific absorption rate (SAR)

■ REVIEW QUESTIONS

1. What is a superficial heat modality?
2. What is a deep heat modality?
3. What is the difference between dry and moist heat? Give examples.
4. What does a "local application" mean? Give examples.
5. What does a "general application" mean? Give examples.
6. What do general dosage terms describe?
7. What are the three general terms used to describe any dosage treatment?
8. What changes in tissue temperature are desired with
    (a) a mild dose?
    (b) a moderate dose?
    (c) a vigorous dose?
9. If a vigorous heat dosage is recommended, what temperature range may maximize the beneficial effects without damaging tissue?
10. What range of tissue temperatures is required to cause a *significant* increase in blood flow to the tissues?

11. What does the term "significant heating" mean?
12. At approximately what temperature do patients begin to perceive pain?
13. What does the term "critical range" mean for colder temperatures? What happens within that range?
14. What is a thermal shock reaction? How can it happen?
15. What is a local reaction? Give examples.
16. What is a systemic reaction?

REFERENCES

1. Lehmann J, Silverman D, Baum B, Kirk N, Johnston V: Temperature Distribution in the Human Thigh Produced by Infrared, Hot Packs and Microwave Applications. *Arch. Phy. Med. and Rehab.* 1966; 47(6):291–299.
2. Borrell R, Parker R, Henley E, Masley D, Repinecz M: Comparison of In Vivo Temperatures Produced by Hydrotherapy, Paraffin Wax Treatment, & Fluidotherapy. *Physical Therapy* 1980; 60(10):1273–1276.
3. Lehmann J, Warren G, Scham S: Therapeutic Heat and Cold. *Clinical Orthopedics and Related Research* 1974; 99:207–245.
4. Sekins K, et al: Local Muscle Blood Flow and Temperature Responses to 915 mHz (MW) Diathermy as Simultaneously Measured and Numerically Predicted. *Arch. of Phy. Med. and Rehab.* 1984; 65:1–7.
5. Moritz A, Henrique F: Studies of Thermal Injury, Part II: The Relative Importance of Time and Surface Temperature in the Causation of Cutaneous Burns. *Amer. J. of Pathol.* 1947; 23:695–720.
6. Licht S, ed: *Medical Hydrology.* New Haven: E. Licht Pub., 1963; 98–99; 102; 242.
7. Hensel H: *Thermal Sensations and Thermoreceptors in Man.* Springfield: Charles C Thomas, 1982; 6; 36; 91–92; 94.
8. Thorman M: The Pathology and Management of Frostbite. *Clin. Management* 1985; 5:12–15.
9. Dyke P, Thomas P, Lambert E, Bunge R, eds: *Peripheral Neuropathy.* Philadelphia: W.B. Saunders 1984; I:453–476; II:1479–1511, 2303–2304.
10. Kottke F, Stillwell G, Lehmann J, eds: *Krusen's Handbook of Physical Medicine and Rehabilitation.* Philadelphia: W.B. Saunders, 1982; 275–350.
11. Kloth L: *Lecture.* Delivered at APTA Combined Section Meeting. Anaheim: February, 1986.
12. Michlovitz S: *Thermal Agents in Rehabilitation.* Philadelphia; FA Davis, 1986;75;193–194.
13. Therapeutic Shortwave and Microwave Diathermy. *FDA Bulletin* 1984; 85–8237, Dec.
14. Krusen F: *Handbook of Physical Medicine and Rehabilitation.* 2nd ed. Philadelphia: WB Saunders, 1971; 261–272.
15. Williamson C, Scholtz J: Time-Temperature Relationships in Thermal Blister Formation. *J of Invest. Dermatology* 1949; 12(1):41–47.
16. Burton A, Edholm O: *Man in a Cold Environment.* London: Edward Arnold Ltd., 1955; 225; 227; 230.
17. Holdcroft A: *Body Temperature Control.* London: Bailliere-Tindall, 1980; 1; 12–26.
18. Lehmann J, ed: *Therapeutic Heat and Cold.* 3rd ed. Baltimore: Williams & Wilkins, 1982; 65; 128–129; 175; 179; 212–213.

7

Thermal Physics

Bernadette Hecox, PT, MA

Heat and the First Law of Thermodynamics

First Law of Thermodynamics

Temperature and Temperature Scales

Heat Transfer

Radiation

Conduction

Convection

Thermal Properties of Substances

State of the Substance

Density and Thermal Expansion

Specific Heat Capacity

Thermal Conductivity

Summary

Key Terms

To understand the amount of heat or cold the patient receives and the resulting therapeutic effects, the physical therapist must become acquainted with basic physical concepts concerning *thermal energy* and with biophysics, the physical relationship to the body and the physiological effects produced. Integrating this information helps the therapist determine which thermal effects are therapeutically beneficial or detrimental. This chapter begins the process by discussing the aspects of thermal physics that are relevant to thermal physical agents.

HEAT AND THE FIRST LAW OF THERMODYNAMICS

Kinetic energy—the movement of molecules or their constituents (atoms, nuclei, and electrons)—is related to the temperature of a substance. Thus, kinetic energy, the internal energy of the substance, is *thermal energy*. As the temperature of a substance increases, the motion of its molecules increases. Movement of the entire molecule is termed translational, and movement of the constituents within the molecule can be either rotational or vibrational. Molecular motion ceases only if the temperature of a substance is absolute zero: ie, it contains no heat.

Assuming that the sun is the initial source of energy, no molecular motion of any substance would occur without solar energy. As long as a substance has some energy, some random molecular motion is present. Thus, the substance contains some heat. With increased input of energy, kinetic energy increases. The increased molecular motion produces more heat and the temperature rises. Because an increase in molecular motion correlates with an increase in heat of a substance, a simple definition of heat could be that *heat* is molecular motion.

TABLE 7–1. PERCEPTION OF COLD AND HOT TEMPERATURE OF WATER FOR A BODY BATH*

°Fahrenheit	Perception	°Celsius
32–55	Extremely cold	1–13
55–65	Cold	13–18
65–80	Cool	18–27
80–92	Tepid	27–33.5
92–96	Neutral	33.5–35.5
96–98	Warm	35.5–36.5
98–104	Hot	36.5–40.0
104–113	Extremely hot	40–46
Maximum tolerance 113–115		Maximum tolerance 45–46

*Adapted from Licht S, ed. *Medical Hydrology.* New Haven, CT: 1963:13, 55, 140, 142, 507.

The words hot and cold are relative terms. One can say that no such thing as cold exists because as long as any molecular motion is present, there is some heat. However, the terms are used for the sake of comparison. If one places a hand previously warmed to 104° F (40° C) in water that is 90° F (32.2° C), the water may feel cold, but if a chilled hand is placed in the same water, the water might feel hot. In each case, the different perception is the result of a different reference point. Thus, cold is not an absolute entity; it is a term used to describe an entity that has less heat, or gives the sensation of less heat, than does another entity. However, in day-to-day terms, we have become accustomed to calling certain temperatures hot or cold for practical purposes. To a snow skier, 50° F (10° C) weather is hot; to a water skier, it is cold. Table 7–1 indicates how various temperatures of water are generally perceived when a person in a temperate ambient temperature immerses a body part in water.

First Law of Thermodynamics

The *first law of thermodynamics* tells us that, with the exception of nuclear effects, energy cannot be created or destroyed but can be transformed from one form to another. Whenever this transformation occurs, some energy is released as heat and thus is considered to be thermal energy. Any activity of chemical, mechanical, or electromagnetic systems always produces some heat. Through such processes, diathermy and ultrasound modalities convert high-frequency electromagnetic or sound energies to heat in the tissue where the original energy is absorbed.[1]

Temperature and Temperature Scales

Temperature is not heat per se, it is a means of measuring or describing heat more specifically than is possible using the relative terms hot and cold. This description is not completely accurate either because two substances (eg, water and melted paraffin) at equal temperatures may not necessarily contain equal amounts of heat energy or feel equally hot.

Temperature can be measured with four different scales. Table 7–2 compares the four scales and notes the temperatures that have special meaning to therapists. Clinically, we use both *Fahrenheit* (F) and *Celsius* (C) (centigrade) *scales*, therefore therapists should be able to quickly convert any information given in either scale to the other. One commonly used conversion formula is

$$°F = (9/5 °C) + 32 \text{ or } °C = 5/9 (°F - 32)$$

The *Kelvin* and *Rankin temperature scales* are used for scientific research. The size of a degree is the same for the Celsius and Kelvin (K) scales and for the Fahrenheit and Rankin (R) scales. The difference between the boiling and freezing

TABLE 7–2. FOUR TEMPERATURE SCALES NOTING SPECIFIC TEMPERATURES PERTINENT TO THERMAL MODALITY TREATMENTS

Rankin[†]	°F		°C (Celsius)	Kelvin*
672°	212	Boiling point of water (steam)	100	373°
	194		90	
	176		80	
	149		65	
	131	Melting point of paraffin	55	
	125.6	Approximate melting point of paraffin-oil mixture	52	
	122		50	
	114.8		46	
	111.2		44	
	107.6		42	
	104.0		40	
	100.4		38	
	98.6		37	
	96.8		36	
	95.0		35	
	77.0		25	
	68.0		20	
	59.0		15	
	50.0		10	
	41.0		5	
492°	32.0	Freezing point of water (ice)	0	273°
0°	−460.00	ABSOLUTE ZERO	−273	0°

*Same as Celsius scale (100° between boiling and freezing point of water).
†Same scale as Fahrenheit (180° between boiling and freezing point of water).

points of water is 100° in both the C and K scales and the difference between these points is 180° (212°–32°) in both the F and R scales. Absolute 0° K equals −273.16° C and absolute 0° R equals −460° F.

HEAT TRANSFER

Heat is always transferred from higher to lower temperature molecules until a state of equilibrium is achieved. This *heat transfer* can occur through radiation, conduction, and convection. Devices using each of these means of heat transfer are available to clinicians. Fig. 7–1 illustrates three thermal modalities that transfer heat by the different mechanisms: heat lamps, hot packs, and fluidotherapy. Therefore, the physical therapist can select the modality with the means of heat transfer that is most appropriate for a particular situation.

Radiation

All objects can give off or take on thermal energy through the process of *radiation*. Energy emitted at infrared frequencies will travel from a warmer substance and be absorbed in a cooler substance. The increase in infrared energy causes the molecular motion in the cooler object to increase, thus increasing its heat. Because infrared rays are synonymous with heat waves, all the physical laws of radiation apply (see Chapter 5).

If you stand in a room and the temperature of your exposed skin is 87° F (30.6° C) and the walls of the room are 65° F (18.3° C), you will radiate infrared energy. That energy will travel from you to the walls, where it will be absorbed; this transfer will continue until you have cooled and the walls have heated so that temperatures

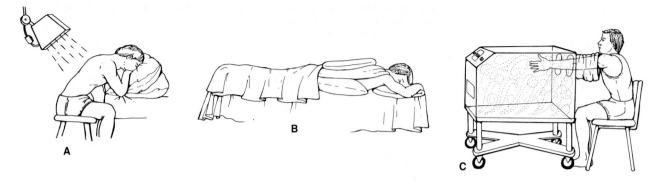

Figure 7–1. Three thermal modalities, each using a different means of transferring heat to the patient. (**A**) A heat Lamp uses radiation; heat energy is beamed through space to the patient. (**B**) A hot pack uses conduction; a moist heat modality is in contact with the patient. (**C**) Fluidotherapy relies on convection; warm air blows over the patient.

of both are equal. Basically, infrared waves are transmitted through space and thus do not heat air. However, some waves are absorbed in dust and other substances that may be in the air. Advertisements for some small-area heaters called quartz heaters explain the concept of infrared heating. These advertisements stress that these heaters are "people heaters," not "space heaters." This is true, because the infrared rays transmitted through space are absorbed into objects and people. But this is just as true for the heated filament units commonly called "space heaters." Both types emit infrared rays; thus, they heat objects rather than the air. The term space heater implies that the heater is effective only within a limited area of space from the heater. Both quartz and filament infrared lamps are used in physical therapy.

Conduction

Conduction is a method of heat transfer from one place to another by successive molecular collisions. Heat transfer by conduction is a slow process. When two objects of different temperatures come in contact—for example, when your warm hand touches a cooler object—the more rapidly moving molecules of the warmer object (your hand) collide with the more slowly moving molecules of the cooler object. The collision causes the more slowly moving molecules to move faster, thus increasing the temperature of that object. But because the warmer object (your hand) gave up some of its energy, its molecules move more slowly after the collision, causing your hand to become cooler.

Paraffin, hot packs, and cold packs use the conduction transfer method. Hot packs and melted paraffin transfer heat from the modality to the body. In the case of a cold pack, however, the rapidly moving, warmer molecules of the body transfer heat to the pack. Consequently, the body cools and the pack becomes warmer.

Convection

Convection is a method of heat transfer in which the heated molecules move from one place to another. This method of heat transfer is more rapid than conduction and occurs in liquids and gases. Increased input of energy into a system increases the energy of some molecules, which produces more forceful collisions and causes the molecules to travel greater distances after colliding. Thus, as the temperature increases, the space between fluid or gas molecules increases, resulting in a less dense heated region. A region of lower density is lighter, but it demands more space, replacing the region of higher density. For example, warm air rises and cool air sinks. Circulation of the air or water takes place as the heated, more buoyant gas or fluid rises.

Fig. 7–2A and B illustrate convection. If the air in a room is initially 50° F (10° C) and a baseboard heater heats the air adjacent to it to 90° F (32.2° C), the warmer air

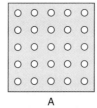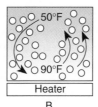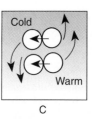

Figure 7–2. In this simplified illustration of the convection process, a baseboard heater is used to heat the air in a room. (**A**) All air in the room is the same temperature (50° F): ie, no convection occurs. (**B**) As the heater begins to heat the room, the temperature of the air near the heater increases to 90° F, the warm air expands (becoming less dense) and therefore rises toward the ceiling, which causes the cooler denser air above to circulate toward the floor. (**C**) As the warmer molecules of air rise, they collide with the cooler descending molecules; during this circulation, some heat transfers from the warmer molecules to the cooler ones.

will expand and the molecules will begin to rise, causing the cooler air nearer the ceiling—because of its greater density—to circulate down toward the baseboard, where it will be heated. However, as rising hot-air molecules pass the descending cool-air molecules, they collide (touch). As a result, some heat is conducted (transferred to the cooler molecules). Thus, the "cool" molecules will be warmer than the initial temperature of the air in the room (50° F) as they near the floor (see Fig. 7–2C).

Nonetheless, as this cooler air, which is now near the floor, is heated, it in turn will rise. The circulatory process will continue until all molecules reach the same temperature. This is analogous to the body's major means of heat transfer between core and surface. As heat is convected in blood flowing through the vascular system some heat is transferred by conduction to adjacent tissues or blood vessels.

The same principles of convection apply to water. With a temperature gradient, water will circulate without any stirring or agitation until all of it reaches approximately the same temperature. For example, suppose you fill one-third of a whirlpool tank with extremely hot water, then add the same amount of cool water. In a few minutes, all the water will be the same temperature via convection even without stirring the water. Of course, agitation hastens this circulating process tremendously.

THERMAL PROPERTIES OF SUBSTANCES

Many properties of substances depend on and vary with changes in temperature and atmospheric pressure. Such properties include (1) the state of the substance (solid, liquid, or gas) (2) its density and thermal expansion, (3) its specific heat capacity (c), and (4) its thermal conductivity (k). Because each substance has a unique molecular structure, no specific temperature or pressure affects the properties of all substances in the same way.

State of the Substance

Heat taken in or given up by a substance does not always change its temperature. Some energy is used in the process of changing a substance from one state to another. The heat required to change a substance from a liquid to a solid is called the *heat of fusion,* and the heat required to change a substance from a solid to a gas is called the *heat of vaporization.*

Heat of Fusion

When water gives up enough heat so that its temperature drops to the freezing point, the next 80 calories per gram of heat (c/g) (336j/g) it gives up will not lower its temperature, they will solidify it into ice. Conversely, as the solid becomes fluid, its temperature will not rise until all the solid has melted, although heat is continually added to the substance. Thus, at approximately the melting point, all substances remain at the same temperature until they have melted completely, although heat continues to be added.

The melting and solidifying temperature points of substances vary. Although the exact temperature at which a substance changes from a fluid to a solid depends on the atmospheric pressure, we usually say that water solidifies at 32° F (0° C), whereas melted paraffin solidifies at approximately 131° F (55° C). Adding mineral oil to paraffin lowers the melting point of the mixture. The exact temperature at which the mixture changes from solid to fluid depends on the amount of mineral oil added. As used clinically, this melting point is approximately 126° F (52° C) (see Table 7–2).

Heat of Vaporization

Water is changed into its gaseous state (steam) at the boiling point. This state requires 540 cal/g (2268 j/g). Thus, at 212° F (100° C) the next 540 c/g (2268 j/g) input of heat into the water does not raise the temperature but converts the water into steam.

The same process occurs with vaporization of sweat—an essential mechanism for cooling the body (see Chapter 8). Fluids do evaporate below 212° F (100° C), growing colder as they do. For example, water left in a dish gradually disappears; the rate of vaporization depends on the humidity of the ambient air. The faster the evaporation of any substance, the more pronounced the cooling effect. Using alcohol, water, or vapor coolant sprays to cool the skin quickly is a clinical example of this phenomenon.

Density and Thermal Expansion

The *density* of a substance refers to the mass of that substance per unit volume (see Fig. 7–3). *Thermal expansion* refers to changes in the density of a substance related to its temperature. How such changes cause heat transfer by convection was discussed earlier.

Nearly all substances expand when their temperatures increase: ie, when the mass per unit volume decreases. Conversely, the density increases when the temperature decreases. The amount of expansion per increase in temperature differs for various substances; for many substances, the amount has been determined and accordingly has been given a specific coefficient of thermal expansion. This coefficient is used to calculate the effects of changes in density per temperature change.

Water is an exception to the rule that density decreases with increases in temperature. Water reaches its greatest density at 39.2° F (4° C). Although it does expand as the temperature increases above that level, it also expands as the temperature drops below that level. Because 0° C ice is less dense than 4° C water, it partially floats above the water level. When the temperature of water in a glass bottle drops to freezing, the bottle may break. The water expands and changes into ice with the decrease in temperature, but the bottle contracts.

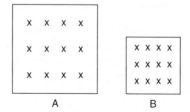

Figure 7–3. An example of how the density of a substance changes as its temperature changes. Both parts of the figure represent a substance with a mass of 12 g (each X represents 1 g). (**A**) As the temperature increases, the substance expands: ie, its density (mass per unit volume) decreases. (**B**) As the temperature decreases, the substance contracts: ie, its density increases.

The mercury and glass thermometer is a good clinical example of different coefficients of thermal expansion. Mercury passes through a narrow glass tube and rises within the tube when placed in a warmer environment. Both the glass and the mercury expand at the higher temperature; however, mercury, having the higher coefficient of thermal expansion, expands more and therefore rises within the glass tube. Incidentally, when the mercury rises, a design feature holds the mercury in the tube as it cools to allow correct reading. Therefore, always "shake down" a thermometer before use to return the mercury to the bulb.

Of more direct concern to clinicians is an understanding of factors that influence the difference in the quantity of heat contained in various modalities at equal temperatures and in the difference in the rate at which each transfers heat to or from the patient. Among the contributing factors are thermal properties inherent to the substance of that particular modality: ie, the *specific heat capacity* of the substance, which influences the quantity of heat in that modality, and the *thermal conductivity* qualities, of the substance, which influence how quickly the substance transfers heat.

Quantity of Heat

Many factors determine the quantity of heat in a specific substance. First, consider the volume. A bathtub one-third full of hot water at any given temperature will not contain as much heat as a tub three-quarters full of water of the same temperature. Thus, if you sit in a tub that is one-third full, your body systems will not be affected as much as if you sat in the fuller tub for the same length of time. In this example, the substance, water; the temperature of the water; and the time of application are equal, but the volume, the amount of the substance, determines the difference in the quantity of heat available for the body to receive.

Next, consider the same substance (water) at different temperatures and volumes. The temperature of a cup of boiling water may contain less heat than a pail full of warm water. Try pouring the water from each container over a block of ice and observe what happens. Ice melts in the area where the cup of boiling water was poured (a local effect) while the remaining block remains much as it was. If the pail of water is poured over the block, the water will melt more of the entire block having a greater effect on the entire object, that is, a more general effect.

Using a clinical example that is relatively analogous, a 20-min local application of heat with a modality such as a towel-wrapped hot pack or hot water bottle at 140° F (60° C), like the cup of boiling water, will produce a noticeable local effect but will produce less systemic change than a 20-minute Hubbard tank treatment at 104° F (40° C) because the quantity of heat available in the Hubbard tank is much greater.

Variations Among Substances

Two different modalities can be of equal mass and temperature; however, if they are not made of the same substance, one modality may contain a much greater amount of heat than the other. The quantity of heat contained in a substance at any given temperature depends on specific physical properties of that substance. Some substances require more energy input than others to achieve similar increases in molecular motion.

In physics the term "quantity of heat" is used to represent the amount of heat (energy) input required to increase molecular motion and thus increase the temperature, or the amount of energy released to reduce the motion and thus the temperature of a substance. Heat is measured in calories or joules or British thermal units (BTU): 1 BTU = 252c (1058.4 J). Note that the lower case c equals calorie; the upper case C used to measure energy relating to food intake equals 1,000 calories. (1 C = 1,000 c).

The quantity of heat required to produce any given change in temperature is determined by (1) the specific heat capacity of the substance, (2) the mass of the substance, and (3) the amount of temperature change desired:

$$Q = SmT,$$

where Q = quantity, S = specific heat capacity, m = mass, and T = temperature change. The constant c or p can sometimes be used instead of S.

Specific Heat Capacity

The ability of a molecule or its constituents to move depends on the structure of the molecule and differs for every substance. Some substances require more energy input than others to increase the internal random motion, thus the temperature. The specific heat input required to raise the temperature of 1 g of a substance 1° C is designated its *specific heat capacity* value. The value given to water is 1 and is used as a basis for comparing the specific heat capacity values of all other substances. Applying the formula Q = SmT to water, 1c is the quantity (Q) of heat input required to change the temperature of 1g of H_2O, the mass (m), 1° C: from 14° C to 15° C. Because the specific heat capacity (S) value for water is 1, the formula can be written as follows:

$$Q = S \times m \times T$$

$$1c = 1 \times 1 \, g \times 1° \, C \text{ (from } 14° \, C \text{ to } 15° \, C\text{).}$$

In British thermal units, quantity = BTU, mass = pounds (lb), and temperature = degrees Fahrenheit. Therefore:

$$1 \, BTU = 1 \times 1 \, lb \times 1° \, F.$$

Table 7–3 gives the specific heat capacity values of substances that are of interest to physical therapists. Note that paraffin, as used clinically, has a specific heat capacity value of 0.65 compared with that of water (1.0).

To clarify the concept of quantity of heat, use the above formula in reverse (SmT = Q) and compare the amount of heat intake required to raise 500 g of water or paraffin 3° C (at no given temperature):

S of water = 1   S of paraffin = 0.65
1 × 500 g × 3° C = 1500 c (6300J)   0.65 × 500g × 3° C = 975 c (4095 J)

Fewer calories (joules) of heat input are required to raise the temperature of the paraffin. Thus, at any given temperature, paraffin contains less heat than does water.

PROBLEM 1

Equal amounts of paraffin and water are put in two pans of identical size; each pan receives equal amounts of heat from a stove burner. The temperature of both pans was the same at the start and both were heated for the same amount of time. At the end of a given time, which substance has the greater increase in temperature? Approximately how great is the increase? Which substance has acquired the greatest amount of additional heat? (See answer page 77)

Thermal Conductivity

Some substances conduct heat more readily than others. Thermal conductivity of a particular substance refers to the ability of that substance to conduct heat. Thermal conductivity properties determine the rate at which heat is taken in or given up by and conducted through the substance.

Generally, metals are good conductors of heat. Stone and sand are moderate heat conductors, and wood is a poor conductor. The following are everyday examples of thermal conductivity. If you are walking barefoot on the beach and the sand is extremely hot, you try to walk on the boardwalk because your feet will not feel as hot. But you would avoid walking on any metal that was lying on the beach. Wood does not give up heat as quickly as sand does, but metal gives up heat much faster than either wood or sand.

TABLE 7–3. CONSTANT VALUES FOR SPECIFIC HEAT CAPACITY AND THERMAL CONDUCTIVITY OF NONBIOLOGIC AND BIOLOGIC SUBSTANCES[*†]

Substance	Constants	
	Specific Heat Value (S)[‡]	Thermal Conductivity Value (k)[§]
Nonbiologic		
Paraffin	0.65	—
Rubber	0.480	0.372
Paraffin and oil	0.45	—
Wood	0.42	0.2
Sand	0.25	93.0
Air	0.24	0.026
Aluminum	0.215	235.0
Plate glass	0.2	2.60
Water	1.0	1.4
Copper	0.0923	401.0
Biologic[‖]		
Skin	0.9	0.898
Muscle	0.895	1.53
Whole blood	0.87	1.31
Average for body	0.86	—
Subcutaneous fat	0.55	0.45
Bone (average)	0.38	2.78

[*]Lehman J, ed: *Therapeutic Heat and Cold*. 4th ed. Baltimore, MD: Williams & Wilkins; 1990:65,128–129,175,179,212–213.

[†]Halliday D, Resnick R: *Fundamentals of Physics*. 3rd ed. New York: John Wiley & Sons; 1988.

[‡]Heat required to raise the temperature of a specific substance: $S = Q/mT$ or $Q = SmT$, where S = specific heat value (constant), Q = quantity (c or BTU), m = mass (g or lb), and T = amount of temperature change ($°F$ or $°C$). Note that S and k are not directly correlated: eg, the k for copper is the highest value given, but the S for copper is lower than that for aluminum.

[§]Speed at which heat transfers through a specific substance: $H = kATG/D$, where H = rate of conduction (c/s), k = value (constant), A = cross-sectional surface area (m^2), T = time (s), G = temperature gradient between hot or cold surfaces on opposite sides of the substance ($t_1 - t_2$) ($°C$), D = thickness (m).

[‖]The values do not represent in vivo tissues; many are simulated models, animal tissues, or in vitro tissues.

Similarly, in an extremely cold environment, if you put your hand on a metal versus a wooden doorknob, the metal knob will feel much colder than the wooden one because it can absorb the heat given off by your hand much faster.

The conductivity of many materials has been scientifically determined and has been given a specific number value for the constant (k). The larger the value of k of a substance, the faster it can transfer heat. Table 7–3 gives the constant values of thermal conductivity for several substances. The constants given indicate that water is a better conductor than wood but not as good a conductor as metal and that paper, cloth, and air are poorer thermal conductors than water. Because they retard the rate of heat transfer, poor heat conductors are considered to be good heat insulators. Table 7–3 also shows the difference in thermal conductivity values for various body tissues. Bone and tissues such as blood and muscle, which have a high fluid content, are the best heat conductors, whereas fat, a poorer conductor, is a good insulator. Thus, when applying thermal modalities, one must consider the amount of subcutaneous fat a patient has. The fat acts to retard heat transfer, by conduction, to or from the deeper body tissues.

Thermal conductivity principles are constantly applied in daily life. For example, imagine two pans of food are heating on the stove. One pan has a wooden handle; the other has a handle made of the same metal as the pan. You could comfortably hold the wooden handle, but not the metal one, without burning your hand. To lift the pan with a metal handle, you would probably use a pot holder made of quilted layers or terrycloth, each with many air spaces. Although air conducts slowly, it is not a perfect insulator. Heat will come through eventually, but less heat over time reduces the possibility of burning your hand. For the same reason, fluffy terry-cloth toweling or other materials with air spaces are used to wrap a hot pack. The heat will then conduct through to a patient at a slower rate.

Most liquids and all gases are poor conductors of heat. Down jackets, fur coats, and thermal blankets, although lightweight, are good heat insulators because air, a poor conductor, is trapped between the feathers, hairs, or in the spaces of thermal fabrics. The air retards the conduction of heat away from the warm body to the outside cold air.

Although good electrical conductors are also good heat conductors, the two uses of the term conductors should not be confused. Both are related to the free electrons of the substance. Electrical conductivity depends on the arrangement of electrons in the atoms of a substance: the attraction of negative ions for positive ions, or a flow of energy along the path of free electrons (see Section IV). Heat conductivity depends on the arrangement of electrons in a molecule and how the electrons react to changes in temperature, not how they react to positive ions or polarity.

PROBLEM 2

You are heating a pan of milk on the stove. You observe that the milk on the surface near the sides of the pan begins to bubble before the milk in the center. Why?

PROBLEM 3

You advise your patients not to touch the sides of the metal paraffin tank. Wooden slats are placed on the bottom of many tanks. Can you explain why?

To differentiate between (1) specific heat capacity, which determines a quantity (how much heat is necessary to raise the temperature of a substance), and (2) thermal conductivity, which determines a rate (how long it takes for heat to conduct through a substance), solve the following problem. (See answer page 77)

PROBLEM 4

If a patient places a hand in liquid paraffin or water, the temperature of which is 128° F, the hand will instantly feel much hotter in the water. Is this the result of the specific heat properties of the substance, its thermal conductivity, or both? (See answer page 77)

To predict the rate of heat transfer in a given time period, many factors must be considered. The rate, ie, how much heat passes through a specific material in a given time, depends on the cross-sectional area, the temperature gradient between the heated surface (t_1) and cooler surface (t_2) to which the heat will transfer ($G = [t_1-t_2]$), the thickness of the material, and the thermal conductivity constant for that substance. The greater the area and the temperature gradient, the faster the heat transfer, and the thicker the material, the slower the transfer. Thus, the following equation can be used to determine the rate of heat conductivity through a substance (see Fig. 7–4) or to predict the rate of heat conduction through body tissues:

$$H = \frac{kATG}{D},$$

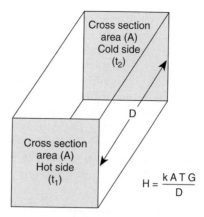

Figure 7–4. Determinants of thermal conductivity. H = Heat passing through the substance in a given time period (the rate). k = Thermal conductivity constant for given substance. A = Cross-sectional Area of the Substance. T = Given time period. G = Temperature Gradient between hot and cold side surface areas ($t_1 - t_2$). D = Thickness of the substance (the slab).

where H = heat, k = constant, A = cross-sectional area, T = time, G = temperature gradient between t_1 and t_2, and D = thickness.

In actuality, the thermal conductivity constant (k) of a tissue is not considered as an isolated factor when determining the conductivity properties of the tissue. Instead, the thermal inertia of the tissue is used: that is, the thermal conductivity, the mass, and the specific heat of the tissue are factored into the equation. But no measurements based on constants are ever precise for body tissues in vivo, primarily because they cannot account for individual variations in circulation.[2]

This brief discussion of heat conductivity formulas represents an attempt to explain the many factors that control the actual rate of heat conduction through a mass of a given substance. An understanding of these factors is useful for developing research projects that investigate heat modalities or for determining why there are differences in the results of other researchers.[4] (See answer page 77)

SUMMARY

This chapter has discussed the physical aspects of treatments with thermal modalities that should be considered. Heat is the kinetic energy of molecules in a substance: ie, the movement of molecules or their constituents. Hot and cold are relative words used to describe heat. Temperature is a numerical means of measuring and describing the amount of heat in a substance; however, temperature is not an accurate measure because different substances can contain different amounts of heat although their temperature is the same. Heat is transferred from one place to another by conduction, convection, and radiation—three completely different methods. However, most heat transfers use more than one of these methods. Changing a substance from a solid to a liquid state or from a liquid to a gaseous state requires energy. Thus, at the point of melting a solid or evaporating a liquid, added heat does not increase temperature until the state of the substance is completely changed.

Every substance has unique thermal qualities, including specific melting points and evaporation points. Some qualities of a substance are described by a given constant for each. The amount of expansion per temperature rise can be determined by the coefficient of thermal expansion of each substance. The amount of heat required to raise the temperature is determined by its specific heat capacity constant (S), and its ability to conduct heat is determined by its thermal conductivity constant (k). These constants can then be used in appropriate equations to determine the heating effects of various substances and modalities. Other factors such as volume, temperature gradient, and time also must be considered.

References to these physical aspects of heat and thermal qualities of substances will constantly accompany the discussion of each treatment modality in later chapters. This should help the therapist understand and select optimal modalities for treatment and also should be helpful when purchasing equipment for clinics. In both cases, the temperature, the heating ability of a modality, and its ability to transfer heat to or from the patient depends on these physical properties.

Equally important, the therapist should understand how these same physical concepts apply specifically to the human body and to its different tissues. These biophysical considerations are addressed in Chapter 8.

■ KEY TERMS

thermal energy
heat
first law of thermodynamics
temperature
  Fahrenheit temperature scale
  Celsius (centigrade) temperature
    scale
  Kelvin temperature scale
  Rankin temperature scale

heat transfer
  radiation
  conduction
  convection
heat of fusion
heat of vaporization
density
thermal expansion
specific heat capacity
thermal conductivity

■ REVIEW QUESTIONS

1. What is the first law of thermodynamics?
2. Explain how hot and cold are relative terms.
3. What is temperature?
4. What are the four temperature scales: Which are used clinically most often?
5. Convert the following temperatures from Fahrenheit to Celsius or vice versa.
   (a) 42° C
   (b) 130° F
   (c) 55° F
6. Explain the three methods of heat transfer:
   (a) radiation
   (b) conduction
   (c) convection
7. Name some properties of a substance that are dependent on or vary with changes in temperature that affect the thermal properties of a substance.
8. What is the heat of fusion?
9. What is the heat of vaporization?
10. What is the melting point of the following? Why do the melting points vary?
    (a) paraffin
    (b) water
11. What is density?
12. What is thermal expansion?
13. What three factors determine the quantity of heat required to produce a given change in temperature?
14. What is 1 c (4.2 J) in terms of specific heat capacity?

REFERENCES

1. Lehmann J, ed: *Therapeutic Heat and Cold.* 4th ed. Baltimore, MD: Williams & Wilkins; 1990.
2. Houdas Y, Ring E: *Human Body Temperature: Its Measurement and Regulation.* New York: Plenum Press; 1982.
3. Licht S, ed: *Medical Hydrology.* New Haven, CT: E Licht; 1963.
4. Halliday D, Resnick R: *Physics.* 3rd ed. extended, New York: John Wiley & Sons; 1988.

ANSWERS TO PROBLEMS

Problem 1. (p. 72) The Specific Heat constant of paraffin is about 1/3 less than water (paraffin-0.65 and water-1.0). Thus, per given time, the paraffin temperature will increase about 1/3 more than the water. Both will have had equal amounts of heat (thermal energy) added.

Problem 2. (p. 74) The Thermal Conductivity constant (k) is much higher for metal than for milk. Thus, the milk on the sides, adjacent to the pan, was heated from that conducted up the sides of the pan as well as that which conducted through the fluid. Thus the milk on the sides reached a boiling point sooner than the milk in the center.

Problem 3. (p. 74) Note on the Heat Determinates Table, (Table 7–3) that the thermal conductivity value (k) for a metal is several hundred times greater than for water which is 1.4. The k value for wood is only 0.2. Obviously, the metal will conduct its heat to the body part much faster than the wood, so touching the metal could be painful while touching the wood is not. The wooden slates on the bottom safely protect the person from touching the metal bottom of the tank.

Problem 4. (p. 74) As mentioned in Problem 1, there is less heat per given temperature in paraffin than in water.

8

Biophysics

Bernadette Hecox, PT, MA

Human tissues, like all substances, are subject to physical laws. Thus, the topics discussed in Chapter 7 apply to human tissues but are complicated by factors beyond those considered in inanimate substances. People, because of their thermoregulatory mechanisms, have a special way of dealing with internal and external thermal conditions. This thermoregulation, under neural control, integrates physiological, psychological, and behavioral adjustments.

THERMOREGULATION

Humans are *homeotherms* (endotherms), commonly referred to as warm-blooded animals. This means that we can maintain a constant internal temperature (constant core temperature) despite considerable variations in environmental temperature. Basically, this *thermal homeostasis* is established by physiological adjustments. Poikilotherms (ectotherms), lower-level creatures such as snakes, cannot make these physiological adjustments. Their survival depends on compensatory behavioral mechanisms when there are marked changes in environmental temperature. For example, they will get out of the sun on a hot day.

Core temperature (or internal body temperature) is usually considered to be the temperature deep within the trunk of the body and is measured either rectally, sublingually, at the tympanic membrane, or near the esophagus; the esophageal measurement is the most accurate.

It is customary to say that the "normal" core temperature is 98.6° F (approximately 37° C). However, normal temperature is not that precise or constant. Many normal variations in body temperature occur. These include diurnal changes (lower temperature in the morning and higher temperature in the afternoon), changes dependent on exercise and food intake, and variations related to sex and age.[1] Older people may have a cooler core temperature—less than 95° F (35° C).[2-4]

Temperature also varies in different areas of the body. For example, the temperature of visceral organs at the center of the body may be higher than the oral temperature. The temperature of muscles at rest is usually lower than the core temperature, but it increases with exercise as muscle metabolism increases.[5]

Variations in temperature are sometimes described in relation to the depth of the tissues (see Fig. 8–1).[6] The outside surface of the body can be referred to as the *shell*. If a resting person is nude and the ambient temperature is 86° F (30° C), the shell will be approximately 92° F (33.5° C), assuming low humidity and minimal air flow.[7] Even the shell temperature varies greatly in different areas of the body. For example, skin temperature is higher in the anxilla and groin areas, where less heat can escape, than on the back and in areas with poor circulation. The various temperatures on the body surface are well defined in color thermographs. They also can be determined by placing a skin thermometer such as a thermistor on several different areas of the skin.

The temperature of the tissues beneath the shell also vary greatly. In general, the deeper the tissues, the higher their temperature, especially in the trunk. For convenience, the variations in temperature in relation to depth have been described as *isotherm layers:* ie, areas with similar temperatures.[6] The temperature of each isotherm layer increases so that the deepest isotherm, the center of the body, is represented as the warmest. However, this is not a completely accurate description. The depth at which tissues are equal in temperature, ie, isothermic, varies

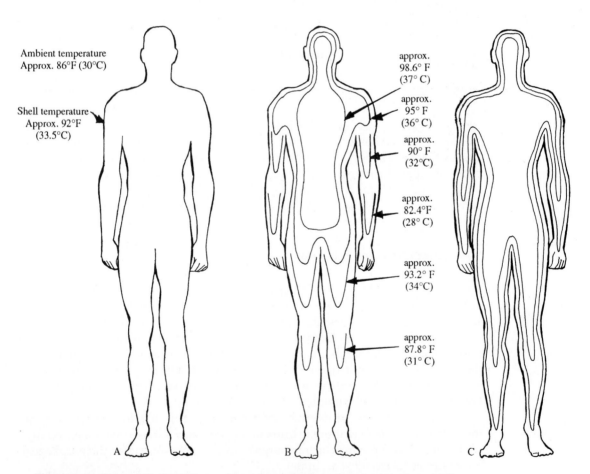

Figure 8–1. Schematic illustrations of an average body surface temperature relative to the ambient temperature and to various depths of tissue in various areas of the body. **(A)** Gradient between ambient temperature and the average temperature of a nude resting man's body surface (shell). **(B)** Variations in tissue temperature (shown in °F and °C) relative to depth and area of the body. **(C)** Illustrations of descriptive isotherm layers. (*Adapted with permission from* Naturwissenschaften (*1958; 45:477–481*).

according to the body size and in different areas of the body.[8] Layers outside the shell, such as clothing, are described as outside isotherm layers.

Ideally, the temperature gradient between the shell and the ambient temperature is approximately 7° F (4° C).[9] Disregarding environmental factors such as wind velocity and humidity, when the ambient temperature is about 77° F (25° C) and the shell is about 84° F (29° C), a nude resting person feels comfortable. (Temperatures vary, depending on the climate one is adjusted to and on individual differences such as age and sex). However, if the ambient temperature drops to 70° F (21° C), a nude person will begin to feel uncomfortably chilly and begin making behavioral adjustments: for example, putting on clothes or moving around a bit to keep warm. This phenomenon has direct application to therapists. When working with a patient in a room where the temperature is 70° F (21° C), the therapist is comfortable and may forget that a partially nude patient lying quietly on a plinth will be uncomfortable. For this reason, a sheet or blanket—an outside isotherm—should be used to cover the patient.

Among the behavioral adjustments people make when the ambient temperature is cold is a preference for warm food and drinks and food with more calories. The opposite behavioral adjustments occur as ambient temperature increases much above 77° F (25° C). People may have the urge to wear fewer clothes and to select cooler foods and drinks. They will also have the urge either to decrease the amount of physical activity or to perform activities more slowly and with less effort.

Because physiological, psychological, and behavioral regulatory mechanisms are integrated with biophysics, separating them from biophysics is impossible. Nonetheless, a focus on thermal physics as it applies to the human body precedes the discussion of the physiological reactions.

HEAT LOSS

Heat, as a by-product of metabolism, is constantly being produced within the body. Because metabolism is a continuous process, heat must be dissipated; otherwise, the body's internal temperature would constantly be increasing. In the ideal environment, the shell is warmer than the environment and the core is warmer than the shell. Because heat transfer is always in the direction of warmer to cooler, this gradient factor allows the body to release heat and maintain a constant internal temperature. The heat leaves the body by the same physical means of heat transfer mentioned in Chapter 7—conduction, convection, radiation—and through the process of evaporation of moisture.

Conduction

Some heat will be conducted from the warmer, deeper tissues to the shell. However, as shown by the thermal conductivity constants in Chapter 7 (Table 7–3), tissues differ in their ability to conduct heat. The thermal conductivity of bone and muscle is high relative to the skin and fat. Thus, skin and subcutaneous fat act as insulators, retarding the rate of heat conduction through tissues to the surface. Although some heat is conducted through tissues to the surface, this conduction is by no means adequate to prevent a rise in core temperature.

Convection

The major means of transferring heat from the deeper areas of the body to the shell is internal convection. Heat is first conducted from the deeper tissues into the vascular system circulating through them. The warmed blood flows through the vessels and is convected toward the shell by the peripheral circulatory system. The circulating blood, just like hot water in the heating system of a building, is transported from the source to a cooler area. This convection, bringing the warm blood to the surface, causes the shell temperature to be warmer than the ambient temperature to which the shell is exposed.

Radiation

If the shell is warmer than the ambient temperature, infrared heat waves will radiate from the warmer skin into the cooler environment. The body gives up its heat in the same way the radiator does in a hot water heating system. Radiation is the main means by which heat escapes until the ambient temperature rises higher than 86° F (30° C). When the skin and ambient temperatures are equal, usually 95°–97° F (35°–36° C), there can be **no heat** lost through radiation[10]. When the ambient temperature is warmer than the shell, radiation takes place in the opposite direction, and the body, in addition to an inability to rid itself of heat, will gain additional heat from the environment. Similarly, when a superficial heat modality is applied, the direction of heat transfer is reversed and the body gains heat. In addition to the heat produced through metabolism, will the core temperature rise with a reversal of heat transfer? Within a limited range of heat application, no, because people have other means of losing heat.

Evaporation

One essential mechanism that enables the body to maintain a constant core temperature is *evaporation of sweat*. In addition to conduction and convection, a large amount of heat can be brought to the body surface in the form of insensible and sensible sweat. The term insensible sweat refers to the constantly occurring diffusion of moisture through the skin. The term sensible sweat refers to the moisture brought to the surface by thermally activated eccrine sweat glands. Regulation of sensible sweating is under neurophysiological control.[11-13] Activation of this sweat mechanism occurs when any increase in core temperature occurs and when the skin temperature rises to approximately 91.4° F (33° C);[14] these increases can be caused by fever, exercise, or an ambient temperature above 85° F (29° C) (see Chapter 15). When local heat is applied, provided that no increase in systemic temperatures has occurred, secretion of sweat is limited to the area where the temperature has increased.

Once sweat is on the body surface, it will evaporate, provided that it is exposed to air and that the moisture content of the air is not too great. This process of evaporation cools the body. When the ambient temperature is greater than the skin temperature and radiation is no longer possible, evaporation is the major means of losing body heat. You may recall that 540 calories per gram (2268 J) is required for vaporization of water to occur (see Chapter 7). Similarly, evaporation of sweat uses heat (calories) to cool the shell. When the air is humid, however, sweat cannot evaporate as easily; it either remains on the body surface or drips off—neither condition assists in cooling the body. It is the process of evaporation that cools and makes one feel more comfortable, even when the ambient temperature hovers around 90° F (32.2° C). This effect accounts for the expression, "it isn't the heat, it's the humidity." It also explains why it is important to consider both the temperature and the humidity, or "apparent temperatures," and to use these apparent temperatures rather than the exact temperature to guide either our patients' or our own activities. When the temperature of the air is 80° F (26.7° C) and the humidity is 40%, the apparent temperature is 79° F (26° C), which is usually safe for disabled people during exercise. With the same temperature and a humidity of 70%, however, the apparent temperature is 85° F (29.4° C); and exercise could be unsafe.

Some evaporation also occurs with respiration. Moisture from the mucous membranes of the respiratory passages can evaporate when passages are open to the environment. In humans, however, this means of heat loss is far less effective than is evaporation of sweat. In an effort to cool off, however, a person may develop a panting like breathing pattern when overheated.

Ambient Air Flow

Air flow contributes significantly to heat loss. When a breeze allows a flow of air molecules that are cooler than the body surface to pass over the body, heat is given up. First, heat is conducted from the warmer molecules on the body surface to the cooler air molecules, thus cooling the surface. Then, the heat is convected, ie, carried away by the moving air molecules. The greater the wind velocity, the greater the cooling effect.

SUMMARY OF BIOPHYSICAL ASPECTS OF HEAT LOSS

Despite the production of heat by metabolism and the heat gained from ambient conditions, a constant internal temperature is maintained by physiological, physical, and behavioral means (eg, modifying one's physical activity, clothing, and eating habits and avoiding environments with extreme temperatures. The body transfers heat from deeper tissues to the surface tissues only minimally by conduction and primarily by convection in the bloodstream and by sweat fluids (sweat). This heat is then released to the environment by infrared radiation, evaporation of sweat, and respiratory moisture or by convection via air flow. Ambient temperature, humidity, and wind velocity influence the body's ability to give off heat.

PROBLEM 1

If the ambient temperature is 93.2° F (34° C), the humidity is 20%, and little wind is blowing, will the core temperature of a nude individual at rest increase or remain stable? Why? (See answer page 90)

PROBLEM 2

If you place a patient in a Hubbard tank with only his head and shoulders above water for a 20-min treatment, and the temperature of the water is 93.2° F (34° C), would you expect his core temperature to increase or remain stable? (See answer page 90)

PROBLEM 3

The ambient temperature is 95° F, the humidity is 80%, and no wind is blowing. Eighty-year-old Ms. Smith, attempting to stay cool, is rocking in her rocking chair and fanning herself vigorously. Will it help? Can you apply this example to a therapeutic situation? (See answer page 90)

HEAT GAIN

Whenever the ambient temperature is higher than the body temperature, heat is transferred to the body. The body gains heat through the same physical processes as it loses heat, but the processes occur in the opposite direction. The effects of exposing the entire body to a warmer environment are discussed under "Generalized Heating" in Chapter 9 and "Ambient Conditions" in Chapter 15. The focus in this section is on the effect of applying heat to one area of the body.

When a superficial heat modality is applied to a local area of the body and the body surface is cooler than the modality, as it usually is, the heat will be transferred from the modality to the local area. This transfer occurs by conduction, radiation, convection, or all of these, depending on the modality used.

Once the local body surface is heated, the specific heat capacity and the *effec-*

tive conductivity of those tissues will influence the amount of tissue temperature rise (TTR) that will occur. Effective conductivity includes both the thermal conductivity properties of the heated tissues described in Chapter 7 and the vascular supply controlling convection. The heat can then be conducted to adjacent tissues. How much and how fast the TTR occurs in adjacent tissues depends on the thermal properties and the effective conductivity of each type of tissue. Although some heat may conduct to subcutaneous tissues, skin and fat layers, the surface tissues are not good conductors, (see Chapter 7, Table 7–3).

Surface Versus Deep Tissues

Because surface tissues are poor thermal conductors, they will retain much of the heat they receive. Some heat may be transferred to adjacent superficial bone and muscle; however, because these tissues are better thermal conductors, they will retain less heat than do skin and fat. Muscle and bone are also deeper than skin and subcutaneous fat and thus farther from the source of heat. The usual explanation is that any heat conducted into blood in the cutaneous vessels will be transported by convection away from the local area of application. This convection, as well as their thermal properties, limits the TTR of superficial muscle and bone. Because the temperature of deeper tissues was originally higher (recall the isotherm layers), it is unlikely that any significant TTR will occur there. Although straightforward, this explanation is an oversimplification.

Some evidence indicates that as the heated blood travels back toward the heart, some heat will be conducted to adjacent tissues and arterial vessels. However, the deep muscles are not likely to be heated by this process. The cutaneous capillaries and their terminal arterioles and venules pass only through the superficial muscles. Blood flow in deep muscle is independent of cutaneous circulation.[15–18] This anatomical distribution of vessels lends support to studies showing that no change in blood flow in deep muscle occurs when superficial heat is applied and to studies showing that the regulation of blood flow in muscle is related to the oxygen demands of the muscles. Only if the temperature of the deep muscles increases, as when deep heat modalities are applied or during exercise, does the blood flow to those muscles increase.[19,20] Fig. 8–2 illustrates the findings of Lehmann's well-executed study showing that local superficial heat modalities produce a modest TTR in tissues that are 1 cm deep but that a significant TTR—higher than 107° F (41° C)—occurs only in surface tissues.[21] The figure also demonstrates the effectiveness of vascular convection. The plateau in the TTR appears to be controlled by the blood flow because, when the flow is obstructed, the surface tissue temperature increases. By comparing Fig. 8–2A and B, one also can see that the peak surface temperature was reached sooner with the Hydrocollator pack than with the infrared lamp, whereas the plateau temperature reached with the lamp was slightly higher. Note that the infrared lamp provides a constant source of heat, whereas the Hydrocollator pack does not.

Many other studies conducted to determine the amount of TTR that can occur in tissues at various depths have produced varying results. One must carefully compare the methods used and the results obtained in these studies. In some of them, all measurements of temperature or circulatory changes were done with instruments that record surface changes; changes in deeper tissues were theorized but not determined. Other studies were done in tissues in vitro (taken out of the body) with their vascular supply abolished; the results of these studies cannot be compared with what occurs in normal (in vivo) human tissues. In studies in which no generalized circulatory changes can occur, the tissue temperature can indeed rise significantly. Although much can be learned about physiological reactions from experiments performed on small animals in vivo, one must remember that the effects of a certain dose of heat that might kill a rat are not directly applicable to humans because the tissue volumes and circulatory capabilities are so different. These studies, however, can be meaningful if a clinician is deciding whether to use heat or cold on tissues with a poor vascular supply.

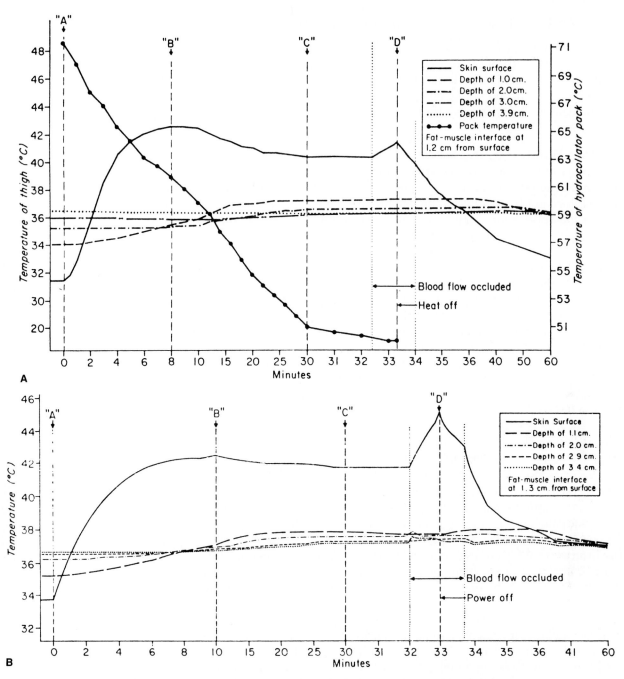

Figure 8–2. Comparison of the effects of two superficial heat modalities on surface and deeper tissues. **(A)** Temperatures recorded in the human thigh during application with Hydrocollator hot packs. **(B)** Temperatures recorded in the human thigh during exposure to infrared radiation from a 250 w Mazda lamp (red bulb) (*Reproduced with permission from* Arch Phys Med Rehab *1966;47:291–299*).

One also must notice how terms are used. For example, the term deeper tissues may mean any subcutaneous tissues, tissues deeper than 1 cm, or tissues deep within a particular part of the body. It is possible to raise the temperature as deep as the joints in small body parts such as the fingers or toes with a superficial modality. To heat joints that are deeper than 1 cm appreciably, however, surface tissue would have to be heated to the point of pain or damage. Fortunately, this is not the case with deep heat modalities. With microwave, shortwave diathermy, or ultrasound, forms of energy other than heat are transmitted to deeper tissues, producing heat where absorbed.

Factors Determining Temperature Rise

The extent to which a local superficial thermal modality will change the tissue temperature significantly or produce heat gain in the body depends on several factors: (1) the ability of the modality to give heat to the body, (2) the physical properties of the specific tissues, and (3) the integrity and response of body systems. For deep heat modalities, the specific absorption rate (SAR) is also a factor (see Chapter 6, Table 6–2).

Factors Related to the Modality

The ability of the modality to give heat to the body depends on (1) the amount of heat the modality can provide, (2) its thermal conductivity properties, (3) the temperature gradient between the patient and the modality, and (4) the duration of the application. Many modalities can provide a large amount of heat. For example, a large amount of heated water or a modality such as an infrared lamp or a heating pad can maintain a constant output of heat for a prolonged period. The large amount of heat these modalities can deliver can cause changes in the body's core temperature, assuming that the vascular system is intact and can convect the heat to the general circulatory system. If the local vascular system is not intact, local tissues can be dangerously overheated by modalities that provide a constant heat output. Thus, such modalities must be carefully monitored. (Table 8–1 outlines the thermal properties of some commonly used superficial modalities). Other modalities, such as hot water bottles and hot packs, provide a limited amount of heat because they are cut off from the source of heating. With these modalities, the amount of heat the body absorbs is limited.

Depending on the thermal conductivity properties and temperature gradient between tissues and the modality, heat can be exchanged quickly or slowly. If the exchange occurs faster than the vascular system can accommodate, the skin temperature may rise quickly. This can occur if a hot pack of 145° F (62.8° C) is placed directly on a patient. If conduction occurs slowly—for example, when several layers of terry cloth are placed between the pack and the patient—the temperature rises gradually over a longer period. Because this gives the vascular system time for convection, it prevents a dangerous change in temperature. However, a slow rise in an area with good circulation may prevent effective changes in local temperature or may require treatment for a longer period to be effective. The importance of using the correct amount of insulators and the correct duration of application cannot be overstated.

It should be noted that heat is transferred from a modality in all directions. For example, unless prevented by some insulated covering, a hot pack may radiate into the environment rather than conduct it into the patient. If one wraps a hot pack with equal toweling on the side exposed to the environment as on the side adjacent to patient, and if the room temperature is 72° F (22.2° C) and the patient's skin is 84° F (28.9° C), more heat will be transferred to the room than to the patient. As the temperature gradient is greater on the room side, the rate of transfer is faster. This illustrates the need to cover packs with good insulators such as plastic and terry cloth covers.

Physical Properties of Tissues

Skin and superficial fat layers are insulators; thus, conduction of heat to deeper tissues is hindered and applied heat remains in cutaneous tissues. Because bone and muscle are better conductors, any heat reaching these tissues is dissipated more easily. The thermal properties of tissues adjacent to bone and muscle and the circulation in the area determine the rate and amount of heat loss. To a great extent, the vascular system controls thermal changes in tissues, primarily by convection of heat from an area where the tissue temperature is increased to an area where the tissue temperature is decreased, thus influencing the local effect of a modality (see Table 8–2).

TABLE 8–1.   THERMAL PROPERTIES OF COMMON SUPERFICIAL HEAT MODALITIES

Hot Pack

- Pack is soaked in and saturated with water that has a relatively high specific heat value (S); thus, much heat is put into the pack to attain a temperature of 145° F or more.
- The pack contains a substance with a lower thermal conductivity constant (k) than water; thus, it conducts heat more slowly—retains heat longer than water alone. Patient's vascular system can normally dissipate the heat readily.
- If a 145° F pack is wrapped in other materials that retard conduction, the temperature reaching the patient is approximately 105° F.
- The hot pack cools down in proportion to the amount of heat given to both the patient and the environment.

Hot Water Bottle

If water is approximately 133° F and the bottle contains approximately 2 quarts of water, compared with water immersion modalities mentioned below, there is relatively little heat contained in the modality. Water is a good conductor, but rubber is an insulator. Thus, the effect on the patient is not the same as direct application of 133° F water. If wrapped in one towel layer, the temperature of the towel may be 122° F. Although the initial rate of heat transfer may be rapid, the initial sensory impression of heat is great, and skin temperature may increase to 110° F, the amount of heat available is limited. Consequently, if the vascular system is normal, there is little additional tissue temperature rise locally.

Immersion

- The quantity of heated fluid is usually larger than the amount of heated substances in the two modalities mentioned above; therefore, it contains more heat/temperature. Actual amount of heat/temperature depends on the specific heat value of the fluid.
- Fluid surrounds the body part; thus, much heat is conducted into the body per temperature of fluid without high intensity per square inch.

Heating Pad

If continuous over time, only an extremely low output can be safely tolerated. If off/on periods are thermostatically controlled and circulation is intact, this modality can give much input to the body, most in general body heating. Only with impaired circulation will it overheat a local area.

Infrared Lamp

- Energy from the lamp radiates to patient and objects. Because of much divergence and reflection of rays, placement of the lamp as well as power output (wattage) determine the intensity.
- A *constant source* of energy output; thus, much heat is available and tissues continue to be heated as long as the lamp is on.

Integrity and Response of Body Systems

To prevent tissue damage, the vascular system must function properly. Any vascular problems will prevent normal protective mechanisms. Vascular control is dependent on both sensory and autonomic nervous systems; thus, these systems also must be intact.

SUMMARY OF BIOPHYSICAL ASPECTS OF HEAT GAIN

Whenever the external temperature is higher than the skin temperature, heat is transferred to the body surface by conduction, radiation, convection, or all of these mechanisms. The greater the gradient between the source of heat and the body, the faster the transfer. The TTR of surface and adjacent tissues is determined by the thermal characteristics and vascularity of the various tissues. Skin and subcutaneous fat are poor thermal conductors; thus, they retain a large amount of heat and conduct little heat to deeper tissues.

Heat conducted to the cutaneous blood supply will be convected away from the heated area. As this blood travels toward the heart, it may conduct some heat to tissues and adjacent arterial vessels. But neither the heat conducted through sur-

TABLE 8–2. BIOPHYSICAL CONSIDERATIONS WHEN HEATING WITH SUPERFICIAL MODALITIES

Cutaneous Skin and Fat Layers

- Good heat insulators.
- Retard conduction of heat to or from deeper tissues.
- Much of applied heat is retained in skin or fat layers.
- If the fat layer is less than 1 cm, some of the applied heat conducts to superficial bone or muscle (temperature rise as high as 6° F).
- If the fat layer is thicker than 2 cm (obese), little heat will conduct through skin or/and fat layers.

Local Vascular Vessels

- Heat is conducted to blood in the cutaneous vessels that permeate the area.
- If the circulation in the area is good, heat is convected to the general body and to adjacent tissues and vessels en route.
- If the circulation in the area is poor, more heat is retained in the surface area where applied and the temperature of these tissues will rise. If temperature rises above 113° F (45° C), damage will occur.

Bone

- Bone is a better conductor than overlying skin or fat. Heat in these tissues can conduct to other tissues.
- Little tissue temperature rise (TTR) occurs if the circulation in the area is good, if the bone underlies muscle, or both.
- The TTR at bony prominences may be great enough to cause discomfort.

Superficial Muscle

- Muscle is a relatively good thermal conductor.
- Some TTR is possible but not significant.
- The vascular supply is usually good; thus, heat is convected from the area.

face tissues or convected in heated blood through tissues is sufficient to produce a significant TTR beneath the surface, although a slight TTR occurs to about 1 cm below the surface.

Superficial heat modalities will not elevate the temperature of deep muscles or increase the amount of blood flow through them. However, deep heat modalities are capable of doing both. Superficial heat modalities, such as a full-body hot water bath or a heat lamp, can transfer enough heat to the body to elevate the core temperature.

Factors that determine the ability of a heat modality to heat body tissues depend on the type of modality, the physical properties of the tissues, and the integrity and responses of the vascular, sensory, and autonomic systems.

Tables 8–1 and 8–2 summarize this discussion as it relates to the thermal effects of superficial heat modalities and their clinical application.

PROBLEM 4

Part 1: Two modalities, A and B, are heating body areas of similar size and contain the same amount of heat, but A has a lower thermal conductivity constant. Which modality will produce less TT change/time? *Part 2:* If the temperature gradient between modality A and the body part being heated is less than the gradient between modality B and the body part, which modality will produce less TT change/time?

■ KEY TERMS

homeotherms

thermal homeostasis

shell

isotherm layers

evaporation of sweat

effective conductivity

REFERENCES

1. Downey J. Physiology of temperature regulation in man. Darling R, ed. *Physiological Basis of Rehabilitation Medicine.* Chap. 7. Philadelphia, PA: WB Saunders; 1971.

2. Collins K: Hypothermic and thermal responsiveness in the elderly. In: Fanger P, Valbjors O, eds. *Danish Build Building Research Inst.* Copenhagen; 1979; 819–833.

3. Collins K, Dore C, Exton-Smith A, et al: Accidental hypothermia and impaired temperature homeostasis in the elderly. *Br Med J.* 1977; 1:353–356.

4. Fox R, Woodward P, Exton-Smith A, et al: Body Temperatures in the Elderly: A National Study of Physiological, Social, and Environmental Conditions. *Br Med J.* 1973; 1:200–206.

5. McArdle W, Katch F, Katch V: *Exercise Physiology.* 2nd ed. Philadelphia, PA: Lea & Febiger; 1986.

6. Aschoff J, Wever R: Kern and Schale in Warmehaushalt des Menschen. *Naturwissenschaften.* 1958; 45:477–481.

7. Houdas Y, Ring E: *Human Body Temperature: Its Measurement and Regulation.* New York: Plenum Press; 1982.

8. Lehmann J, ed: *Therapeutic Heat and Cold.* 3rd ed. Baltimore, MD: Williams & Wilkins: 1982.

9. Astrand P, Rodahl K: *The Physiology of Work.* New York: Taylor & Francis; 1989.

10. Folk G Jr: *Textbook of Environmental Physiology.* 2nd Ed. Philadelphia, PA: Lea & Febiger; 1974; 44: 88–132.

11. Frisancho A; *Human Adaptation: A Functional Interpretation.* St. Louis, MO: CV Mosby; 1979. pp. 44–45.

12. Sloan A: *Man in Extreme Environment.* Springfield, MO: Charles C Thomas; 1979: 9.

13. Slonim NB, ed: *Environmental Physiology.* St. Louis, MO: CV Mosby; 1974. 94; 102–103.

14. Holdcroft A: *Body Temperature Control.* London, UK: Baillière-Tindall; 1980. p. 1; 12–26.

15. Dentry J-M, Brergelmann G, Rowell L, et al: Skin and muscle components of forearm blood flow in directly heating resting man. *J App Physiol.* 1972; 32:506–511.

16. Downey J: Physiological effects of heat and cold. *Phys Ther.* 1964; 44:713–717.

17. Weinbaum S, Jiji LM, Lemons D: Theory and experiment for the effect of vascular microstructure on surface tissue heat transfer: pt I. Anatomical Foundation and Model Conceptualization. *J Biomech Eng.* 1984; 106:321–330; 333–341.

18. Weinbaum S, Jiji LM, Lemons D: Theory and Experiment for the Effect of Vascular Microstructure on Surface Tissue Heat Transfer: Part II Model Formulation and Solution. *J Biomech Eng.* 1984; 106:331–341.

19. Rowell L: Reflex control of the cutaneous vasculature. *J Invest Dermatol.* 1977; 69:154–166.

20. Rowell LB, Shepherd J, Abboud F. Cardiovascular adjustment to thermal stress. In: *Handbook of Physiology.* Bethesda, MD: American Physiological Society. 3: (Sect. 2, pt. 2), 967–1023.

21. Lehmann J, Silverman D, Baum B, Kirk N, Johnston V: Temperature Distribution in the Human Thigh Produced by Infrared, Hot Packs and Microwave Applications. *Arch Phys Med Rehabil.* 1966; 47:291–299.

22. Licht S, ed: *Medical Hydrology.* New Haven, CT: E. Licht; 1963.

ANSWERS TO PROBLEMS

Problem 1. The core temperature will remain stable if the patient's sweating mechanism is functioning.

Problem 2. Assuming that the temperature of the body shell is 84° F (29° C) and the temperature of the water is 93° F (34° C), heat will be conducted into the body. The metabolic process increases because of the input of heat. Little heat is being given off. Core temperature may rise.

Problem 3. Although the fan may circulate air, the temperature of the air is dangerously high. The rocking and fanning exercise may increase Ms. Smith's metabolic rate, producing more internal heat and raising her core temperature. Thus, her fanning will probably be more damaging than helpful, although she may gain some relief from the air movement across her face. An electric fan, of course, would be more helpful. Similarly, attempting to ask Ms. Smith to exercise vigorously in such ambient conditions also could be dangerous.

Problem 4. *Part 1.* A is the answer. *Part 2.* Again, the answer is A. The lower the temperature gradient, the slower the rate of heat exchange. Any TTR is lower because the heat is convected from the area in the vascular system.

9

Physiological Responses to Local Heat Gain or Loss

Bernadette Hecox, PT, MA

W henever the body gains or loses heat, regardless of cause, physiologic adjustments occur in an effort to preserve homeostasis. This chapter discusses the physiologic responses that are related to (1) the application of heat or cold modalities, (2) the metabolic rate related to physical activity, and (3) ambient conditions. Although the emphasis is on the application of heat or cold modalities, the interrelationship of all three factors must be considered. For example, a treatment program consisting of a heat modality and therapeutic exercise, given in hot weather, may cause physiologic changes that would not occur in cooler weather. Some individuals—the very old or very young or those who are medically compromised—may be unable to tolerate the combination of effects of a heat modality, hot weather, and therapeutic exercise, although they might be able to tolerate any one factor.

Under what circumstances might one omit the therapeutic exercise or the heat modality? When would it be feasible to substitute a cold modality for a heat modality? To answer such questions, therapists must understand both the local and systemic physiological responses resulting from local application or general body exposure to heat or cold. These responses include the effects on specific types of body tissues and on the functions of the body systems. For example, vigorous heat may be indicated for a patient with a chronic ankle sprain problem because the effect of heat on local tissues and sensory nerves may reduce pain and increase range of motion. However, if the patient also has diabetes and poor circulation, vigorous heat would be contraindicated because the vascular system would be unable to make the adjustments necessary to remove excessive heat or metabolic wastes.

The focus of this chapter is on the physiological responses to locally applied thermal modalities, although much of the information pertains to all thermal treatments. The effects of full body exposure to heat and cold are discussed further in Chapter 15 and Chapter 16.

MECHANISMS CAUSING RESPONSES TO HEAT AND COLD

The body responds to thermal changes to protect tissues from damage from excessive heat and cold and to maintain a constant core (internal) temperature (thermal homeostasis). Some local responses may be related to the effects that heat or cold have on substances found naturally in tissues, that modulate microcirculatory blood flow. Such vasoactive substances include the prostaglandins, histamine, bradykinin, and serotonin.[1] In turn, these substances can directly affect the activity of the sweat glands in the skin or the local blood vessels.[2]

In general, however, local and systemic responses are under neural control. Free nerve endings that respond to warm, cold, and thermal pain are situated in the skin and probably in many deep body sites. Other thermal sensors are located in the central nervous system (CNS). Information received from the cutaneous receptors travels through afferent pathways to the hypothalamus and also to the cortex, where conscious awareness of heat and cold sensations occur. Within the hypothalamus are sensor sites that monitor the temperature of the blood flow through the capillaries at the hypothalamus itself.[3]

Although extrahypothalamic deep body sensors appear to exist, in general the hypothalamus integrates information received from the receptors, then mediates appropriate responses through neural efferent pathways. Some evidence indicates that areas that trigger activities to prevent temperature rise are situated in the anterior hypothalamus, and those that prevent cooling are situated in the posterior hypothalamus. A well-balanced integration of neurotransmitter substances probably mediates these efferent pathways.[4]

Because both local and systemic thermal responses depend on information initiated by receptors, receptors (especially those in the skin) and their afferent pathways must be intact for appropriate physiologic responses to occur when thermal modalities are applied. In addition, the patient's ability to report excessive heat or cold depends on those receptors. Fig. 9–1 illustrates the frequency of firing of warm, cold, and thermal pain fibers at various temperatures. Note that the frequency of firing, as shown in the figure, approximates the temperatures given in Table 7–1 for perceptions of cold, heat, and thermal pain and for marked changes in tissue function. For example, the firing of warm fibers decreases and that of heat-pain fibers begins at approximately 109° F to 113° F (43° C to 45° C), the temperature above which tissue damage can occur. Similarly, cold fibers decrease and cold-pain fibers increase firing at temperatures below about 59° F (15° C), the temperature at which tissues and physiological functions are endangered.[3]

The responses triggered by the peripheral sensory input are the safety mechanisms that protect against tissue damage. There is a range of about 50° F (30° C)

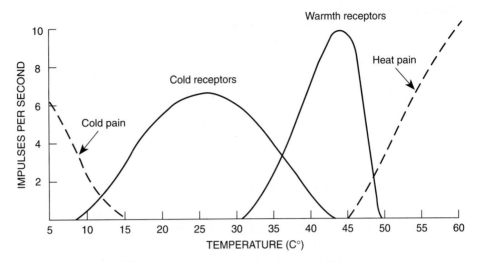

FREEZING COLD	COLD	COOL	INDIFFER-ENT	WARM	HOT	BURNING HOT

Figure 9–1. Frequencies of discharge of (1) cold-pain receptors, (2) cold receptors, (3) warmth receptors, and (4) heat-pain receptors. Note that the frequencies of firing shown in this figure approximate the temperatures at which pain related to hot and cold are perceived as shown in Table 7–1. (*Adapted with permission from* Human Physiology and Mechanisms of Disease. *A Guyton. 6th ed. 1981) 1881, WB Saunders. Drawn from original data collected in separate experiments by Zotterman, Hensel, and Kenshalo*)

within which one can usually tolerate changes in tissue temperature, but pain is perceived when the temperature rises toward 109° C (43° C) or when it falls below 59° F (15° C). This pain is a warning that tissues are in danger. Depending on the length of time that the temperatures of tissues is beyond the safe range, damage or necrosis can occur (see Table 6–1).

To maintain a constant internal temperature, systemic responses occur that are triggered at the thermoregulatory center of the CNS. However, relatively little is known about the central processing of thermal afferents.[5,6] Various thermoregulatory systems probably operate from *set points,* which are not necessarily identical for all systems.[7] The control of the activities of these systems has been compared with the control of the temperature of a room by a thermostat that acts from a set point. When the temperature of a room rises above the point at which the thermostat is set, the heater switches to "off." When the temperature drops below that point, the heater switches to "on" again. Because the regulation of body temperature appears to occur primarily in the hypothalamic region, it is sometimes called a hypothalamic thermostat.

The body strives to maintain an internal temperature of about 98.6° F (37° C) and a mean skin temperature of about 91.4°–94° F (33°–34.5° C) for men and about 90°–95° F (32.2°–35° C) for women. The information about these temperatures is integrated at the hypothalamus.[6] When either the skin or internal temperature changes or the relative difference between the two temperatures varies, the thermoregulatory centers trigger appropriate responses to reestablish the set-point temperatures.

Although the set-point theory is useful to explain how humans maintain thermal homeostasis, it is open to criticism and leaves many questions unanswered. For example, experiments have shown that thermoregulatory responses are elicited by changing the temperature of the spinal cord, although the hypothalamic temperature remains constant. However, changes as small as 0.2° C in the temperature of blood passing near the hypothalamus can cause systemic responses proportional to the temperature change, that act to restore homeostasis.[8]

IMMEDIATE RESPONSES

When either a heat or cold agent is applied to the skin, specific reactions relative to the temperature gradient between the modality and the skin may occur before any appreciable change occurs in tissue temperature. Fig. 9–2 illustrates these responses. The immediate reactions caused by the thermal sensory experience of either hot or cold may be similar. However, other responses to heat differ from those to cold because they are appropriate for preventing tissue injury from opposite problems: either excessive heating or cooling. Thus, this discussion of immediate responses proceeds as follows: (1) thermal sensory reactions to hot and cold, (2) other responses to tissue temperature rise, and (3) other responses to tissue cooling.

Responses to Thermal Sensory Experiences

Sometimes called *thermal shock reactions,* reactions to *thermal sensory experiences* occur whenever the skin comes in contact with something that is hotter or colder than the skin.[9] The specific response depends on the size of the surface area and the temperature gradient between the skin and the modality. More precisely, the reaction depends on the temperature change at the site of the cutaneous thermal receptors.[5] Fig. 9–1 indicates that the frequency of firing of thermal neurons is stable at any given temperature (a static response). However, with a change in temperature at the receptor sites, the rate of firing changes (a dynamic response). Depending on the amount and rate of temperature change, the frequency of neuron firing at first overshoots, then settles at the predictable frequency for any given temperature. These immediate responses will differ according to the area experiencing the thermal change: the smaller the area, the less response. The individual's perception of and attitude toward such changes in thermal sensation also will influence the reaction.

An initial sensation of mild heat or coolness may produce an analgesic effect in the area of application. Mild warmth or coolness applied to a local area can reduce local pain and/or muscle spasms and promote general relaxation.[10] If the temperature of a modality is such that one experiences a greater sensation of hot or cold, other reactions occur. A moderate temperature change may serve as a general stimulant that produces an arousing, invigorating effect.[11] For example, a hot or

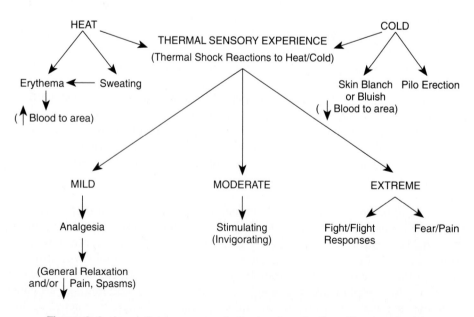

Figure 9–2. Immediate responses to the local application of heat and cold.

cold shower often helps one get going in the morning. However, if the temperature change is perceived as too hot or too cold, one may experience pain or fear. Fight-or-flight responses of eye dilation and changes in facial and skin color, blood pressure, and pulse may be observed. If the temperature of the modality is within the therapeutic range, these reactions subside quickly as one adapts to the temperature change: ie, as the rate of neuron firing stabilizes.

Other Responses to Heat

Local sweating and erythema also increase in immediate response to the local application of heat. Although the erythemal response is clearly observed, the reasons for it are not clearly established. It may be related to a spinal reflex. It also has been theorized that because sensory axons have many branches, the excitation of hot, cold, or noxious afferent neurons may result in action potentials that travel back to the area of stimulation through another branch of the same sensory axon, causing release of a vasodilatory substance—possibly a hormone, histamine, or acetylcholine. These substances produce a local capillary dilation, thus erythema. Because this is an event that is separate from any action potentials reaching the spinal cord, it is termed *axon reflex*.[12,13] Fig. 9–3 illustrates this axon activity. However, current researchers believe that an axon reflex is improbable.

Temperature increases may act directly on smooth muscles of blood vessels and on the sweat glands. Immediate local sweating has been shown to release bradykinin, which in turn causes erythema.[1]

Other Responses to Cold

In addition to the thermal shock reactions, other immediate responses to cold include local vasoconstriction, with blanching of the skin and local piloerection. Some investigators believe that the cold inhibits the release of histamine; thus blanching occurs.[14,15] Others explain the vasoconstriction as being part of the initial reaction of the body to maintain core temperature—an autonomic neural response acting to prevent that part of the body from giving up heat to the colder environment. Whatever the cause, vasoconstriction restricts the rate of blood flow. It thus decreases the amount of warm blood arriving at the site of the cold application and enhances the ability of applied cold to lower the local tissue temperature.[11]

In animals, piloerection, also an autonomic neural response, causes body hair to stand up. This increases air space between hairs, producing insulation that pre-

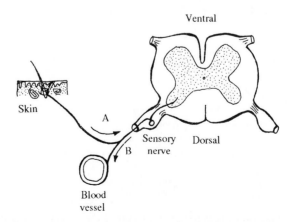

Figure 9–3. An axon reflex. (**A**) A cutaneous sensory receptor is stimulated, which sends impulses along the axon toward the spinal cord. (**B**) Theoretically, the impulses could then travel on another branch of the axon back to a capillary, where it could release vasodilatory substances. (*Adapted from A Guyton*[12].)

vents body heat form escaping. Goose bumps in humans are a remnant of this response, but because we have little hair, it is ineffective.

Summary and Therapeutic Implications

The correlation between the afferent input resulting from firing of cutaneous thermal receptors, the sensory perception, and the thermoregulatory responses is based primarily on information derived from animal studies.[5] The immediate responses occurring with the application of a thermal modality may be caused by the direct effect of temperature change on the activity of sweat glands, vessels, nerves, or mediator substances in the treated area; from central control of information from skin receptors; by the conscious recognition of a noticeable temperature gradient between skin and the thermal agent; or by any combination of these factors.

Many beneficial results attributed to the use of thermal modalities—for example, decreased pain, general relaxation, or both—may be the result of effects of the perceived sensations. However, other benefits are the result of physiologic responses caused by the actual changes in tissue temperature, as the next section will show.

PHYSIOLOGIC RESPONSES TO A RISE IN TISSUE TEMPERATURE

A series of physiologic changes occur whenever tissue temperature rises. These changes will be discussed step-by-step as they relate to localized tissue temperature rise (TTR). Fig. 9–4 indicates that an applied heat initially increases the tissue temperature. Vertical and horizontal arrows indicate reactions produced as a result of TTR.

The viscosity of blood is temperature related. As the temperature increases, the viscosity decreases; the blood becomes more fluid. Increase in local tissue temperature also causes an increase in local sweating.[16]

As indicated by the two-way arrows in Fig. 9–4, a feedback system exists between an increase in tissue temperature and metabolic rate. Metabolism is an ongoing cellular activity; its rate is related to the tissue temperature. The process speeds up as the temperature increases and slows down as the temperature decreases. As a general estimate, for every 10° C rise in body tissue temperature, the metabolic rate may increase two- or three-fold, depending on the type of tissues.[17] This change in metabolic rate per 10° C is referred to as the $Q_{10}Ratio$. Centuries ago, van't Hoff presented information relating tissue temperature to metabolic rate, which was the basis for future investigations in this area. Consequently, the terms *van't Hoff's law* or *van't Hoff effect* are sometimes used when referring to the relationship between tissue temperature and metabolic rate.[18]

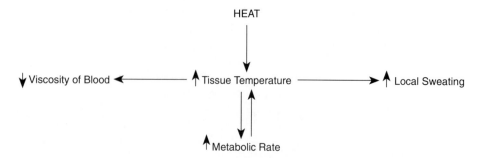

Figure 9–4. Physiologic responses to an increase in tissue temperature. The rise in tissue temperature leads to decreased blood viscosity, increased local sweating, and increased metabolic rate. Because metabolism produces heat, an increased metabolic rate, in turn, increases the tissue temperature, which then increases the metabolic rate and so on in a cyclic pattern.

The metabolic activity itself, the oxygen consumption and chemical interactions that synthesize body proteins, produce heat as well as an accumulation of acids and other metabolic wastes as by-products. When metabolic activity increases, both heat production and waste accumulation increase. Thus, the feedback system operates: that is, TTR increases the metabolic rate, which increases heat production, thus an additional TTR. The metabolic wastes are cleared through sweat, urine, and blood, thus, a normal pH balance is maintained.

Metabolic Responses

Fig. 9–5 indicates two interrelated reactions that are produced with the increase in metabolic rate. The diagonal arrow indicates an increase in phagocytosis. The normal inflammatory process for healing tissues involves activity of the leukocytes and phagocytes of white blood cells. An increase in metabolic rate will increase this activity, which in turn may hasten the healing process and the restoration of damaged tissues. (See the discussions about inflammation in Chapters 1 and 13.)

The vertical arrow indicates the beginning of vascular changes— arteriolar dilatation. As the metabolic rate increases, the activity of the vascular system, acting through its neuronal and hormonal controls, also increases. Arteriolar dilatation increases blood flow at the heated site. This increased flow is essential to provide the white blood cells for the stepped-up leukocytic and phagocytic activity and the nutrients needed to meet the increased demands of the metabolic process. Because the metabolic process uses O_2 and increases production of CO_2, acids, and other by-products, the tissues must have a constant and sufficient flow of arterial blood to bring oxygenated blood to the heated area. A sufficient venous flow is also needed to remove the metabolic wastes and retard increases in tissue temperature because heat is convected away from the site through the venous flow. The fact that stepping-up the metabolic rate increases phagocytic activity and local circulation explains why the application of local heat is indicated to hasten the healing of damaged tissues and the clearing of interstitial exudates resulting from inflammation, hemorrhage (hematomas), or edema. The erythema observed, which continues as long as the tissues are heated, is an indication that this process is occurring.

In addition to localized healing effects, the application of a superficial heat before exercise often enables a person to move better. Some people mistakenly believe that this improvement occurs because they have "warmed up their muscles" and, consequently, have increased muscle metabolic rate and blood flow. A deep heat modality could possibly increase the metabolic rate and blood flow in muscle in a local area, but as Rowell[19] emphasized, even the most intense heating of skin does not increase blood flow to underlying muscle.[20–22] In general, exercise physiologists believe that a "warm-up"—increasing one's general metabolic rate and blood flow in muscles in preparation for strenuous activity—should be attained through activity rather than a passive heat application. Nonetheless, local modalities, either superficial or deep, are used before the active warm-up for both therapeutic and athletic exercise and do appear to enhance movement. The benefits must be the result of some other effects of heating, such as analgesic or relaxation effects, but not the increase in general muscle metabolism.

Precautions Related to Increased Tissue Temperature and Metabolic Rate. When tissues are heated within the therapeutic range, the accumulated by-product (meta-

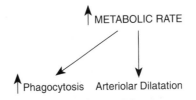

Figure 9–5. Effects of an increase in the metabolic rate in relation to a rise in tissue temperature.

bolic acids) can escape with body fluids and homeostasis is maintained. This includes an increase in uric acids excreted in urine and lactic acids excreted in sweat. Thus, vascular, renal, and sweat balance mechanisms all come into play. If any of these mechanisms is compromised, the pH balance may be upset and unfavorable reactions may occur. Therefore, vigorous heat modalities should be used with caution with patients with Addison's disease, metabolic problems, or any deconditioned people whose systems cannot meet the required demands.

When the tissue temperature rises above 113° F (45° C), tissue damage can occur. If the metabolic rate increases beyond its capacity to function, enzymes are denatured and proteins are destroyed. Above this temperature, the rate of chemical activity decreases.

Vascular Responses

As was stated earlier, the viscosity of blood decreases and arteriolar dilation occurs as blood temperature increases; thus, flow to the capillaries increases. Fig. 9–6 indicates the vascular responses that then occur in the capillary region. The increased blood flow to the capillary beds increases the capillary pressure, perhaps increasing the number of patent (open) channels and the permeability of the capillary membranes (see Chapters 2 and 3).

In general, the vasodilation in a local heated area allows more blood to flow through the area, resulting in (1) an increase in nutrients and leukocytes that enhances tissue healing, (2) an increase in the rate of clearing of metabolites, which decreases pain or muscle spasms caused by the accumulation of lactic acid or other wastes, and (3) an increase in the amount of cooler blood arriving at the area and warmer blood being carried away, which helps prevent tissue damage from excessive heating. All of these effects are beneficial. Conversely, increase in blood flow may cause bleeding to increase or resume at injured tissue sites or lead to hemorrhage in patients with conditions such as ulcers and hemophilia.

The precise means by which substances are transported between the blood and interstitium, including the causes and effects of increased capillary pressure and permeability, are still being investigated. It may be that an increase in capillary permeability permits more wastes and fluids to be reabsorbed into the bloodstream from the extracellular space, thus enhancing tissue healing and clearing of exudates, including long-standing edema. Conversely, an increase in permeability allows more fluids to flow from the bloodstream to the extracellular space, thus encouraging the formation of edema.

On the basis of these responses, heat treatments may at times be beneficial and at other times may increase problems; therefore, they should not be used indiscriminately. With patients whose conditions suggest the possibility of edema or

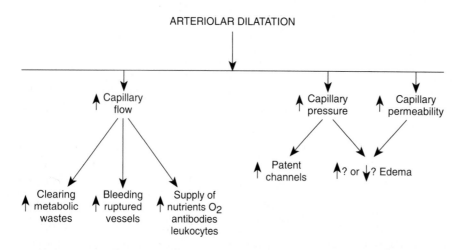

Figure 9–6. Vascular responses resulting from a rise in tissue temperature.

bleeding, only mild heat, if any, is advised. To prevent edema, the body parts to be heated should be elevated to encourage flow of fluid away from the area toward the heart. Frequently, when bleeding or edema is anticipated, eg, after an acute injury, many therapists prefer to avoid applying any heat for at least 24 to 72 hours, substituting with ice, compression, and elevation (ICE).

Finally, the integrity of the vessels must be considered. It is important for vasodilatation to occur to enable more arterial blood flow to the tissues to meet their increased metabolic demands. In conditions such as arteriosclerosis, arterial wall compliance is compromised, limiting dilatation. If local heat is applied and the increased demand for blood cannot be met, tissue damage, ischemia, or necrosis may occur.

Other vascular considerations include local vascular shunting and reflex heating. These are discussed below.

Local vascular shunting. Some researchers have hypothesized that when overheating endangers the superficial tissues, the branching of the peripheral system that usually supplies blood to the muscles or other tissues underlying the heated tissue may constrict, shunting usual blood flow of the system to the cutaneous area in need.[23] This shunting occurs at the expense of temporary deprivation of blood to the underlying tissues. If this is the case, superficial heat modalities not only would be ineffective in enhancing blood flow to deep muscles, they also would be decreasing such flow. However, because the circulation to deeper muscles is independent of that to cutaneous tissues, this hypothesis cannot be supported (see Chapter 2).

Application of even vigorous superficial heat may have no effect on blood flow to deep muscles, and a superficial heat modality cannot be expected to cause a significant TTR of any tissues at a depth greater than 1 cm. However, if a deep heat modality is used, that actually heats these deeper tissues, blood flow to deeper tissues may increase.

Reflex Heating. The term *reflex heating* refers to a technique involving the application of heat to one area of the body that results in an increase in cutaneous circulation and other reactions in another area. Because the effect occurs almost immediately—that is, before systemic changes have the opportunity to be an influencing factor—it is called reflex heating. This technique also is termed consensual heating, remote heating, or—since the studies by Landis and Gibbons first called attention to the phenomena—the Landis-Gibbons reflex.[24]

Many studies have reported that heat applied to one body part, either by local modalities or by immersion in hot water, results in increased cutaneous circulation, sweating, and hyperemia in other parts of the body.[10,25,26] These include reactions on (1) the leg or arm opposite to the one heated, (2) the ipsilateral upper extremity when the lower extremity is heated, and (3) the lower extremity when heat is applied to the back or abdomen.

A reflex heating technique may be useful for patients with circulatory problems such as diabetes or peripheral vascular diseases, especially if dermatological conditions such as stasis ulcers are present. These patients could benefit from increased blood flow to their extremities, but they cannot tolerate a great increase in tissue temperature in those extremities. Heating an extremity when the circulation cannot meet its metabolic needs or dissipate the added heat may cause tissue damage. In such cases, heating another part of the body may reflexively increase the cutaneous blood flow to the involved extremity. An extremity with poor circulation that initially appeared blanched and cool will appear pinker and the skin temperature will increase. This response, however, only lasts for a brief period.[27]

It was reported by Bisgard and Nye that visceral changes occur beneath the area where superficial heat is applied. These visceral changes include a decrease in gastrointestinal activity, relaxation of gut muscles, and a decrease in periastalis. Thus, a time-honored household remedy, placing heat on the abdomen to decrease stomach or menstrual cramps, is verified.[28]

Whether superficial or deep heat modalities are more effective in producing remote changes needs more investigation. One unpublished study showed that a hot pack applied to the back for 20 minutes produces significantly greater changes in the skin temperature of the foot than does a 10-minute ultrasound treatment to the same area.[29] There is no evidence that deep circulation improves with any remote techniques.

Systemic Responses

Recall that when the temperature of the blood near the site of thermal integration in the hypothalamus rises or when the normal difference between skin and core temperature changes, the CNS activates body heat loss mechanisms to maintain thermal homeostasis. These are not local responses but reactions that affect the entire body. General vasomotor and sudomotor (sweat control) systems respond to bring heat to the body surface to be released by radiation and evaporation. These systemic reactions will occur regardless of the cause of the rise in the circulating blood temperature. General heating from ambient conditions, physical exercise, general heat modalities, such as whirlpools and Hubbard tanks, or even a local heat modality can provoke systemic reactions if their intensity and duration is sufficient to increase the temperature of the blood in the peripheral system.

Cardiovascular responses. With any increase in general body temperature, the responses are (1) generalized vasodilation of cutaneous vessels to allow more heat to reach the surface, (2) a drop in peripheral blood pressure caused by the dilation, which could cause a temporary decrease in peripheral blood flow until the body responds to the drop in pressure, by (3) an increased heart rate. With increased heart rate, cardiac output is maintained, and peripheral blood flow is increased. The clinical signs that occur with increased core temperature (for example, a fever) signify these changes: The skin will be warm and have a pink flushed color, and the pulse rate will be increased.

However, the body's regulators may overshoot their mark slightly when adjusting to different temperatures in a manner that resembles a room thermostat, as explained earlier. A slight temperature rise above or a drop below the "set point" is needed to stimulate the reactions of regulators. As the heart rate increases, it overshoots slightly, resulting in an increase in blood pressure. The heart rate then drops. This decrease in heart rate may cause a drop in blood pressure below its set point; thus, the heart rate will increase again. These temporary fluctuations during adjustments to temperature changes are normal, but eventually the blood pressure can be expected to stabilize with a slightly higher heart rate, which maintains the increase in peripheral blood flow. Fig. 9–7 summarizes these reactions.

It is interesting to observe these fluctuations occurring in normal adults. If one monitored several young healthy adults sitting waist deep in a hot tub in which the water is 105° F, each person might have rises and drops in both pulse and blood pressure. However, the duration and amount of fluctuation would differ for each person, as would the recovery time.

Systemic vascular responses may produce therapeutic effects. The increase in cutaneous blood flow may, in addition to cooling the body, bring additional nutrients to the skin. But unwanted effects such as increased bleeding also may occur. A drop in blood pressure resulting in less blood flow to the brain may cause fainting. It is not uncommon for debilitated people to faint as a result of systemic responses to a rise in temperature. Patients in moderately heated hydrotherapy pools or those receiving prolonged heat from a constant output source such as infrared or diathermy must be monitored carefully.

Systemic vascular shunting. Shunting to protect tissues in a localized area from excessive changes in temperature was discussed in Chapter 2. Systemic shunting occurs when the internal temperature is high. In an effort to cool the body, blood may be shunted from deep circulatory systems, such as the renal system, to the peripheral system.[30] Thus, more blood reaches the surface to give off heat to the environment. Of course, only a temporary reduction of blood flow from these sys-

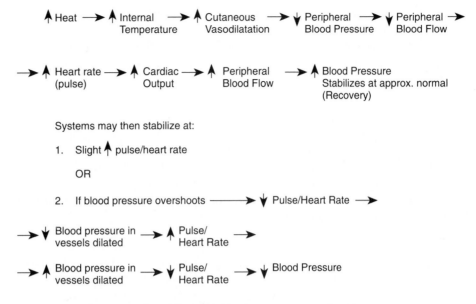

Figure 9–7. Cardiovascular responses when applied heat is sufficient to increase the internal (core) temperature. (*Based on data in J Hales:* Thermal Physiology. *New York: Raven Press; 1984.*)

tems can be tolerated without serious damage to those organs because they, too, need their blood supply.

Sudomotor responses. Central thermoregulators also control the *sudomotor systems.* Sensible sweat resulting from activation of eccrine sweat glands begins when the skin temperature rises above approximately 91.4° F and with virtually any rise in core temperature above normal. Some eccrine sweat glands, primarily those located in the palms of the hands and soles of the feet, react to emotional stress, but most of the eccrine glands throughout the body are thermoregulators. These sweat glands, controlled by the autonomic nervous system, may be activated by adrenal activity or by epinephrine, norepinephrine or both circulating in the bloodstream.[3] As was mentioned in Chapter 8, insensible water loss through the skin is an ongoing activity that preserves thermal homeostasis. All sweat acts to prevent an increase in body temperature as follows: (1) the heat is brought to the surface in the fluid, (2) if exposed to the air, the fluid may then evaporate, using calories of heat to vaporize the sweat and thus cool the surface, (3) heat may transfer from sweat molecules on the body surface to adjacent cooler air molecules, then be removed by air flow, ie convection.

Normally, the salt concentration in sweat is low, as little as 5 mEq/L, and most of one's salt intake is reabsorbed by the body. However, unless a person is acclimatized, the salt concentration in sweat will increase as sweating increases. With profuse sweating, the salt concentration may be as high as 60 mEq/L and the body supply may be greatly diminished. Problems related to excessive salt loss are discussed in Chapter 15. Sweat also contains potassium ions, urea, and lactic acid. With profuse sweating, the lactic acid concentration in sweat also increases. Thus, the excess lactic acid, produced by the increase in metabolism, escapes and helps to maintain homeostasis. Fig. 9–8 summarizes this process. The concentration of other ions also will increase with increased sweating, but not markedly so.[3]

Respiratory responses. The warm air given off by breathing rids the body of some heat. The expired air is saturated with moisture. Evaporation of the moisture in this air and from the moist mucous membrane of the respiratory passages contributes to the body cooling. When resting in a neutral environment, as much as a

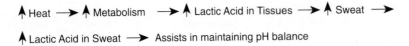

Figure 9–8. Sudomotor responses to generalized heating when applied heat increases the internal (core) temperature.

third of the evaporative heat loss is through the respiratory tract. Panting is an effective means of heat loss in many animals, but not in humans, although humans do maintain this mechanism. If a person is extremely hot, a "panting" exhalation, a response to metabolic acidosis, may be observed. This is a signal that heat or exercise treatments should be terminated. Vigorous, prolonged heat is not advised for any cardiopulmonary patients.

Renal responses. Some heat, but not a significant amount, is lost during urination. Of greater significance is the increase in the phosphate and acid concentration in the urine that occurs and when excreted, serves to rid the body of the increase in these metabolic by-products. Thus, to prevent acidosis, patients with renal disease or urine retention problems should not receive prolonged or frequent heat treatments, which would increase the internal temperature.

Summary and Therapeutic Implications

Table 9–1 summarizes the physiologic responses to local heat gain. The responses include both local and systemic initial neurophysiologic responses to the sensation of hot or cold and changes resulting from a rise in tissue temperature, core temperature, or both. The TTR causes an increase in the metabolic rates which in turn produces changes in arteriolar blood flow and capillary activities. Under certain circumstances, these reactions may have therapeutically beneficial effects; in other circumstances, the effects may be detrimental. Local application of superficial heat may cause physiologic changes in other areas of the body, such as a temporary increase in cutaneous blood flow or a decrease in deep smooth muscle activity.

TABLE 9–1. SUMMARY OF PHYSIOLOGIC RESPONSES TO APPLIED HEAT AND THEIR CLINICAL SIGNIFICANCE

Physiologic Response	Effects	Clinical Significance
Thermal sensory experience (thermal shock).	Mild: analgesic/sedative. Moderate: autonomic responses. Severe: fight or flight responses.	Decreases pain spasms, and aids relaxation. Invigorating general stimulant. Pain and fear.
Changes in skin color.	Observable sign is erythema.	Usually increases blood flow.
Increased metabolic rate.	Increased healing and waste production.	Increases heat production and tissue temperature.
Increased blood flow.	Increase bleeding.	Increase healing (increases nutrients to and waste removal from the area).
Reflex response.	Increased cutaneous blood flow in areas of body other than where heat applied.	Effect is transitory.
Increased capillary permeability.	Increase (or decrease) interstitial fluid.	Increased (or decreased) edema.
Increased sweating.	Increased cooling.	Decreases fluid/salt balance in body.
Fluctuations in cardiovascular (CV) activity.	Changes in heart rate/blood pressure.	Stresses CV system and/or can cause fainting if excessive.
Increased respiration.	Little value in maintaining thermal homeostasis.	Indicates heat distress.
Decreased joint stiffness.*	Increase speed and freedom of joint movement.	Increases agility.
Increased extensibility of nonelastic tissues.*	Assist in elongating or stretching tendons, scar.	Increases range of movement of any body segment.
Increased peripheral nerve conduction velocity and motor nerve activity.*		Increases speed and motor function.

*Indicates responses that are discussed in Chapter 10.

This procedure is termed remote, reflex, or consensual heating. Blood also may be shunted from other channels to the cutaneous vessels when damage from externally applied heat may occur and from other circulatory systems as a response to an excessive rise in core temperature. However, blood flow in deep muscles acts independently of cutaneous circulation. Local heating, either superficial or deep, may enhance the movement of individual joints, but it is not an appropriate warm-up for strenuous exercise. Such general warm-ups should involve active, not passive, heating of the body.

Thermoregulatory sites in the body integrate information from skin and deep receptors. Whenever these sites receive information that the internal temperature has risen above normal, systemic changes occur to preserve thermal homeostasis. Depending on the severity of the heat, cardiovascular, sudomotor, respiratory, and renal systems may react to prevent a rise in internal temperature. Any person with systemic problems or indications that any of these systems cannot adapt may not tolerate vigorous heat. Therefore, dosages and pathologies must always be considered when applying heat.

RESPONSES TO A DECREASE IN TISSUE TEMPERATURE

Local Application of Cold. When cold is applied locally to the body surface, one might expect reactions to be just the opposite of those occurring with heat, but this is not always the case. In general, the metabolic responses are the opposite but the vascular responses are not.

As with heat, the ability of a cold modality to affect local and systemic changes depends on (1) the temperature of the cold, (2) the skin-modality temperature gradient, (3) the duration of application, (4) the vascular supply to the area, and (5) the thermal conductivity and thickness of each tissue layer. A modality cooled to 59° F (15° C) may initially draw heat from the body, although not as rapidly as a colder modality and, as the skin temperature decreases and the modality becomes warmer, there will be no significant gradient between them. Various forms of cold packs represent this type of modality. Ice slush pots, ice water, or other modalities remaining just about 32° F (0° C) can be more effective in cooling superficial tissues because the skin-modality temperature gradient is greater, and the temperature remains near freezing until the ice melts.[31] However, the danger of cold related tissue damage is also greater.[32] When super cooling modalities are used (ie, modalities below freezing), there may be more marked cooling effects, but there also will be more danger of damaging tissues.[33] (See Table 6–18 for critical cold temperatures.)

The immediate responses to cold were discussed earlier in this chapter. These immediate responses are related to the thermal sensory experience (thermal shock) caused by the increase in the frequency of the firing of cold sensory receptors. The amount of increase in the frequency of firing is related to the temperature gradient between the skin and the modality. In addition to these immediate responses, which are related to the sensation of cold, are those related to the lowered tissue temperature.

Initial Vascular and Metabolic Responses

Fig. 9–9 summarizes the *initial* responses that can occur in tissues cooled by cryotherapy modalities. As the tissue temperature decreases, both local blood flow and metabolic rate decrease. The local cutaneous vessels constrict, increasing resistance in the vessels proximal to the capillaries and causing the fall in capillary perfusion (blood flow).[9] The viscosity of the blood increases slightly as the tissue temperature begins to drop, and it increases markedly should the tissue temperature fall below 80° F (27° C).[34,35] These temperature-related changes in blood flow can reduce

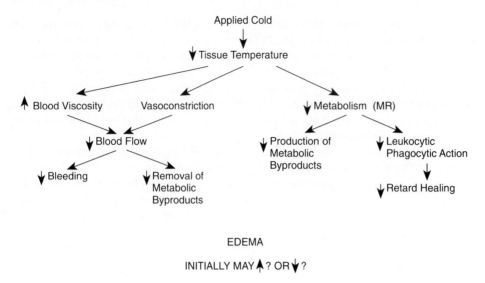

Figure 9–9. Initial physiologic responses when applied cold lowers the tissue temperature.

bleeding or hemorrhage. The reduced flow of warmer blood to the cooled area enhances the effect of a cold modality. The slower rate of flow of cooled blood away from the local area back toward the core serves to prolong the local cooling effect[36] and to prevent a decrease in core temperature as well. This initial vasoconstriction response is only transitory, lasting approximately 10–30 minutes.

However, this decrease in incoming arterial blood results in less oxygen and other nutrients being brought to the cooled area. The decrease in venous flow from the area results in increased retention of metabolic wastes and CO_2. The increased content of CO_2 in the blood accounts for the blue color of cooled skin.[3]

Evidence has been presented suggesting that the retardation of wound healing that occurs when tissues are cooled may be related to the hypoxia caused by this decrease in blood flow.[37] Because metabolic rate is temperature dependent, it, too, will decrease at the site of the cooled tissues, as will the heat produced as a metabolic by-product.

With a decreased metabolic rate, there is less demand for O_2 and other nutrients and less production of, or need to rid the area of, metabolic wastes. But this slower metabolic rate also may contribute to the retardation of the healing process, as the inflammatory process—ie, the action of leukocytes and phagocytes—is decreased. Lundgren et al. showed that the wounds of animals placed in a cooler environment took longer to heal than did the wounds of animals placed in a warmer environment. These investigators suggested that the retardation in healing might be caused by the decrease in nutrients at the wound area related to the decrease in blood flow but that it was more likely that the decreased metabolic rate caused the slower healing. Such evidence suggests that cold should not be applied after the acute or subacute phases of injury, when bleeding has stopped and swelling subsided.

It is commonly accepted that cooling tissues for 10–30 minute periods prevents or diminishes formation of posttraumatic edema in the acute phase. However, some studies have shown that cold may actually increase rather than decrease edema or that, even if diminished during application, edema may increase as tissues rewarm.[38–40]

Schmidt et al.[4] studied the effects of heat and cold on the edema resulting from artificially induced inflammation in rats and found that the effects of cold on swelling varied with the type of chemical mediator used to cause the inflammation. Like posttraumatic edema, inflammation induced by mediators such as histamine and serotonin could be inhibited significantly during the acute stage (as long as 24 hours) but other forms of inflammation, particularly those mediated by prostaglandins, could be aggravated by cold.[40]

A more recent study compared the effects of heat, cold, and contrast baths on posttraumatic edema.[41] This study used common clinical duration parameters: 20 minutes for the heat or cold modalities and, for the contrast baths, immersion for 3 minutes in hot water followed by 1 minute in cold water with these alternations continuing for 20 minutes. On Day 3 the edema treated with cold had decreased slightly, whereas it had increased with the other two modalities. But on Days 4 and 5, the edema increased with all three modalities, although the increase with cold was significantly less than with the other modalities.

The preceding studies exemplify the importance of having clinicians not only keep abreast of the literature but also carefully consider whether and how the findings of published studies may or may not have direct implications. Findings of studies in which the duration of cold applications ranged from 1 hour to days may not be directly applicable to a 10–30 minute clinical treatment. However, studies such as the one by Schmidt et al[40] may have direct significance. Their findings suggest that all rheumatic conditions should not be treated the same way because the chemical mediators of the swelling related to various rheumatic conditions may not be similar.

Intensity as well as duration influence the effect of the applied cold. In their experiments, Schmidt et al[40] used deep-frozen gel packs for 1 hour. They suggested that extremely brief applications of cold (eg, ice massage) cannot suppress any inflammation effectively and that cooling to 53.3° F (12° C) is not a true cold treatment, as are frozen gel packs or ice. Other investigators reported an immediate increase in edema when a cold compress, soaked in 53.3° F, (12° C) was applied.[39] This suggests an immediate response of increased inflammation.

The conflicting results of various studies may be attributed to the differences in the duration and temperature of the modality used in the investigations. The results of cryotherapy used with patients also may depend on these factors. The intensity of the cold per duration should be considered carefully for each condition and for each patient treated. Individual patients may react differently to any one dosage.

Responses of Peripheral Nerves

Both motor and sensory peripheral nerves are affected by cooling. Cold fibers fire minimally at temperatures as high as 109° F (43° C). The rate of firing peaks at about 77° F (25° C), gradually decreasing and ceasing at approximately 47° F (8.5° C). Cold-pain fibers begin firing at approximately 59° F (15° C), and the rate increases as their temperature lowers to approximately 40° F (4.7° C). Thus, between 59° F and 47° F (15° C–8.5° C), the sensation of cold diminishes as cold-pain increases.[3] Fig. 9–1 illustrates the firing temperature of the thermal neurons.

As the temperature lowers, the firing of all pain and tactile neurons gradually decreases. At a temperature near freezing, all sensory neuron activity ceases. Based on these neural changes, the sensations one may feel as tissues become colder may first be cold, then painfully cold, then less cold and more pain, which is sometimes perceived as warmth or burning. Eventually, numbness and anesthesia occur.[6,42] During ice massage, patients often report sensory changes in this sequence. The motor nerves also are affected by cold. Both the excitation and nerve conduction velocity of these neurons decrease relative to the temperature. Obviously, this has an effect on motor performance.

Responses of Deeper Tissues

It is generally agreed that a superficial cold modality can affect the temperature of tissues to a greater depth than can a superficial heat modality.[11] There are several reasons for this. First, the temperature gradient between the modality and the skin is greater. Recall that heat always transfers from the hotter to the cooler substance and that the rate of transfer depends on the temperature gradient. If a superficial heat modality at 110° F (43.3° C), which is about as hot as is tolerable, is applied to skin that is 85° F (29.4° C), there is a 25° F (13.9° C) temperature gradient. But if a cold modality at 45° F (7.2° C) is applied, there is a 40° F (22.2° C) temperature gradient. Thus, the rate of heat transfer **from** the body surface to the cold modality is much more rapid than is the rate **to** the body from the heat modality.

Second, heat is not convected from the area as rapidly. Recall that because heat modalities increase superficial circulation, much of the heat is quickly convected from the site, deterring conductive transfer to the deeper tissues, and only superficial tissues are heated significantly. But with a cold modality, the vasoconstriction deterring **convective** heat transfer to the cooled site prolongs the surface cooling and allows more time for heat from deeper tissues to **conduct** toward the cooled surface. Thus, the increased temperature gradient—increasing the rate of heat transfer and decreasing the rate of blood flow—increases the ability of cold to change the temperature of deep tissues more than heat.

Other factors that influence the depth at which tissue cooling is effective include the thickness of the subcutaneous fat layer and the vascular status in the area. Because fat is a heat insulator, heat transfer from the deeper tissues by conduction is related to the thickness of the subcutaneous fat layer. Studies have shown that with application of ice, muscles at a maximum depth of 2 cm will cool approximately 3.4° F (2° C) in 10 minutes if the subject's fat layer is less than 1cm thick. But if the subject has more than 2 cm of subcutaneous fat, tissues even 1 cm deep are scarcely cooled at all in 10 minutes; more than 30 minutes are required to achieve a temperature change similar to those obtained in subjects with less than a 1 cm thick fat layer in 10 minutes.[43] However, after deep tissues are cooled, because fat is a thermal insulator, the fat layer and any vasoconstriction caused by cold help prolong the time that tissues remain cool. Consequently, one can assume that if a modality with a temperature of 50° F (10° C), (a less intense cold with less gradient than ice) is applied for 15–20 minutes, it is unlikely to cool deeper tissues significantly. The relief obtained when cold at approximately 50° F (10° C) is applied for purposes such as relief of deep muscle spasms may be related to effects other than the change in the temperature of those muscles.

Vascular factors also influence the depth at which cooling occurs. Some heat conducted from arterial vessels to tissues along the route to the cooled site and to adjacent outgoing venous blood via counter-current heat exchange (see Chapter 2 and a later section of this chapter) lowers the temperature of blood arriving at the cooled site. Consequently, incoming blood is less able to warm the tissues. In areas with a poor blood supply, the effect of cooling is enhanced even more, perhaps dangerously, because less blood flows to the area. Pugh et al[43] theorized that constriction of superficial vessels may shunt incoming blood to deeper branches, thus supplying underlying tissues with an increased volume of warmer blood and retarding the cooling of these deeper tissues.[44] This theory, if true, discourages the use of cold to prevent bleeding of deeper tissues but makes cold beneficial for nourishing them; however, this kind of reciprocity in blood flow is questionable. The theory may, in part, be based on misinterpretation of published reports.[22,45]

Reports conflict about the amount of temperature change per depth and per duration of application of cold modalities. They also conflict about the length of time tissues remained cool after treatment. One investigation found that tissues that were 2 cm deep were cooled in 5 minutes, but cooling was minimal thereafter.[46] Another study which also reported that tissues 2 cm deep were cooled (4.1° C, approximately 7.3° F) in 5 minutes. Continuing the ice massage for 10 minutes longer cooled the deep tissues an additional 1.1° C, but the skin temperature reached maximum cooling in the first 5 minutes. This study also found that when a similar ice massage was applied to calf muscles and posterior thigh muscles the temperature changes at the same depth were different.[47]

Investigators using supercooling at 20° F (−7° C) for 20 minutes were able to cool deep muscles much more. Although they found considerable variation among subjects regarding both the time required for cooling and for fluctuations in temperature that occurred over time, they reported an important finding: Supercooling **decreased the spasticity** in all of their subjects who had multiple sclerosis.[34]

Considering the findings of the investigations just described, it appears that ice can reduce the temperature of tissues that are 2 cm deep about 7° F (4° C) in 5 minutes with little or no further decrease in the next 5 minutes. A "super cool" modality applied for a longer duration, 20 minutes, can cool deeper muscles markedly. Similar dosages do not achieve similar results in all subjects or in different muscle tissues.

Secondary Vascular Responses

If the duration of application or exposure to intense cold is prolonged, tissue damage can occur. Fortunately, unless the cold is excessive, when the local tissue temperature drops significantly, secondary responses occur, which act to prevent damage. After 15–30 minutes, depending on the vascular status of the area, blood flow to the endangered tissues increases.[48]

Current theories suggest that the vessels are no longer constricted because neuronal transmission controlling vasoconstriction has diminished or ceased below a critical temperature and because arterioventricular (A-V) shunts open.[15] (See Chapter 2 for a description of these shunts.)

Fig. 9–10 illustrates the A-V shunt mechanism, as reported in a famous study by Lewis in 1930.[48,49] In this study, a finger was immersed in crushed ice. As expected, with time the skin temperature decreased and the finger looked blue, indicating that the vessels had constricted and the amount of blood flowing through the capillaries had decreased. After the temperature had dropped to approximately 2.5°–4° C (36°–39° F), the temperature began to increase and the normal pink/red skin color returned. Because there was no flow through local capillary beds, this warming of tissues was attributed to the opening of the shunts. When the tissue temperature rose above 4°–10° C (39°–50° F), depending on the subject, the temperature again began to decrease and the blue color of the skin returned, indicating that the shunts had closed down. The alternating of skin temperature and color continued for up to 2 or 3 hours, gradually diminishing over time. This alternation in blood flow is referred to as the "hunting reaction" or *Lewis' hunting phenomenon.* Although the underlying mechanisms are unknown, severe cold may affect the interaction of adrenergic neuroeffectors in the cutaneous vessels.[15] The

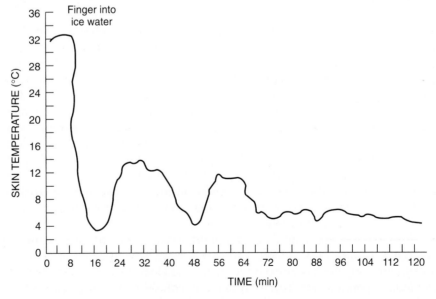

Figure 9–10. Fluctuation in the skin temperature of a finger immersed in crushed ice for a prolonged period. (*Modified from T Lewis, ed.*[48].)

actual tissue temperature and time required for these shunts to open and close are highly variable, depending to some degree on the acclimatization of each person. Snow skiers and other people who have spent much time outdoors in extremely cold weather are familiar with the changes that occur in color of the skin on cheeks and fingers. Blue cheeks and fingers indicate vasoconstriction and closed shunts. Then, after a few minutes, although still exposed to the cold, the cheeks and fingers turn red, indicating that the shunts are open. These alternations in skin color continue throughout the period of exposure, provided that the exposure time is not prolonged. Depending on the individual, after 1–3 hours of exposure to extreme cold, this shunting mechanism will cease to function and tissue damage may occur.

Systemic Responses

Systemic responses, which act to maintain the body's constant internal temperature, are based on integration of information received from the superficial cold receptors (free nerve endings) and centrally located thermoreceptors and on the temperature of the blood in the general circulation. Responses are activated when the temperature of blood passing the central sites of integration (primarily the hypothalamus) falls below normal. Theoretically, the responses that occur depend on the amount of temperature change from an original set point. To conserve body heat, there will be generalized cutaneous vasoconstriction. To increase internal temperature, three mechanisms commence: nonshivering thermogenesis, unconscious tension of muscles, and shivering. Nonshivering thermogenesis refers to the production of internal heat by sympathetically controlled, cold-induced chemical reactions that increase the rate of cell metabolism. This means of heat production is not related to shivering.[6,12,50] Although several sites in the body contribute to nonshivering thermogenesis, its effectiveness appears to be related to brown fat content, which is more prevalent in animals and in infants than in adult humans. Thus, it may be a more important factor in the thermoregulation of infants than of adults. Shivering is a tremorlike continuation of brief muscle contractions throughout the body, an exhausting form of exercise. This exercise, which increases the metabolic rate and the production of heat, is a metabolic response to preserve homeostasis.

Counter-current exchange (CCE) Sufficient exposure to cold can cause a decrease in the temperature of the blood in the general circulation, resulting in a lower core temperature and systemic responses. But because of the exchange of heat by conduction between vessels and the tissues through which they pass and, to a lesser extent, from arteries to their adjacent veins through the process of counter-current exchanges (CCE), the temperature of the cutaneous venous blood is warmed before returning to the general circulation. Although it appears that the heat exchange occurs predominately between the vessels and the tissues, the CCE theory, for purposes of simplification, is used to explain how internal temperature is preserved.[51] Fig. 9–11 is a theoretical example of how, disregarding all other heat exchange procedures, CCE acts to preserve core temperature. Fig. 9–11A indicates how markedly venous blood could cool, and consequently lower core temperature, if CCE did not exist. The blood at approximately core temperature would travel from the deeper body to the skin. In a cold environment, a considerable temperature gradient would exist between the temperature of the blood and the environment. Consequently, as blood reached the surface, it would give up its heat to the environment rapidly. The venous blood returning to the general circulation would be considerably cooler than under normal ambient conditions and cause the internal temperature to drop below normal.

Fig. 9–11B illustrates the CCE. Proceeding distally toward the periphery, the temperature of the arterial blood gradually lowers, having given off heat to the parallel, returning venous blood. By the time the blood reaches the body surface, the blood temperature has dropped to some extent. With this lower temperature of blood in surface tissues and capillaries, the gradient between the body surface and the cooler environment is decreased. This, in turn, decreases radiation and the rate

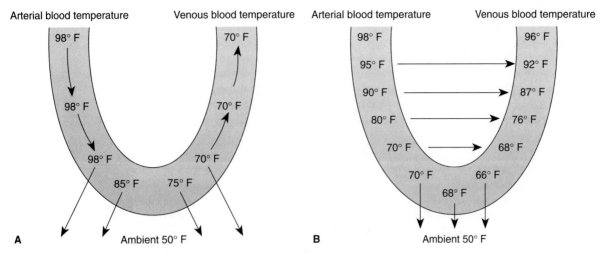

Figure 9–11. Schematic illustration of heat convection through the vascular system from deep in the body to the skin and return (ambient temperature, 50° F). (**A**) Hypothetical blood temperatures without countercurrent exchange. At an ambient temperature of 50° F, if the blood flowing to the skin remained at approximately core temperature, there would be a temperature gradient of approximately 40° F that would encourage rapid heat transfer from the blood. The blood returning to deeper circulation would be considerably cooler. If a large area of the body was exposed to this condition, a considerable drop in core temperature could occur. (**B**) Hypothetical blood temperatures with countercurrent exchange. Arteriole blood gradually gives heat to the returning venous blood, which results in a lower gradient between the blood and ambient temperatures and a gradual increase in the temperature of the returning venous blood.

of heat transfer to the environment. Of course, some heat is given off to the cooler environment, so the venous blood is cooler than its adjacent arterial blood; however, it gains heat as it moves toward the heart until an equilibrium with arterial temperature is reached.[51] Although less than formerly presumed in humans, this mechanism, even when one is exposed to great temperature changes, helps the core temperature to remain constant. The heat exchange occurring between vessels and adjacent tissues and between tissues and the environment is similar.

Sometimes the goal of cold treatments is to lower core temperature: for example, if a patient has a dangerously high fever. Generally, when treatments are given by physical therapists the goal is to lower *local* tissue temperature *without lowering core temperature.* DonTigny and Sheldon[52] suggested that when cold is applied to one part of the body, application of heat to another part of the body will prevent a drop in core temperature that might initiate undesirable shivering, tensing of muscles, or both.

Tissue Damage

As with heat modalities, tissue damage may occur with cold modalities, depending on the duration or intensity of the exposure as well as on the sensory and vascular condition of the area being cooled. With prolonged cooling, even if the temperature is not low enough to freeze tissues, injuries can occur.[32] Chilblains, a mild injury, causes redness, swelling, tenderness, and itching. It occurs primarily in fingers and toes and is most commonly seen in people with peripheral vascular deficiencies such as Raynaud's disease and syringomyelia.[53]

Tissue damage resulting from cold can be divided into stages according to severity and is related to both the temperature (at or near freezing) and to the duration of exposure. The reader is referred to articles by Thorman[54] for a good overview and to Meryman[55] for a more comprehensive discussion of cold injuries. Table 9–2 categorizes cold injuries according to their severity: ie, the depth of tissue damage.[18,56]

TABLE 9–2. CLASSIFICATION OF COLD INJURIES*

Classification	Type of Damage
First-degree damage	Tissues appear red, inflamed, with perhaps a mild edema.
Second-degree damage	Marked edema, blisters, or both.
Third-degree damage (frostbite)	Necrosis and a blue-gray skin color are probably the result of the formation of ice crystals in tissues. These crystals can damage blood vessels and cause dehydration in interstitial spaces.
Fourth-degree damage (severe frostbite)	Gangrene and neurological complications.

*Modification of Hardy's classification, from J Lehmann[18] and B Washburn.[56]

Although one usually associates cold injuries with prolonged exposure to cold ambient conditions, the possibility of injury occurring with treatment does exist. It is not unusual to be treating patients with peripheral vascular deficiencies, with whom any intense cold should be avoided, or, when treating some conditions such as spasticity to apply ice wraps for up to an hour, striving to cool deep tissues. The authors know of a group of physical therapy students who were piercing each others' ears. Knowing that ice could anesthetize, some of the students sandwiched their ear lobes between two ice cubes long enough to cause first degree damage.

In the past, it was believed that the best emergency treatment for frostbite was slow rewarming. However, experience has shown that rapid rewarming is more successful in preventing permanent tissue damage. Thorman has suggested immersing the part in a whirlpool bath at 104°–110° F (40°–43.3° C).[54]

Other adverse reactions can occur with cold. Many people are hypersensitive, and the neurochemical activity caused by cold can result in severe local or systemic reactions or both. Patients with certain systemic diseases are especially prone to hypersensitive reactions. Related specific precautions and contraindications are given in chapter 14.

Summary and Therapeutic Implications

When cold modalities are applied to the body, local and systemic physiological changes can occur. The physiologic effects of cold can be categorized as those resulting from (1) changes in the firing of cold sensory receptors, (2) a decrease in tissue temperature—initial responses lasting about 10–30 minutes followed by secondary responses, and (3) a decrease in internal body temperature. The amount of physiologic change is related to dosage (ie, the temperature gradient between the body surface and the modality); the intensity of the cold, which is generally measured by the temperature of the modality; the duration of application; and the size of body surface area to which it is applied.

Each of these effects has therapeutic implications. Based on the skin-modality temperature gradient, the firing frequency of sensory neurons will be altered. These changes in thermal sensory experience may result in general relaxation, a "hyperstimulating analgesic" (counterirritant) effect, or general arousal invigorating effects. Any of these effects may decrease pain and spasms. Local vasoconstriction and piloerection also may occur; the latter has no therapeutic value. As the tissue temperature falls, the viscosity of blood increases and, initially, superficial vessels constrict for as long as 30 minutes. The vasoconstriction causes a fall in capillary perfusion at the cooled area, thus decreasing bleeding and, probably, the formation of edema. After the initial period, cutaneous blood flow increases, which tends to increase the tissue temperature. This increase in cutaneous circulation may be caused by the opening of A-V shunts, by dilatation of the constricted vessels, or both. The latter occurs because cold has inhibited the function of the neurotransmitters that affected constriction. If this secondary response is not desired, for example after an acute injury, cold application should be limited to 10–30 minutes.

As the tissue temperature declines, the metabolic rate also decreases, resulting

TABLE 9–3. SUMMARY OF PHYSIOLOGICAL RESPONSES TO APPLIED COLD AND THEIR CLINICAL SIGNIFICANCE.

Physiologic Response	Effect	Clinical Significance
Thermal sensory experience (thermal shock).	Mild: analgesic/sedative.	Decreases pain and spasms and promotes relaxation.
	Moderate: autonomic responses.	Invigorating general stimulant.
	Severe: fight or flight responses.	Pain and fear.
Initial superficial vasoconstriction.	Decreased superficial bleeding.	May not alter or may increase deep blood flow.
Secondary vasofluctuations.	Blood flow varies accordingly.	Protects tissues from cold injury.
Observable change in skin color.	Initial: blanching.	Decreases superficial blood flow.
	Secondary: redness.	Increases superficial blood flow.
Increased blood viscosity.	Decreased blood flow.	Retards bleeding/hemorrhage.
Decreased metabolism.	Decreased inflammation; may decrease edema.	May retard healing.
Rapid muscular contractions (shivering).	Increased metabolic rate.	Mechanism to maintain thermal homeostasis.
Piloerection—contraction of muscles of skin hair.	Skin hair rises to an erect position (goose bumps).	Ineffectual mechanism for maintaining thermal homeostasis.
Decreased extensibility of nonelastic tissue.*	Decreased ability to elongate tissues e.g. tendons and joint capsules.	Decreased range of motion and increased probability of rupturing soft tissue fibers.
Decreased peripheral nerve activity.*	Decreased firing and conduction of motor and sensory nerves.	May decrease spasticity.
Possible decreased temperature of joint tissues and fluids.*	Increased joint stiffness.	Decreased speed of joint motion.
	Decreased activity of fluid enzymes.	May decrease destruction in degenative joint disease (e.g. Rheumatoid arthritis).

*Indicates responses that are discussed in Chapter 10.

in a decrease in the inflammatory process. This may decrease the production of edema, retard the healing process or both; however, the effect of cold on edema needs further investigation. As the temperature decreases, a decrease in the firing of sensory neurons may cause numbness and anesthesia. Eventually, all sensory and motor activity ceases.

If the application of intense cold is prolonged or is applied to much of the body, the core temperature may fall. Countercurrent exchange and the transfer of heat from adjacent tissues to the circulating blood help prevent applied cold from decreasing the core temperature, and the accompanying shivering or other heat producing mechanisms act to increase internal temperature. A heat modality applied proximal to the cold also may help prevent a decrease in core temperature.

Superficial cold modalities can affect tissue temperature to a greater depth than superficial heat modalities can and the temperature change is more prolonged. The effects of cold on deeper tissues are not yet completely understood. The vascular supply, the amount of subcutaneous fat, as well as the intensity and duration of application are all factors to be considered. Cold can reduce spasticity. This effect can be attributed to a cold-induced decrease in the activity of various neurons or contractile elements of the muscles. Table 9–3 outlines physiologic effects and therapeutic implications.

Application of cold may cause tissue damage, the severity of which depends on the intensity and duration of the application. At present the recommended treatment is rapid rewarming. Cold well above freezing can cause tissue inflammation and damage. Therapists also must be aware that cryotherapy can cause adverse reactions in patients who are hypersensitive to cold and that certain systemic diseases increase an individual's hypersensitivity. Such conditions, with precautions and contraindications, are discussed in Chapter 14.

■ KEY TERMS

set points
thermal sensory experience
Q_{10} ratio

van't Hoff's Law / van't Hoff Effect
reflex heating
sudomotor systems

■ REVIEW QUESTIONS

1. What does thermal homeostasis mean?
2. In general, what controls local and systemic responses to thermal modalities?
3. What part of the brain appears to regulate body temperature?
4. Why should thermal modalities be avoided if a patient's heat receptors are not intact? Give two reasons.
5. At what temperature range do heat-pain fibers begin firing?
6. Below what temperature do cold-pain fibers begin firing?
7. What damage can be caused by high tissue temperatures? By low tissue temperatures?
8. Explain the set point theory of the thermoregulatory system.
9. What internal temperature does the body strive to maintain?
10. What mean skin temperature does the body strive to maintain for
    (a) men?
    (b) women?
11. In addition to thermal shock, what are the other two immediate reactions to local application of
    (a) heat?
    (b) cold?
12. How does an increase in local tissue temperature affect
    (a) blood viscosity?
    (b) local sweating?
    (c) the metabolic rate?
13. Define the Q_{10} ratio or the van't Hoff effect.
14. An increase in metabolic rate also increases phagocytosis. What is the effect of this phagocytosis?
15. An increase in metabolic rate also increases arteriolar dilatation. What is the effect of this increased dilatation?
16. How long does the initial vasoconstriction response last during the application of a cold modality?
17. What are the negative effects of vasoconstriction?
18. How are motor nerves affected by cold?
19. Why can superficial cold modalities change the temperature of deep tissues more than heat modalities can change them?
20. How can fat affect the effectiveness of a cold modality?
21. How can poor vascular status affect the effectiveness of a cold modality?
22. Approximately how long does ice take to cool the temperature of tissues that are 2 cm deep?
23. Approximately how long do supercooling modalities take to cool the temperature of tissues that are 2 cm deep? Is this constant?
24. What happens approximately 15–30 minutes after the tissue temperature drops significantly? Why?

REFERENCES

1. Fox R, Hilton S. Bradykinin formation in human skin in heat vasodilatation. *J Physiol (Br)*. 1958; 142:219–232.
2. Baez S. Microcirculation. *Ann Rev Physiol*. 1977; 39:391–415.
3. Guyton A. *Textbook of Medical Physiology*. 6th ed. Philadelphia, PA: WB Saunders; 1981:323,623,894.
4. Ogawa T. Regional differences in sweating activity. In: Hales J, ed. *Thermal Physiology*. New York: Raven Press; 1984:229–234.

5. Hensel H. *Thermoreception and Temperature Regulation.* New York: Academic Press; 1981:199.

6. Hensel H. *Thermal Sensations and Thermoreceptors in Man.* Springfield: Charles C Thomas; 1982:6,36,91–92,94.

7. Mekjavic IB, Sundberg CJ, Linnaisson D. Core temperature "Null zone". *J App Physiol.* 1991; 71:1289.

8. Downey J. Physiological effects of heat and cold. *Phys Ther.* 1974; 44:714.

9. Licht S, ed. *Medical Hydrology.* New Haven: Elizabeth Licht; 1963:98–99,102.

10. Kottke F, Lehmanns, eds. *Krusen's Handbook of Physical Medicine and Rehabilitation.* 4th ed. Philadelphia, PA: WB Saunders; 1990:261–272.

11. Hartviksen K. Ice therapy in spasticity. *Acta Neurol Scand.* 1962; 38 (suppl 3):79–84.

12. Guyton A. *Function of the Human Body.* 3rd ed. Philadelphia, PA: WB Saunders; 1969:311–312.

13. Pieriau Fr-K, Mizutani M, Taylor D. Do dichotomizing afferent nerve fibres transmit the axon reflex? In: Hales J, ed. *Thermal Physiology.* New York: Raven Press; 1984:17–20.

14. Berne R, Levy M. *Cardiovascular Physiology.* 4th ed. St. Louis, MO: CV Mosby; 1981:224.

15. Vanhoutte P, Leusen I, eds. *Vasodilatation.* New York: Raven Press: 1981:263–271.

16. Holdcroft A. *Body Temperature Control.* London: Baillière-Tindall; 1980:12–26.

17. Brooks G, Fahey T. *Exercise Physiology.* New York: John Wiley & Sons; 1984:20.

18. Lehmann J, ed. *Therapeutic Heat and Cold.* 3rd ed. Baltimore, MD: Williams & Wilkins; 1982:65,128–129,175,179,212–213.

19. Rowell L. Reflex control of the cutaneous vasculature. In: *Invest Dermatol.* 1977; 69:154–166.

20. Astrand P, Rodahl K. *Textbook of Work Physiology.* New York: McGraw-Hill; 1977:563.

21. Berger P. *Applied Exercise Physiology.* Philadelphia, PA: Lea & Febiger; 1982:199–201.

22. Morehouse L, Miller A. *Physiology of Exercise.* 7th ed. St. Louis, MO: CV Mosby; 1976:236–238.

23. Davies C, Young K. Effect of temperature on contractile properties and muscle power of tricep surae in humans. *J App Physiol.* 1983; 55(1):191–195.

24. Gibbons J, Landis E. Vasodilatation in the lower extremities in response to immersing the forearm in warm water. *J Clin Invest.* 1932; 11:1019.

25. Bennett R, Hines E.A., Krusen F. Effect of SWD on the cutaneous temperature of the feet. *Am Heart J.* 1941; 21:490.

26. Lota M. Optimal exposure time for development of acclimatization to heat. *Fed Proc.* 1965; 22:704.

27. Downey J, Darling R. *Physiological Basis of Rehabilitation Medicine.* Philadelphia, PA: WB Saunders; 1971.

28. Bisgard J, Nye D. Influence of hot and cold application upon gastric and intestinal motor activity. *Surg Gyn Obstet.* 1940; 71:172–180.

29. Schulman L. *A Comparative Study of the Effects of Ultrasound vs. Hot Packs on Increasing Cutaneous Blood Flow to the Lower Extremities Utilizing the Reflex Heating Technique.* New York: Columbia University; 1983. Master's thesis.

30. Henrikien O, Bulow J, Kristensen J, et al. Local tissue temperature: an important factor for regulation of blood flow in peripheral tissues during indirectly induced hyperthermia. In: Hales J, ed. *Thermal Physiology.* New York: Raven Press; 1984:255–258.

31. McMaster W, Liddle S, Waugh T. Laboratory evaluation of various cold therapy modalities. *Am J Sports Med.* 1978; 6:291–294.

32. Burton A, Edholm O. *Man in a Cold Environment.* London, UK: Edward Arnold; 1955:225–230.

33. Mai J, Pedersen E, Arlien-Sobory P. Changes in afferent discharge during cooling. In: Koni P, ed. *Biomechanics-VA.* Baltimore, MD: University Park Press; 1976:171–175.

34. Popovic V, Popovic P. *Hypothermia in Biology and in Medicine.* New York: Grune & Stratton; 1974:66.

35. Rand P, LaCombe E, Hamilton E, et al. Viscosity of normal human blood under normothermic and hypothermic conditions. *J Applied Physiol.* 1964; 19(1):117–122.

36. Michlovitz S. *Thermal Agents in Rehabilitation.* Philadelphia; PA: FA Davis; 1986:75,193–194.

37. Lundgren C, Muren A, Zederfeldt B. Effect of cold- vasoconstriction on wound healing in rabbit. *Acta Chir Scand.* 1959; 118(1):1–4.

38. Marek J, Jezdensky J, Ochononsky P. Effects of local cold and heat therapy of traumatic oedema of the rat hind paw. *Acta Univ Palack Olomucensis.* 1973; 65–66:203–266.

39. Matson F, Questa K, Matson A. The effect of local cooling on postfracture swelling. *Clin Orthop Rel Res.* 1975; 109:201–206.

40. Schmidt K, Ott V, Rocher F, et al. Heat, cold and inflammation. *Zeit Rheumatol.* 1979; 38:391–404.

41. Coté D, Prentice W Jr, Hooker D, et al. Comparison of three treatment procedures for minimizing ankle sprain swelling. *Phys Ther.* 1988; 68:1072–1076.

42. Fox P. Local cooling in man. *Br Med Bull.* 1961; 17(1):14–18.

43. Pugh L, Edholm O, Fox R, et al. A physiological study of channel swimming. *Clin Sci.* 1960; 19:257–273.

44. Coles D, Cooper K. Hyperaemia following arterial occlusion of exercise in the warm and cold human forearm. *J Physiol Br.* 1959; 145:241–250.

45. Abdel-Sayed W, Abbourd R, Cavelo M. Effect of local cooling responsiveness of muscular and cutaneous arteries and veins. *Am J Physiol.* 1970; 219:1773–1778.

46. Lowdon B, Moore R. Determinants and nature of intramuscular temperature changes during cold therapy. *Am J Phys Med.* 1975; 54:223–233.

47. Waylonis G. The physiologic effects of ice massage. *Arch Phys Med Rehabil.* 1967; 48(1):37–42.

48. Lewis T, ed. Observations upon the reaction of the human skin to cold. In: *Heart.* London, UK: Shaw & Son; 1929/31; 15:177–208.

49. Frisancho A. *Human Adaptation: A Functional Interpretation.* St. Louis, MO: CV Mosby; 1979:44–45.

50. Stanier MW, Mownt LE, Bligh J. *Energy Balance & Temperature Regulation.* Cambridge, UK: Cambridge University Press; 1984:292.

51. Slonim NB, ed. *Environmental Physiology.* St. Louis, MO: CV Mosby; 1974:94.

52. DonTigny R, Sheldon K. Simultaneous use of heat and cold in treatment of muscle spasms. *Arch Phys Med Rehabil.* 1962; 43:235–237.

53. Wyngaarden J, Smith L Jr, eds. *Cecil's Textbook of Medicine.* 17th ed. Philadelphia, PA: WB Saunders; 1985:358,2229,2304–2306.

54. Thorman M. The pathology and management of frostbite. *Clin Management.* 1985; 5:12–15.

55. Meryman H. Tissue freezing and cold injury. *Physiol Rev.* 1957; 37:233–251.

56. Washburn B. Frostbite. *N Eng J Med.* 1962; 2:266, 974.

10

Clinical Effects of Thermal Modalities

Bernadette Hecox, PT, MA

Effects on Soft Tissue

Nonelastic Tissue

Contractile Muscle Fibers

Muscle Spasms with Pain

Effects on Joints

Joint Stiffness

Intra-Articular Structures and Fluid

Neuronal Activity

Peripheral Nerves: Sensory and

Motor Firing

Nerve Conduction Velocity

Central Nervous System

Muscle Performance

Effects on Visceral Tissues

Abnormal Tissues: Hematomas and Malignant Tumors

Summary

D ecisions regarding which thermal modality to use for specific treatment programs should be based on an understanding of which modalities can improve the condition of the involved tissues or systems most effectively. For example, the functional problem, limited range of motion of a joint, may be caused by several conditions, including edema, soft-tissue contractures, muscle tension, pain/spasms, peripheral nerve damage, and spasticity or other conditions involving the central nervous system (CNS). Because some of these conditions may respond better to superficial heat and others, to deep heat or cold, the practice of automatically applying a favorite modality is unacceptable.

For some conditions, the relative values of heat and cold are supported by consistent findings in scientific studies. For others, studies are either lacking or the reported results are inconsistent. If the rationale for choosing a specific modality is based on objective findings, one can assume that the results obtained will be relatively predictable. For example, at the site of a wound, the blood flow will predictably increase if heated and decrease if cooled. When objective findings are lacking, clinical judgments must be based on the information available, which may be theoretical or based on subjective clinical observations or patients' reports of benefits. In an effort to help the physical therapist make intelligent selections and uses of thermal modalities, this chapter summarizes the information that is currently available regarding some frequently treated pathological conditions.

EFFECTS ON SOFT TISSUE

Nonelastic Tissues

If limited range of motion or nerve compression is the result of shortened collagen tissues, the value of heat is well documented.[1-3] A study comparing the effects of a sustained load on rat tendons at room temperature, 78.8° F (26° C), and at 113° F (45° C) showed that, at the higher temperature, the extensibility of the collagen tissues was increased.[2] Nonelastic fibrous tissues, joint capsules, and or scar tissue as well as tendons will yield to a prolonged stretch when heated, but similar results are not obtained if the stretch is applied after the tissues have been cooled.

Warren and colleagues[3,4] demonstrated that although a prolonged low-load stretching procedure produced some residual elongations of tissues at 98.6° F (37° C), better results and less damage occurred when tissues were heated before beginning the stretch. These investigators recommended the use of the highest possible therapeutic temperature with low-force load and the maintenance of the stretch for a few minutes after the heat is removed to achieve the greatest lengthening of collagenous tissues. They attributed the elongation of the tissue to organizational changes in the collagen fibers and to changes occurring in the viscoelastic properties of the tissues. If the involved tissues, eg, ligaments and capsules, are deeper than 1 cm, only deep heat modalities can increase their temperature sufficiently. Ice packs are sometimes applied immediately after the heat is removed to help stabilize the elongation just achieved, but evidence of the value of this procedure is limited.[5]

Contractile Muscle Fibers

Wessling and associates[6] showed that the effect of a passive stretch procedure for increasing range of ankle dorsi flexion was enhanced when heat (ultrasound) was applied to the tricep surae muscle before and during the procedure. They focused the ultrasaound more on the belly than the tendon portion of the muscle and suggested that the heat contributed to the overall increase in joint range by increasing the plasticity of the muscle belly rather than by altering the viscoelastic properties of the tendons.

When muscles remain in a shortened position for a prolonged period, the number of contractile units (sarcomeres) in the muscle fiber decreases. This factor may influence the reduced range of joint motion. Although prolonged stretch may increase the number of sarcomeres, evidence that direct application of thermal modalities enhances the changes in the sarcomeres is lacking.

Muscle Spasms With Pain

Both heat and cold have been shown to be effective for reducing pain and for relaxing muscle tension and spasms. Fountain, Gersten, and Sengir[7] compared the effects of ultrasound, hot packs, and infrared radiation on the relief of pain and spasms in subjects with "spasms of the neck" and on subjects who were polio patients with tight, painful hamstrings and found that all three modalities produced subjective relief. They also found that the three modalities reduced the spasms, as determined by a significant reduction in the amount of force required to initiate movement. The maximum decrease in spasms was apparent 10 to 15 minutes after termination of treatment. Both of the superficial modalities were significantly more effective than ultrasound for the subject with neck spasms, whereas hot packs were significantly more effective than the other two modalities for the subjects with tight hamstrings. These investigators suggested that the intense sensory stimulation provided by hot packs might play a significant role in the greater relaxation that was apparent. However, before concluding that hot packs are best, the clinician must note the following dosage factors.

Hot packs were *changed every 5 minutes for a 20-minute period.* For neck spasms, the ultrasound (1 MHz frequency at either 0.95 w/cm^2 or 1.5 w/cm^2) was applied to painful tendon sites of both the upper and middle trapezius using a continuously moving head for a total of **5 min.** A 1000 w infrared lamp was positioned 16 in. from the skin surface. This study was published in 1960.

One might assume that all three modalities, if applied using methods and dosages similar to those used by Fountain and colleagues, would produce similar subjective and objective benefits. But one hot pack left on a patient for 20 minutes—a procedure commonly practiced in clinics—may not demonstrate the same results. If ultrasound had been applied to the upper and middle trapezius muscles for 5 min each, more closely approximating a clinically recommended area per time, (5 sq in for 3–5 min) the results might have been more effective.

Prentice[8] investigated the value of combining ice packs or hot packs with either static or proprioceptive neuromuscular facilitation stretching techniques to determine which combination would decrease spasms best: ie, elicit the greatest muscle relaxation, as determined by a decrease in Electromyographic (EMG) activity. Each modality was applied for 20 min. All experimental groups as well as a control group displayed some decrease in EMG activity. However, *the group treated with ice packs and static stretch* was the only one that differed significantly from the control group. Consider that the temperature gradient between an ice pack and skin is great; a less intense form of cold might not produce the same results.

EFFECTS ON JOINTS

Joint Stiffness

Thermal modalities can affect the freedom with which a joint moves. In general, joint freedom refers to the amount of time and force required to move through a given range. Heat enhances this freedom (less force and time are required), whereas cold increases stiffness.

Wright and Johns[9,10] showed that when skin is heated to 113° F (45° C) the underlying joint moves about 20% more freely than when the skin temperature is 91.4° F (33° C). When the skin is cooled to 64.4° F (18° C), the stiffness increases 10–20%. They believed that the stiffness is caused by "tension in the peri-articular structure rather than by the changes in the viscous properties of the joint."

Backlund and Tiselius[11] also showed that stiffness increases with cold and decreases with heat. However, they found that marked changes occurred with cold—when hands were placed in water at 50° F (10° C) for 10 minutes—whereas the changes occurring with heat were slight—when hands were placed in water at 109.4° F (43° C) for 10 min. Note that the study using the more intense heat increased the joint freedom more effectively, whereas the one using intense cold increased stiffness more.

Wright,[12] in his review of research on joint stiffness, reported that Ingpen and Kendall found that "wax baths" caused fingers to move faster. This supports the use of paraffin baths for reducing joint stiffness. Wright also reported that studies on the knee joint showed increased stiffness when the knee was immersed in "ice water" (50° F, 10° C) compared with 91.4° F (33° C) conditions. Interestingly, Wright reported that although shortwave diathermy reduced stiffness about 20%, the effect was transient: it disappeared about 10 min after treatment. Although the testing methods and specific findings of these studies differ, all indicate that heat is the preferred modality for decreasing joint stiffness.

Intra-articular Structures and Fluid

In general, the application of heat tends to increase the temperature within a joint and cold decreases the temperature. However, Hollander and Hovath[13] found that when hot or cold packs were applied to knee joints, a temporary, paradoxical phenomenon occurred. Hot packs increased the temperature of the skin but reduced the temperature of the underlying joint, whereas cold packs increased the temperature of the joint. They attributed this phenomenon to a reflex reaction in which the circulation in the joint opposed the circulation at the surface. However, with other heat modalities, the intra-articular temperature increased. Some increase was observed with infrared radiation, more was observed with paraffin wraps, and the most was observed with deep heat.

Although either heat or cold can be used to relieve symptoms, which in turn permits an increase in joint range of motion, and heat is preferred to gain freedom of joint movement, the therapeutic value of applying heat modalities to joints affected by rheumatoid arthritis has been questioned. Evidence indicates that increasing the temperature of synovial fluid may increase the proteolytic enzyme activity and thus the destruction in a rheumatoid joint.[14,15]

Because metabolic activity is temperature related and enzyme activity decreases as temperature declines, presumably the destructive enzyme activity that occurs in joints will also decrease. At present, no studies have conclusively verified this assumption. However, this assumption, plus the fact that some patients are relieved of symptoms when cold is applied, suggests the positive effects of cold. Nonetheless, the use of heat also should be considered.

Both the heat modality being used and the location of the joint must be taken into account. Only ultrasound or a diathermy such as 915 MHz microwave, not commonly found in clinics, can be expected to raise the temperature significantly in deep seated joints. However, the temperature of wrist or finger joints could be elevated with even superficial heat.[16] Of interest is a study by Mainardi,[17] in which one hand of a patient with rheumatoid arthritis was placed in an electric mitten heated to 104° F (40° C) and the other hand acted as a control. The study failed to show that daily heating had any effect on progression of the disease. Lehman and DeLateur[18] pointed out that some investigators [15,19,20] did not study temperatures higher than 105.8° F (41° C) and that at temperatures between 102.2°–105.8° F (39°–41° C) the rate of enzyme activity *decreased*. Lehmann[21] suggested that bringing the temperature of a joint into the range of 105.8°–113° F (41°–45° C) "may in fact inactivate destructive collagenase, as at higher temperatures the protein component is denatured." Obviously, the final answer concerning the effects of heat versus cold on intra-articular structures is not yet in. However, Lehmann[21] suggested that because arthritic joints may be stiff and have contractures that require stretching, the use of heat may be appropriate but should be used cautiously. This is especially true with a modality such as ultrasound, which is most likely to heat joint fluids.

NEURONAL ACTIVITY

Peripheral Nerves: Sensory and Motor Firing

The activity of peripheral nerves varies with changes in temperature. Some factors of interest are mentioned in this section. As shown in Chapter 9 (Fig. 9–1), the rate of firing of the receptors of warm fibers peaks at approximately 109° F (43° C) and declines rapidly at higher temperatures. Heat-pain fibers begin firing at a temperature of 113° F (45° C), which is only slightly higher than the temperature at which the firing of warm fibers peaks, and their rate of firing increases as the temperature increases.

Cold-pain fibers begin firing at a temperature only slightly lower than the one at which the firing of warm fibers peaks. The temperature at which the firing rate of cold fibers peaks is approximately 77° F (25° C) and their firing stops at approximately 46.4° F (8° C). The firing of cold-pain fibers begins at approximately 59° F (15° C), and the rate increases until the temperature reaches 40° F (4.7° C). Thus, firing of the warm and cold fibers overlaps with their respective pain fibers, with the rate of firing of the pain fibers increasing as the temperatures reach those at which the tissues are endangered.

Impulses conveyed by thermal fibers are fed into the CNS, where they are integrated with information from the internal environment. Cutaneous receptors set up mechanisms to protect local tissues and preserve thermal homeostasis. The face has a large number of clusters of thermal receptors, cold spots, and hot spots; the forehead is especially sensitive to cold.[22,23] Thus, there is a valid rationale for the common practice of placing cool compresses on the forehead to reduce the physiological effects of and relieve the discomfort caused by excessive heating.

Temperature affects the activity of all peripheral nerves, both sensory and motor.[24] De Jong et al[25] found that when a neuron is stimulated electrically, the threshold for the firing of an action potential increases as the temperature decreases below 73.4° F (23° C): ie, the current intensity (amperage) required to evoke an action potential increases. However, above that temperature, the threshold for firing remained constant. This study suggests the value of cooling tissues if a decrease in neuronal activity is desired. Tissues are often heated before treatment with electrical stimulation so that less voltage is required to excite the neurons. This is not done specifically to lower the threshold for firing of action potentials; it is done because the increase in sweat and blood at the heated tissue site (usually skin) lowers the electrical impedance of the tissue.

Nerve Conduction Velocity

The conduction velocity of both sensory and motor nerves increases and their conduction latency decreases when the temperature is increased. These neuron conduction parameters are discussed in Section IV. The rate of change in nerve conduction velocity is approximately 2 m/s per degree centigrade change in temperature. However, investigators do not agree about the exact rate of change, probably because of variations in testing procedures.[26] In the temperature ranges studied by de Jesus et al[27] for each 1° C change in temperature, the conduction velocity of motor nerves changed 2.4 m/s and the conduction velocity of sensory nerves changed 2.0 m/s. Studies also have shown that cold receptor neurons conduct faster than warm receptor neurons and that humans react faster to cold than to warm stimuli.[28,29] These results support the use of cold over heat as a neurofaciliatory technique.

Nerve conduction velocity is related to the diameter of the fibers. However, the decrease in velocity relative to cooling does not appear to be based solely on fiber size. Douglas and Malcolm[30] studied the effects that localized cooling has on retarding the activities of cat nerve fibers of various sizes. They found that the small myelinated A fibers, both motor and sensory, required less lowering of the temperature to retard their activity than did the large myelinated A fibers. Furthermore, the small nonmyelinated C fibers were least susceptible; they required the greatest lowering of temperature to block conduction.

On the basis of these findings, Till[31] suggested cooling toward 32° F (0° C) if the primary goal is to reduce pain traveling via C fibers. If the goal is to decrease pain or spasms in conjunction with muscle reeducation, however, cold must be less intense to avoid slowing the conduction of motor nerves, the myelinated A fibers. Till regarded modalities at 53.6° F to 59° F (12°–15° C) as ideal.

Evidence pertaining to cat nerve fibers cannot be applied directly to humans. Some studies of human nerve fibers have found that changes in nerve conduction velocity per temperature change are the same for all fibers regardless of size.[27]

Brown[32] attributed the alterations in neural activity to changes in "sodium channels: kinetics", the lower the temperature, the slower the opening of the sodium channels of the membrane. He believed this accounted for the slower rise time and prolonged duration of an action potential that is known to occur with decreases in temperature. Brown also suggested that the slower conduction velocities resulted from depolarization taking longer to occur at the next Node of Ranvier.

Cold decreases pain. Theories suggest that the increased stimulation required to activate the pain fibers, the reduced velocity along the pathways, or both diminish the pain. As the temperature continues to decrease, electrical activity decreases and numbness or anesthesia is produced, which in turn may reduce the pain. All nerve conduction velocity ceases at approximately 48° F (9° C).[33]

Application of either heat or cold reduces both tension- and pain-related muscle spasms and CNS-related spasticity.[34-36] Both superficial and deep heat (hot packs and inductance diathermy), each applied for 20 minutes on trigger point areas, have been shown to be effective in relieving pain.[37]

Central Nervous System

Many investigators have studied the effects of temperature on neuromuscular activity, attempting to determine why the changes in muscle tone occur.[35,38-40] For example, Mense[35] studied muscle spindle activity and found that with warming, the rate of firing of primary ending (I-A) fibers increased (as did Golgi tendon organs, I-B fibers) but that the firing of spindle secondary ending (II) fibers decreased. More recent neurological theories and evidence suggest that although fusimotor activity accompanies skeletal muscle activity, excessive fusimotor activity may not be involved in either spasticity or Parkinson rigidity.[41] If this is true, other factors, rather than changes in muscle spindle activity, may be altering spasticity when heat is applied. In spite of ample clinical evidence and countless anecdotal reports indicating that both heat and cold reduce spasms and spasticity, conclusive explanations of why this occurs are not yet available.

Although both heat and cold can reduce spasticity, the effects of heat last for only a brief period, whereas the effects of cold have been shown to last from a few minutes to as many as 90 min. Lehmann and DeLateur[18] suggested that the decreased blood flow in cooled tissues permits the effects of cold to last longer.

When treating spasticity, Scholz and Campbell's[42] advice is worth considering. "A therapist cannot assume that a particular technique will be effective by virtue of the fact that it has worked with similar patients. . . . Clinical research under controlled therapeutic conditions, in concert with modern neurodiagnostic techniques for lesion characterization is needed to document: 1) effectiveness of specific techniques, 2) variations in responses under different parametric conditions and 3) variation in response in different pathological conditions."

MUSCLE PERFORMANCE

When the temperature of muscles increases, the speed of movement increases.[43] When a muscle is cooled, a twitch response is prolonged; thus, a decreased rate of action potential firing is required to produce a tetanic contraction. This muscle reaction is consistent with findings regarding changes in action potential responses—slow rise time and prolonged duration—when peripheral nerve fibers are cooled. Studies relating muscle strength and performance to temperature have seldom been duplicated, and the results are so inconsistent that few conclusions can be reached. For these reasons none of these studies are cited here. Reviews and summaries of many of the investigations are available.[18,44,45] It may be that with ordinary treatment dosages and clinical conditions, one modality is not consistently more effective than the others in affecting muscle strength, or it may be an oversimplification to relate a motor activity to muscle temperature alone.

Of interest is the work done by Asmussen et al,[46] who compared the height of a jump starting from a squat when the muscle temperature was 89.6° F (32° C) versus 98.6° F (37° C). They found that the jump was higher at the higher muscle temperature. But when the upward jump was preceded by a downward jump from an elevated level (0.4m) the upward jump was higher at the cooler muscle temperature. These findings suggest that other factors interact with muscle temperature to affect muscle function.

EFFECTS ON VISCERAL TISSUES

Application of thermal modalities on the surface of the abdomen appears to have a paradoxical effect on visceral tissues. Evidence indicates that a superficial heat applied on the abdomen reduces blood flow to the mucous membranes of the stomach and intestines and decreases gastric acidity. Such heat also decreases exaggerated peristaltic actions (stomach cramps), whereas an ice pack aggravates peristalsis.[47]

The effects of a Sitz bath also have been studied (see, also, Section III). A significant decrease in internal anal pressure occurred when subjects were immersed in water at 104° F (40° C).[48] But when the temperature was cooler or cold, this did not occur. Because this change in pressure appears to reduce pain, immersion in hot water is recommended for hemorrhoidal disease or fissures and after childbirth or anorectal surgery.[48]

EFFECTS ON ABNORMAL TISSUES: HEMATOMAS AND MALIGNANT TUMORS

Local deep heat modalities are known to modify abnormal deep structures. The time required to resolve hematomas can be reduced significantly when a deep heat modality is applied daily.[49] Deep heating alone or in conjunction with radiation has been used in therapy for malignant tumors. The treatment is highly specialized, requiring the temperature of the tumor to be raised to an extremely high level without damaging normal adjacent tissues.[18]

SUMMARY

We hope that the information provided in this chapter will help the clinician select appropriate thermal modalities for treatments. For some conditions, strong evidence has been presented to support the selection of certain modalities. For other conditions, especially neurologically related problems, investigations continue because the results of various studies do not agree. Thus, the choice of modality for these conditions must be based on clinical evidence and observation.

Heat is definitely the thermal modality of choice for lengthening collagen tissues and reducing joint stiffness. However, for the treatment of joints affected by rheumatoid arthritis, only superficial heat is advised, and controversy exists regarding the possibility that heating joint fluids may cause further destruction of the joints. Some evidence indicates that heat reduces stomach cramps and internal anal pressure and that cold has the opposite effect.

Both heat and cold may reduce spasms and pain. The fact that the results of various comparative studies conflict may be caused by differences in the methods used, including the intensity of the heat or cold. Although both heat and cold appear to reduce spasticity, cold seems to be more effective and for a longer period. Cold is also recommended for neuromuscular facilitation.

With regard to muscle function, cold is more effective for producing tetanic (ie, holding) muscle contractions, whereas heat is more effective for increasing speed of movement. The effectiveness of heat versus cold on muscle strength requires further investigation. Table 10–1 summarizes the clinical effects of thermal modalities as they relate to information gathered from scientific investigations, empirical observations, or clinical experience.

TABLE 10–1. GUIDELINES FOR SELECTING HEAT AND COLD FOR CLINICAL PROBLEMS

Clinical Problem	Responses Desired or Expected	Is Heat Recommended?	Is Cold Recommended?
Pain	Analgesia by hyperstimulation (counter-irritant).	Yes.	Yes.
	Anesthesia.	No.	Yes.
Muscle spasms	Reduction of pain by clearing metabolites.	Yes.	No.
Upper motor neuron spasticity	Affects motor nerves (mechanism is not clearly established).	Yes. May decrease spasticity for a brief period.	Yes. May decrease spasticity for up to 90 min, but neurological "rebound" may follow.
Bleeding, hemorrhage	Retardation of blood flow to affected area (vasoconstriction).	No. May increase flow.	Yes. May decrease flow for initial period (15–30 min), but flow may increase after initial period or when cold is removed.
Edema	No clear evidence of effectiveness of either heat or cold.	May increase acute edema. May decrease chronic edema.	May decrease formation of acute edema, but edema may increase if treatment is prolonged.
Wound healing	Increased blood flow and metabolism at wound site.	Yes. Hastens healing	No. Retards healing.
Frostbite	Hastened healing, as indicated by clinical observation.	Yes.	No. See Chap. 9, 15.
Orthostatic hypotension	Vascular reaction	No. May enhance the problem	Yes. See Chap. 14
Joint stiffness	Increased mobility of periarticular structures.	Yes.	No.
Inability to perform *skilled* movements	Increased neuron firing and nerve conduction velocity. Increased mobility of tissues.	Yes.	No.
Arthritic joints osteoarthritis and non-acute rheumatoid	Decreased pain and joint stiffness	Yes.	Yes. May reduce pain.
	Increased mobility and function.	Yes.	No. Will increase joint stiffness.
Acute rheumatoid arthritis	Reduced enzyme activity of joint fluid. Decrease pain.	Superficial heat, yes. Mild or moderate heat will not increase enzyme activity significantly. Deep heat, no. May increase enzyme activity.	Yes. May reduce enzyme activity.
Shortness of soft tissues	Increased extensibilty of non-elastic tissues.	Yes.	No.
Any need for general stimulation or relaxation	Response of stimulation or relaxation due to mild or moderate sensory stimulation.	Yes.	Yes.
CNS Problems	Increased firing and NCV of sensory neurons to neurologically facilitate movement	Yes. Less than cold.	Yes.

■ REVIEW QUESTIONS

1. Which treatments, heat or cold, have been well documented as the best treatments for
   (a) limited range of motion caused by shortened collagen tissues?
   (b) joint stiffness caused by osteoarthritis?
   (c) joint stiffness caused by rheumatoid arthritis?
2. Why has the therapeutic value of applying heat modalities to joints affected by rheumatoid arthritis been questioned?
3. Why is placing a cool compress on the forehead often effective in reducing the effects of a fever?

4. Why do humans react more quickly to cold than to warm stimuli?
5. In what way are the conduction velocities of sensory and motor nerves changed by
   (a) an increase in temperature?
   (b) a decrease in temperature?
6. Is heating or cooling suggested if the desired effect is to reduce the sensation of pain traveling along small nonmyelinated C fibers? What temperature is recommended?
7. Is heating or cooling suggested if the desired effect is to reduce pain or spasms in conjunction with muscle reeducation? What temperature is recommended?
8. At approximately what temperature does nerve conduction velocity cease?
9. Compare the effects of heat and cold when treating spasticity. Which effects last longer? Why?
10. What is the effect of increased temperature on the speed of muscle movement?
11. What is the effect of reduced temperature on the speed of muscle movement?
12. How are stomach cramps affected by
    (a) superficial heat?
    (b) superficial cold?
13. For what conditions can a hot Sitz bath be helpful? Why?
14. How can treatment with deep heat modalities affect hematomas?

REFERENCES

1. Gersten J: Effects of ultrasound on tendon extensibility. *Am J Phys Med.* 1955; 34:362–369.
2. Lehmann J, Masock A, Warren C, et al: Effect of therapeutic temperatures on tendon extensibility. *Arch Phys Med Rehabil.* 1970; 51:481–487.
3. Warren C, Lehmann J, Koblanski J: Elongation of rat tail tendon: Effect of load and temperature. *Arch Phys Med Rehabil.* 1971; 52:465–474; 484.
4. Warren C, Lehmann J, Koblanski J. Heat and stretch procedures: an evaluation using rat tail tendon. *Arch Phys Med Rehabil.* 1976; 57(3):122–126.
5. Sapega A, Quedenfeld T, Moyer R, et al: Biophysical factors in range-of-motion exercise. *Physician Sports Med.* 1981; 9(12):57–65.
6. Wessling K, DeVane D, Hylton C: Effects of static stretch versus static stretch and ultrasound combined on tricep surae muscle extensibility in healthy women. *Phys Ther.* 1987; 67:674–679.
7. Fountain F, Gersten J, Sengir O: Decrease in muscle spasm produced by ultrasound, hot packs, and infrared radiation. *Arch Phys Med Rehabil.* 1960; 41(7):293–298.
8. Prentice W Jr: An electromyographic analysis of the effectiveness of heat or cold and stretching for inducing relaxation in injured muscle. *J Ortho Sports Phys Ther.* 1982; 3(3):133–140.
9. Wright V, Johns R: Physical factors concerned with the stiffness of normal and diseased joints. *Johns Hopkins Hosp Bull.* 1960; 106:229.
10. Johns R, Wright V: Relative importance of various tissues in joint stiffness. *J Appl Physiol.* 1962; 17:824–828.
11. Backlund L, Tiselius P: Objective measurements of joint stiffness in rheumatoid arthritis. *Acta Rheum Scand.* 1967; 13:275–288.
12. Wright V: Stiffness: a review of its measurements and physiological importance. *Physiotherapy.* 1973; 59(4):107–111.
13. Hollander JL, Horvath M: The influence of physical therapy procedures on the intra-articular temperature of normal and arthritic subjects. *Am J Med Sci.* 1949; 218:543–548.
14. Febel A, Fast A: Deep heating of joints: a reconsideration. *Arch Phys Med Rehabil.* 1976; 57:513–514.
15. Harris E Jr, McCroskery P: The Influence of Temperature and Fibril Stability on Degra-

dation of Cartilage Collagen by Rheumatoid Synovial Collagenase. *N Engl J Med.* 1974; 290(1):1–6.

16. Borrell R, Parker R, Henley E: Comparison of in vivo temperatures produced by hydrotherapy, paraffin wax treatment, & fluidotherapy. *Phys Ther.* 1980; 60:1273–1276.

17. Mainardi C, Walter J, Spiegel P: Rheumatoid arthritis: failure of daily heat therapy to affect its progressions. *Arch Phys Med Rehabil.* 1979; 60:393–399.

18. Lehmann J, DeLateur B: Therapeutic Heat in: *Therapeutic heat and cold.* 4th ed. Baltimore: Williams & Wilkins; 1990. Chap. 9.

19. Kottke F, Stillwell G, Lehmann J, Eds: (1982) *Krusen's Handbook of Physical Medicine and Rehabilitation.* Philadelphia, PA: WB Saunders; 1982; 275–350.

20. Castor C, Yaron M: Connective tissue activation: VIII. The effects of temperature studies in vitro. *Arch Phys Med Rehabil.* 1976; 57:5–9.

21. Lehmann J: *Arch Phys Med Rehabil.* 1977; 58:232–233. Letter to the Editor.

22. Clark R, Edholm O: *Man and His Thermal Environment.* London: Edward Arnold; 1985; 136:155.

23. Noback C, Demarest B: *The Human Nervous System.* New York: McGraw-Hill; 1981: 87–88.

24. Holdcroft A: *Body Temperature Control.* London, UK: Baillière-Tindall; 1980: 1, 12–26.

25. DeJong R, Hershey W, Wagman I: Nerve conduction velocity during hypothermia in man. *Anesthesiology.* 1966; 27:805–810.

26. Currier D, Kramer J: Sensory nerve conduction: heating effects of ultrasound and infrared. *Physiother Can.* 1982; 34:241–246.

27. De Jesus P, Housmanowa-Petrusewicz I, Barchi R: The effect of cold on nerve conduction of human slow and fast nerve fibers. *Neurology.* 1973; 23:1182–1189.

28. Fruhstorfer H, Guth H, Pfaff U: Thermal reaction-time as a function of stimulation site. *Pflug Arch* 1972; 335:49.

29. Zotterman Y, Ed: *Sensory Function of the Skin: Primates.* Oxford, UK: Pergamon Press: 1976; 331–353.

30. Douglas W, Malcolm J: The effects of localized cooling in conduction in cat nerves. *J Physiol (Br).* 1955; 130(1):53–71.

31. Till D: Cold therapy. *Physiotherapy.* 1969; 55:461–466.

32. Brown W: *The Physiological and Technical Basis of Electromyography.* Boston: Butterworth; 1984; 26–27, 385–388.

33. Clark R, Edholm O: *Man and his thermal environment.* London: Edward Arnold; 1985.

34. Bishop B: Spasticity: its physiology and management: IV. Current and projected treatment procedures for spasticity. *Phys Ther.* 1977; 57:396–401.

35. Mense S: Effects of Temperature on the Discharges of Muscle Spindles and Tendon Organs. *Pflug Arch Eur J Physiol.* 1978; 374(suppl):159–166.

36. Petajan J, Watts N: Effects of cooling on the triceps surae reflex. *Am J Phys Med.* 1962; 41:240–251.

37. McCray R, Patton N: Pain relief at trigger points: a comparison of moist heat and short wave diathermy. *J Ortho Sports Phys Ther.* 1984; 5:175–178.

38. Hartviksen K: Ice therapy in spasticity. *Acta Neurol Scand.* 1962; 38 (suppl 3):79–84.

39. Knutsson E: Topical cryotherapy in spasticity. *Scand J Rehabil Med.* 1970; 2:159.

40. Miglietta O: Action of cold on spasticity. *Am J Phys Med.* 1973; 52:198–205.

41. Burke D: Critical examination of the case for or against fusimotor involvement in disorders of muscle tone. In: Desmedt J, ed. *Motor Control Mechanisms - Health and Disease—Advances in Neurology.* New York: Raven Press; 1983; 39:133–150.

42. Scholz J, Campbell S: Muscle spindles and the regulation of movement. *Phys Ther.* 1980; 60:1416–1424.

43. Fox R: Local cooling in man. *Br Med Bull.* 1961; 17(1):14–18.

44. Chastain P: The effect of deep heat on isometric strength. *Phys Ther.* 1978; 58:543–546.

45. Kowal M: Review of physiological effects of cryotherapy. *J Orth Sports Phys Ther.* 1983; 5(2):66–73.

46. Asmussen E, Bonde-Peterson F, Jorgensen K: Mechano-elastic properties of human muscles at different temperatures. *Acta Physiol Scand.* 1976; 96:83–93.

47. Bisgard J, Nye D: Influence of hot and cold application upon gastric and intestinal motor activity. *Surg Gynecol Obstet.* 1940; 71:172–180.

48. Dodi G, Bogoni F, Infantino A: Hot and cold in anal pain? *Dis Colon Rect.* 1986; 29:248–251.

49. Lehmann J, Dundore D, Esselman P: Microwave diathermy: effects on experimental muscle hematoma resolution. *Arch Phys Med Rehabil.* 1983; 64(3):127–129.

11

Superficial Heat Modalities

Diana Fond, PT, MA and
Bernadette Hecox, PT, MA

T he previous chapters discussed the physics, biophysics, and physiologic effects of heat as well as evidence supporting or refuting the value of the available methods of heating. This chapter briefly reviews the physiologic effects of local heating. The general indications and contraindications that are common to all local superficial heating modalities are provided before presenting each individual modality and its specific effects, indications, contraindications, and treatment procedures.

PHYSIOLOGIC EFFECTS OF SUPERFICIAL HEATING: A REVIEW

Any addition of heat to the body may trigger certain physiologic responses. For example, local application of *superficial heat* in the form of *hot packs*, paraffin, *Fluidotherapy*, and infrared radiation, can lead to many beneficial local physical changes and may or may not affect systemic factors such as the core (internal) temperature.

Some physiologic responses to heat are increases in tissue temperature, local metabolism, and blood flow. In addition, heat causes both analgesia and sedation (relaxation), which are helpful in chronic conditions. Local heating also leads to increased nerve conduction velocity.[1] Fig. 11–1 summarizes some of the physiological and therapeutic effects of local heating.

Heat has been used throughout history to soothe aches and pains. Many people enjoy sitting in the sun more for the heat and relaxation benefits they receive than for its tanning effects. Most households have a heating pad in a closet for use at some future time.

Both the sun and the heating pad are forms of superficial heat: that is, they heat the surface of the body or the underlying tissue to a depth of a few millimeters. Any transfer of heat that takes place is a result of radiation, conduction, or convection.[1]

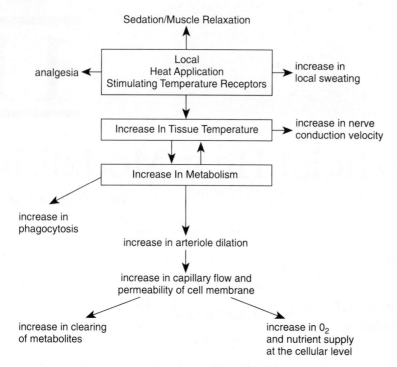

Figure 11–1. Summary of the physiological and therapeutic effects of local superficial heating.

The decrease in muscle spasm and the decrease in pain resulting from local heating are closely interrelated. Sometimes a patient "guards" a painful affected part and increases muscle tension in that area. If this cycle can be broken by local heating, then the part can be treated easily with massage, exercise, or other modalities. Local heating also may help reduce skin resistance, thus making this modality desirable to use before other modalities such as electrical stimulation are applied.

Heat is not recommended during the first 24 to 36 hours after an injury if a hemorrhage is present, but it can be used subsequently to hasten healing, alleviate local edema, and aid in resorption of a hematoma. As was mentioned in earlier chapters, vigorous heating should not be used if a patient has severe edema caused by renal or cardiac failure or has severely impaired circulation and therefore an impaired thermoregulatory system.

INFORMATION COMMON TO ALL SUPERFICIAL HEAT MODALITIES

General Indications

Superficial heating modalities are useful in the following situations; remember, however, that superficial heating will only affect superficial tissue—that the effects on deeper tissues such as muscle are minimal or nonexistent.[2] However, if vigorous or prolonged, superficial heating can cause systemic changes.

1. Before active exercise because of their analgesic and sedative effects.
2. Before passive range of motion (stretching) exercises because they promote relaxation and provide greater extensibility of soft tissue.[3]
3. Before electrical stimulation because they reduce skin impedance.
4. Before traction because they promote general relaxation and decreased tension in muscles in area receiving traction.
5. Before massage because they increase local blood flow and relax the tissue.
6. In the presence of muscle spasm because they help relax the patient.

7. Before ultrasound because they relax the patient and warm the local superficial tissue.
8. Before joint mobilization procedures because they relax the patient and improve the extensibility of superficial soft tissue.[4]

General Contraindications

The contraindications listed below are relative to the intensity of the heat: vigorous heat will cause greater reactions than mild heat.

1. If an injury is at a stage where bleeding or edema may still be present, the heat could exacerbate both problems.
2. In the presence of deep vein thrombophlebitis, increased heating and blood flow could dislodge a clot and cause more serious problems such as a stroke or blockage of a coronary artery.
3. In areas with poor circulation, eg, in peripheral vascular disease, the body cannot dissipate heat.
4. If a patient has dysesthesia and therefore cannot discern excessive heat, he or she may sustain a burn.
5. In areas where sensation is reduced, eg, in scarred areas, a burn may occur.
6. If a patient is very old or very young, he or she may not tolerate heat modalities because of an inability to control body temperature easily.
7. If a patient cannot report heat sensations accurately, eg, because of senile dementia, a burn may occur.
8. In the presence of skin or lymphatic cancer, superficial heat may be contraindicated because the safety of its use in the presence of cancer has not been determined.

INFORMATION REGARDING THE USE OF SPECIFIC MODALITIES

Most clinics have the following superficial heat modalities available: hot packs (chemical-silica gel), paraffin, Fluidotherapy®, and infrared lamps. The general procedures listed below should be followed before any superficial heat modality is applied:

1. Have the patient remove any heavy clothing that may induce generalized sweating or temperature rise.
2. Explain the purpose of the treatment to patients and tell them what to expect, especially the type of heat sensation they will experience.
3. Prepare patients by positioning and draping them properly for the treatment.
4. Inspect the area to be treated to note any blemishes, discolorations, open wounds, or indicators of circulatory problems.
5. Cleanse the area to ensure that no oils, liniments, or analgesic balms that may increase skin reactions to heat are present.
6. Make certain that the patient can respond normally to changes in temperature.

Hot Packs

Chemical hot packs, a frequently used superficial heat modality, transmit moist heat to body tissues by conduction. The patient should experience a sensation of pleasant warmth.

Duration
The usual duration of treatment is 20–30 minutes.

Equipment

Hot packs consist of silica gel in a canvas cover that has many stitched divisions so that the pack can be placed over body parts with different contours. The packs are immersed in a stainless steel tank containing water that is between 165° F and 175° F (73.9°–79.4° C). New packs should be left in the tank for at least 24 hours to absorb as much moisture as possible and achieve the desired temperature. Between treatments, the packs should be left in the tank for at least 20 to 30 minutes. Many clinics have a rotation system for the packs so that therapists know which ones are the hottest.

Hot packs come in many different sizes and shapes. Those most commonly used are the standard or low back packs and the cervical packs (Fig. 11–2).

Hot pack covers and terry cloth towels are also needed (Fig. 11–3).

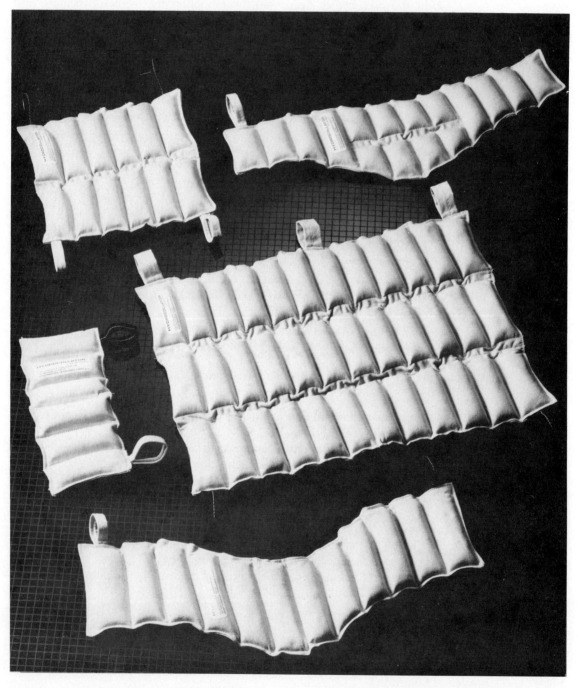

Figure 11–2. This photograph shows a variety of hot packs shaped to conform to specific parts of the body. In the top row are the standard "low back" and "cervical" styles. (*Reproduced with permission from GE Miller, Inc., Yonkers, NY.*)

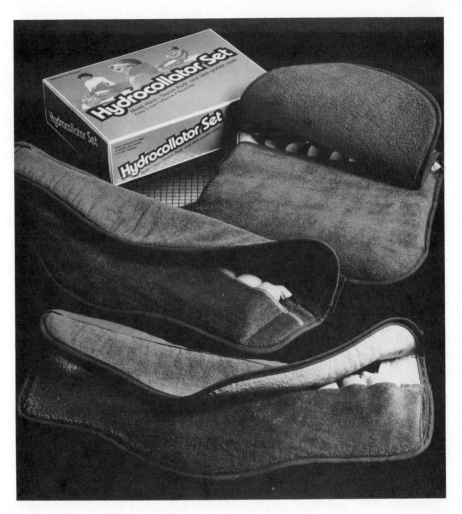

Figure 11–3. Hot packs placed in commercially made terry cloth "envelopes" to prevent rapid heat loss. (*Reproduced with permission from GE Miller, Inc., Yonkers, NY.*)

Technique of Application

The hot-pack method of heating is *not* a constant source of heat (unlike a heating pad). The temperature of a hot pack drops quickly once the pack is removed from the tank.[4] Therefore, the more quickly the pack is covered and placed on the patient, the warmer it will be during the treatment.

The procedures listed below are followed when using a hot pack:

1. Remove the hot pack from the tank with metal or wooden tongs, allow the excess water to drip off, and place it immediately in a terry cloth cover or towel. At least 6 to 12 layers of toweling or the equivalent should be placed between the hot pack and the patient. A hot pack cover (envelope), when new and fluffy, is equivalent to about three layers of toweling (five layers if the envelope contains a sponge insert). So that the cover does not require laundering after each use, at least one extra towel layer of toweling must be placed between the pack and the patient's skin. Additional toweling can be added to achieve the required number of layers. More or less toweling may be necessary, depending on the patient's physical condition and heat tolerance, the fluffiness of the cover and the towels, and the actual temperature of the hot pack.

2. Place the pack on the appropriate body area and secure it firmly to prevent it from slipping off the area. Hot pack covers are equipped with velcro straps for this purpose.

3. Cover the pack with a rubber sheet or plastic (eg, materials such as those used for incontinent patients) to prevent loss of heat to the surrounding environment. (Some envelopes have a plastic top layer.) The patient should then be properly draped with a sheet to prevent a chill if the air in the room is cool. Although it is preferable not to do so, if a patient must lie on top of a hot pack, more toweling must be used between the patient and the pack. Because the pressure and weight of the body or body part will increase the contact with the heat source, less heat can dissipate to the environment and more heat will conduct to the body, which increases the danger of burns and can elevate the core temperature.
4. Always provide patients with a method of calling should they experience any discomfort. It is always necessary to explain to a patient that if the therapist is not immediately available and the pack feels too uncomfortably hot, the patient can remove the hot pack.
5. The skin should be inspected after 5 minutes to ensure that no extremely hot red areas or burns have developed. The therapist should continually check with the patient to make certain that no severe discomfort is felt.
6. It is advisable to have timers in each treatment room so that the duration of treatment can be monitored.

Posttreatment Procedures

After the treatment is completed, the therapist must do the following:

1. Dry and inspect the patient's skin.
2. Replace the drape sheet or clothes to avoid the patient's becoming chilled.
3. Replace the pack in the tank.
4. Hang the covers and toweling to dry.
5. Put the towel layer that was next to the patient's skin in the laundry hamper.

Indications

Hot packs are often used before or in conjunction with other techniques to achieve relaxation and sedation or when moist rather than dry heat is more comfortable for a patient. If the hot pack is an adjunct to subsequent techniques (modalities or exercise), remember to begin those treatments as soon as possible after the pack is removed so that the treated area does not cool down.

Contraindications

When a patient has a local infection that could be exacerbated by moist heat, a hot pack should not be used. Furthermore, some dermatologic conditions may respond adversely to heat and moisture; therefore, the use of hot packs should be avoided.

Precautions

Although a hot pack is not a source of constant heat, do *not* let the patient fall asleep on it. Make certain that the patient is aware of the true heat of the pack and will speak up if more toweling is required. Burns must be avoided.

Some patients cannot tolerate the weight of a hot pack. In such a case, another superficial heat modality should be used.

Keep in mind that hot packs heat only the superficial structures significantly. However, a study by Lehmann et al[4] did show a slight rise in TT at a depth of 1 centimeter and even a slight rise at a depth of 2 centimeters.

Paraffin

Paraffin is another superficial heating method used to treat chronic joint disorders. This modality also transfers heat by conduction. Initially, the patient will experience a hot, but not painful sensation of heat, but the sensation will be one of pleasant warmth after about 3 to 5 minutes.

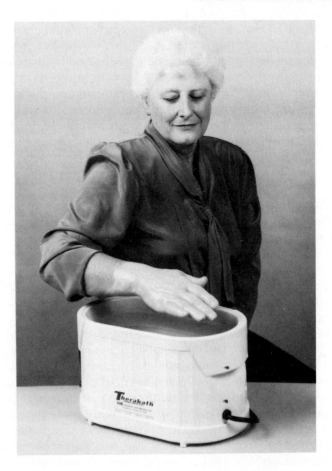

Figure 11–4. A patient whose hand has been just been removed from a paraffin bath. (*Reproduced with permission from WR Medical Electronics Co., Stillwater, MN.*)

Duration

The treatment usually lasts 15 to 20 minutes. Because the paraffin solution is in the fluid state, its use is especially practical when treating distal joints that are difficult to heat evenly.

Equipment

A mixture of paraffin wax and mineral oil in a ratio of about 6 to 1 or 7 to 1 is melted in a tank.[5] The oil helps lower the melting point of the paraffin and make it easily removable after treatment. The tank contains a built-in heating unit thermostat that should maintain the temperature at about 126° F to 135° F (52.2°–57.2° C). for upper extremities and 113° F to 126° F (45° C to 52° C) for lower extremities.[6,7] The temperature of the paraffin must be checked with a thermometer immersed in the solution before each treatment. Some tanks have thermometers that remain permanently inside (see Fig. 11–4). The tanks currently used in beauty salons are similar to those used in clinics but are set at lower temperatures and the premixed paraffin mixtures used must contain more oils to lower the melting point.

Insulated wrapping material (eg plastic bags, aluminum foil, toweling, or commercially available paraffin) must be available and near the tank.

Techniques of Application

Because the skin temperature of the part being treated is lower than the temperature of the paraffin in the tank, a solid layer of paraffin forms on the skin when the part is immersed in the tank. This layer insulates the part, and the air trapped between each additional layer of paraffin also acts as an insulator. Therefore, the patient should be instructed not to move the part to avoid cracking the insulating layers. Even if the part remains in the tank, as is prescribed in one method, it will have the beneficial effects of the paraffin.

Before treatment the patient's skin should be checked for discolorations associated with circulatory problems, for open wounds or infections, and for a lack of thermal sensory "integrity." If any of these conditions are present, the patient should **not** be treated with paraffin. If a wound is minor, it should be protected with gauze and a nonpermeable material such as a plastic strip. The part to be treated should be washed and dried before the treatment because the tank is used by many people. All rings and jewelry should be removed.

Note that care must be taken to check the temperature of the paraffin **before** each use. It is best to leave a thermometer in the tank for accurate, satisfactory readings. If the thermostat is not checked, the patient could be severely burned by paraffin that is too hot. Thermometers that can be held and dipped into the tank for temperature readings are available.

Paraffin can be applied by three different methods: (1) the "glove" technique, (2) the dip-immersion technique, and (3) the brush technique. The most commonly used method is the glove technique, which involves dipping the relaxed body part, eg, the hand, into the tank several times. The fingers of the hand should be slightly abducted, if possible, to allow the fluid to surround them. Before the part is dipped into the paraffin, however, the patient must be instructed not to move or crack the layers of the paraffin glove or touch the metal bottom or sides of the tank because they will feel hot. (Remember, metal is an excellent conductor of heat.) After the part is dipped into the paraffin, it is immediately removed and the paraffin solidifies. This dipping is then repeated 8 to 10 times so that a glove of paraffin layers forms. The part should not be held out of the tank for more than a few seconds between dips to minimize heat dissipation. After the final dip, the treated part is immediately placed in a loose-fitting plastic bag, wax paper, plastic wrap, or aluminum foil, then wrapped in a mit or several layers of towels to help maintain the heat. Finally, the patient rests for 15 to 20 minutes with the treated part in a comfortable position.

In the second method, the dip-immersion technique, following the procedure, the part is immersed into the tank and allowed to remain there for about 15 minutes. With this method, much more heat is transferred to the body.

With the third method, the brush technique, an angular or difficult-to-reach part such as the elbow is painted with multiple layers of paraffin, wrapped as described in the glove technique, and covered with towels for about 20 minutes.

Posttreatment Procedures.

With all three methods, the wax should be removed over the tank or a protective covering so that wax does not get on furniture or floors. Ask the patient to move the part so that the wax cracks, then peel it off as if removing a glove or stocking. Encourage the patient to exercise the part immediately while it is still warm. Wipe the part to remove excess oil and perspiration or use the oil to massage the part.

The three techniques just described heat only superficial tissues; however, one method described in the literature[7] claimed to achieve heating of deeper tissues (the joint capsule) without having a detrimental effect on superficial tissues. This method involved a seven-dip immersion method lasting for 30 minutes. The hand was then removed and wrapped in plastic and toweling for an additional 30 minutes.

Advantages

Because of its fluid nature, paraffin can heat areas that are difficult to reach because of bony prominences or uneven contours, eg, the hand. The paraffin-oil mixture softens the skin and prepares the part for massage or other modalities. The immersion technique of paraffin evenly heats the part being treated and therefore is useful for treating arthritic joints of the hands or feet.

Paraffin is indicated for the patient with pain because of its soothing, comfortable heating properties.

Disadvantages

A part with open wounds should never be treated in the paraffin tank because the wound and the tank can become contaminated. Some joints of the body are not accessible for immersion techniques. Although the brush method can be used, other heating methods may be more advantageous and easier to apply. Paraffin can be a messy procedure if the wax is not removed directly over the tank or protective covering.

Home Use

Small, relatively, inexpensive home units are available for patients with chronic pain who cannot come to the clinic often or have been discharged from the physical therapy department. The following alternative can be used if the patient has someone to help at home, but it is far less efficient or safe. Blocks of premixed paraffin and oil, or ingredients for the paraffin mixture (5 to 7 pounds paraffin to 1 pint of mineral oil) can be purchased.[8] The ingredients are placed in the top part of a double boiler so that the paraffin is not too close to the heat source (Remember, paraffin is flammable). The mixture is heated until it reaches a temperature of about 125° F (51.7° C) (A candy thermometer can be used to measure the temperature). Then the mixture is removed from the heat source. If no thermometer is available, the wax should be cooled until a thin white coating appears on top. Dip the hand as described previously. A simpler method is to use a crock-pot, as long as the correct temperature can be determined.

Studies on the value of paraffin treatments are few; one was mentioned in Chapter 10. Studies on the temperature of skin and underlying tissues after a 20-minute treatment would help substantiate the value of this method of treatment that is used so often by physical therapists. An in vivo study comparing paraffin treatment with Fluidotherapy and hydrotherapy found that paraffin treatment raised the temperature of the small joint capsule of the hand 13.5° F (7.5° C) at a depth of about 0.5 centimeters below the skin.[4]

Fluidotherapy

Another form of superficial heating available to physical therapists is Fluidotherapy, which can be used as an alternative to paraffin or hydrotherapy in some instances or when dry heat is desirable. This modality transfers heat by convection.

Fluidotherapy has been in existence since the 1970s, but the construction of the unit has changed slightly over the years. Extremely small solid particles are heated and suspended by circulating air, thus producing an effect similar to circulating warm liquid. The thermal conductivity and specific heat of the particles and air allow the temperature of the unit to be higher than that of water used therapeutically. That is, the patient can safely tolerate a higher temperature. The feeling produced by the unit resembles that produced by placing a hand in a small enclosed sandbox with heated, air-blown sand.

Duration

The duration of treatment is usually 20 minutes.

Equipment

The machine stands 3 feet high (see Fig. 11–5) and contains a heating element, an air compressor, tiny silicon or corn-cob particles in an enclosed see-through container into which the limb is inserted, a timer, a temperature gauge, and a mesh sleeve. The sleeve can be closed snugly around the proximal portion of the arm or leg, thus preventing the circulating particles from blowing into the room. There are usually four openings for the insertion of a limb: two on the top of the unit, which are best for a hand, and two on the side for hand or foot. In addition to this limb unit, larger units are available to accommodate the lower back and thigh areas. All the information that follows refers to the smaller units.

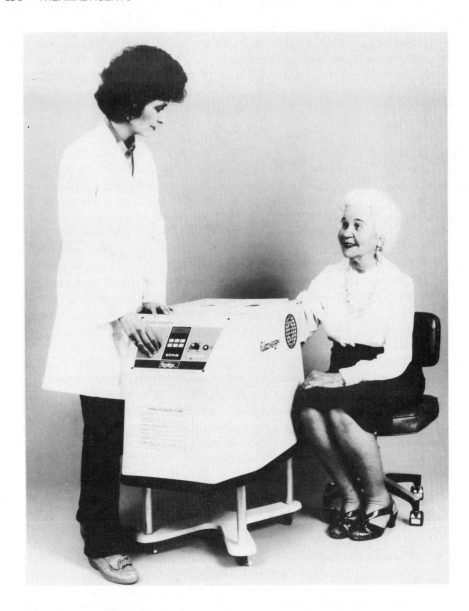

Figure 11–5. A patient whose hand is immersed in a Fluidotherapy limb cabinet. (*Reproduced with permission from Henley International, Sugarland, TX.*)

Technique of Application

As is the case for other superficial heat modalities, before initiating the following procedures, the therapist must inspect the part for skin integrity, good circulation, and sensitivity to heat:

1. Wash and dry the part to be treated because other patients will be using the same container.
2. Remove all jewelry from the part being treated.
3. Check the part for open wounds. The manufacturer recommends that if an open wound is present, the part should be placed in a plastic bag or large rubber glove so that no particles enter the wound.
4. Insert the part into the sleeve and close it snugly around the more proximal portion of the limb so that particles do not come out once the blower is turned on.
5. Set the thermostat at the desired temperature (usually between 115° F and 123° F (46.1°–50.6° C), depending on the patient's tolerance.

6. Turn the timer on (usually for 15 minutes).
7. Instruct the patient about how to exercise or stretch (or help the patient perform these activities) during the treatment if these activities are appropriate for the condition being treated. If a patient's hand is being treated through the side opening, the therapist can insert his or her hands through the top openings to help the patient exercise. The therapist also can watch what is going on.

Posttreatment Procedure

When the treatment is finished, loosen the sleeve. Before removing the limb from the unit, help the patient remove all the particles from the part so that the treatment area remains clean and few particles are lost from the tank. Then, inspect the part once again and continue with other treatments as necessary.

Advantages

The remarkable aspect of Fluidotherapy treatment is that the circulating, air-blown, warmed particles give the patient the feeling of lightness and surrounding warmth provided by a whirlpool bath. In addition, because the limb is free to move, active exercise is possible. As mentioned above, the therapist can insert his or her hand or hands through a separate access sleeve to perform passive range of motion or stretching procedures to the part being treated or to assist the patient exercise.

A limb can be inserted in the unit and positioned in the horizontal plane, thus minimizing the effects of gravity. Remember the dependent position can lead to edema. Because this is a dry heat method, the patient can tolerate a higher temperature than in a hydrotherapy treatment. Like paraffin or water, the circulating particles can surround uneven, bony parts. Finally, because the unit does not require a water source, it can be placed anywhere in the physical therapy department.

Disadvantages

The limb units are too small to accommodate more than a distal limb; thus, they cannot be used to treat a back, hip, or shoulder. The larger units have a nylon cloth on which a patient can lie if the lower back or thigh are treated. Open wounds cannot be treated unless they are protected. Furthermore, wounds cannot be debrided (unhealthy tissue removed) as in the whirlpool.

As is the case with other superficial heat treatment techniques, more studies must be done to validate the effects of this modality on the tissues being treated. Studies performed by Henley[9] indicated that Fluidotherapy treatment did, in fact, increase the temperature, blood flow, and metabolic rate in the treated area. In another study, Valenza et al[10] found that a maximum increase in the temperature (measured with a thermistor) of the medial capsule of the first metatarsophalangeal joint occurred at the temperature provided by Fluidotherapy (115°–123° F, 46.1°–50.6° C) compared with a 102° F (38.9° C) hydrotherapy treatment and a 126° F (52.2° C) paraffin (glove) treatment, all of which were performed for 20 minutes.

An in vivo study by Borrell et al[3] compared the glove method of paraffin treatment (126° F, 52.2° C) with hydrotherapy (102° F, 38.9° C) and Fluidotherapy (118° F, 47.8° C). Fluidotherapy appeared to raise the temperature of the small joint capsule the most; however, this study has been criticized for not using the optimal methods for the paraffin treatment or hydrotherapy (We would have recommended higher temperatures for the hydrotherapy and the immersion technique for the paraffin treatment).

Alcorn et al[11] described a study using Fluidotherapy and exercise for patients in crisis from sickle cell anemia. The authors reported that the results were positive: The treatment reduced the length of the patients' hospital stays and need for analgesics.

Infrared Radiation

Infrared radiation, the final type of superficial heat discussed in this chapter, is an extremely useful modality for providing superficial heat. The physical laws governing radiated energy are discussed in Chapter 5, which contains a graphic representation of various waves of electromagnetic energy in ascending order of wavelength (see Fig. 5–2). Infrared rays are a portion of the electromagnetic spectrum and are just beyond the red portion of visible light. As is discussed in Chapter 5, the depth of penetration to which electromagnetic energy is absorbed depends on the wavelength.

When a material is heated, it gives off electromagnetic rays in the infrared ranges (the result of electrons vibrating in their orbits). The range of infrared rays for heating superficial tissue is divided into *near infrared* (770–1500 nanometers) and *far infrared* (1500–150,000 nanometers).

Certain principles must be understood before a discussion of the clinical uses of infrared energy can proceed. When rays strike the skin or travel from one tissue to another, they can either be absorbed or be reflected (turned back) toward the source. The proportion of rays reflected depends on the angle at which they strike the surface, the type of surface they encounter, and the actual wavelength of the rays. According to the cosine law (see Chapter 5), optimal absorption will occur when the rays strike perpendicularly (at a right angle to a surface). Even then, however, some rays may be reflected.

This concept is important to consider during positioning of an infrared lamp over a body part because energy must be absorbed to have any effect. It is important to place the lamp parallel with the body part being treated so that the rays hit the body surface as close to a 90° angle as possible. When the angle of incidence is not 90°, reflection will be greater and absorption will be less (the Grotthus-Draper law).

According to the inverse square law, the intensity of rays from a point source varies inversely with the square of the distance from the source. The farther away from the body part the infrared lamp is placed, the less intense the heat will be per given area (by geometric proportions). For example, if you hold a flashlight 2 feet from a piece of paper, then 4 feet from the paper, what do you see? The rays are more dispersed when the light is 4 feet from the paper. Because equal energy is dispersed over a larger area, the intensity per area is diminished. Similarly, the patient will receive **four** times as much heat per area from an infrared lamp at a distance of 2 feet than at a distance of 4 feet, providing that the rays reach the patient at a 90° angle (obeying the cosine law).

Duration

Treatments last about 20 minutes for maximum heating. However, treatment time depends on the intensity desired and the distance of the lamp from the part. The distance should be increased if the skin turns more than a rosy pink or if the patient complains of too much heat.

Equipment

Two types of therapeutic infrared instruments are available: luminous and nonluminous. The *luminous instrument* produces mainly near infrared rays and the *nonluminous instrument* produces mainly far infrared rays. As determined by their specific wavelengths, the near rays penetrate to subcutaneous tissue, whereas the far rays are absorbed primarily by the superficial epidermis.[12]

Luminous (near) rays are produced by an incandescent tungsten and carbon filament encased in a quartz tube (similar to a light bulb). Nonluminous (far) rays are often produced by a metal spiral coil around a nonconducting material such as porcelain. As electricity flows through the coil, it encounters resistance, thus producing heat. Most machines used in clinics radiate electromagnetic energy in the near, far, and visible light ranges of the spectrum. Even the nonluminous lamps give off a minimal glow, indicating the presence of some visible light.

Both luminous and nonluminous machines have a reflecting hood designed to reflect the rays downward, thus evenly radiating the energy directly under the lamp (Fig. 11–6). This method of reflection minimizes the focal points of heat, thus minimizing the possibility of spot burns (areas of concentrated heat energy). Coverings must be available to protect eyes, hair and the skin areas not to be treated.

Techniques of Application

Again, before initiating the following procedures, the therapist must inspect the part for skin integrity, good circulation, and sensitivity to heat:

1. The therapist should allow a few minutes for the nonluminous instrument to warm up before beginning the treatment. The luminous lamp can be used immediately.
2. The patient should be placed in a relaxed, comfortable position with the part to be treated properly exposed and devoid of all creams, ointments, and the like.
3. Position the lamp between 18 and 36 inches from the part being treated. (luminous unit, 18–24 inches; nonluminous unit, 29–36 inches). Depending on the patient's tolerance to heat, condition (ie, the competency of the patient's vascular system), and the specifications of the particular piece of equipment, the distance between the part and the machine can be increased. Do not change the height of the lamp while it is above the patient because the lamp may fall on the patient while bolts or other parts are loosened. Make certain the lamp is aligned with the body part being treated to avoid reflection and to allow as much absorption of rays as possible (Fig. 11–7).
4. All jewelry in the area must be removed or, if not removable, covered with reflecting tape to avoid burns. If an area near the face is being treated, covering the eyes with cotton balls, gauze or goggles may be advisable.

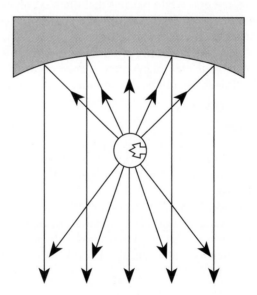

Figure 11–6. A diagrammatic representation of a reflecting hood on an infrared lamp showing that energy is radiated most evenly to the area of the body directly beneath the lamp.

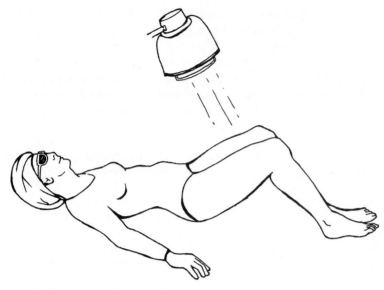

Figure 11–7. An infrared lamp aligned parallel with the body part being treated so that direct rays are at a 90° angle for maximum absorption.

Cover hair (it can dry out) and all of the body other than the treatment area with reflecting material such as white sheets or pillow cases.

5. During treatment, the therapist should periodically check the patient's skin and wipe off perspiration so that spot burns do not develop. Some therapists place a single layer of thin toweling over the part being treated to absorb perspiration; however, the skin must be checked for redness in any case.

Posttreatment Procedure

Turn off the lamp and move it away from the patient. Then check the patient's skin immediately. Mottling, red and white patches that often occur, can indicate that the superficial dermis has been pushed to its maximum with respect to heat control. If this has occurred, a temporary paralysis of the nerves to the arterioles may occur, resulting in vasodilation that could take a number of hours to resolve. With repeated intense treatments, Erythema ab igna, skin pigmentation, may occur from overexposure to infrared radiation. Treatments should be discontinued in the above cases.

Special Techniques

If the therapist wants to use a moist heat treatment, but hot packs or whirlpools are unavailable or cannot be tolerated, a Turkish towel that has been moistened and wrung out can be used in conjunction with infrared. The towel should be placed over the part to be treated.

When prolonged mild heat is indicated and the heat cannot be applied directly to the skin—for example, in cases of drying out pressure sores (decubitus ulcers) or trying to increase circulation in that area—infrared radiation can be used at a greatly reduced intensity. For example, a 150-watt lamp at a distance of 40 inches for 30 minutes.

Precaution

If the patient lacks sensation in the treated area, burns can occur. As was noted earlier, if mottling is already present in the area, it signals that the superficial dermal heat control mechanism is being pushed to its maximum. (Refer to the general contraindications for superficial heat.)

Advantages

Infrared treatment may be used to treat a larger body part, such as the lumbar and thoracic back area, that cannot always be covered completely by a hot pack. Patients who cannot tolerate the direct contact or weight of another modality such as a hot pack or ultrasound may feel comfortable during an infrared treatment. Because the heat from infrared lamps is so soothing and gentle, patients who are extremely tense may become more relaxed and ready for treatment.

Disadvantages

Infrared radiation dries the skin more than other modalities. In addition, burns may occur when an irregular or bony body part such as the shoulder is treated if the machine is too close or if the treatment time is not closely monitored. Thus, patients must be watched closely to ensure that the skin is not becoming too red. Finally, some patients may find that dry heat is agitating and irritating.

Although infrared is a superficial heat source, Kramer[13] compared the heating effects of continuous ultrasound and infrared radiation with placebo and found that both the conduction velocity of the ulnar nerve (distal humeral segment) and the temperature of the subcutaneous tissue increased with both modalities.

SUMMARY

This chapter has presented the various types of superficial heating available in most clinical settings. The therapist must be able to evaluate the patient's problem and determine which of the four modalities is the best choice. A patient may require a deeper heating modality or no heat at all; in fact, as we have pointed out, heat may be contraindicated for some patients.

Physical therapists should try to keep abreast of the most recent studies involving the available modalities. They also may wish to do research to compare the effects of one superficial heat modality with another. Finally, because we need to be certain that we are actually achieving our intended goals with each modality that we use, more studies need to be done on what actually occurs in patients' tissues during treatment.

■ KEY TERMS

superficial heat
hot packs
Fluidotherapy
near infrared

far infrared
luminous infrared instruments
non-luminous infrared instruments

■ REVIEW QUESTIONS

1. If a patient has an open cut on the hand that requires treatment for arthritis, which superficial heat modality would you select? Why?
   (a) a hot pack
   (b) paraffin
   (c) an infrared lamp
   (d) Fluidotherapy
2. Should heat be used on an acute injury?
3. Name some contraindications for the use of local heating.
4. After an injury, how much time should elapse before local heating is used?

5. How long is the usual treatment time for the following modalities?
   (a) hot packs
   (b) paraffin
   (c) Fluidotherpy
   (d) infrared radiation
6. What is the optimal temperature range for the following modalities?
   (a) hot packs
   (b) paraffin
   (c) Fluidotherapy
7. What method of heat transfer does each of the following modalities use?
   (a) hot packs
   (b) paraffin
   (c) Fluidotherapy
   (d) infrared radiation
8. Which of these four superficial heat modalities offers the best heating around small bony joints?
9. When one places a hot pack on a patient, approximately how many layers of toweling should be used in addition to the hot pack cover?
10. On what part of the body other than the neck might you use a cervical hot pack? Explain.
11. What sanitary precautions need to be taken with hot packs? With paraffin?
12. Should paraffin be used on the hot, swollen hand of a patient who has rheumatoid arthritis? Why?
13. Describe the glove, dip-immersion, and brush methods of paraffin application.
14. Briefly explain the cosine law and how it applies to infrared treatment.
15. Is it important to place the infrared lamp directly in parallel with the part to be treated? Why?
16. Why should the therapist check the skin and wipe off the patient's perspiration during infrared treatments?
17. Should infrared radiation ever be used to treat decubiti? Why?
18. What is the inverse square law? How does it apply to infrared treatments?
19. To what level does each of the following infrared treatments penetrate?
    (a) luminous rays
    (b) nonluminous rays

REFERENCES

1. Lehmann JF, ed: *Therapeutic Heat and Cold.* 4th ed. Baltimore, MD: Williams & Wilkins; 1990.
2. Borrell RM, Parker R, Henley RJ, et al: Comparison of in vivo temperature produced by hydrotherapy, paraffin wax treatment, and Fluidotherapy. *Phys Ther.* 1980; 60:1273–1276.
3. Lehmann JF, Massock AJ, Warren CG, et al: Effect of therapeutic temperature on tendon extensibility. *Arch Phys Med Rehabil.* 1970; 51:481–487.
4. Lehmann JF, Silverman DR, Baum BA, et al: Temperature distribution in the human thigh produced by infrared, hot pack, and microwave applications. *Arch Phys Med Rehabil.* 1966; 47:291–99.
5. Krusen FH, ed: *Krusen's Handbook of Physical Medicine and Rehabilitation,* Philadelphia, PA: WB Saunders; 1982.
6. Griffin JE, Karselis TC: *Physical Agents for Physical Therapists,* 3rd ed. Springfield, IL: Charles C Thomas; chap 5, 1988; 212.
7. Abramson DL, Tuck SI, Chu LSW, et al: Effects of paraffin bath and hot formentations on local tissue temperature. *Arch Phys Med Rehabil.* 1964; 45:87–94.
8. Hayes K: *Manual of Physical Agents.* 3rd ed. Chicago, IL: North Western University Medical School, Program in Physical Therapy; 1984.
9. Henley EJ: Engineering and medicine—Fluidotherapy® *Chemtech.* April 1982; 215–220.

10. Valenza J, Rossi C, Parker R, et al: A clinical study of a new heat modality—Fluidotherapy®. *J Am Podiat Assoc.* 1979; 69:440–442.

11. Alcorn R, Bowser R, Henley E, et al: Fluidotherapy and exercise in the management of sickle cell anemia: a clinical report. *J Am Phys Ther Assoc.* 1984; 64:1520–1522.

12. Forster A, Palastangan N, eds: Clayton's Electrotherapy, Theory and Practice. 8th ed. Baltimore, MD: Williams & Wilkins; 1981.

13. Kramer JP: Ultrasound: evaluation of its mechanical and thermal effects. *Arch Phys Med Rehabil.* 1984; 65:223–227.

12

Diathermy

Mary Joan Day, PT, MS

D iathermy, from the Greek meaning "through heat" is a physical agent used "most frequently" to increase temperature in deeply positioned tissues in order to (1) increase delivery of nutrients to the area by increasing blood flow, (2) diminish pain, or (3) increase the extensibility of tissues in musculoskeletal disorders. *Diathermy* utilizes nonionizing electromagnetic energy from the radio-frequency portion of the electromagnetic spectrum.

The popularity of diathermy as a therapeutic agent used by physical therapists has ebbed and flowed throughout this century; nevertheless, it remains a viable form of patient treatment. Therefore, to determine whether its application in patient management is theoretically and therapeutically sound, it is important to understand the effects of diathermy along with its scientific basis.

Three major types of diathermy (longwave, shortwave, and microwave) have been used by physical therapists to increase the temperature in tissues below the surface of the skin. Each is named for its respective position in the radio-frequency portion of the electromagnetic spectrum (see Chapter 5). Within the radio-frequency range, the Federal Communication Commission (FCC) has authorized the use of three specific bands for shortwave and two for microwave diathermies. At present, the following bands are used most commonly: shortwave—frequency, 27.12 MHz; wavelength, 11 m; and microwave—frequency, 2450 MHz; wavelength, 12 cm.

The electromagnetic energy generated by devices available to physical therapists is assumed to travel at a constant velocity (about 300×10^6 m/s). Thus, the wavelength of electromagnetic energy—ie, the distance between the apex of two successive waves—is inversely related to the frequency of its output. The longer the wavelength, the lower the frequency; the shorter the wavelength, the higher the frequency. Of the forms of electromagnetic energy used for their thermal effects, diathermy, with its longer wavelength and lower frequency, penetrates more deeply than does infrared, which has shorter wavelengths and higher frequencies.[1] Because diathermy is characterized by long wavelengths (approximately 3 cm to 300 m), theoretically its most potent thermal effect is not on skin and subcutaneous tissues but on the underlying musculature and associated connective tissues.

BIOPHYSICS AND PHYSIOLOGIC EFFECTS

Longwave Diathermy

The wavelength of *longwave diathermy* (300–30 m) is greater than shortwave (30–3 m) and microwave diathermy (3–.03 meters) and is the most penetrating of the three types. However, longwave diathermy has fallen into disfavor because it has been associated with the production of potentially harmful electrical burns[1] and because it interferes with radio transmissions.[2] Consequently, it has not been used clinically for many years and thus will not be discussed further.

Shortwave Diathermy

The thermal effects of *shortwave diathermy* were investigated by Esau as early as 1925.[3] However, its development as a therapeutic tool evolved most rapidly during World War II. During this developmental period, shortwave diathermy replaced longwave diathermy as the principal physical agent used to increase the temperature of muscle tissue safely. More recently, the fact that the application of shortwave diathermy can lead to therapeutically useful elevations of deep-tissue temperature has been well documented.[1,4–6]

The shortwave diathermy unit can be viewed as having a primary and a secondary circuit. The primary circuit is connected to the power supply and is also called a machine or power circuit. The secondary circuit is connected to the patient and thus is also called the patient circuit. Usually, the machine circuit consists of (1) a power supply, (2) a step-up and step-down transformer, (3) a rectifier, (4) oscillating circuits, and (5) a radio-frequency power amplifier designed to modify the output of the unit to levels required by the patient circuit. The machine circuit converts 110 V–60 Hz house current into high-voltage, high-frequency, low-amp current to be used in the patient circuit (see Fig. 12–1). This high-frequency energy is induced from the primary oscillating circuit of the machine circuitry into a secondary oscillating circuit in the patient circuitry. As the name implies, the patient circuit containing the secondary oscillating circuit transfers the energy to the patient.

The tissue type, the position of the body part, and the position of the diathermy electrodes influence the oscillation frequency in the patient circuit. For maximum efficiency, the oscillating frequency of the patient circuit must be in res-

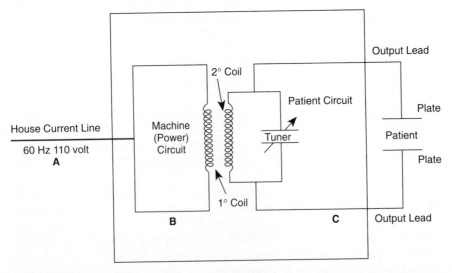

Figure 12–1. A simplified diagram of a shortwave diathermy unit with a patient positioned between condenser plates. **(A)** A representation of AC house current for the machine circuit. **(B)** The machine circuit which includes the transformers, rectifier, power amplifiers and primary (1°) radio-frequency oscillator of the machine circuit. **(C)** The patient circuit, which includes the secondary (2°) transformer coil, the tuner, high-frequency output leads, and condenser plates.

onance with that of the machine circuit. This is achieved by matching the frequency of the patient circuit with that of the machine circuit. The outcome is similar to what occurs when a radio is tuned to receive a clear signal from a specific station.

Some diathermy equipment is designed so that tuning is adjusted automatically, whereas other equipment is tuned manually. When manually tuning diathermy equipment, the therapist can determine whether the two circuits are in resonance (ie, tuned) by visual inspection of an **Output Indicator.** With the **Power Output** control remaining at a fixed position, the readout of the Output Indicator will be at the maximum point when the two circuits are "in tune" (resonance). The Output Indicator on shortwave diathermy units also indicates the average current passing through the patient circuit or the Power Output (in watts) of the unit. However, the indicator does not accurately indicate the amount of energy actually passing through the treated body parts.

When the oscillating frequency of the patient circuit is in resonance with that of the machine circuit, the resultant output is high-frequency (> 10 MHz), low-amp electromagnetic energy. As a consequence of this extremely high frequency, nerve depolarization does not occur because the rapid rate of change in current direction does not allow ions to flow across the nerve membrane. Instead, the electromagnetic energy is absorbed, primarily by fatty and muscle tissue, and is converted into heat.

Shortwave diathermy is subdivided into condenser (or capacitor) field diathermy and induction field diathermy. Condenser field and induction field diathermy are distinguished by the predominant type of energy emitted and the type of electrode used during a diathermy application.

Condenser Field Diathermy

In *condenser field diathermy*, a high-frequency alternating current generator emits electromagnetic energy from a pair of oppositely charged electrodes called *condenser* or *capacitor plates,* part of the secondary oscillating circuit. The charge on each electrode alternates in accord with the frequency of the alternating current. As a result, a strong electrical field is generated between the plates. Fig. 12–2 is an illustration of this strong electrical field. Note that the strength of the field is not

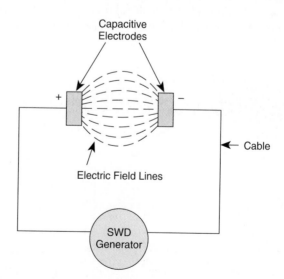

Figure 12–2. With condenser field diathermy, an electric field occurs between two oppositely charged electrodes (dashed lines). The distance between lines indicates the relative strength of the field. Note that the field is stronger near each electrode. (*Modified from HHS Publication FDA 85–8237. Kloth L, Morrison MA, Ferguson BH: Therapeutic Microwave and Shortwave Diathermy: A Review of Thermal Effectiveness, Safe Use, and State of the Art: 1984. December 1984) 1984, Food and Drug Administration, U.S. Department of Health and Human Services.*)

homogeneous; it is strongest near the plates but spreads or diverges farther from the plates. Because the strength of the field is greatest near the plates, it might overheat skin and subcutaneous fat if placed too close. Thus, the condensers are positioned a slight distance from the skin (about 2–3 cm) to allow divergence before contact with the skin. When a body part is positioned properly between the oppositely charged condensers—ie, within the electric field of the plates—the electrical energy will cause ions and dipole molecules within the tissues (molecules that behave as if they had oppositely charged ends) to change direction every time the charge on the plates and the direction of the electric field change. The faster the current changes direction (ie, the higher its frequency), the smaller the actual movement of the particles from their original position. The frequency of the back and forth oscillation of the ions matches the output frequency of the generator.

Ordinarily, dipole molecules tend to be randomly situated within tissue; however, when subjected to the energy emitted from the diathermy unit, they rotate in the direction dictated by their polar charge (see Fig. 12–3). The rate of rotation is tightly coupled with the frequency of the energy emitted from the diathermy unit.[3] Thus, the high-frequency oscillatory movement of ions and dipoles results in sharp increases in molecular kinetic energy, which results in increased tissue temperature.

The tissue response to the high-frequency oscillatory field is somewhat analogous to the response of any conductor when electrical current passes through it. According to Joule's law, the amount of energy converted to heat (H) is proportional to the square of the intensity of current (I^2), the impedance of the conductor (R), and the duration of current flow (t). This law is often expressed as

$$H = I^2Rt.$$

By applying this law and assuming that the strength of the current is equal throughout the tissues within the electric field, it is theoretically possible to predict the location of the tissues having the greatest temperature increases. If the condenser field plates and the tissues are arranged in series with one another (see Fig. 12–4), the heat produced will be proportional to the impedance of the tissue (see Chapter 17 for a more detailed discussion of series circuits). Because the current intensity is the same in all parts of a series circuit, the temperature of the tissue having the greatest impedance to the molecular activity is elevated to the greatest degree. For example, fat has a significantly higher impedance than does muscle or

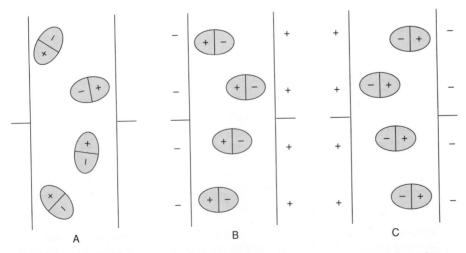

Figure 12–3. Dipole molecules. **(A)** Random arrangement when condenser plates are not charged. **(B, C)** Direction toward which dipoles rotate according to the change in polarity of the plates. The positive end of the dipole is always toward the negatively charged plate. (*Modified from* Clayton's Electrotherapy Theory and Practice. *Forster A, Palastanga N. 9th ed. 1985, Bailliere Tindall.*)

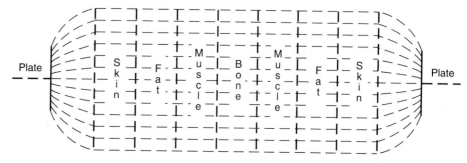

Figure 12–4. Theoretical example of an high-frequency oscillatory field, assuming that the strength of the electric current is uniform through the tissues within the electric field. The condenser plates are in series with the cross-section of a body part. Note the field spread in the space between the plates and the skin, indicating that the field density is less at the skin than it would be if the plates were on the skin.

bone; therefore more heating occurs in fatty tissue than occurs in more conductive tissues such as muscle.[7]

The relative heating pattern is similar to that depicted in Fig. 12–5.[8,9] This heating pattern of the tissues can be changed so that the temperature of muscle is elevated but the entire cross-section of the part is *not,* as it is when plates and tissue are in series with each other (see Chapter 17). This is accomplished by positioning the body part so that deeper tissues are **in parallel** with more superficial tissues. This configuration is easily achieved by placing the part to be treated under, rather than between, the two condenser plates (see Fig. 12–6). In this configuration, the heat produced is more dependent on the intensity of current because the density of the current varies throughout a parallel circuit. In a parallel circuit, the current has a "choice" of paths it can follow, but it will always follow the path of least resistance. To the extent that this parallel position of plates produces a parallel circuit, more current will flow through tissues of low impedance and more heat will be generated in those tissues.

Muscle tissue has low impedance properties and thus will be heated selectively when the two plates are placed parallel to the body part to be treated. This application may be useful when treating areas such as the mid and low back (see Fig. 12–7). This more selective heating of muscle is clearly advantageous when treating problems of muscular origin.

In clinical practice, both arrangements of condenser plates are used. *Contra-planar positioning* (also called transverse positioning) of plates uses the "series" arrangement, whereas *coplanar positioning* of plates uses the "parallel" arrangement. Although the analogy of series versus parallel electrical circuits is useful to explain the heating patterns of shortwave diathermy clinically, the situation is more complex.

Essential differences exist between electrical line circuits and body tissues in series. Within the body, the strength of the electric field, and therefore the amount

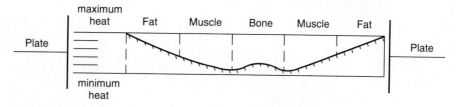

Figure 12–5. In this schematic rendition of inner tissues of a body part, with the tissues in series with the condenser plates, note that although the temperature of the entire cross-section has increased, the temperature of the fatty tissue is higher than that in muscle tissue when the condenser plates are in series. (*Adapted with permission from* Introduction to Shortwave and Microwave Therapy. H Thom 1966, Charles C Thomas.)

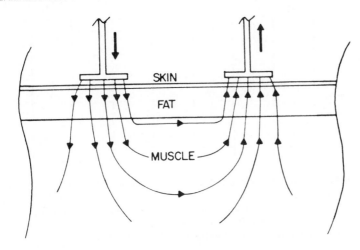

Figure 12–6. Schematic drawing of condenser plates in parallel with a longitudinal section of a body part. (*Modified with permission from* Therapeutic Heat and Cold. *Lehmann J, ed. 3rd ed. 1982, Williams & Wilkins Co.*)

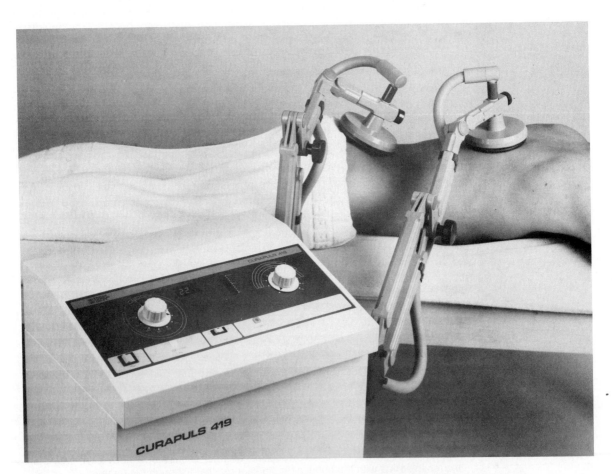

Figure 12–7. Condenser plates positioned in the parallel position to treat muscle in the mid and lower back. Although not shown, one thin layer of toweling over the skin is recommended to absorb moisture. (*Reproduced with permission from Henley International, Sugar Land, TX.*)

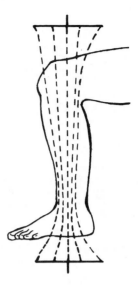

Figure 12–8. The field must converge when in a narrow part of the body such as the lower leg.

of current flow, is not uniform throughout. The lines of force of the electric field diverge with increasing distance from the plates and according to the electrical properties of the various tissues. For example, there is less divergence in fat than in tissues with a higher fluid content such as muscle. In narrow body parts such as an ankle or a wrist, the lines of force converge and the field is much stronger (see Fig. 12–8). In addition, unlike "phantom model" tissue layers, tissues in the body are seldom found in precisely layered arrangements.

Although coplanar positioning is comparable to parallel electrical circuits, this electrode positioning, in fact, produces within the body a combination of series and parallel circuits. All current must first pass through the skin and fat layers in series before selecting the course of least resistance through deeper tissues (see Fig. 12–6). With either series or parallel plate positioning, any metal on or within the body, or metal anywhere within the electric field, will alter the heating pattern. The field can concentrate in metal and may overheat adjacent tissues.

Induction Field Diathermy

The second type of shortwave diathermy is referred to as induction (coil field) *diathermy.* The principal difference between condenser field and *induction field diathermy* is that, with induction field diathermy, a strong magnetic field is produced by the patient circuit, which then induces an electrical current within the body part. In condenser field diathermy, the body part is positioned in an electrical field generated by two condenser plates. The single induction field electrode is made of metal, which is shaped into a coil (Fig. 12–9) and has properties of high conductivity. Fig. 12–10 shows the typical arrangements of coils: the monode, with the coil basically arranged in one plane, and the hinged diplode, which permits the electrode to be positioned on one-to-three sides of a body part. When high-frequency electrical energy is applied to the coil, a fluctuating magnetic field is generated around the coil. As with any current conducting wire, a coil shape increases the strength of the magnetic field along the concave side. The direction of the magnetic field changes with each change in the direction of current.

When a low impedance conductor such as a body part is placed within the magnetic field, electric currents are induced within that conductor. Within the body part, these are small *eddies* or circular-shaped currents that alternate in direction in concert with the changes in the direction of the magnetic field.

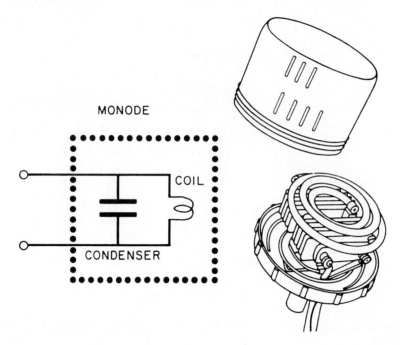

Figure 12–9. Inductive shortwave diathermy electrode (monode); arrangement of preshaped coils used for induction shortwave diathermy. (*Reproduced with permission from* Therapeutic Heat and Cold. *Lehmann J, ed. 3rd ed. 1982, Williams & Wilkins Co.*)

Although the strength of the magnetic *field* fluctuates in phase with the high-frequency current that produced it, the strength is uniform throughout the various tissues at any given distance from the inductor. Thus, one can reasonably assume that the greatest current density—ie, the greatest eddy current activity—occurs in the low impedance tissues. Consequently, in accordance with Joule's law, the greatest heat generated is within low impedance tissues. The higher the electrolyte content of the tissue, the lower the impedance. Blood has the highest electrolyte content of all tissues (0.9%); therefore, muscle, which is rich in blood, can be heated more easily than fat, bone, or collagen tissues.[2,3,8,9] This pattern of heat distribution is shown in Fig. 12–11. It should be noted that the magnetic field is strongest near

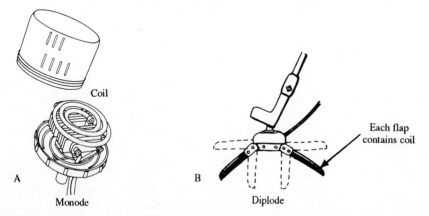

Figure 12–10. Inductive shortwave diathermy (drum) electrodes. Two arrangements of preshaped coils used for induction shortwave diathermy. **(A)** The monode sends energy to tissues in the same plane as the surface of the drum. **(B)** the diplode has coils in each flap. The three-section hinged arrangement permits heating at various angles around three sides of the body part or in one plane. (*Modified with permission from* HHS Publication FDA *85–8237.* Kloth L, Morrison MA, Ferguson BH: *Therapeutic Microwave and Shortwave Diathermy: A Review of Thermal Effectiveness, Safe Use, and State of the Art: 1984. December 1984 Food and Drug Administration, U.S. Department of Health and Human Services.*)

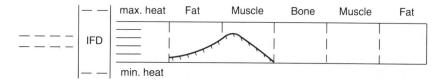

Figure 12–11. Pattern of depth of heat distribution in induction field shortwave diathermy (IFD). The temperature in muscle is elevated to a greater degree than the temperature in fatty tissue, but no temperature change occurs in bone. (*Adapted with permission from* Introduction to Shortwave and Microwave Therapy. *H Thom 1966, Charles C Thomas.*)

the coil; thus, skin and subcutaneous tissues also are affected, but not as much as muscle. In general, the heating that occurs depends on the type of tissue and its depth.

Similar heating patterns, relative to depth, are developed with either the induction field method or the condenser field method when the plates are positioned parallel to the body part. Deeper muscle temperature change is not significant with either method. Although superficial muscle layers can be heated with both methods, the relative difference in magnitude of change in muscle temperature between these two methods is unknown. However, there are some differences in heat distribution between these two methods. The condenser field method produces more heat than the induction field method in the superficial skin and fatty layer (see Figs. 12–6 and 12–11).

Again, metal on or implanted in tissues must be considered. Because metal is a better electrical conductor than body tissues, the magnetic flux will induce more eddy currents in the metal. Thus, in accordance with Joule's law, the metal will heat, and may overheat, adjacent tissues.

Pulsed Shortwave Diathermy

On the basis of the belief that benefits other than thermal ones can be derived from high-frequency electromagnetic energy, some advocate the use of *pulsed shortwave diathermy.* Units are available that permit "on-off" cycles so that the energy is absorbed in the tissues but the blood flow during the "off" cycle prevents tissue temperature rise. There are many "convincing" anecdotal clinical reports of the positive wound healing effects of this mode. However, the many scientific attempts to demonstrate its therapeutic value have failed to produce sufficient evidence to support the clinical use of the pulsed mode of shortwave diathermy.[4]

Microwave Diathermy

Microwave diathermy is the other major type of diathermy in current use. The microwave diathermy unit that is available in the clinic most often is distinguished by the presence of a high-frequency electrical generator called a *magnetron oscillator.* To function efficiently, the magnetron oscillator requires a brief warm-up period; however, it does not require manual tuning. The electromagnetic energy generated in the magnetron has a relatively short wavelength (about 12 cm) and an extremely high frequency (about 2450 MHz). Energy with waves of this length cannot be conducted by conventional cables without loss of substantial quantities of energy. Therefore, to minimize this leakage, the energy is transmitted through a coaxial (shielded) cable to a microwave director, which is an antenna mounted in a reflector. The director is used to transmit radiated energy to the body part, where the energy is converted to heat, principally by dipole movement. Tissues having properties of high conductivity contain numerous dipole molecules.

In general, muscle tissue contains more dipole molecules than does fatty tissue. This should lead to a significant rise in muscle temperature when microwave diathermy is used. However, subcutaneous fatty tissue may be heated even more than muscle. A possible explanation for this heating follows.

Microwave energy is radiated from the director and, like other forms of radiated energy, follows the cosine and inverse square laws (see Chapter 5). Most important, it follows the laws of optics; thus microwave energy can be refracted, reflected, absorbed directly, or all of these. Consequently, when microwave energy is passing through fatty tissues, some energy is absorbed directly, some is reflected back into the fatty tissue at the fat-muscle interface, and the remainder passes through the interface and is absorbed by muscle.[10] The energy reflected back into fatty tissue is then absorbed by that tissue. The combined quantities of energy absorbed by fat lead to a heating pattern in which the temperature of fatty layers may be equal to or even exceed that of muscle when the fatty layer is thicker than 20

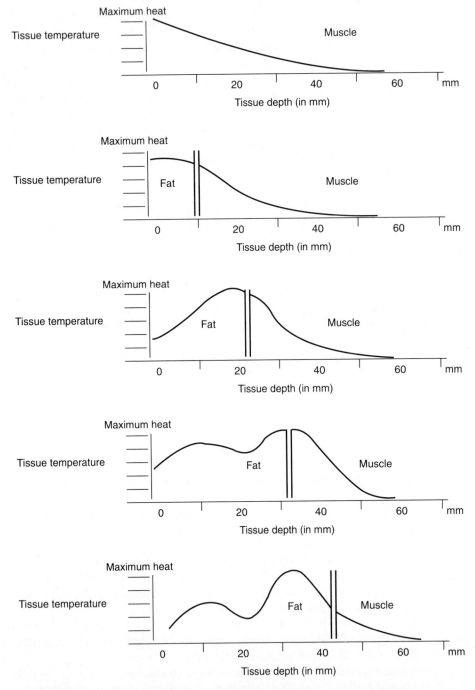

Figure 12–12. Influence of the thickness of the fat layer on heat distribution in muscle and fat during microwave diathermy. As the thickness of the fatty layer increases, its absorption of the heat increases and the absorption of heat by muscle decreases. (*Adapted with permission from* Introduction to Shortwave and Microwave Therapy. *H Thom 1966, Charles C Thomas.*)

mm. The actual ratio of fat:muscle temperature depends to a degree on the thickness of the two layers of tissue. This can be seen in Fig. 12–12.[3] Because of the danger of overheating fat, the power output must be limited. Thus, the depth to which 2450 MHz microwave diathermy heats tissues is slightly less than with shortwave diathermy.

Precautions must be taken when metal is in the area of therapeutic microwave radiation. Just as in microwave ovens, most metals will reflect the rays. If this occurs outside of the body, the rays may reflect back to the director or to other people and objects in the environment. When the metal is within the body, the reflected rays may overheat the adjacent tissues.

In 1984 a survey of clinical facilities conducted by the Food and Drug Administration (FDA) revealed that the facilities were using shortwave less than 6 hours per week and microwave even less.[2] This low usage may in part be justified because it has been well known for years that 2450 MHz microwave diathermy is less effective than it is at lower frequencies. For example, a frequency of 915 MHz is capable of deeper heating, and an even lower frequency (750 MHz) is under investigation.[4]

Another disadvantage of the 2450 MHz microwave unit is that the director is placed a distance from the body and energy is emitted into the surrounding environment, whereas the power output must be limited so that skin and fat will not be overheated. The 915 MHz unit is now designed to permit surface contact, thus decreasing energy leakage, while forced cool air cools the skin. With these units it has been shown that significant heating can occur in muscle that is 4 cm deep while the temperature of subcutaneous fat rises considerably less than that of muscle.[4] Using these units on rabbit joints, Fadilah et al[11] compared the TTR in skin, muscle, cartilage, and joint capsules and found that the only significant temperature rise occurred in the capsule. Such studies indicate that deep tissue can be heated with air cooled 915 MHz microwave units without overheating the superficial tissues. However, these units are similar in frequency to cellular telephones (840–880 MHz), and it has been suggested that tumor growth may be associated with the use of these telephones.[12] But the results of systematic investigations of the effects of microwaves at low frequencies are controversial, mixed, and inconclusive.[13] Current and future research should help establish whether exposure to low-frequency microwaves alters cell growth.

TREATMENT CONSIDERATIONS

Preparation of the Patient

Before initiating the treatment, the therapist should carry out the following steps.

1. Remove all clothing, jewelry, coins, and electronic devices from the area. Magnetic fluctuation may demagnetize watches or other electronic devices such as hearing aids.
2. Inspect the area to be treated, checking carefully for any metal on or around the patient, and ask the patient whether any metal (eg, prosthetic implants, sutures, intrauterine devices) are within the body.
3. Cleanse the area to remove all dirt and oils.
4. Place the patient in a seated, prone, supine or side-lying position, depending on the particular condition or body part to be treated. The patient should be relaxed and comfortable.
5. Elevate an extremity to be treated to encourage fluid drainage.
6. Position the patient so that the musculature in the area to be treated is at the physiologic resting length or slackened whenever possible, unless the goal is to increase the extensibility of tissues during heating. In such cases position to encourage elongation of involved tissues.
7. With shortwave diathermy, cover the part with one layer of toweling to

absorb and prevent pooling of perspiration. With microwave diathermy, keep the area exposed so that perspiration can evaporate.

8. Instruct the patient about the heat sensation he or she should expect. Tell the patient to notify you or pull the emergency switch in case of any discomfort or if "it gets too hot."

9. Instruct the patient not to move after the unit is positioned for treatment because any changes in the arranged position may increase or decrease the amount of heat received. (With shortwave diathermy, movement can change the tuning, either improving or reducing the frequency resonance between primary and secondary circuits. With microwave diathermy, movement may alter the distance or direction of the rays.)

The patient must not be positioned on a metal bed or plinth, on a mattress with metal springs, or in a metal chair such as a wheelchair when receiving a diathermy treatment. In addition, the presence of any indwelling metal devices in the effective field represent contraindications. In short, any metal in the effective area of the diathermy unit must be removed or diathermy is contraindicated because the heat generated can burn tissues or objects.

When preparing for shortwave treatments, turkish toweling is applied to body surfaces for sanitary purposes and to absorb perspiration. If perspiration is allowed to accumulate, it may cause a strong concentration of energy leading to excessive heating of the skin and possible burns. Absorbent material should be inserted whenever two skin surfaces such as the axilla are likely to make contact. In the case of microwave diathermy, no toweling is placed directly on the skin to allow perspiration to evaporate. However, the patient should be watched carefully, and perspiration should be removed periodically.

With diathermy, as with other electrical devices, the patient should be positioned so that he cannot touch anything connected to the ground (eg a radiator, a water pipe or an electrical outlet). Although the energy in the patient circuit was induced from the primary circuit, thus is "ground free", dangerously excessive current may flow through the body should the patient become grounded.

Dosage

Because the actual amount of energy the patient receives during treatment cannot be monitored directly, the patient's own subjective sensation of heat is the most important indicator. A dose that produces a mild but pleasant sensation of heat is believed to be beneficial for subacute inflammatory processes, whereas chronic conditions respond to a more vigorous dose that leads to a sensation of heat that is just below the patient's maximum tolerance.[4,12] Clinicians generally assume that the sensation of heat on the skin is correlated with the degree of heating in deeper-lying tissues. Obviously, the patient must be alert and able to report sensations of heat reliably. If the integrity of the peripheral nervous system is suspect, the therapist must test the patient's sense of temperature before initiating treatment.

In addition, it is prudent in a first treatment to take the extra precaution of using slightly lower intensities. A more subtle point is the need to monitor the patient's reports of heat sensation at the initial phase of treatment and again during the treatment. When the output of the diathermy unit is adjusted, a "lag" of several seconds occurs between the time the output is changed and the time the patient will be aware of a change in the sensation of heat. Therefore, the patient must be given sufficient time to perceive this change before further adjustments are made.

The duration and frequency of treatment depend on the treatment goals (decreased pain or increased tissue extensibility) and the status of the condition treated (subacute or chronic). Investigators have shown that 20 to 30 minute treatments are usually long enough to be therapeutically beneficial. It may take 3 to 8 minutes for the tissue temperature to rise to desired levels. When the temperature reaches the plateau caused by increased blood flow, 10 to 20 additional minutes should be sufficient to achieve therapeutic gains. The TTR time is an important consideration when the goal is to elongate tissues at high temperatures. For example, if the intent is to heat and stretch for 20 minutes and the TTR requires 8 minutes, the treatment should continue for about 30 minutes.[4] The specific absorption rate (SAR) of electromagnetic energy in tissues can be used to determine dosage factors. Information about SAR and guidelines for dosages based on the SAR are given in Chapter 6 and Table 6–2).

Techniques of Application

The therapist should be familiar with and follow the manufacturers' recommendations for the proper application of specific diathermy units. This section presents general recommendations for condenser and induction-field shortwave and microwave diathermy.

Condenser field diathermy. Placing the condenser plates parallel to the body part to be treated is recommended to heat superficial muscle. If this is not possible, or if it is desirable to treat two sides of a body part such as a shoulder, knee, or ankle; the plates should be placed in series with the body part to be treated. The plates themselves, usually located within plate guards, can be moved a predetermined distance to vary the spacing between plate and skin. The guard can contact the skin or overlying towel, but the **metal plate** itself **must not contact the towel or skin.** Power output (dosage) is dictated by the patient's subjective sensation of heat. At any given energy output, the closer the plates are to the skin, the greater the sensation of heat. As the distance between the plate and the skin increases, the sensation of heat decreases; thus, the power output can be increased, and more energy can be provided to promote greater heating of deeper-lying tissues.[1] A plate-skin distance of 1 inch is suggested to provide maximum heating at maximum depths with minimum risk to the patient (see Figs. 12–7 and 12–13).[13]

Induction or coil field diathermy. Depending on the manufacturer, the current conductor may be preshaped into a coil (sometimes referred to as a drum) designed as a diplode or monode. (see Fig. 12–10) If the conductor is not preshaped, the therapist can coil the conductor cable manually. The space between the coiled conductor and the surface of the drum is fixed so a single layer of toweling laid on the body part provides adequate spacing (see Fig. 12–14). If the therapist coils the cable, there must be one inch of spacing between all parts of the cable and an inch of toweling between the patient and all parts of the cable. Although effective, the manually coiled technique is seldom used because a safe, efficient position is difficult and time consuming to achieve.

Microwave diathermy. The microwave electrodes, called directors, vary in shape and size (see Fig. 12–15). The choice of shape is usually determined by the site and shape of the body part and the extent of the area to be treated. The circular-shaped microwave director provides a doughnut-shaped pattern of heat distribution, with minimum heating occurring in the central area. This director is preferred for treating an area with a bony prominence, a superficial joint, or both because the central part of the director can be positioned over the area requiring less heating. In contrast, when rectangular-shaped directors are used, the predominant heating occurs in the central area (see Fig. 12–15).[4]

Unlike shortwave electrodes, the microwave director can be positioned several inches away from the skin. The amount of tissue area heated is proportional to the distance from the director to the skin. Because the body's contours are uneven, the distance from the highest point of the skin surface to the director should be measured when determining the proper director-to-skin distance and dosage. In addition, the effect of the heating will diminish over surfaces that are not perpendicular to the rays; the relative effect of the heating can be determined by the cosine law (see Chapter 5). The minimum distance between the skin and the director is approximately 1 inch, but this distance can be increased when treating a larger area, assuming that the power output (intensity) is increased accordingly. Ordinarily, the manufacturer of a particular piece of equipment provides a guide for deter-

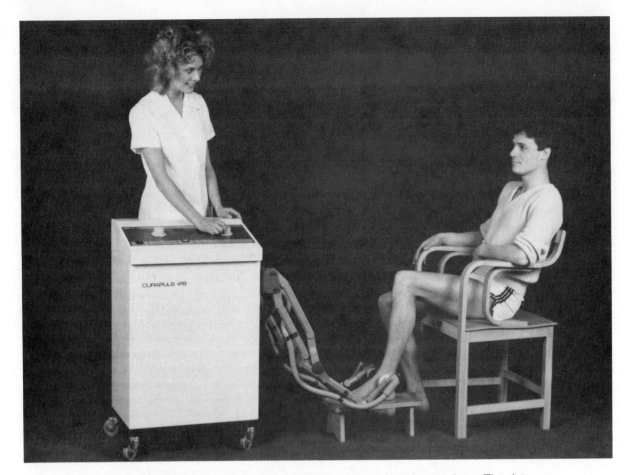

Figure 12–13. Contraplanar (transverse) position of condenser plates. The plates are in series with body tissues. (*Reproduced with permission from Henley International, Sugar Land, TX.*)

mining the proper wattage output for each director used at specific director-to-skin distances.

Indications and Contraindications

Diathermy has been used to help *clear* inflammatory exudates in subacute conditions. However, it is most frequently used in the treatment of musculoskeletal disorders.

It is especially useful when treating tissues and joints that lie close to the surface[4,17] and when treating secondary muscle spasms or pain associated with pathologies such as degenerative joint disease, sprains and strains. Furthermore, the extensibility of collagenous tissue is increased when the tissue temperature is elevated. Therefore, when stretching is the goal of the physical therapy program, positioning that elongates the tissues to be stretched, during the diathermy treatment and stretching or exercising the part while the temperature is still elevated will enhance the results of the stretching techniques.[18-20]

When treating these disorders, selection of a heating modality depends on the depth of the penetration of each modality, the depth of the tissue to be treated, the size of the area to be treated, and the amount of heating required. The depth of penetration of shortwave and microwave diathermy is greater than the infrared modalities and less than ultrasound. The size of the body part that can be heated can be a small circumscribed area or a relatively large area, depending on the type of diathermy and electrodes used. When diathermy is applied to deep-seated joints covered by a thick layer of tissue (eg, the hip joint) the temperature of that joint

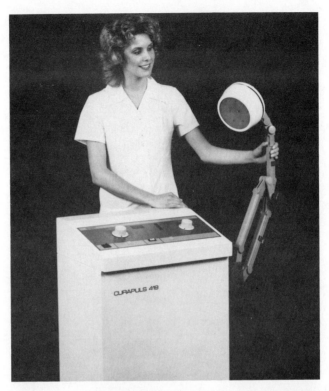

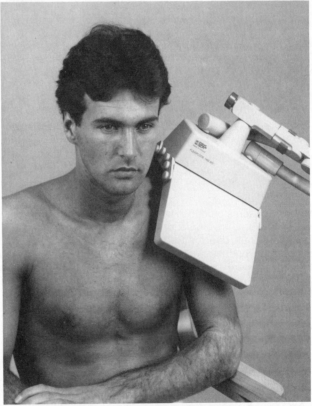

Figure 12–14. (A) Monode and **(B)** diplode inductance units. These drums are designed with adequate space between the coil and the drum. However, a layer of toweling over the skin is recommended for absorption of moisture and sanitary purposes. (*Reproduced with permission from Henley International, Sugar Land, TX.*)

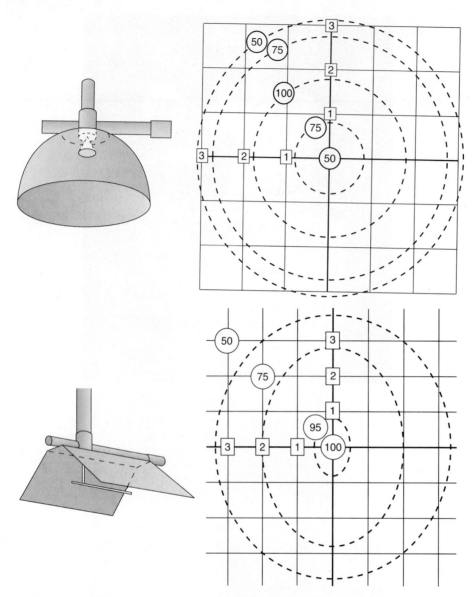

Figure 12–15. Field patterns produced by microwave directors. **(A)** A circular director "A" head and the field pattern it produces. The maximum intensity (100%) occurs beneath the periphery of the director (Zone 2); it diminishes to 50% at the center and gradually diminishes beyond the periphery of the director. **(B)** A rectangular director "C" head and the field pattern it produces. In this case, the maximum intensity (100%) occurs beneath the center of the director. (*Modified with permission from* Therapeutic Heat and Cold. *Lehmann J, ed. 3rd ed. 1982, Williams & Wilkins Co.*)

does not increase appreciably. The highest temperatures occur in the more superficial musculature.

When treating joints with minimal soft-tissue coverage, such as the knee or ankle, diathermy can significantly elevate the temperature in the musculature surrounding the joint. If the condenser field electrodes and the joint are in series, the temperature within the joint may be elevated as well. As always, the clinician should consider the desirability of heating within a joint in light of a patient's specific condition. Fadilah et al[11] suggested that if therapeutic heat to joints is a desired treatment, air-cooled 915 MHz microwave diathermy has the advantage of heating only the target area, the synovium for example, and sparing adjacent tissues. However, heating synovial fibroblasts to 42° in vitro may induce cellular stress responses.[16] More information is needed to determine the short- and long-range effects of vigorously heating joint synovium.

The general contraindications associated with any modality that elevates tissue temperature should be observed. The application of diathermy should always be avoided if inflammation is acute, hemorrhage is likely, the vascular system is compromised, the patient cannot perceive or report heat sensation accurately, or the patient has a fever.

The contraindications associated specifically with diathermy are numerous. As was mentioned earlier, any metal in the field is clearly a contraindication. Furthermore, cardiac pacemakers or other pacing devices are of special concern because their presence is a contraindication in itself. In addition, however, the energy emanating from the diathermy unit may disrupt the operation of a pacer in any person in the proximity of the diathermy unit.[1,15]

In addition, because the application of diathermy to the low back has been reported to increase menstrual flow, menses may represent a contraindication in some cases. Although there is no evidence that high-frequency current has a negative effect on the pregnant uterus when the low back or abdomen are treated, pregnancy remains a contraindication to diathermy. Furthermore, Lehmann and De Lateur[4] recommend that pregnant therapists avoid operating the unit. It is always wise to avoid direct diathermy heating of the testes, the area near the eyes, and the epiphyses in growing children. Direct heating of malignancies is contraindicated because the increased vascularity may increase blood flow to the extent that metastases may occur.[7] Although hyperthermia is a form of cancer therapy, the diathermy equipment and the techniques used for cancer therapy are not the same as the equipment and techniques commonly used in physical therapy clinics.[21]

The evidence that stray radiation from diathermy units constitutes an occupational hazard is equivocal. Silverman[22] and Michaelson[23] reviewed studies on the possible deleterious effects of microwaves and concluded that the results of the studies were not compelling.[22,23] Two separate groups of investigators studied the effects of exposure to shortwave and microwave diathermy respectively.[24,25] Both groups concluded that ordinary prudent practice (remaining within 1 meter of an operating unit for only short periods) makes it unlikely that therapists would be exposed to harmful levels of radiation. Hamburger,[26] on the other hand, reported an association between heart disease in male physical therapists and the use of shortwave diathermy. However, of the 3004 male therapists who responded to the survey, only 73 reported heart disease, and most of them were in the age group frequently associated with heart disease. In addition, information about smoking habits, alcohol consumption, and the like was not gathered. Thus, more rigorously designed studies are needed.

SUMMARY

At the frequencies commonly found in clinics, both shortwave and microwave diathermies can, if properly applied, increase the temperature of skeletal muscle. The greatest elevations in temperature will occur in skeletal muscle that is close to the surface, while virtually no changes in temperature occur in muscles surrounding a deep-seated joint such as the hip joint. Like other modalities, diathermy will result in some transference of heat to other tissues by conduction and by local circulation of warmed blood, but its greatest effect is mild-to-moderate heating of superficial musculature. The distribution pattern of temperature resulting from a diathermy treatment is influenced by the type of diathermy and the method of its application. If properly executed, treatment with condenser field, induction field, and microwave diathermy can increase temperatures in skeletal muscle. The actual amount of energy absorbed by specific tissues and the dosage required to elicit maximum therapeutic benefits have not been elucidated. More investigations similar to those undertaken by Lehmann and associates[27] are needed. With further research, physical therapists can make more precise decisions about the efficacy of this modality and other modalities in the management of musculoskeletal disorders. As with any modality, the decision to use diathermy for a particular treatment situation depends on a number of variables: the depth of penetration of the modality, the depth of tissue to be treated, the size of the area to be treated, whether vigorous, moderate, or mild heating is desired,[4] and whether the primary treatment goals include tissue nutrition, extensibility, and pain relief.

■ KEY TERMS

diathermy
longwave diathermy
shortwave diathermy
   condenser (capacitor) field diathermy
   condensers
   capacitor plates

contraplanar positioning
coplanar positioning
induction field diathermy
pulsed shortwave diathermy
microwave diathermy

■ REVIEW QUESTIONS

1. The Federal Communication Commission assigns specific high-frequency bands for medical purposes. The band for shortwave diathermy used most often in clinics in the United States is approximately
   (a) frequency, 13 MHz; wavelength 22 m
   (b) frequency, 27 MHz; wavelength 11 m
   (c) frequency, 48 MHz; wavelength 7.3 m
   (d) any FM radio band

2. "Lines of Force" is a term used to describe the strength of magnetic or electric fields; the lines are more concentrated where the field is stronger. On the basis of this model, it is true to say
   (a) the electric field in the body tissues between two condenser plates of a shortwave diathermy machine is strongest directly beneath the plates; thus, subcutaneous fat will be heated more than underlying muscles.
   (b) the ability to produce molecular activity, thus heat, will be greater in regions where the lines of force "spread" than were they are concentrated.
   (c) spacing between plates and body tissues enables some "spreading" of the lines of force between plates and the skin; thus, fields strong enough to produce more heat in deep tissues can be tolerated.
   (d) both a and c are true.

3. Which statement (or statements) about shortwave diathermy is (are) true?
   (a) The output indicator placed in the resonating circuit indicates the amount of current that the patient is receiving. Thus, it can accurately predict the amount of increase in tissue temperature.
   (b) The "tuner" is used to establish resonance between the oscillating circuits in the machine and *patient* circuits.
   (c) When the condenser technique is used, heat is conducted from the pad into the patient's tissues.
   (d) Induction rather than condenser plate shortwave is established by variations in the components of the "machine" circuit.

4. With the condenser method of shortwave diathermy,
   (a) there is a rapid alteration of negative and positive charges on the condenser pads.
   (b) heat is produced within the body because of the rapid back and forth vibration of ions.
   (c) heat is produced within the body because of the rapid rotations of dipole molecules.
   (d) all the above statements are true.

5. Induction field diathermy can increase the temperature of
   (a) superficial muscles
   (b) deeply positioned joints
   (c) deeply positioned bones
   (d) all of the above
6. If the inductance method of shortwave diathermy is completely inductive (ie, the tissues are not within an electric field):
   (a) the patient is part of the circuit.
   (b) the changing magnetic field produced by the high-frequency current influences the body tissues.
   (c) the greatest number of eddy currents will be in the tissues with the least electric conductivity.
   (d) the heating is uneven and fatty tissues become overheated.
7. Concerning microwave diathermy, which one of the following statements is true?
   (a) Most metals reflect rather than absorb microwave energy; thus, metal within the body would not be heated. However, body tissues near the metal might become overheated.
   (b) Tissues containing numerous dipoles such as fat heat most readily when microwave energy is absorbed in them.
   (c) The 2450 MHz units usually produce a significant tissue temperature rise in muscles 4 cm deep, and the rise in subcutaneous fat is only one-third that of muscles.
   (d) When a circular director is used, most heating occurs in the center of the area being radiated.
8. Three indications for which deep heat might be more helpful than superficial heat are
   (a) ligamentous injuries, general relaxation, and deep muscle ruptures.
   (b) general "warmup" before therapeutic exercise, low back pain of unknown etiology, and adhesive capsulitis.
   (c) deep muscle ruptures, ligamentous injuries, and warmup before stretching nonelastic tissues such as tendons or capsules.
   (d) all of the above

REFERENCES

1. Griffin JE, Karselis TC. *Physical Agents for Physical Therapists.* Springfield, IL: Charles C Thomas; 1982.
2. Kloth L, Morrison MA, Ferguson BH. *Therapeutic Microwave and Shortwave Diathermy: A Review of Thermal Effectiveness, Safe Use, and State of the Art: 1984.* Food and Drug Administration, U.S. Department of health and Human Services; December 1984. HHS Publication FDA 85–8237.
3. Thom H. *Introduction to Shortwave and Microwave Therapy.* Springfield, IL: Charles C Thomas; 1966.
4. Lehmann JF, De Lateur BJ. Diathermy and superficial heat laser, and cold therapy. In: Kottke FJ, Lehmann JF, eds. *Krusen's Handbook of Physical Medicine and Rehabilitation.* Philadelphia, PA: WB Saunders; 1990.
5. Guy AW. Biophysics of high frequency currents and electromagnetic radiation. In: Lehmann JF, ed. *Therapeutic Heat and Cold.* Baltimore, MD: Williams & Wilkins; 1990.
6. Guy AW, Lehmann JF, Stonebridge JB. Therapeutic application of electromagnetic power. *Proc IEEE.* 1974; 62:55–75.
7. Lehmann JF, Guy AW, Stonebridge JB, et al. *Review of Evidence for Indications, Techniques of Application, Contraindications, Hazards, and Clinical Effectiveness of Shortwave Diathermy.* Food and Drug Administration, U.S. Department of Health and Human Services; 1974. Report No. FDA/HFK–71–1.
8. Paetzold J. Physical laws regarding distribution of energy for various high frequency methods applied in heat therapy. *Ultrasonics Biol Medi.* 1964; 9(3):58–67.

9. Kebbel W, Krause W, Paetzold J. Composition of energy distribution in fat muscle layers of long decimeter waves and hi-frequency waves. *Elektromedizin Band.* 1964; 9:171–179.

10. Lehmann JF, McMillian JA, Brunner GD, et al. Heating patterns produced in specimens by microwaves of the frequency of 2,456 megacycles when applied with the "A", "B" and "C" directors. *Arch Phys Med Rehabil.* 1962; 43:538–546.

11. Fadilah R, Pinkas J, Weinberger A, et al. Healing rabbit joint by microwave applicator. *Arch Phys Med Rehabil.* 1987; 68:710–712.

12. Avery WR. Cell membranes: the electromagnetic environment and cancer promotion. *Neurochem Res.* 1988; 13:671–677.

13. Shore RE. Electromagnetic radiations and cancer. *Cancer.* 1988; 62(suppl):1747–1754.

14. Kloth L, Ziskin M. Diathermy and pulsed electromagnetic fields. In: Michlovitz S, ed. *Thermal Agents in Rehabilitation.* Philadelphia, PA: FA Davis; 1990.

15. Hayes K. *Manual for Physical Agents.* Norwalk, CT: Appleton & Lange; 1993.

16. Evans C, Brown TD. Role of physical and mechanical agents in degrading the matrix. In: Woessner JK, Howell DS, eds. *Joint Cartilage Degradation: Basic and Clinical Aspects.* New York: Marcel Dekker; 1993.

17. Cassvan A. Rehabilitative measures in arthritis and related conditions. *Osteopath Ann.* February 1977; 78–87.

18. Lehmann JF, Masock AJ, Warren CG, et al. Effects of therapeutic temperatures on tendon extensibility. *Arch Phys Med.* 1970; 51:481–487.

19. Warren CG, Lehmann JF, Koblanski JN. Elongation of rat tail tendon: effect of load and temperature. *Arch Phys Med.* 1971; 52:465–474.

20. Lehmann JF, Warren CG, Scham SM. Therapeutic heat and cold. *Clin Orthop Rel Res.* 1974; 99:207–245.

21. Shimm DJ, Gerner E. Hyperthermia in treatment of malignancies. In: Lehmann JF, ed. *Therapeutic Heat and Cold.* Baltimore, MD: Williams & Wilkins; 1990.

22. Silverman C. Epidemiologic studies of microwave effects. *Proc IEEE.* 1980; 68:78–84.

23. Michaelson SM. Bioeffects of high frequency currents and electromagnetic radiation. In: Lehmann JF, ed. *Therapeutic Heat and Cold.* Baltimore, MD: Williams & Wilkins; 1990.

24. Stuchly MA, Repacholi MH, LeCuyer DW, et al. Exposure to the operator and patient during short wave diathermy treatments. *Health Physics.* 1982; 42:341–366.

25. Moseley H, Davison M. Exposure of physiotherapists to microwave radiation during microwave diathermy treatment. *Clin Phys Physiol Meas.* 1981; 2:217–221.

26. Hamburger S, Logue JN, Silverman PM. Occupational exposure to non-ionizing radiation and as association with heart disease: an exploratory study. *J Chron Dis.* 1983; 36:791–802.

27. Lehmann JF, McDougall JA, Guy AW et al. Heating patterns produced by shortwave diathermy applicators in tissue substitute models. *Arch Phys Med Rehabil.* 1983; 64:575–577.

13

Ultrasound

Ronald W. Sweitzer, PT, MS

Ultrasound, a form of acoustic energy, is often used by physical therapists because of its deep-heating and pain-relieving effects. In 1980 Stewart et al[1] estimated that 15 million ultrasound treatments are given each year in hospital settings alone. The frequent use of this modality is probably related to its large number of indications and few contraindications or detrimental effects, its relative ease of application, and its clinically reported success. A thorough understanding of ultrasound as a physical agent is necessary to ensure safe and effective treatments. The purpose of this chapter is to educate the reader not only in the basic physics and physiological effects of ultrasound but also in specific techniques and clinical applications of this modality.

Sound waves are mechanical pressure waves that are described in terms of their frequency. Audible sound has an approximate frequency range of 20 to 20,000 cycles per second or Hertz.[2] Ultrasound waves have frequencies greater than 20,000 Hz. The most common frequency used in therapeutic ultrasound is 1 MHz (1 million Hertz), although other frequencies, such as .98 MHz, are currently being introduced. Ultrasound units with a lower frequency (.87 MHz) are believed to be more effective in treating deeper tissues, whereas units with a higher frequency (3 MHz) are believed to be more effective in treating more superficial tissues. Dual-frequency ultrasound generators are sold at a higher price than are single-frequency units. It would be advantageous for all clinics to have at least one dual frequency generator to allow greater variability of treatment parameters and a subsequent improvement in the ability to treat a larger number of conditions and tissues. Throughout this discussion, the term ultrasound refers to clinical units that generate 1 MHz unless stated otherwise. These units should not be confused with diagnostic units, which are used as an evaluative tool in medicine.

INSTRUMENTATION AND BIOPHYSICS

A basic description of how ultrasound is produced will introduce the reader to the physical characteristics of ultrasonic energy. The ultrasound generator uses common house current, 60 Hz at 110 volts, as a power source. The conversion of this electrical energy to ultrasonic energy occurs in the following steps: (1) a transformer boosts the voltage from 110 to 200 to 300 volts, (2) an oscillating circuit converts the incoming frequency to the desired higher frequency, (3) the modified electrical energy is transmitted through a coaxial cable to the transducer, and (4) the transducer converts the high-frequency electrical energy to ultrasonic energy.

Transducer

Ultrasound is delivered to the patient through the sound head or applicator. In most units, the applicator consists of a metal face plate with a piezoelectric crystal cemented to it. The crystal is a transducer, a device that converts one form of energy into another: in this case, from electrical energy to ultrasonic energy. This conversion occurs through a reverse piezoelectric effect. A piezoelectric effect is the phenomenon of developing an electric charge on certain crystals by applying mechanical pressure to them. The reverse piezoelectric effect is the production of mechanical energy by imposing electric charges across a crystal. When a direct current voltage is applied across a crystal, the crystal is deformed in one direction. The crystal will remain deformed as long as the current flows continually in that direction. The degree of deformation is proportional to the amount of voltage applied across the crystal. When alternating current is applied, such as in the generation of ultrasound, the crystal deformation changes direction as the flow of current changes direction. The crystal becomes thicker during one-half of the AC cycle and thinner during the other half of the cycle as the current changes direction. The reverse piezoelectric effect allows the use of mechanical vibrations of the crystal.

These oscillations produce pressure waves that are known as ultrasound waves (see Fig. 13–1).

Synthetic ceramic crystals of lead zirconate titanate or barium titanate are used most commonly because of their lower cost and lower voltage requirements. Quartz crystals, which require 2000–3000 volts for activation, were originally used because of their natural piezoelectric properties.

Characteristics of Ultrasound Waves

The frequency of ultrasound waves is predetermined by the frequency of the modified current delivered to the soundhead from the oscillating circuit. A natural relationship exists between the frequency and the velocity, as defined by the formula

$$V = \lambda f,$$

where V is velocity, f is frequency, and λ is wavelength. Once the frequency of the energy waves is established, the energy is propagated throughout a medium at that frequency. The velocity of sound waves (1) is related to the physical properties of the medium through which it travels and (2) changes as the densities of tissue change. Acoustic energy travels best through a solid medium and cannot be transmitted through a vacuum. The average velocities for sound waves through different media include the following: 3360 meters/second in bone, 1500 meters/second in water and soft tissues, and 330 meters/second in air at sea level.[3]

Ultrasound travels poorly through air. Air transmits the vibratory energy from the transducer so poorly that the excessive, nondispersed, mechanical energy may cause physical damage to the crystal or to the seal around it if the ultrasound is directed into the air rather than into body tissue or another medium. To prevent this from occurring, a coupling medium is needed between the transducer and the skin. The couplant, usually a gel or water, replaces the air that lies on the skin and in the pores. The couplant also acts as a surface lubricant to allow the applicator to glide easily.

The primary mode of propagation of ultrasound in soft tissues is the longitudinal, or compressional wave. This type of wave produces movement of molecules in the same direction as the flow of energy. Therefore, the flow of activated molecules will be parallel to each other and to the flow of energy. The analogy of a piston moving forward and backward may help to illustrate the concept of a piezoelectric crystal expanding and contracting to produce a longitudinal wave. Imagine a piston at one end of a closed tube containing a fluid medium. If the piston is at rest, the fluid density should be uniform throughout the tube. The piston now moves forward, causing compression of adjacent molecules, which actually increases the density in this area. The molecules are actually pushed forward, exert-

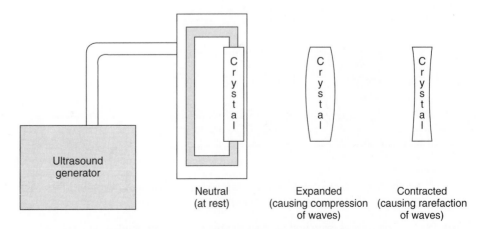

Figure 13–1. The production of ultrasound waves.

ing compressive force on the molecules lying in their paths. Now withdraw the piston to its starting point; this removes the compressive force and produces a decreased density or rarefaction of molecules in the immediate area. The cycle is repeated and another wave of compression and rarefaction occurs (see Fig. 13–2).

The waves will be propagated in the medium until the energy is absorbed. Consider the ultrasound crystal as the piston oscillating back and forth 1 million times per second. When in contact with a patient, compression and rarefaction of the molecules of the body occur. This molecular flow that occurs parallel to the direction of wave propagation can be referred to as microstreaming of molecules. One can create a similar, but visible, streaming effect by holding the ultrasound applicator just below the surface of water in a basin. Direct the ultrasound waves parallel to the surface and gradually increase the intensity. Notice a streaming and rippling effect, which increases as the intensity is raised. Ultrasound is transmitted in a straight line, as if in a cylinder, when it first leaves the transducer. This area of the ultrasound beam closest to the transducer is referred to as the near field or Fresnel zone. As the energy travels farther from the transducer, the waves begin to diverge. This point of divergence is the start of the far field or Fraunhofer zone (see Fig. 13–3).

Another type of ultrasound wave that may occur in the body is the shear or transverse wave, which causes particle oscillation perpendicular to the direction of the wave propagation. Shear waves are produced by frictional forces of molecules contacting other molecules as they pass by. Production of shear waves can occur effectively only in solid media. It is the solid state of a substance rather than its chemical composition that allows propagation of shear waves. Ice can conduct shear waves, whereas water cannot. Solids have strong three-dimensional intramolecular bonding, which allows transverse forces to be transmitted. Williams[4]

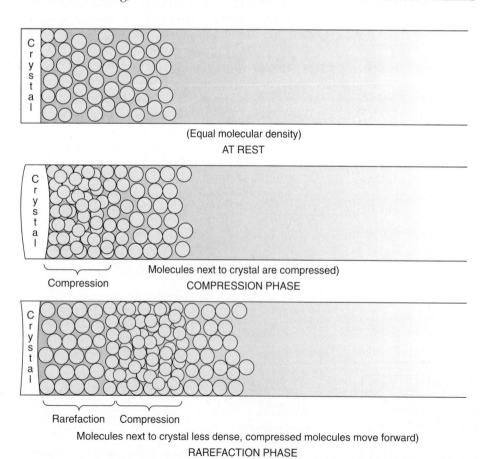

(Equal molecular density)
AT REST

Compression — Molecules next to crystal are compressed)
COMPRESSION PHASE

Rarefaction   Compression
Molecules next to crystal less dense, compressed molecules move forward)
RAREFACTION PHASE

Figure 13–2. The compression and rarefaction phases of the longitudinal wave. The cycles repeat as the piezoelectric crystal continues to expand and contract.

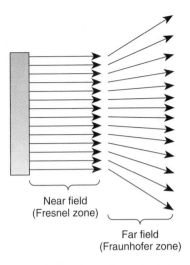

Near field
(Fresnel zone)

Far field
(Fraunhofer zone)

Figure 13–3. The Fresnel and Fraunhofer zones. When ultrasound first leaves the transducer, it is transmitted in a straight line in the area known as the near field (Fresnel zone). As the energy travels farther from the transducer, the waves begin to diverge in the area known as the far field (Fraunhofer zone).

gave the following example: If you hold a steel bar at one end and twist it, the other end will also twist. If you put your hand into a cylinder of water and try to twist the water, no twisting will occur at the opposite end of the column. Liquids, with their weaker intramolecular bonds, are ineffective transmitters of shear waves. The shear wave is not considered to transmit ultrasonic energy or produce heating in the soft tissue of the body.[5] In the body, the shear wave has a role in heating bone, particularly when striking the bone from an oblique angle of incidence.[6]

Biophysical Characteristics

Ultrasound has some of the same characteristics as radiant energy. It can be transmitted, absorbed, reflected, and refracted. The type of tissue that the energy affects and the angle of incidence of the energy will determine the nature of each characteristic.

Ultrasound is transmitted most effectively through a homogeneous medium. A highly homogeneous and dense medium such as steel will transmit ultrasonic energy in a relatively straight pathway at a high velocity. A less homogeneous and low-density medium such as water will allow less transmission at a lower velocity. Transmissiveness is directly related to depth of penetration. If an adequate power supply is available, a highly transmissive medium will allow for a deep penetration. The effective depth of penetration for therapeutic ultrasound is generally considered to be from 3–5 cm.[7,8]

Depth of penetration is inversely related to the frequency of the ultrasonic energy. The lower the frequency, the deeper the penetration. As the frequency increases, more attenuation occurs and consequently less energy will be available for penetration to the deeper tissues. Griffin and Karselis[8] reported that 90 KHz ultrasound penetrated soft tissue twice as far as 1 MHz. They found a penetration of 10 centimeters versus 5 centimeters, respectively. Conversely, 6 MHz ultrasound will not penetrate beyond the depth of the skin.[9] It appears that the 1 MHz frequency of the commercially available ultrasound generators allows adequate depth of penetration to treat most soft-tissue problems without posing the potential risks associated with the greater penetrating abilities and cavitational potential of the low-frequency generators. The dangers of cavitation will be discussed later.

Attenuation refers to the combination of absorption and scattering of ultrasonic energy as it passes through a medium. Scattering refers to the production of spherical waves that radiate the reflected ultrasound in all directions. As ultrasonic energy strikes a tiny reflecting surface such as a cell nucleus, which is smaller than the wavelength of the incident energy, scattering occurs. Scattering occurs in all living tissues because of the nonhomogeneous composition of different cellular structures. Tiny blood vessels or cell nuclei are examples of scattering structures within living tissue. Attenuation coefficients have been determined for various substances. Two substances may have similar attenuation coefficients but may possess different proportions of absorption and scattering. Attenuation coefficients increase as the frequency of the ultrasound increases. Therefore, as the frequency of ultrasound increases, absorption and scattering occur at a higher rate, resulting in less energy being available for penetration to the deeper tissues.

Depth of penetration also is inversely related to the coefficient of absorption of the medium. If energy is absorbed, it is no longer available for penetration. According to Piersol et al[10] the tissue with the highest protein content demonstrates the highest absorption of ultrasonic energy. These authors have listed several body tissues according to their absorption coefficients. Wells[11] compiled a similar list of absorption coefficients showing that tissues with a high collagen content demonstrate the highest absorption. Both sources list the following tissues in order from highest to lowest in their ability to absorb ultrasound: bone, peripheral nerve, skeletal muscle, fat, blood, and water. Frizzell and Dunn[12] added cartilage and tendon to the list between bone and skeletal muscle. The clinical significance of this information is that ultrasound will be transmitted relatively well through water and fat with little absorption of the energy. For heating to occur, the ultrasound must be absorbed. A more detailed discussion of heating will follow.

Reflection and Refraction

Reflection and refraction occur when ultrasound is transmitted from a material of one density to material of another density. The angle of reflection equals the angle of incidence. If a wave has a 60° angle of incidence from the left, it will be reflected at a 60° angle to the right. If the angle of incidence is perpendicular to the surface, reflection will occur directly toward the source (see Fig. 13–4).

If the ultrasound source is stationary, energy waves can be cyclicly transmitted and reflected to and from the source. When energy waves overlap, summation of the energy occurs when the waves are in phase. If overlapping ultrasonic energy waves reach equilibrium, they become standing waves. Standing waves are poten-

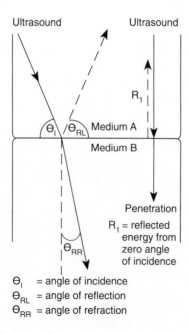

Θ_I = angle of incidence
Θ_{RL} = angle of reflection
Θ_{RR} = angle of refraction

Figure 13–4. Reflection and refraction of sound waves.

tially hazardous to biological tissues because high concentrations of energy are produced when multiple waves are in phase.

Refraction, the deflection of energy waves, depends on the changes in velocity and wavelength that occur when ultrasound passes from one medium to another. When ultrasound is transmitted from a high-density medium to a lower-density medium, the velocity and wavelength decrease while the angle of refraction becomes less than the angle of incidence (see Fig. 13–4). In the body, reflection, refraction, and attenuation occur largely at tissue interfaces. These interfaces include (1) fat to muscle, (2) muscle to fascia, (3) tendon to periosteum, and (4) ligament to periosteum. The proportion of reflection to refraction depends on the acoustic impedances of the materials or tissues on each side of the interface. Acoustic impedance (z) is the product of the density (ρ) of a material and the velocity (v) of the sound waves in it. Thus,[4]

$$z = \rho v.$$

For a more detailed description of acoustic impedance, the reader is referred to Williams.[4]

Thermal Responses

Ultrasound is used primarily for its deep heating effects. For heating of tissues to occur, the energy must be absorbed. The absorption of the high-frequency vibrational energy results in the production of heat. Transmission, reflection, and refraction are means by which the ultrasonic energy is distributed to the various tissues in different patterns; they should not be confused with heat production. However, if standing waves are produced because of reflection at an interface—for example, between bone and ligament—a greater energy concentration is available for absorption by the tissue between the transducer and the reflecting surface. However, not all reflections result in standing waves. If a tissue has a high concentration of ultrasound energy and a relatively high absorption coefficient, it has the potential to produce a strong thermal response. This is the case at the myofascial or tenoperiosteal interfaces. Fat, on the other hand, is a homogeneous tissue with a low absorption coefficient; therefore, it transmits ultrasound effectively without being heated significantly. This low heat-producing ability in fat is considered an advantage of using ultrasound rather than the electromagnetic diathermies to heat deep tissues.

One should not assume that the tissue with the highest absorption coefficient will be the hottest. Although thermal energy can be produced in the tissue, the following factors also contribute to the total tissue temperature rise (TTR): (1) the rate at which energy is applied and the length of time it is applied, (2) the thermal conductivity, and (3) the rate of perfusion of blood to tissue.

The rate at which energy is applied is controlled by the *intensity adjustment* and the *mode of application* of the ultrasound. If the intensity of ultrasound is too low, energy required to produce a significant TTR will be inadequate. If the energy is applied at an extremely high intensity, the local thermal response may be so great and sudden that pain from overheating will occur before heat can be conducted away from the local area to produce a more general TTR. Lehmann et al[13] demonstrated this result in a study of human thighs exposed to ultrasound. The results of the study indicated that for ultrasound to heat the soft tissue adjacent to the bone effectively, the energy level must be (1) kept low enough to allow the energy to heat the bone and soft tissue to a safe, pain-free level, (2) high enough to allow adequate depth of penetration, and (3) applied long enough to allow for conduction of the heat away from the bone into the surrounding tissue. While this conductive heating is occurring, time will also be available for more energy absorption and thus conversive heating directly into the soft tissues. If the energy is applied too quickly, heat production will be so rapid that the thermal nocicepters of the body will be stimulated. The patient's painful response will require a withdrawal of the ultrasound before a general TTR in the surrounding soft tissue can be produced.

The second consideration is thermal conductivity. For example, bone has a higher thermal conductivity than surrounding tissues. With its high absorption coefficient, bone does not become proportionately hotter than the muscle or tendon lying next to it. As the energy is absorbed, the heat produced is quickly dissipated throughout the bone to the cooler, nonsonated areas. Another reason that excessive bone temperatures are not observed is that about 20% to 30% of the incident energy striking bone is reflected into the surrounding tissue.[14] This reflected energy is available to be absorbed by the soft tissue rather than the bone.

The third consideration is the rate of blood perfusion in the tissues. If a local body tissue with an impaired circulation is heated, it may not be able to dissipate the excess heat. Therefore, the risk of thermal injury to the tissue is higher than it would be if the circulation were normal. For example, a healthy muscle belly will be less likely to suffer thermal injury than would a poorly vascularized tendon. The vascularity of tissue must be considered when determining the dosage level for ultrasound.

Nonthermal Responses

Suggested nonthermal effects of ultrasound include (1) micromassage, (2) increased membrane permeability, (3) arteriolar vasoconstriction or dilation, and (4) cavitation. Nonthermal effects, sometimes described as mechanical effects, are changes that are not related to heat production.

Micromassage. The term *micromassage* refers to the microscopic movement or oscillations of the body fluids and tissues as a result of exposure to ultrasound. The term was used as early as 1942 to describe the action of ultrasound.[15] The other nonthermal effects of ultrasound are probably produced as a result of this micromassage to the body tissues.

Increased membrane permeability. Acoustic streaming has been described as a mechanism that induces changes in diffusion rates and *membrane permeability.*[7] The ultrasound causes a stirring effect in the fluid near a biological membrane. This agitation of the ions increases the ionic concentration gradient, thereby accelerating the diffusion rate. These mechanical effects were similarly documented by analyzing membrane potentials that were altered by exposure to ultrasound.[16]

Lota and Darling[16] demonstrated that the membrane permeability of erythrocytes to potassium increased because of mechanical rather than thermal effects. Dyson et al[17] suggested that streaming might be an important mechanism in tissue regeneration because of its effect on weak secondary bonds in the tissue. They hypothesized that the making and breaking of these bonds, which are important to enzyme activity necessary for tissue repair, are enhanced by the types of stresses placed on them during streaming. So far, the scientific documentation for this theory is inadequate.

Further evidence supports changes in membrane permeability during exposure to ultrasound. Coble and Dunn[18] observed changes in frog skin that suggested changes in membrane permeability. Mortimer and colleagues, in a series of experimental studies,[19–21] confirmed changes in membrane transport by documenting changes in the action potential of cardiac muscle and increased oxygen transport through frog skin and silastic membranes. In the last study the changes occurred in the absence of a temperature rise or transient cavitation. This further confirms the non-thermal effect of ultrasound on membrane transport.

Arteriolar vasoconstriction or dilation. The nonthermal effect of arteriolar vasoconstriction or vasodilation is not clear. Hogan et al[22] used pulsed ultrasound at supraclinical intensities of 5–10 W/sq cm with a stationary technique to demonstrate vasoconstriction of the smallest arterioles of rat cremaster muscle. They later used pulsed ultrasound at a clinical intensity to demonstrate arteriolar vasodilation and increased opening of capillary beds in chronically ischemic muscles.[23]

These results were obtained in the absence of thermal responses. The mechanism that produced the above reactions is unknown. Results from these reports may encourage clinicians to use nonthermal ultrasound in the clinical intensity range. However, much more research is needed before any conclusions can be reached.

Cavitation. Cavitation, the most widely known of the nonthermal responses, refers to the formation and collapse of gas- or vapor-filled cavities in liquids.[24] It occurs within the biologic system when small gas pockets, (bubbles) are subjected to the compression and rarefaction cycles of ultrasound. As the bubble grows to a stable size, characteristic of the resonant frequency, it pulsates in the sound field and is considered to be a stable cavity. This stage is not destructive but, with further sonation, induced microstreaming may produce increased cellular stress and disruption. As the bubble or cavity grows larger, the tissue membrane becomes thinner and more fragile. If a compression wave causes a collapse of the cavity, transient cavitation has occurred. Transient cavitation causes spotty cell destruction and tissue damage. It should be noted that cavitation occurs much more readily in vitro than in vivo. That is, transient cavitation will occur at therapeutic intensities in a suspension of cells in a laboratory but not in intact tissues.[25] Cavitational thresholds are much more attainable when using low-frequency ultrasound. For example, at a frequency of 10 KHz, cavitation may occur in vitro at 0.1–1 W/sq cm; at a frequency of 1 MHz, however, 100 W/sq cm may be required to produce the same level of cavitation. Most research states that transient cavitation will not occur in the body using a 1 MHz frequency at therapeutic frequencies of less than 3 W/sq cm.[4]

Williams[4] agreed that transient cavitation has not been convincingly demonstrated in vivo at therapeutic intensities and frequencies. However, he cautioned that stable cavitation has been documented within the therapeutic range. Nonacoustic factors, such as muscular exercise and muscular contraction induced by electrical stimulation, enhance the formation of gas bubble. Williams implied that it may be more hazardous to apply the combination treatment of ultrasound with electrical stimulation than to apply each treatment individually. Therefore, to justify the use of electrical stimulation with ultrasound, further research is needed to show that the combination treatment is more effective then the individual techniques.

CLINICAL USES

Ultrasound is used clinically to treat various conditions. For clarity, the effect of ultrasound on inflammation, pain, edema, tissue healing, circulation, and extensibility of collagen tissue are discussed separately. However, the goal, when possible, should be to restore tissue function rather than to treat symptoms alone.

Inflammation

Following an injury, the body tries to repair itself. The first stage of this process is acute inflammation. The area of damage becomes walled off, and the flow of fluid into the extracellular space eventually ceases. The tissue remains swollen because the excessive extracellular fluid and waste products have not been reabsorbed by the body. Next, the body must begin to lay down collagen tissue to strengthen the weakened area. However, if the acute inflammation becomes excessive, tissue damage and scarring occur as a result of uncontrolled edema. Frequently, the collagen tissue, commonly called scar tissue, is distributed in a manner that impairs the normal function of the tissue.[15] The end result for the patient is a chronic condition resulting from periodic microtearing and further scarring. Ultrasound is widely used to treat conditions related to the effect of inflammation on tissue. With its dual effect (thermal and mechanical), ultrasound may prevent the development of chronic conditions. The fact that ultrasound should not be used at an intensity that would produce a temperature rise in the acute inflammatory process should be obvious. However, one can consider the use of ultrasound at extremely low intensities or in the pulsed mode during the acute phase of inflammation. The non-thermal micromassage and alteration of tissue permeability may be beneficial to enhance reabsorption of interstitial fluid. Enhanced reabsorption from ultrasound was demonstrated by Reid et al[26] in their treatment of experimentally produced hematoma in rabbit's ear.

Pain and Nerve Conduction Velocities

The concept of pain remains elusive and has been described differently by many authors (see Chapter 4). Wyke[27] described pain as "an abnormal emotional state that is aroused by unusual patterns of activity in specific afferent systems." This emotional situation is created by activation of a nociceptive afferent system. However, many factors are involved in interpreting a patient's report of pain. Although it is important to relieve a patient's pain to allow for increased function, one must not assume that because pain is absent, healing has occurred. The pain may be temporarily masked.

Numerous clinical studies describe the effectiveness of ultrasound in relieving the pain of bursitis, tendonitis, osteoarthritis, and other musculoskeletal conditions. In addition to considering the direct effect of ultrasound on an injured tissue, the reader should examine the effect of ultrasound on nerves to understand the mechanisms of pain that are possibly related to ultrasonic therapy. Pain relief is often associated with an increase in temperature. Ultrasound was shown to raise pain thresholds in human subjects similar to the level produced by raising tissue temperature by other means.[28]

Szumski[29] summarized the effects of ultrasound on nervous tissue as follows: (1) it selectively heats peripheral nerves, (2) it may alter or block impulse conduction, (3) it may increase membrane permeability, and (4) it may increase tissue metabolism. He pointed out that any of these mechanisms may occur from heating and may effect pain relief. Pain impulses are transmitted by small-diameter axons. Anderson et al[30] established that B and C type fibers are more sensitive to ultrasound than is the A type. Perhaps this selective absorption by smaller fibers allows for decreases in pain transmission (see Chapter 4).

On the basis of studies on the effect of ultrasound on the conduction velocities of motor and sensory nerves, some authors have suggested a relationship between changes in nerve conduction velocities and pain. This relationship may or may not be explained by the thermal effects of ultrasound alone. Some initial studies of motor nerve conduction velocities (MNCV) showed that when certain intensities of ultrasound were applied over peripheral nerves, a reduction in nerve conduction velocity occurred, whereas an increase in MNCV occurred at other intensities. Zankel[31] found no significant reduction of ulnar MNCV at 1 W/sq cm applied for 5 minutes to the flexor forearm but did find a significant decrease in MNCV after 10 minutes or by applying 2 W/sq cm for 5 minutes. Farmer[32] found a decrease in MNCV when the intensity range was 1–2 W/sq cm, but found an increase in MNCV when 3 W/sq cm was applied to the ulnar nerve. These results can not be explained but indicate that there is more than just a thermal effect on nerve. Although the above authors did not report changes in tissue temperature, one would expect an increase at the intensities of 1–2 W/sq cm.[33] Why the above differences occurred is not understood.

Studies performed on sensory nerves are more supportive of a parallel relationship between increased temperature and increased sensory nerve conduction velocity (SNCV).[34] This has been supported by several studies on SNCV. Currier et al[35] exposed the lateral cutaneous branch of the radial nerves of five men to 1.5 W/sq cm for 5 minutes and found that the speed of conduction increased as the subcutaneous temperature increased. Similarly, Halle et al[36] demonstrated an increase in conduction of superficial radial nerve associated with an increase in subcutaneous temperature. Consentino et al[37] attempted to clarify the previous findings with a study on the sensory fibers of the median nerve. However, they were unable to show any significant difference between the control group and the experimental groups, which received ultrasound at 0.5, 1, or 1.5 W/sq cm for 10 minutes.

The studies reported here have been presented as evidence that changes in nerve conduction velocity do occur. One can only hypothesize that these changes, whether through thermal or nonthermal mechanisms, may reduce pain in patients.

Edema

Subacute inflammatory edema can be treated by the physical therapist in the following ways: (1) compression, (2) massage, (3) ice, (4) electrical stimulation, (5) heat, and (6) ultrasound for its thermal and nonthermal effects. Middlemast and Chattergee[38] reported better reduction of swelling, tenderness, and pain in soft-tissue lesions by using ultrasound rather than other forms of heat such as short-wave diathermy, infrared radiation, and paraffin baths.

Tissue Healing

Ultrasound has been found to enhance tissue repair in both subcutaneous injuries and open wounds. Vanharant et al[39] had limited success in producing a long-term rise in glycosaminoglycan (GAG) metabolism in normal adult rabbit knees after 5 days of treatment with ultrasound through water at 1 W/sq cm for 5 minutes. GAG is a product of connective tissue cells and can be used as an indicator of metabolic activity. Concentrations in articular cartilage, menisci, and collateral ligaments were unaltered one day after the last treatment. The only significant finding—an increase in radioactivity in the medial collateral ligament in the treated knees—reflects increased metabolic activity. These authors evaluated the response in normal rather than pathological tissue.

Stratton et al[40] discovered an increase in the number of tissue repair cells—macrophages, lymphocytes, fibroblasts, endothelial cells, and myoblasts—in sonated rat thighs. Collagen, required for tissue strengthening, also was increased in the sonated group. The significant number of healing cells was present only in the group sonated with continuous ultrasound at 1.5 W/sq cm. Lower intensities and pulsed ultrasound were ineffective. Young and Dyson[41] used lower intensities of 0.1 W/sq cm at 0.75 MHz and 3 MHz to increase the responsiveness of macrophages in vitro. They also used 0.5 W/sq cm at 0.75 MHz and 3 MHz to increase granulation tissue and fibroblasts in the first 5 days after experimentally produced full-thickness lesions in rat skin. They suggested that ultrasound is useful in accelerating the inflammatory and early proliferative stages of repair.[42] Young and Dyson's study may support the use of higher intensities to promote healing after the acute stages.

Open wounds also may benefit from treatment with ultrasound. In 1960 Paul et al[43] reported clinical success in completely healing 13 of 23 pressure sores and significantly improving 5 others. Since then, various controlled studies have documented the effectiveness of ultrasound in wound repair. Shamberger[44] summarized several studies demonstrating that tissue healing increased after treatment with ultrasound as compared with a control group. Some studies measured wound size; others measured tensile strength or fibroblast proliferation. Dyson and colleagues[17,45] documented increased tissue regeneration in rabbit ears and in chronic varicose ulcers in humans as the result of treatment with ultrasound. They theoretically attributed the increased rate of healing to ultrasound-induced protein synthesis and perhaps to the vibrational micromassaging effect, which may reduce edema and thus facilitate repair. Dyson and her colleagues used 3 MHz ultrasound rather than the common 1 MHz clinical frequency. In a clinical report, Ferguson and Noel[46] described the use of pulsed ultrasound, 0.5 W/sq cm at 1 MHz for 3 minutes, in the treatment of episiotomy wounds on the first and second postoperative days. They claimed that hematomas were resolved more quickly and that patients reported a soothing effect on the pain.

Not all studies have confirmed accelerated healing as a result of ultrasound exposure. Eriksson et al[47] found no significant difference in the proportion of area of healed chronic leg ulcers between an experimental group and a placebo group. They used 1 MHz ultrasound at 1 W/sq cm by direct contact for 10 minutes. Compared with the results of Vanharanto et al's[39] underwater technique, the effective intensity was higher and the exposure time was longer in Eriksson et al's study. Their study also was done on chronic human ulcers rather than on fresh animal lesions.

Enwemeka's research[48] supports the use of ultrasound to promote tendon healing. He emphasized that identification of all correct parameters of application must be addressed for successful results. In 1989 he treated rabbit Achilles tendons in deionized water with 1 MHz continuous ultrasound at 1 W/sq cm for 5 minutes with a moving sound head technique. The ultrasound was applied daily for the first nine postoperative days. The results showed an increase in overall tensile strength of the tendons because of increased cross-sectional area in the sonated tendons. In 1990 Enwemeka et al[49] repeated these studies using 0.5 W/sq cm of continuous ultrasound instead of 1 W/sq cm and produced greater increases in tensile strength and capacity for energy absorption after sonation. Jackson et al[50] also found increased breaking strength and collagen synthesis in rat Achilles tendons in the first 5 to 9 days of treatment with ultrasound. They treated puncture wounds and used 1.5 W/sq cm of continuous ultrasound with a stationary sound head technique under water for 4 minutes. Although these authors obtained favorable results, a stationary technique should not be used in the clinic.

The studies on tendon healing just described emphasize the effectiveness of clinical doses of ultrasound for tendon repair immediately after the injury. Prolonged use of ultrasound may be of no value or even harmful. Turner et al[51] found no significant difference between treated and untreated tendons after 5 weeks of treatment given three times a week. Roberts et al[52] demonstrated reduced strength and healing in surgically repaired tendon after treatment with pulsed ultrasound of 0.8 W/sq cm at 1.1 MHz after 5 minutes per day for 6 weeks.

Circulation

Ultrasound-induced heating has been shown to increase local circulation by both direct and reflex means. In 1953 Bickford and Duff[53] reported an increase in blood flow after ultrasound at intensities high enough to heat tissue. This finding was supported by other investigators.[54-56] Abramson et al[57] demonstrated increased blood flow 26 minutes after the termination of experimental ultrasound treatments. Lota[58] not only demonstrated that as tissue temperature increases, so does blood flow, but also demonstrated that a reflex vasodilation may be initiated by the application of ultrasound. He sonated the sympathetic lumbar ganglia in human subjects to produce an increase in superficial circulation to the big toe.

Extensibility of Collagen Tissue

Collagen tissue is an effective absorber of ultrasonic energy. Ligaments, joint capsules, and tendons (all high in collagen composition) are common sites of pathology for which ultrasound is indicated. These structures often lie deeper than the effective heating range of the diathermies and superficial heating modalities. Ultrasound may be the only clinical modality that can produce a TTR in these deeper structures, which are heated effectively because of their close proximity to bone and their high absorption coefficients. Lehmann et al[59] demonstrated the effectiveness of a stroking technique of continuous ultrasound at 1.5 W/sq cm for 5 minutes in heating intra-articular menisci and joint capsules in the knees of hogs. Lehmann et al[60] also studied the effect of heating on the extensibility of rat tail tendon. They found that the greatest increase in tendon length occurred when heat and sustained stretch were simultaneously applied and the stretch was maintained during the cool down period. This experimental model provides a rationale for using ultrasound and stretching for tight joints.

Ultrasound can be applied locally to the sites of small fibrous lesions to produce relaxation of the scar tissue. Griffin and Karselis[8] reported the relaxation of polypeptide bonds after the application of ultrasound. Relaxation of collagen tissue bonds would allow increased extensibility of the scar, which in turn would permit normal function of the joint, tendon, or muscle and subsequent pain reduction. While administering the ultrasound, the therapist also can stretch the tissue, which will further break up the scar.

Phonophoresis

Phonophoresis is the use of ultrasound to drive medications into body tissues. Hydrocortisone, dexamethasone, and lidocaine are the medications commonly administered by phonophoresis.[61] Williams[4] described the phonophoretic effect as a synergistic interaction of ultrasound and drugs. He documented the positive effects of phonophoresis with viricidal ointments, such as increased tissue regeneration in rabbit corneal ulcers following penicillin phonophoresis. The synergistic effect was also demonstrated by the increased clinical effectiveness of sonating soft tissue after injection of anti-inflammatory or analgesic medications. After the physician injected the drug into the inflamed periarticular structure, the physical therapist applied an ultrasound treatment over the same area. The ultrasound was assumed to have distributed the drug through the inflamed tissue and enhanced its absorption.[62,63]

Ultrasound also has increased penetration and absorption of topical medications into deeper tissues.[62,64] Griffin and colleagues[65,66] reported that phonophoresis was effective in driving hydrocortisone through the skin of pigs by measuring the cortisol levels in muscle and nerve. Griffin et al[67] later studied the effectiveness of hydrocortisone phonophoresis in patients with periarticular conditions. Sixty-eight percent of the subjects treated with phonophoresis showed significantly improved range of motion and decreased pain compared with only 28% who improved with ultrasound and a placebo instead of hydrocortisone.

The technique for phonophoresis is the same as a routine ultrasound treatment except that the medication is placed on the skin immediately over the target structure. The hydrocortisone should be combined with an aqueous base to form a 10% concentration. This must be prescribed by a physician and formulated by a pharmacist. Kleinkort and Wood[68] demonstrated the superiority of a 10% hydrocortisone preparation over a 1% mixture in the treatment of 285 patients with a variety of inflammatory conditions. The medications must be rubbed onto the skin before the normal coupling agent is applied. Effective clinical results have been achieved using intensities in a mid to high range of 1 W/sq cm to 2 W/sq cm.[67,68] However, phonophoresis of low intensity and long duration proved to be more effective in driving cortisol into pig muscle and nerve in a study involving only 10 subjects.[69] In contradiction to the above studies, Benson et al[70] failed to demonstrate enhanced absorption of benzydamine through phonophoresis. Additional studies are needed to document the most efficient mode of application for this noninvasive alternative to injection of medication into painful and inflamed structures.

INDICATIONS, CONTRAINDICATIONS, AND PRECAUTIONS

Indications

Ultrasound is indicated for the treatment of many musculoskeletal conditions. Only the most common indications are mentioned below. Many of these conditions have already been discussed in the text. Additional information is supplied for some conditions for which the treatment may not be obvious.

Contracture: Joint capsules or adhesive scars. Tightness and scarring of periarticular structures have a variety of causes. Adhesive scars result from excessive proliferation of collagen, which may occur secondary to a laceration, incision, or burn or may occur insidiously. Success in treating Dupuytren's contracture has been documented. Increased range of softening of the fibrous tissue has been accomplished with ultrasound.[71,72] In other conditions of fibrous hypertrophy, pain is a factor. Ultrasound has been reported to be effective in relieving pain, reducing curvature of the penis, and altering the consistency of the fibrous plaque in Peyronie's disease.[73,74]

Chronic arthritis. The pain of osteoarthritis and rheumatoid arthritis may be relieved by ultrasound, probably because of its deep heating ability.[75]

Periarticular conditions. The symptoms of bursitis, tendonitis, and ligamentous sprains may be relieved by ultrasound because of its thermal and possibly nonthermal effects.[76,77]

Muscular problems. The symptoms and decreased function of strains, spasm, fibrosis, myositis, and hematoma may be relieved by ultrasound.[78]

Neuromas. The pain of neuromas may be relieved by ultrasound because of its effects on nervous tissue. Griffin[8] stated that pain relief might be a result of relaxation of excessively proliferated connective tissue.

Sympathetic nervous system disorders. The reflex dystrophies, such as causalgia and Sudek's atrophy, can be treated by paravertebral sonation of the involved segments or underwater over the segment of hyperpathia.[79]

Plantar warts. Several authors reported success with the elimination of pain or the wart itself after exposure to ultrasound.[80–82] Vaughn,[80] in particular, reported excellent results with the direct contact technique at a mean intensity of 0.69 W/sq cm for 15 minutes. These findings are from clinical reports rather than controlled studies, however.

Open wounds. Refer to the discussion earlier in this chapter about pressure sores and tissue repair studies. Ultrasound can be administered to open wounds with a water immersion technique or with a direct contact technique using a sterile couplant.

Chronic systematic peripheral arterial disease. Griffin and Karselis[8] advocated sonation directly over vessels affected by vasospasm or sonation of the sympathetic nervous system. **Warning:** If signs of thrombophlebitis are present, direct sonation is contraindicated.[4]

Contraindications

There are relatively few contraindications for therapeutic ultrasound. Any condition for which a TTR is contraindicated will also be contraindicated for the use of ultrasound in a manner that will produce a thermal response. Refer to the list of contraindications to therapeutic heat in Chapter 11.

Cardiac pacemakers. If a pacemaker or its surrounding tissue is exposed to the ultrasound field, it may malfunction. Note that the use of ultrasound is not excluded for a distal part of the patient's body, where the sound field will not affect the pacemaker.[83]

Pregnancy. The effects of therapeutic ultrasound on the fetus are not known. Therefore, if pregnancy is suspected, avoid sonating the abdomen, pelvis and lumbar-sacral areas. Diagnostic ultrasound is not included in this contraindication.

Tumors. Whether a tumor is malignant or benign, sonation of the tumor is probably best avoided because the heat and mechanical energy may encourage metastasis. (**Note:** Ultrasound is being used experimentally to induce hyperthermia for destruction of tumor cells.[84]) It has also been used successfully to produce regression of psoriatic lesions, which are caused by benign hyperproliferative disease.[85]

Thrombophlebitis. The mechanical energy may disrupt a clot, resulting in the formation of an embolus that may travel to the brain, heart, or lungs.[83]

Infected areas. Ultrasound may promote the spread of infection.

Areas with a tendency to hemorrhage. Increased blood flow and capillary permeability produced by ultrasound may encourage bleeding.

Epiphyses of growing bone. Ultrasound has been shown to cause bone growth disturbances in experimental situations.[86]

In conjunction with deep x-ray, radium, or radioactive isotopes. There may be an interaction effect of low intensity ultrasound and ionizing radiation on surface tumor cells. Six months should pass after termination of radiation treatment before ultrasound treatment begins. Routine diagnostic x-rays are not included in this contraindication.[83]

Cardiac disease. Ultrasound over the cervical ganglia, stellate ganglia, or heart area may stimulate a coronary reflex that might be hazardous to a person with cardiac disease.[83]

Over the eyes. Ultrasound in this area may have a cavitational effect because of the fluid medium.[6]

Over the spinal cord in areas without adequate protection. In cases of laminectomy or other conditions that reduce the normal bony and muscular protection of the spinal cord, ultrasound may cause cavitation or overheating of the spinal fluid.[6]

Precautions

Unhealed fracture sites. Although Griffin and Karselis[8] stated that ultrasound over unhealed fractures is contraindicatory, they were unable to find further documentation. The effect of low-intensity ultrasound has been found to produce fibula osteotomies in rabbits. Pilla et al[87] used 1.5 MHz ultrasound delivered in 200 microsecond bursts at a burst frequency of 1 Khz and an intensity of about 30 mW/sq cm for 20 minutes from postoperative Day 1 to Day 28. Until further research is completed, however, routine clinical intensities over recent fractures should be avoided.

Primary repair of tendon or ligament. This also may include a partial tendon rupture in the early stages. (Refer to the section on tissue healing.)

Osteoporosis. Use ultrasound with caution over osteoporotic bones until research is available to rule out its detrimental effect on the already demineralized bone.

Plastic implants. High-density plastics used for joint replacements have high coefficients of absorption of ultrasonic energy. Theoretically, this factor would pose a potential risk. Although the risk has not been documented in any controlled studies or clinical reports, direct sonation over plastic implants should be avoided until it can be proved to be safe.[7]

Metal implants. Lehmann et al[88] investigated the acoustical properties of various metals used for surgical implants and found that a large amount of ultrasonic energy was reflected at the tissue-metal interface, thus creating standing waves of increased intensity in front of the metal. In addition, little penetration of sound occurred through the metal. Other studies using animal or human tissues have shown that no appreciable temperature rise occurred in the metal implant and that the soft tissues surrounding the isolated metal implant were actually heated less than if the bone had been present.[89,90] The most probable explanation relates to the high thermal conductivity of metal, which is able to transmit the heat generated at the metal tissue interface away from the sonated area more quickly than the heat can be produced.

Metal plates and screws are commonly used for the internal fixation of fractures. Does ultrasound have detrimental nonthermal effects on the strength of internal fixation? Skoubo-Kristenson and Sommer[91] implanted metal plates fastened by three cortical screws into the femura or humeri of dogs. After 2 weeks, half of the dogs were treated with low intensity (0.5 W/sq cm) ultrasound and the other half were treated with high intensity (3 W/sq cm) ultrasound for 5 minutes a day for 14 days. The authors found no significant difference in the torque used to insert the screws with the torque needed to remove the screws in the sonated and control groups. Thus, they supported the notion that internal fixation does not contraindicate the use of ultrasound therapy.

CONSIDERATIONS REGARDING THERAPEUTIC MODE AND DOSAGE

Continuous- Versus Pulsed-Wave Mode

Continuous wave ultrasound, as the name implies, is acoustic energy transmitted without interruption from the time the transducer is energized until the intensity control is returned to zero. *Pulsed-wave ultrasound* is acoustic energy with brief cyclical breaks in transmission throughout its application. These breaks in transmission reduce the overall amount of energy available to the patient for a given time interval compared with ultrasound at the same peak intensity. If 1 W/sq cm of pulsed ultrasound is applied for 1 minute, the patient receives less energy than if continuous ultrasound is applied at 1 W/sq cm for 1 minute. How much less energy depends on the ratio of on-time to off-time. This will be discussed in the section on intensity.

Many clinicians use the rationale that pulsed ultrasound produces only nonthermal effects because of the interruptions in transmission of energy. It would be more accurate to say that less heating occurs with pulsed ultrasound than with continuous ultrasound at similar peak intensities. It should be noted that similar thermal effects can be obtained if the same time average intensities are used. Lehmann et al[6] stated that there is no evidence that the use of pulsed ultrasound is more advantageous than is continuous ultrasound. The clinician can use extremely low intensities of continuous ultrasound to minimize its thermal effects. Perhaps the mode of ultrasound is less important than the average intensities and power used. However, the depth of penetration is a factor when choosing the pulsed or continuous mode. If the nonthermal effects of ultrasound are required in a deep tissue, a low duty cycle (20%) and a high spatial average intensity will allow the energy to penetrate to the deep target tissue without heating it.

Physical therapists must understand the characteristics of quantification of ultrasonic energy for several reasons: (1) to ensure the selection of the safe and appropriate intensity for the patient's condition, (2) to apply a consistent dosage from treatment to treatment, and (3) to keep accurate clinical records so that more reliable and meaningful descriptive information can be obtained about the clinical success and failure of ultrasound techniques. To be meaningful, these considerations require regular calibration of the ultrasound unit. The many inconsistencies in reports of clinical trials are probably related to lack of calibration and accurate documentation of dosages and techniques. Even with calibration, the dosage the patient receives at similar meter readings from different ultrasound units varies. This variation is the result of the fact that the meter reading represents the energy in the unit before it reaches the transducer and does not represent the net ultrasonic energy output of the transducer. The manufacturers of newer machines are addressing this issue.

The clinician must review the specifications dealing with power efficiency and accuracy and beam nonuniformity, not just price, when considering which new ultrasound unit to buy. We suggest setting priorities that would include the reliability and accuracy of the instrument. This may enhance the scientific base of the profession rather than perpetuate the trial-and-error type of practice resulting from the inconsistencies of instruments and techniques.

Power, measured in watts, is the amount of acoustic energy in the radiating beam per unit of time. The power value is the only indicator of the total amount of ultrasonic energy a patient receives. If a therapist treated a patient one day with an intensity of 1.5 W/sq cm with a 10 sq cm transducer, the patient would receive 15 watts of energy. If, on a subsequent day, the therapist treated the patient at 1.5 W/sq cm using an ultrasound unit with a 7 sq cm transducer, assuming the treated area is the same, the patient would receive only 10.5 watts of energy (1.5 W/sq cm × 7 sq cm), which may have produced a less effective second treatment. This example demonstrates the need to record both power and intensity in the patient's record. The term *time average power* is sometimes used with pulsed ultrasound generators to represent the total watts applied to the patient during a treatment.

Intensity

Intensity (I) is the term used most frequently when discussing ultrasound dosage. The more accurate term is *spatial average intensity*, which is the acoustic power (W) divided by the effective radiating area (ERA) (sq cm) of the transducer. In medical ultrasonics, the units are watts per square centimeter (W/sq cm). If 15 watts of acoustic energy is radiated from a crystal, the area of which is 10 square centimeters, the intensity is 1.5 W/sq cm, or

$$I = W/sq\ cm.$$

Intensity represents the strength of the acoustic energy at the point of application. The effective radiating area is not necessarily the same size as the metal face of the sound head, but rather the size of the radiating surface of the crystal within. The ERA should be stated in the specification list of each ultrasound generator. In general, the more acute the condition, the less the intensity should be.

Forrest and Rosen[92] demonstrated that the temperature of pig extensor tendon did not rise to nearly the same degree when sonation was done under tap water compared with sonation by direct contact. Because of the reduced efficiency of energy transmission by the immersion technique, these authors suggested an increase in dosage. Hayes[93] recommended an increase of 0.5 W/sq cm in the intensity for immersion versus direct contact. This is only a general guideline. The ultimate guide is the patient's response and clinical signs. Patients should not experience discomfort at any time. If they complain of an ache or a sudden stabbing pain, the intensity should be reduced or the sound head should be moved more quickly.

Duty Cycle

When pulsed ultrasound is used, the duty cycle must be considered to determine the overall amount of energy the patient receives. *Duty cycle* is a percentage or ratio of the pulse duration (on-time of the pulse) to the pulse period (the sum of the on- and off-time of the pulse during each cycle). Fig. 13–5 shows two different pulse modulations being applied at the same spatial average intensities. The raised rectangles represent the flow of energy, the on-time; the return to baseline begins the rest period, the off-time.

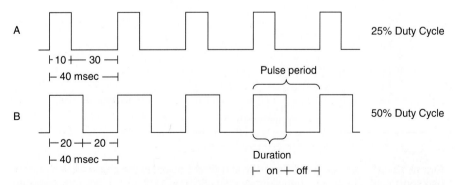

Figure 13–5. Pulse modulation of ultrasound energy. Modulation B provides twice as much energy as modulation A because its on-time is twice as long.

In Fig. 13–5, which modulation is providing the most ultrasound to the patient? How much more energy is modulation B providing than is modulation A during the same time period? Modulation B is providing twice as much energy as modulation A, although only half as much as if it were continuous ultrasound at the same spatial average intensity. Note that in both A and B in Fig. 13–5, the complete cycles are 40 milliseconds in duration. Pulsed ultrasound intensities should be stated as time averaged and spatial averaged intensities so that both the time and area are specified.

Beam Nonuniformity Ratio

The spatial average intensity represents the intensity averaged over the area of the beam of energy. This implies that the ultrasonic energy is not distributed evenly throughout the beam. In some areas within the beam, the intensity is much higher than it is in the adjacent areas. The *beam nonuniformity ratio* (BNR) is a numerical value that represents the ratio of the highest intensity in the ultrasound field (peak intensity) to the spatial average intensity indicated on the ultrasound meter.[94]

Fig. 13–6 represents the variation in intensity at different points in the cross-section of a near ultrasonic field. The spatial average intensity is the average of the shaded area under the curve. In this example, the BNR is 6 to 1 and the peak intensity is 12 W/sq cm in a field of spatial average intensity of 2.0 W/sq cm. Therefore, if a patient is treated with an intensity of 2.0 W/sq cm, as indicated by the ultrasound meter, the beam will create a hot spot with an intensity of 12 W/sq cm if the sound head remains stationary.

The BNR should be considered when purchasing an ultrasound unit. Examine the specifications and an ultrasonic beam diagram showing the relatively even energy distribution with low BNR. The therapist must be aware that many ultrasound units currently in service are inaccurate. Stewart et al[95] tested 56 different units and found that 20% of them emitted at least 20% more energy than the power meter indicated. Fyfe and Parnell[96] further confirmed the inaccuracy of power output and effective radiation surface. Only 5 of 18 transducers tested met the required plus or minus 15% of power expected according to the manufacturers' data.

Irradiation Time and Surface Area

In addition to power, intensity, and duty cycle, the total amount of time the patient is treated must be noted. Logically, if a patient receives 10 watts of ultrasound for 2 minutes, twice as much energy has been administered than if the patient had received 10 watts for only 1 minute.

The other major consideration when determining dosage is the size of the surface being treated. Assuming the same total watts and time, the larger the area sonated, the smaller the amount of energy available per unit of tissue. Consider

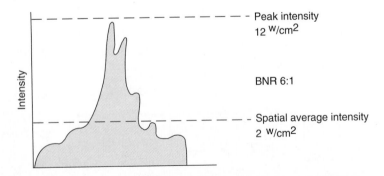

Figure 13–6.   The variation in intensity at different points in the cross-section of near ultrasonic field. The beam nonuniformity ratio (BNR) is 12:2, or 6:1, the ratio between the peak intensity and the spatial average intensity. If kept stationary, the sound head will create a hot spot of 12 watts per square centimeter.

this example: A physical therapist treats the right lumbar paravertebral muscles of a patient at 2 W/sq cm for 5 minutes. The effective radiating area of the transducer is 10 sq cm. Thus, the therapist administers a total of 20 watts at 2 W/sq cm for 5 minutes to the 50 sq cm area. On the other hand, if the therapist decides to include more of the musculature and doubles the length and width of the sonated area, the surface area quadruples (see Fig. 13–7). In other words, the exposure time of each section of tissue is reduced to one-fourth the amount of energy that would be received if the smaller area were heated.

In this example, only 10 sq cm of each section can be sonated at any point in time. During the course of a 5-minute treatment, each portion of tissue can receive only 1 minute of ultrasonic energy if the treatment area is 50 sq cm. If the 5-minute treatment is distributed over a treatment area of 200 square centimeters, each section of tissue receives only 15 seconds, or one-fourth the previous amount of ultrasound. In this example, one would not expect a significant TTR in the larger area of treatment because the exposure time per unit area of tissue would be inadequate.

METHODS OF APPLICATION

Three techniques of applying ultrasound are available: (1) direct contact, (2) immersion, and (3) fluid-filled bag. Each technique can be performed using a stationary or a moving sound head.

Stationary Procedure

The stationary procedure involves directing the ultrasonic transducer so that the only area sonated is directly under the sound head. This technique is generally not recommended because of its potentially detrimental effects. Stewart et al[97] reported on the studies of Barth and Wachsman, which indicated that bone damage in dogs was produced by a stationary transducer at 0.5 W/sq cm to 1 W/sq cm compared with about 3 W/sq cm for a moving sound field. One might argue that treating with only low dosage (below 0.5 W/sq cm) should produce no detrimental effects. Unfortunately, the intensity of power indicated on many power meters is inaccurate.

Another disadvantage of the stationary technique is the development of "hot spots"—areas within the ultrasound field that are exposed to higher intensities than the surrounding tissue within the same sound field. (Refer to the preceding discussion of BNR.) Haar[98] emphasized the nonuniformity of the ultrasound field or beam. There are areas of peak intensity that are considerably higher than would be indicated by the space average intensity on the power meter. Haar recommended using a moving sound head technique so that no section of tissue is exposed to the peak intensity for a significant amount of time. Similarly, Allen and Barrye[99] and the U.S. Department of Health and Human Services,[94] recommend using the moving sound head to compensate for the lack of uniformity of the ultrasound field.

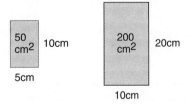

Figure 13–7. A comparison of ultrasound treatment areas. If the same amount of power and time are used for both areas, the larger area will receive only 25% of the energy per unit of tissue compared with the smaller area because the larger area is four times as big.

Another reason to abandon the stationary technique is the possibility of impairing blood flow. Dyson and Pond[100] produced blood cell stasis in chick embryos exposed to therapeutic levels of ultrasound by the stationary sound head procedure. This only occurs during the exposure period in vessels lying parallel to the direction of ultrasound propagation. This mechanism is believed to be associated with the production of standing waves that accompany the stationary technique. The stasis can be avoided by using a moving sound head.

We recommend avoiding the stationary technique for the above reasons. It should be noted, however, that others have used the technique at extremely low intensities. Griffin and Karselis[8] recommended this technique for treating small localized areas of pain, spasm, or organized hematoma. They recommended intensities of 0.02 to 0.1 W/sq cm for 5 minutes or more. However, they cautioned that even at these extremely low intensities, overheating, particularly of the periosteum, can occur because one small area receives all the energy. Thus, a hot spot might develop within that area.

Moving Sound Head Procedure

Technique. When using the moving procedure, the sound head must be moved over the treatment area in a smooth rhythmical pattern. It is important to keep the rhythm constant throughout the treatment and during each consecutive treatment. If the sound head is moved slowly, the patient will be unable to tolerate as high an intensity. A consistent movement is required to insure the even distribution of energy and to avoid hot spots. The choice of movement pattern is based on the contour of the area treated. The pattern can be either small overlapping circles or small overlapping strokes. The circular technique is desirable when treating an area with irregular contours; either technique can be used when treating a large flat area.

The circular method requires the therapist to make circles of small diameter, about the size of the sound head, that glide just far enough for the subsequent circle to overlap the preceding circle by half. The stroking method requires the therapist to glide the sound head slowly and longitudinally in one direction, then slide it laterally one-half the width of the sound head before returning longitudinally. The pattern chosen is repeated over the involved area for the desired treatment time. Some authors have recommended that when treating a large area, the area should be treated in subdivisions so that the energy covers the area long enough to have an additive effect. For example, Lehmann[101] suggested exposing the area no more than 75 sq cm at one time to allow for effective heating. Oakley[102] recommended treating sections about 1½ times the size of the transducer for 30-second periods. This procedure is repeated over the entire treatment area until the total prescribed treatment time is reached.

Coupling Agents. A coupling agent must always be used between the sound head and the patient to enhance transmissivity. Most clinicians use a commercially prepared thixotropic gel for applications involving direct contact. Although thixotropic gel is the most expensive type of coupling agent, it is the most convenient to use. Warren et al[103] compared the degree of transmissiveness of four commercially available coupling agents—gels, mineral oil, glycerine, and degassed water—and found that, except for glycerine, which had the lowest transmissiveness (60%), the mean levels of transmissivity were within 10% of the reference: degassed water. Transmissiveness was measured through 1 mm films of the couplant, similar to the amount used in applications involving direct contact.

Tepid degassed water is the ideal medium for the immersion technique because it does not allow the formation of bubbles that can interfere with transmission. Tap water is used most commonly because of its ease of access and low cost. According to Griffin,[104] water transmits ultrasound more efficiently than does glycerin or mineral oil. If glycerin or mineral oil is used, it must be kept cooler than water. The coolness reduces the amount of surface heating that seems to impair deep heating by ultrasound when the immersion technique is used. Lehmann et al[105] suggested that water is an effective coupling medium at 75° F (24° C) but mineral oil is not. Mineral oil may be no warmer than 64° F (18° C) to allow for heating at the level of a deep-set joint capsule.

Direct-Contact Procedure

Technique. The most common, convenient, and efficient method of applying ultrasound is by direct contact. Very simply, the sound head glides directly on the surface of the skin.

Three basic requirements must be met to use this technique correctly. First, the contour of the part being treated must allow for good contact of the sound head for the duration of the treatment. If total contact does not exist, the area of the transducer that is in contact with the air will be unable to dissipate its energy, and the transducer may overheat. Partial contact also will reduce the total amount of energy the patient receives.

Second, the skin or soft tissue must not be so sensitive to pressure that moving the sound head along the skin causes pain. This condition can be minimized by 5–7 minutes of ice massage immediately before the ultrasound. In our experience, the icing reduces the sensitivity of the skin without impairing the responsiveness of the deeper thermal receptors that are needed to prevent overexposure.

Third, the skin must be intact. If skin eruptions, blisters, or infection are present in the treated area, the movement of the sound head may irritate the area further or spread the infection. Therefore, ultrasound should not be applied over these areas.

Preparation for treatment. Before the treatment is initiated, the following procedures must be carried out:

1. The ultrasound unit, a coupling agent, and toweling should be placed in an area that is easily accessible to the therapist but does not interfere with the patient.
2. Explain the procedure in a manner appropriate for each patient's intellect and interest. Inform patients that a mild sensation of warmth is acceptable but that they must tell the therapist if they feel even the slightest degree of heat, pain, or discomfort so that the intensity of the treatment can be reduced.
3. Position the patient so that the area to be treated is exposed, the patient is relaxed and comfortable, and stretching can be done if desired.
4. The sound head, which should not be turned on at this point, can be used to spread the coupling agent over the area to be treated. The couplant should cover the entire area with a thin film. (**Note:** If the patient reports a prickling, tingling, or superficial burning sensation during the treatment, the cause may be an inadequate amount of couplant. If this occurs, reduce the intensity to zero and apply more couplant before continuing the treatment. If the patient continues to feel these sensations, check the machine.)
5. Switch the unit on with the power switch or by turning on the timer. Adjust the timer to include the time required to bring the intensity to the desired level.
6. Check the meter to insure that the intensity is at zero and that the desired mode (continuous or pulsed) has been selected.
7. Place the sound head firmly on the patient and glide it firmly on the patient. Move the sound head back and forth, maintaining total contact with the skin as the intensity gradually rises to the desired level. The sound head *must be moved continuously;* if not, the patient may report a sudden strong ache or a stabbing pain that resembles being struck by a needle as the intensity of the dose increases. These sensations are probably caused by periosteal overheating or a too rapid rise in temperature in the local soft tissue. This is obviously not the way to establish good rapport with

and gain your patient's confidence. At no time should the sound head be exposed to the air while the power is on.

8. At the end of treatment, the timer should run out and stop the output of power. Turn the intensity control to zero before removing the sound head from the patient. Wipe the couplant from the sound head and place the head in its holder. Remove the couplant from the patient's skin with soft toweling. Most coupling gels are water soluble and do not stain clothing. If necessary, alcohol can be used to cleanse the skin.

Immersion Procedure

Technique. The next most common method of applying ultrasound is to immerse the body part in a fluid medium. This technique is indicated when none of the three criteria for the direct contact method are met. The immersion procedure is especially useful for treating small irregular surfaces such as joints of the hands and feet. It is also indicated for treatment of areas that are too sensitive to be touched or have broken skin.

Preparation for treatment. The therapist must carry out the following preparatory procedures before initiating treatment:

1. Prepare the immersion medium and position the ultrasound unit in an easily accessible position.
2. Explain the procedure to the patient.
3. Position the patient so that the area to be treated is exposed and the patient is comfortable and relaxed.
4. Immerse the non-energized sound head in the basin and direct it toward the treatment target about ½ to 1 inch from the skin.
5. Begin a slow rhythmic pattern of movement similar to the one described for the direct-contact procedure and slowly raise the intensity to the desired level. It is extremely important to direct the ultrasound waves perpendicular to the skin surface to reduce surface reflection. As the angle of incidence increases, less energy will be directed to the target structure and be available for penetration and absorption. Air bubbles on the skin or sound head also will increase reflection and reduce transmission. If air bubbles develop during the treatment, simply brush them away from the sound head or skin with a quick light stroke using a piece of gauze attached to a tongue depressor.
6. When the treatment is finished, reduce the intensity to zero before removing the sound head from the medium, then dry the head before replacing it in its holder.

Precautions. The ultrasound generator should be plugged into a receptacle that is protected by a ground fault interrupter (GFI). This will protect both the patient and the therapist from a potential shock associated with leakage of low-level current that would not trip a standard circuit breaker. The GFI is recommended for use in areas where large amounts of moisture accumulate. The National Electrical Code requires a GFI for all newly built outdoor structures, bathrooms, and garages where electrical appliances are used.[106]

The therapist should avoid placing his or her hands in the path of the direct or reflected ultrasound waves. Poor technique will expose the therapist's hands to excessive amounts of ultrasound during repeated immersion treatments.

Fluid-Filled Bag or Cushion Procedure

Technique. The fluid-filled bag or fluid cushion procedure, although not widely used, provides an alternative method of treating areas that have irregular contours or are overly sensitive. This procedure is more practical than the immersion procedure for treating a proximal body part such as a shoulder, scapula, or trochanter, which would require a large tank. The technique requires only a thin-membraned bag, such as a condom or a surgical glove, and a coupling medium such as degassed water, mineral oil, or glycerine. It is important to use degassed water rather than tap water in this procedure because clearing bubbles that form within the bag is difficult.

Preparation for treatment. Before initiating the treatment, the therapist must carry out the following procedures:

1. Fill the condom or surgical glove with the fluid and put the mouth of the bag around the sidewalls of the sound head. Squeeze the bag gently to force out the air until the sound head is in full contact with the fluid. Seal the bag with a rubber band or tape. Remember that air between the sound head and fluid will reduce transmission.
2. Apply the bag to the patient. Ideally, the medium used in the bag should be used on the skin and the outside of the bag to ensure good contact and to eliminate air bubbles from the skin surface.
3. With the bag in firm contact with the skin, begin moving the sound head within the bag rhythmically and gently as the intensity increases to the desired level. Keep the sound head at a 90° angle to the treatment surface and avoid sliding the bag on the skin.

A variation of this procedure is the use of a fluid cushion, made by filling a bag with fluid and sealing it. The cushion is placed on the body part with a coupling medium between the bag and skin and between the bag and the sound head. While firmly holding the bag over the part, slowly stroke the top surface of the bag with the sound head. The major drawback of this technique is that it creates an extra interface between the sound head and the skin. Even the fluid-filled bag procedure creates one more interface than does the direct contact method. The membrane of the bag and the couplant form an interface that attenuates sound waves.

TREATMENT PROTOCOL

The treatment protocol for ultrasound is established by (1) the size of the area to be sonated, (2) the duration of the treatment, and (3) the intensity used. The frequency and total number of treatments also must be considered.

Size of the Area and Duration of Treatment

The therapist determines the size of the area to be sonated. This determination is based on the area required to produce a healing effect or relief of pain.

In determining the duration of treatment, the therapist should consider the following guidelines: (1) the first treatment should be shorter than subsequent treatments, (2) acute conditions should be treated for shorter periods than are chronic conditions, and (3) smaller areas require less time than do larger areas. To produce a maximally safe thermal response, the same intensity can be applied for a longer period to prolong the physiologic response.

These general principles have been stated because no definitive, objective standard exists for the duration of treatment. We suggest the following formulas for determining the duration of treatments. The formulas are general guidelines based on values recommended by others[7,13,14] and by clinical experience. (ERA = effective radiating area.)

For subacute conditions:

$$\frac{\text{Area be treated}}{1.5 \times \text{ERA}} = \text{Minutes of ultrasound}$$

For example, if you are treating an area of 50 square centimeters with a transducer that has an ERA of 10 square centimeters,

$$\frac{50 \text{ cm}^2}{1.5 \times 10 \text{ cm}^2} = \frac{50}{1.5 \times 10} = 3.3 \text{ minutes}$$

For chronic conditions:

$$\frac{\text{Area to be treated}}{1 \times \text{ERA}} = \text{Minutes of ultrasound}$$

For example, if you are treating an area of 50 square centimeters with a transducer that has an ERA of 10 square centimeters,

$$\frac{50 \text{ cm}^2}{1 \times 10 \text{ cm}^2} = \frac{50}{1 \times 10} = 5 \text{ minutes of ultrasound}$$

For maximal thermal effect:

$$\frac{\text{Area to be treated}}{0.8 \times 10 \text{ ERA}} = \text{Minutes of ultrasound}$$

For example, if you are treating an area of 50 square centimeters with a transducer that has an ERA of 10 square centimeters,

$$\frac{50 \text{ cm}^2}{0.8 \times 10 \text{ cm}^2} = \frac{50}{0.8 \times 10} = 6.2 \text{ minutes}$$

Intensity of Treatment

When determining the intensity of treatment, the therapist should consider the following guidelines:

- A superficial lesion, including one near a bony prominence, should be treated with a lower intensity than is the case for a deep lesion.
- A subacute lesion, or any lesion where thermal effects are undesirable, should be treated with a lower intensity than is the case for a chronic lesion.
- A slightly lower-than-estimated "ideal" intensity should be used for the first treatment so that the patient's response can be assessed.
- The patient's feedback should be obtained both during and after the treatment to determine the appropriate intensity. (If the therapist decides to treat a patient with deficient sensory or thermal awareness, only a low intensity should be used);

In the absence of any other deficits such as circulatory impairment, ultrasound can be applied to the part with the sensory deficit after establishing a safe dosage. This can be done by determining the dosage the patient can tolerate on the similar contralateral body part. Patients can tolerate (1) a higher intensity of pulsed ultrasound than continuous ultrasound and (2) a higher intensity during an immersion procedure than a direct-contact procedure.

It is difficult to prescribe precise values for different situations. Part of the problem relates to the individual differences in the output of the many ultrasound units in use. The power output of many units is extremely inefficient, and many demonstrate inaccurate metering. Thus, clinicians must be familiar with the characteristics of their ultrasound units.

Although estimates of treatment intensities are based on a scale of 0 to 2 W/sq cm, the key rule is to rely on the patient's response and clinical signs. If the patient experiences pain during the treatment, reduce the intensity immediately.

Patients may report several types of pain or discomfort. A sharp, stabbing pain is usually a sign of periosteal overheating caused by moving the sound head directly onto a bony prominence or stroking it slowly over bone. This type of pain can be prevented by (1) reducing the intensity, (2) avoiding direct sonation over bony prominences, or (3) moving more quickly over bony prominences. A dull, aching pain is probably the result of an intensity that is too high, which causes a too rapid TTR from prolonged application. In the latter case, treatment should be terminated.

A prickling, tingling, stinging, or vibrating sensation under the sound head may indicate an inadequate amount of couplant or inadequate contact with the skin. This can be corrected by (1) applying more couplant, (2) repositioning the part to allow adequate skin contact, or (3) changing to the immersion or fluid-filled bag procedure.

The following suggestions for determining intensity are based on an ultrasound generator with a range of 0 to 2 watts per square centimeter on continuous mode using a moving sound head and the direct-contact procedure:

- For acute conditions, use 0.1–0.5 watts per square centimeter to reduce the production of thermal effects. The patient should feel no warmth. The therapist must be discreet and cautious when treating an acute condition.
- For subacute conditions, use 0.5–1.0 watts per square centimeter. If minimal thermal effects are desired, the patient should feel no warmth or only minimal warmth on the skin.
- For chronic conditions, use 1.0–2.0 watts per square centimeter. If maximal safe thermal effects are desired, the patient should feel a strong sensation of warmth but no discomfort.

The above suggestions represent a common sense perspective derived from a review of studies on the physiologic effects of ultrasound and from clinical experience. At any given frequency, the tissue adjacent to the sound head will receive more sound energy than will deeper tissue; therefore, if the lesion is superficial (eg, an acromioclavicular sprain), the intensity should be at the lower end of the suggested range of intensity. If the lesion is deep (eg, a piriformis spasm), the intensity should be at the higher end of the range.

Frequency and Number of Treatments

The documentation regarding the optimal frequency and number of treatments is inadequate. However, the following suggestions have been fairly well accepted in clinical practice:

- Ultrasound is commonly applied once a day or every other day.
- The course of treatment depends on how quickly the desired effects are obtained.
- Treatment should be discontinued (1) when complete relief of symptoms and restoration of function is achieved, (2) if no positive results are achieved after three or four treatments, and (3) after a course of 12 to 15 treatments. (After 12–15 treatments, which in most cases produce the desired effects, the patient should be observed for 2 weeks without ultrasound. If the condition regresses during that period, another series of ultrasound treatments should be initiated. In special cases, eg, Dupuytren's contracture, treatments may continue for many months but with only one or two treatments per week.)
- The treatment should be modified immediately if the patient reports an exacerbation of symptoms. The symptoms must be evaluated carefully to determine the cause of the exacerbation and to make the appropriate modifications in treatment.

Clinical experience indicates that a significant number of patients may report a mild increase in symptoms several hours after the first or second ultrasound treatment. This discomfort lasts for only a few hours, and the original symptoms improve by the following day. This pattern does not indicate that ultrasound should be discontinued. It appears to be a type of "treatment soreness" that may be the result of increased activity in the tissue. The patient should be informed in advance that this soreness may occur and can be relieved by applying ice. This information should be presented to the patient in a manner that will not cause alarm. However, if the patient's symptoms increase immediately after the treatment and persist for 24 to 48 hours after the treatment, ultrasound should be discontinued. If ultrasound treatments are reinitiated later, they should be given at a lower intensity and only after the symptoms have subsided.

Discontinuation after 12–15 treatments is recommended to reduce the possible risk factor of excessive exposure to ultrasound. Only one case of clinical overexposure has been documented in the scientific literature. In this case, a woman who treated herself, unsupervised, over multiple body parts several times a day had many physical complaints that may or may not have been aggravated by the ultrasound.[107] Therefore, the recommendation to limit exposure to ultrasound is made from a perspective of caution. An ethical issue also may be involved. If a patient has not made significant progress after several treatments, another form of treatment should be considered. Another related issue is psychological addiction to ultrasound. Certain patients become dependent on ultrasound because of its immediate soothing effect. The therapist is responsible for discouraging or eliminating this dependency.

CLINICAL EXAMPLE

The following clinical problem is presented with a diagnosis and some pertinent clinical information. Keep in mind that this example simply serves as a guide for establishing treatment parameters; it does not rule out other approaches to the same problem. When a patient appears in the clinic, many factors may have to be considered. The solutions proposed here are not intended to serve as recipes for clinical prescriptions; they are intended to enhance understanding and promote the intelligent, rational selection of treatment procedures. Assume that the ultrasound generator used has a maximum intensity of 2 watts per square centimeter and that the transducer has an ERA of 10 square centimeters.

A 25-year-old woman with *chondromalacia patellae* is referred to the clinic for physical therapy. She noticed pain and "puffiness" around the right patella about 1 week ago. She currently has pain when she rises from a sitting position and climbs stairs. She has mild crepitus and tenderness of the medial articular facet of the right knee. She has been resting and icing the knee for the past week.

Goals. Eliminate the patients pain and reduce her mild edema.

Technique. The direct-contact procedure using a small sound head or the immersion procedure if a whirlpool bath is available and feasible.

Position. If the articular facets are the target areas, the knee is placed in the neutral position so that the patella can be displaced medially. If the ultrasound is applied in a normal manner, ie, it follows the regular contours of the knee, the peripatellar structures will be treated but the articular facets will not. When the patella is displaced medially, the lateral facet is accessible and the sound beam can be focused toward it. When the patella is displaced laterally, the medial facet is accessible.

If the lateral articular condyle of the femur is the target area, the knee is placed in a flexed position. It should be maintained in a relaxed, flexed position of at least 90° so that the condyle is exposed for sonation.

Sequence. Ultrasound and other treatments should be administered in the following sequence:

1. Mild exercise—straight leg raises and no quadricep groups.
2. Gentle patellar distraction mobilization.
3. Ultrasound to provide pain relief and nonthermal effects.
4. Ice massage to provide pain relief and reduce risk of postexercise inflammation.

Mode. Continuous and pulsed.

Size of area. Moderate (100 sq cm), although the medial facet is the most painful area, the patient is experiencing general circumferential pain and mild edema as well.

Time. Five minutes.

Intensity. Continuous-wave mode, 0.5–1 watt per square centimeter; pulsed-wave mode, 1–1.5 watts per square centimeter at a 50% duty cycle (this dosage was selected because the area treated was about 10×10 centimeters (4 inches $\times$ 4 inches) and the tissue to be treated was superficial).

■ KEY TERMS

attenuation	pulsed-wave ultrasound
micromassage	time average power
membrane permeability	spatial average intensity
cavitation	duty cycle
phonophoresis	beam nonuniformity ratio (BNR)
continuous-wave ultrasound	

REFERENCES

1. Steward HF, Absug JL, Harris GR: Considerations in ultrasound therapy and equipment performance. *Phys Ther.* 1980; 60:425.
2. Halliday D, Resnick R: *Physics.* New York: John Wiley & Sons; 1990.
3. Schwan HP: *Therapeutic Heat and Cold.* Elizabeth Licht; 1965.
4. Williams AR: *Ultrasound: Biological Effects and Potential Hazards.* New York: Academic Press; 1983.
5. Carlin B: *Ultrasonics.* 2nd ed. New York: McGraw-Hill; 1960.
6. Lehmann J, Warren C, Guy A: *Ultrasound: Its Applications in Medicine and Biology.* New York: Elsevier Scientific; 1978.
7. Lehmann JF: *Therapeutic Heat and Cold.* Baltimore, MD: Waverly Press; 1972.
8. Griffin J, Karselis T: *Physical Agents for Physical Therapists.* Springfield, IL: Charles C Thomas; 1982.
9. Allen KGR, Battye CK: Performance of ultrasonic therapy instruments. *Physiotherapy.* 1978; 6:176.
10. Piersol GM, Schwan HP, Penwell RB, et al: Mechanism of absorption of ultrasonic energy in blood. *Arch Phys Med Rehabil.* 1952; 33:327.
11. Wells PNT: Ultrasonics in medicine and biology. *Phys Med Biol.* 1977; 22:629–669.
12. Frizzell LA, Dunn F: *Therapeutic Heat and Cold.* Baltimore, MD: Williams & Wilkins; 1982.
13. Lehmann JF, DeLateur B, Stonebridge J, et al: Therapeutic temperature distribution produced by ultrasound as modified by dosage and volume of tissue exposed. *Arch Phys Med Rehabil.* 1967; 664–666.
14. Lehmann JF, Johnson EW: Some factors influencing the temperature distribution in thighs exposed to ultrasound. *Arch Phys Med Rehabil.* 1958; 39:346.
15. Licht S, Kamenetz H: *Therapeutic Heat and Cold.* 2nd ed. Baltimore, MD: Waverly Press; 1972.
16. Lota M, Darling R: Changes in permeability of the red blood cell membrane in a homogeneous ultrasound field. *Arch Phys Med Rehabil.* 1955; 36:282–287.
17. Dyson M, Pond JB, Joseph J, et al: The stimulation of tissue regeneration by means of ultrasound. *Clin Sci.* 1968; 35:238.
18. Coble AJ, Dunn F: Ultrasonic production of reversible changes in the electrical parameters of isolated frog skin. *J Acoust Am.* 1976; 60:225–229.
19. Mortimer AJ, Bresden B, Forester GV, et al: System for measurement of the effects of ultrasound on the membrane properties of the myocardium. *Med Biol Eng Comp.* 1984; 22:22–27.
20. Mortimer AJ, Trollope BJ, Villeneuve EJ: Ultrasound enhanced diffusion of oxygen through isolated frog skin. *J Med Ultrasound.* 1988; 6(suppl):
21. Mortimer AJ, Dyson M: The effect of therapeutic ultrasound on calcium uptake in fibroblasts. *Ultrasound Med Biol.* 1988; 6:499–506.
22. Hogan RD, Franklin TD, Fry FJ: The effect of ultrasound on microvascular

hemodynamics in skeletal muscle: effect on arterioles. *Ultrasound Med Biol.* 1982; 8(1):44–55.

23. Hogan RD, Burke KM, Franklin TD: The effect of ultrasound on microvascular hemodynamics in skeletal muscle: effects during ischemia. *Microvas Res.* 1982; 23:370–379.

24. Carlin B: *Ultrasonics.* 2nd ed. New York: McGraw-Hill; 1960.

25. Wells PNT: *Biomedical Ultrasonics.* London, UK: Academic Press; 1977.

26. Reid PC, Redford SB, King P: *Training: Scientific Basic and Application.* Springfield, IL: Charles C Thomas; 1972.

27. Wyke B: *The Lumbar Spine and Back Pain.* London, UK: Sector Publishing; 1976:188.

28. Lehmann JF, Brunner GD, Stow RW: Pain threshold measurements after therapeutic application of ultrasound. *Arch Phys Med Rehabil.* 1958; 39:560.

29. Szumski AJ: Mechanisms of pain relief as a result of therapeutic application of ultrasound. *Phys Ther Rev.* 1960; 117.

30. Anderson TP, Wakim KG, Herrick JF: An experimental study of the effects of ultrasonic energy on the lower part of the spinal cord and peripheral nerves. *Arch Phys Med Rehabil.* 1951; 32:71.

31. Zankel HT: Effect of physical agents on motor conduction velocity of the ulnar nerve. *Arch Phys Med Rehabil.* 1966; 47:787–792.

32. Farmer W: Effect of intensity of ultrasound on conduction velocity of motor axons. *Phys Ther.* 1968; 48:1233–1237.

33. Paul WD, Imig CJ: Temperature and blood flow studies after ultrasonic irradiation. *Am J Phys Med Rehabil.* 1955; 34:370.

34. Abramson DI, Clier LSW, Tuck S: Effect of tissue temperature and blood flow on motor nerve conduction velocity. *JAMA.* 1966; 198:10:156–162.

35. Currier DP, Greathouse D, Swift T: Sensory conduction: effect of ultrasound. *Arch Phys Med Rehabil.* 1978; 59:181–185.

36. Halle JS, Scoville CR, Greathouse D: Ultrasound's effect on the conduction latency of the superficial radial nerve in man. *Phys Ther.* 1981; 61:345–350.

37. Consentino AB, Gross DL, Harrington RJ: Ultrasound effects on electroneuromyographic measures in sensory fibers of the median nerve. *Phys Ther.* 1983; 62:1788–1792.

38. Middlemast S, Chatterjee DC: Comparison of ultrasound and thermotherapy for soft tissue injuries. *Physiotherapy.* 1978; 64:331–332.

39. Vanharanta H, Eronen I, Videman T: Effect of ultrasound on glycosaminoglycan metabolism in the rabbit knee. *Am J Phys Med Rehabil.* 1982; 61:221–228.

40. Stratton SA, Heckmann R, Francis RS: Therapeutic ultrasound: its effects on the integrity of a non-penetrating wound. *J Ortho Sports PT.* 1984; 5:278–281.

41. Young SR, Dyson M: Macrophage responsiveness to therapeutic ultrasound. *Ultrasound Med Biol.* 1990; 8:809–816.

42. Young SR, Dyson M: Effect of therapeutic ultrasound on the healing of full-thickness excised skin lesions. *Ultrasonics.* 1990; 28:175–180.

43. Paul BJ, Lafratta CW, Dawson AR: Use of ultrasound in the treatment of pressure sores in patients with spinal cord injury. *Arch Phys Med Rehabil.* 1960; 39:439–440.

44. Shamberger RC, Talbot T, Tipton H: The effect of ultrasonic and thermal treatment on wounds. *Plast Reconstr Surg.* 1981; 68:860–870.

45. Dyson M, Suckling J: Stimulation of tissue repair by ultrasound: a survey of mechanisms involved. *Physiotherapy.* 1978; 64(4):105–108.

46. Ferguson N: Ultrasound in the treatment of surgical wounds. *Physiotherapy.* 1981; 67(2):43.

47. Eriksson SV, Lundebert T, Malm M: A placebo controlled trial of ultrasound therapy in chronic leg ulceration. *Scand J Rehabil Med.* 1991; 23:211–213.

48. Enwemeka CS: The effects of therapeutic ultrasound on tendon healing. *Am J Phys Med Rehabil.* 1989; 6:283–287.

49. Enwemeka CS, Rodriquez O, Mendosa S: The biomedical effects of low-intensity ultrasound on healing tendons. *Ultrasound Med Biol.* 1990; 8:801–807.

50. Jackson BA, Schwane JA, Starcher BC: Effect of ultrasound therapy on the repair of Achilles tendon injuries in rats. *Med Sci Sports Med.* 1991; 2:171–176.

51. Turner SM, Powell ES, Ng CS: The effect of ultrasound on the healing of repaired cockerel tendon: is collagen crosslinkage a factor? *J Hand Surg.* 1989; 4:428–433.

52. Roberts M, Rutherford JH, Harris D: The effect of ultrasound on flexor tendon repairs in rabbits. *Hand.* 1982; 14(1):17–20.

53. Bickford RH, Duff RS: Influence of ultrasonic irradiation on temperature and blood flow in human skeletal muscle. *Circ Res.* 1953; 1:534.

54. Paul WD, Imig CJ: Temperature and blood flow studies after ultrasonic irradiation. *Am J Phys Med Rehabil.* 1955; 34:370.

55. Buchan JB: The use of ultrasonics in physical medicine. *Practitioner.* 1970; 205:319.

56. Imig CJ, Randal BF, Hines HM: Effect of ultrasonic energy on blood flow. *Am J Phys Med Rehabil.* 1954; 3:100–102.

57. Abramson DI, Burnett C, Bell Y: Changes in blood flow, oxygen uptake and tissue temperatures produced by the therapeutic physical agents, I. Effect of Ultrasound. *Am J Phys Med Rehabil.* 1960; 39:51.

58. Lota M: Electronic plethsymographic and tissue temperature studies of effect of ultrasound on blood flow. *Arch Phys Med Rehabil.* 1965; 44:315–322.

59. Lehmann JF, DeLateur BJ, Warren CG: Heating of joint structures by ultrasound. *Arch Phys Med Rehabil.* 1968; 49:28–30.

60. Lehmann JF, Masock AJ, Warren CG: Effect of therapeutic temperature on tendon extensibility. *Arch Phys Med Rehabil.* 1970; 51:481–487.

61. Moll MJ: A new approach to pain: lidocaine and decadron with ultrasound. *USAF Med Serv Digest;* May 8–11, 1977.

62. Newman M, Kill M, Frompton G: The effects of ultrasound alone and combined with hydrocortisone injections by needle or hypospray. *Am J Phys Med Rehabil.* 1958; 37:206–209.

63. Mune O: Ultrasonic treatment of subcutaneous infiltrations after injections. *Acta Orthop Scand.* 1963; 33:346.

64. Novak FJ: Experimental transmission of lidocaine through intact skin by ultrasound. *Arch Phys Med Rehabil.* 1964; 64:231–232.

65. Griffin JE, Touchstone JC: Ultrasonic movement of cortisol into pig tissues. *Am J Phys Med Rehabil.* 1963; 43:77–85.

66. Griffin JE, Touchstone JC, Liu AC: Ultrasonic movement of cortisol into pig tissues, II. movement into paravertebral nerve. *Am J Phys Med Rehabil.* 1965; 44:20–25.

67. Griffin JE, Echternach JL, Price RE, et al: Patients treated with ultrasonic driven hydrocortisone and with ultrasound alone. *Phys Ther.* 1967; 47:594–601.

68. Kleinkort JA, Wood F: Phonophoresis with 1 Percent Versus 10 Percent Hydrocortisone. *Phys Ther.* 1975; 12:1320–1324.

69. Griffin JE, Touchstone JC: Low-intensity phonophoresis of cortisol in swine. *Phys Ther.* 1968; 12:1336–1344.

70. Benson HAE, McElnay JC, Harland R: Use of ultrasound to enhance percutaneous absorption of benzydamine. *Phys Ther.* 1989; 69:113–118.

71. Markam DE, Wood MR: Ultrasound for Dupuytren's contracture. *Physiotherapy.* 1980; 66:2:55–58.

72. Bierman W: Ultrasound in the treatment of scars. *Arch Phys Med Rehabil.* 1954;35:209.

73. Miller H, Ardrizzone J: Peyronie disease treated with ultrasound and hydrocortisone. *Urology.* 1983; 21:584–585.

74. McBride A, Varghese G, Arthur D: Peyronie's disease: treatment with long-term ultrasound. *Arch Phys Med Rehabil.* 1982; 63. Abstract.

75. Lehmann JF, et al: Comparison of ultrasonic and microwave diathermy in the physical treatment of periarthritis of the shoulder. *Arch Phys Med Rehabil.* 1954; 35:627.

76. Echternach JC: Ultrasound: an adjunct treatment for shoulder disability. *Phys Ther.* 1965; 45:865.

77. Bearzy HJ: Clinical applications of ultrasonic energy in the treatment of acute and chronic subacromial bursitis. *Arch Phys Med Rehabil.* 1953; 34:228.

78. Fountain FP, et al: Decrease in muscle spasm produced by ultrasound, hot packs and infrared. *Arch Phys Med Rehabil.* 1960; 41:294.

79. Portwood MH, Lieberman JS, Taylor RG: Causalgia of the foot: successful management by simple conservative measures. *Arch Phys Med Rehabil.* 1981; 62:502. Abstract.

80. Vaughn DT: Direct method versus underwater method in the treatment of plantar warts with ultrasound. *Phys Ther.* 1973; 53:396–397.

81. Cherup N, Urben J, Bender LF: Treatment of plantar warts with ultrasound. *Arch Phys Med Rehabil.* 1965; 44:602–604.

82. Rowe RJ, Gray JM: Ultrasound treatment of plantar warts. *Arch Phys Med Rehabil.* 1965; 46:600.

83. Oakley EM: Dangers and contra-indications of therapeutic ultrasound. *Physiotherapy.* 1978; 64(6):173–174.

84. Marmour JB, Pounds D, Hahn N, et al: Treating spontaneous tumors in dogs and cats by ultrasound induced hyperthermia. *Int J Radiat Oncol Biol Phys.* 1978; 4:967–973.

85. Orenberg, Deneau DG, Farber EM: Response of chronic psoriatic plaques to localized heating induced by ultrasound. *Arch Dermatol.* 1980; 116:893–897.

86. DeForest RE: Effects of ultrasound on growing bone: experimental study. *Arch Phys Med Rehabil.* 1953; 34:21.

87. Pilla AA, Mont MA, Nasser PR, et al: Non-invasive low-intensity pulsed ultrasound accelerates bone healing in the rabbit. *J Ortho Trauma.* 1990; 3:246–253.

88. Lehmann JF, Lane KE, Bell JW, et al: Influence of surgical metal implants on the distribution of the intensity in the ultrasound field. *Arch Phys Med Rehabil.* 1958; 39:756–760.

89. Lehmann JR, Brunner GD, McMillan J: Influence of surgical metal implants on the temperature distribution in thigh specimens exposed to ultrasound. *Arch Phys Med Rehabil.* 1958; 37:692–695.

90. Gersten JS: Effect of metallic objects on temperature rises produced in tissues by ultrasound. *Am J Phys Med Rehabil.* 1958; 37:75–82.

91. Skoubo-Kristensen E, Sommer J: Ultrasound on internal fixation with a rigid plate in dogs. *Arch Phys Med Rehabil.* 1982; 63:371–373.

92. Forrest G, Rosen K: Ultrasound: effectiveness of treatments given under water. *Arch Phys Med Rehabil.* 1989; 70:28–29.

93. Hayes KW: *Manual for Physical Agents.* 2nd ed. Evanston, IL: Northwestern University Medical School, Program in Physical Therapy. 1979.

94. Ferguson B: A practitioner's guide to the ultrasonic therapy equipment standard. *HHS Publication*No. 85–8240; 1985.

95. Stewart HF, et al: Survey of use and performance of ultrasonic therapy equipment in Pinellas County, Florida. *Phys Ther.* 1974; 54:707–714.

96. Fyfe MC, Parnell SM: The importance of measurement of effective transducer radiating area in the testing and calibration of "therapeutic" ultrasonic instruments. *Health Phys.* 1982; 43:377–381.

97. Stewart HF, Abzug J, Harris G: Considerations in ultrasound therapy equipment and performance. *Phys Ther.* 1980; 60:427.

98. Haar GT: Basic physics of therapeutic ultrasound. *Physiotherapy.* 1978; 64(4):102.

99. Allen KGR, Barrye CK: Performance of ultrasonic therapy instruments. *Physiotherapy.* 1978; 64(6):179.

100. Dyson M, Pond JB: The effects of ultrasound on circulation. *Physiotherapy.* 1973; 59:284–287.

101. Lehmann JF, McMillan JA, Brunner SD, et al: Comparative study of the efficiency of shortwave, microwave and ultrasonic diathermy in heating the hip joint. *Arch Phys Med Rehabil.* 1959; 40:510.

102. Oakley EM: Application of continuous beam ultrasound at therapeutic levels. *Physiotherapy.* 1978; 64(6):170.

103. Warren GC, Koblanski JN, Sifelmann R: Ultrasound coupling media: their relative transmissivity. *Arch Phys Med Rehabil.* 1976; 57:218–222.

104. Griffin J: Transmissiveness of ultrasound through tap water, glycerin and mineral oil. *Phys Ther.* 1980; 60:1010–1016.

105. Lehmann J, DeLateur BJ, Silverman DR: Selective heating effects of ultrasound in human beings. *Arch Phys Med Rehabil.* 1966; 47:331–339.

106. Frankel W: *Basic Wiring.* Chicago, IL: Time-Life Books; 1980.

107. Levenson JL, Weissberg MP: Ultrasound abuse: case report. *Arch Phys Med Rehabil.* 1983; 64:90–91.

14

Cryotherapy

Diana Fond, PT, MA and
Bernadette Hecox, PT, MA

*C*ryotherapy or cold therapy has been used in medicine over the centuries. The Greek word "cryos" means cold. The physical and physiological effects of cooling of localized tissues or generalized body cooling have already been discussed in detail in Chapters 7 through 10. The purpose of this chapter is to introduce the reader to the clinical aspects of cryotherapy as used in physical therapy. Physical therapists frequently use cold in the treatment of various orthopedic, neurological and other disorders.

COMMON CONSIDERATIONS

Tissue temperature can be reduced by (1) applying a low-temperature solid (ice), liquid, or slush directly to the skin (heat transfer by conduction), (2) immersing a body part in cold or ice water (heat transfer by conduction and convection), (3) blowing a volatile liquid (eg, Fluori-Methane) on the part being treated (heat transfer by evaporation), and (4) blowing cold air on a part being treated (heat transfer by convection), a method not used often in physical therapy. Because heat always travels from the hot to the cold, the tissues are cooled because they transfer their heat to the cold modality. The cold does not transfer to the body.

Cryotherapy in its various forms is recognized as an important treatment because it can reduce pain and spasms,[1-4] thereby breaking the cycle of pain, spasms, and ischemia.[5] It can also decrease the inflammatory process, bleeding and hemorrhage, and possibly traumatic edema. Cold also can diminish the effects of central and peripheral nerve disorders. Spasticity such as that caused by a stroke or spinal cord lesion can be diminished for brief periods,[6] and motor responses in patients can be facilitated by using specific techniques: for example, the quick icing technique described by Rood.[7] Some patients may experience a "rebound phenomenon" with increased spasticity from 30 min to a couple of hours after removal of the cold.

Numerous methods of treatment with cold are available, including ice massage, chemical cold packs, ice towels, ice packs, vapocoolant sprays, quick icing, cold combined with compression, and cold immersion (baths). Before applying any form of cryotherapy, the therapist should do the following:

1. Inspect the patient's skin before applying the cold to determine if any rashes or discolorations are present.
2. Test a small area of skin (not on the part to be treated) to determine whether the patient is hypersensitive to cold.
3. Verify that the circulatory status of the body part is good.
4. Make certain that the patient has not had frostbite in the area to be treated.
5. Make certain that the patient has never previously experienced an exacerbation of spasticity when cold was used.
6. Make sure that the patient is positioned comfortably and draped well to avoid any chilliness during the treatment.

FORMS OF TREATMENT

Ice Massage

Ice massage, the stroking of ice on a body part, is generally used to anesthetize the skin. Longer exposure is required to lower intramuscular temperature. When the therapist is performing an ice massage, the size and the amount of fat of the area being treated must be taken into account[8] (See Chap. 9).

Equipment

Ice massage can be performed in three ways. The therapist can use (1) ice that has been frozen in an insulated cup and touch a rounded area of the ice to the patient, (2) a "lollipop," a small cylindrical container with a small tongue depressor frozen in the middle, or (3) an ice cube wrapped in a few paper towels or a washcloth. In the first two techniques, the container helps form a smooth rounded surface. With the ice cube, however, the therapist must round the end of the cube so the patient does not feel a sharp edge. In all three techniques, the therapist's hand is protected from the cold either by the insulation of the cup, by holding the tongue depressor, or by the paper towels or washcloth (Fig. 14–1). Extra towels should be available to absorb water dripping from the melting ice.

Technique

The therapist should describe to the patient the sensations he or she is most likely to feel during an ice massage: first cold, then burning, then aching, and finally numbness. In addition, the therapist should inform the patient that the part being treated may become pale and eventually red. Color changes are the result of the "Hunting reaction" described in Chapter 9. If the normal responses mentioned above are not explained properly, the patient may want to end the treatment because of discomfort or fear.

The ice should be applied in circular, smooth, rhythmical strokes over the treatment area, reducing the size of the circles as the massage proceeds. Because water from the melting ice can be uncomfortable for the patient, it should be wiped up with extra towels. The therapist should try to avoid bumping into bony prominences because this, too, can be uncomfortable.

Duration

To anesthetize an area, the treatment should last from about 3 to 10 min or more, depending on the size of the area being treated. For example, the lateral aspect of the ankle might be treated for only 3 min, whereas 10–20 min might be required to

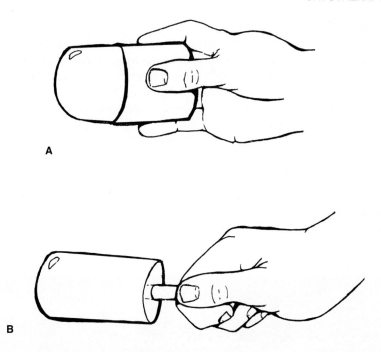

Figure 14–1.   Ice massage modalities. Ice is frozen in a cylindrical container. **(A)** Ice frozen in a paper cup. The top half of the cup is cut away so the ice will come in contact with the patient. The therapist holds the lower part of the cup while stroking the ice over the part to be treated. **(B)** The "lollipop" technique. A tongue depressor is frozen in the center of the container, the ice is then removed from the container, and the therapist uses the tongue depressor as a handle.

treat the hamstrings. Of course, the treatment time may vary, depending on the patient.

Advantages

Because ice massage anesthetizes the skin easily in a short time, a painful technique such as deep friction massage can be performed without causing discomfort to the patient. Ice is colder than the chemical cold packs that will be discussed next. Small areas near bony prominences can be treated easily without directly affecting the surrounding skin and underlying tissues. Ice in some form is usually readily available.

Disadvantages

The disadvantages are few, except for the drips of cold water that can cause the patient discomfort. The therapist's hands must be protected from the cold by the insulation of the cup or the paper towels or the tongue depressor. Because the ice may cause frostbite, the therapist must always check the color of the patient's skin. If the skin turns blue, the ice should be removed immediately.

Chemical Cold Packs

Three types of **chemical cold packs** are available. The clinical type of cold pack has a durable plastic cover around a silica gel (similar to a hot pack) and is stored in a refrigerator tank. The second type is similar to but smaller than the clinical cold pack; these can be purchased in most pharmacies and can be stored in the freezer of a home refrigerator. The third type must be activated by breaking an inner seal that mixes the chemicals within. This type must be disposed of after one use because the ice pack will warm up once the chemical reaction has taken place; these cold packs are usually readily available at health spas or gymnastic and other sports events for immediate emergency use. This section focuses on the chemical cold packs available in most clinics: for example, Hydrocollator or Col-Pack.

Equipment

Chemical cold packs are stored in a refrigeration tank resembling the one used for chemical hot packs. A thermostat maintains the temperature at about 10°–15° F (−12.2°–9.4° C). The cold packs should remain in the tank at least 24 hrs before the first use and at least 30 min between subsequent uses. The chemical cold packs, like hot packs, are available in different sizes and shapes, the most common are those for the cervical and low back areas (see Fig. 14–2).

Technique

The chemical cold pack should not be placed directly on the patient's skin, not only for hygiene, but also to prevent irritation. Many therapists advocate using a wet, well wrung out towel or cloth (cold or warm, depending on the patient's tolerance of cold). The wet towel hastens the cooling of the part being treated because the moisture increases the rate of thermal conductivity. Some therapists choose to use

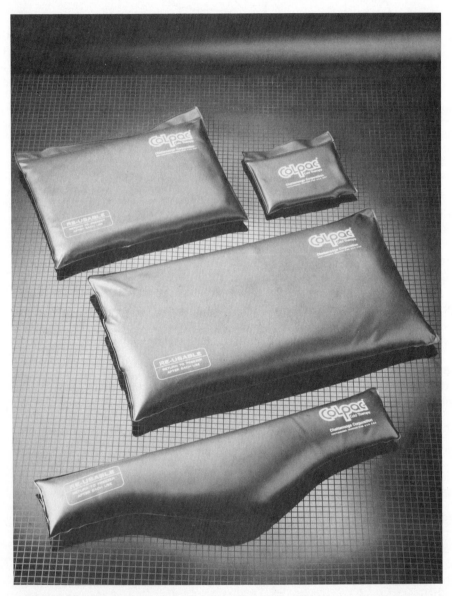

Figure 14–2. Chemical cold packs. Packs of different sizes and shapes can be molded easily around various body parts. For example, the pack at the bottom of the photograph conforms well to a cervical area, a shoulder, or a knee. (*Reproduced with permission from the Chattanooga Corp, Chattanooga, TN.*)

a dry towel to enhance the patient's comfort; the cooling effect is slower and permits the patient to adjust gradually to the cold temperature. The pack should be insulated by covering it with a towel or rubber mat, thus preventing the pack from being warmed by the ambient air. The patient should be draped with a sheet or light blanket to prevent chilling. The therapist should check the skin after 5 min to make sure that it is not bluish. If it is, the pack should be removed immediately.

Duration
The cold pack should be kept on the part for 10–15 min. Once again, the duration of treatment depends on the amount of subcutaneous fat and the desired depth of cooling. By the end of 15 min, the temperature of the pack will have increased substantially.

Advantages
Chemical cold packs are found in almost all physical therapy facilities and, as mentioned earlier, come in different shapes and sizes to fit the contours of many different body parts. These packs are reusable. If the patient can tolerate a cold pack, the therapist can leave the patient and work with another patient if the facility is extremely busy. These cold packs can be used immediately after injuries such as sprains or fractures.

Disadvantages
The cold offered by some chemical cold packs may be less intense than that provided by an ice massage or ice pack (this topic will be referred to later). Chemical cold packs, as mentioned above, must be kept in the refrigeration unit at least 30 min before reusing, whereas ice can be used immediately.

Ice Towels

Ice towels are towels containing ice shavings. They can be used if chemical cold packs and their refrigeration units are not readily available.

Equipment
Terry cloth towels and a bucket of ice water with ice shavings are the only necessary equipment. The ice shavings are caught in the nap of the towel, allowing a substantial cooling effect.

Technique
A terry cloth towel should be thoroughly soaked in the water and ice-shaving mixture. The towel is then wrung out and applied to the part being treated. Because the ice shavings melt quickly, the procedure should be repeated every few minutes to achieve the greatest cooling possible.

Duration
As with cold packs, the treatment time should last about 10 to 15 min.

Advantages
The equipment required is available almost anywhere. No special refrigeration unit is required, as it true of cold packs, although some type of freezer to make ice or ice shavings must be available.

Disadvantages
The main disadvantage of ice towels is that the therapist must keep changing the towels. In addition, because ice water can wet the floor, it must be cleaned up so that no one slips or falls.

Ice Packs

Equipment
Ice packs are simply plastic bags filled with ice cubes or crushed ice. As this definition implies, all that is required is a heavy plastic bag filled with ice or crushed ice.

The crushed ice is preferable because the bag will be more easily molded to the part being treated. Towels also must be available.

Technique

The bag should be filled with ice or ice shavings and be sealed well to prevent melting ice from leaking on the patient or the floor. The technique is the same as that for chemical cold packs. It is usually preferable to place a warm, damp towel between the plastic bag and the patient's skin, mainly for comfort. As is the case for all other treatments, the patient should be placed in a comfortable position and draped well to keep him or her warm if the ambient air is cold.

Duration

The ice pack should remain in place from 5–15 min, depending on the amount of fat in the treated area and the depth of cold penetration desired. In some cases of spasticity, when striving to cool deeper muscles, the time can be extended to 20–40 min (see Chapter 9).[9]

Advantages

The ice pack is quite useful since it can be molded around the part being treated and usually allows the subcutaneous areas to get much colder than a chemical cold pack application does.

Disadvantages

The plastic bag can leak, making it uncomfortable for the patient and dangerous for people in the area if the floor becomes wet. Furthermore, the therapist must continuously check the patient's skin because the ice can cause frostbite.

Vapocoolant Spray

Vapocoolant spray is a method of cooling the skin by the evaporation of a substance sprayed on the skin. Travell[9] used Kraus's method of spraying ethyl chloride on a sprained joint of the middle finger of a young patient and found that the joint was less painful after the spraying and that the normal range of motion was restored quickly. Travell developed the "stretch and spray" technique for treating trigger points. The etiology of trigger points is discussed in Chapter 4. Theoretically, through cooling and desensitization, the pain cycle can be broken. However, some authors believe that counterirritation is the means by which pain is alleviated[10,11]: ie, stimulation of cold or touch can diminish transmission of pain signals.

Equipment

Two vapocoolant sprays are available: ethyl chloride and Fluori-Methane. Today, ethyl chloride is used less often than previously because it is highly flammable or explosive when heated and may cause general anesthesia in patients who inhale large amounts. Ethyl chloride places pressure (as does any aerosol spray) on its container when at room temperature and can explode if dropped. In clinical physical therapy, the use of Fluori-Methane® has replaced ethyl chloride. When sprayed from an inverted bottle, the liquid begins evaporating. Upon contact with the skin of the part being treated, the liquid continues to evaporate, thus cooling the skin for a brief period.

Technique

The area to be treated should be exposed, and the other parts should be covered for warmth and comfort. The patient should be draped and positioned so that the eyes are protected. The bottle of Fluori-Methane must be held in an inverted position to ensure flow of the liquid. According to Travell,[9] the liquid should be sprayed at a 30° angle, 18 inches away from the skin, moving at a rate of 4 inches per second (see Fig. 14–3).

Travell[9] advises beginning at the origin of pain and continuing out over the area of referred pain, spraying the entire length of the muscle once it is in a position

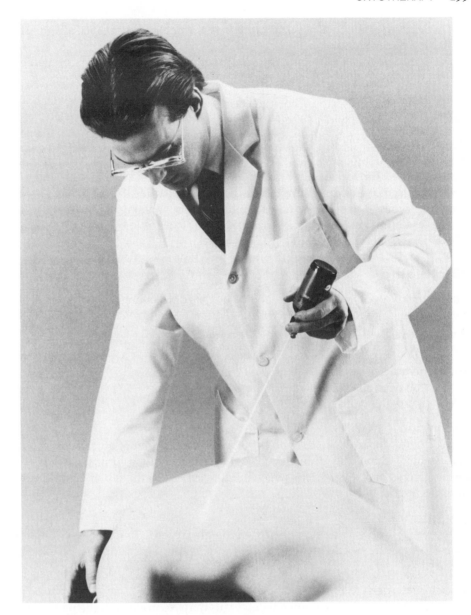

Figure 14–3. Vapocoolant spray. The container is held approximately 18 inches away from the skin in a position that allows the spray to be directed toward the treatment area at an angle of about 30 degrees. (*Reproduced with permission from the Gebauer Company, Cleveland, OH. The trademark Fluori-Methane is the property of that company.*)

of stretch. The muscle is stretched passively before and during spraying. This pattern of spraying is repeated a couple of times. Note that the speed of spraying depends on the patient's condition and response to the technique.

Duration
Spraying should not exceed 6 seconds so that frosting of the skin can be avoided. Should frosting occur, a quick, light massage to the area will help defrost it.

Advantages
Vapocoolant spray offers a quick reaction for immediate reduction of pain. It has also been cited in the treatment of

- joint sprains to relieve pain and swelling and possibly lead to early restoration of motion,[9]

- thermal burns to decrease pain, erythema, and blistering (especially in first-degree burns), and[12]
- painful areas in acute myocardial infarction to replace some pain medications.[13]

Travell[9] advises placing a hot pack briefly over the area after treatment with stretch and spray to avoid subsequent muscle soreness.

Disadvantages

The therapist must be careful not to spray the patient's eyes; therefore, the patient must be draped carefully to protect the face when treating the anterior cervical musculature, for example, As mentioned earlier, frosting of the skin should be avoided because it can lead to ulceration. When using ethyl chloride, the therapist must take extreme care not to drop the bottle because it could explode.

Quick Icing

Quick icing involves the use of three to five swipes of ice along an area to be facilitated. Although this special technique of facilitating muscle contractions is used primarily in patients with central nervous system disorders, it can certainly be used on patients with peripheral nerve injuries.

Equipment

An ice cube held in a paper towel or gauze (see "Ice Massage") and towels to absorb water are the only equipment necessary.

Technique

According to Margaret Rood,[7] who developed this technique, quick swipes with an ice cube over the belly of the involved muscle must be performed three to five times to have a facilatory effect, which might occur immediately or 27 to 42 minutes after application.

Advantages

A motor response may be seen—in a hemiplegic patient, for example—once the patient is past the flaccid stage. The technique is not uncomfortable or dangerous.

Disadvantages

A response may not be seen immediately. This may frustrate both the patient and the therapist.

Combination Treatment: RICE Therapy

In the acute stages of trauma such as a sprain, strain, or fracture, cryotherapy can be combined with compression and elevation of the involved part to reduce or prevent pain, bleeding and swelling. Cold packs, ice towels, ice packs, or *Cryo/Temp* (ie, the coldest form of cryotherapy available) should be used. The technique is known by the acronym RICE because it includes the following:

- Rest (removing weight-bearing pressure and temporarily immobilizing the part).
- Ice (or another cold modality).
- Compression (usually with an ace bandage or an air splint).
- Elevation of the involved limb as much as possible for the first 24–48 hr.

If Cryo/Temp is used, a modality combining cold and compression (discussed in Chapter 28) the therapist must take great care not to apply pressure sufficient to increase bleeding or inflammation in an already painful, sensitive area. Treatment should be limited to about 20 minutes and can be repeated after about 30 minutes to one hour.

GENERAL INDICATIONS AND CONTRAINDICATIONS

Indications

As was stated earlier in the section on the physiological effects of cold, ice and cold can affect tissues in many ways. The uses of cryotherapy are numerous:

1. *Reduction of acute pain.* The mechanisms are not certain; however, the following are possibilities: slowing nerve conduction velocity, anesthetizing the area, or acting as a counterirritant.
2. *Reduction of local bleeding and swelling.* In the acute stages of trauma such as sprains, strains or fractures, cold application can reduce inflammation, bleeding, and swelling.
3. *Reduction of spasm.* Because spasm can be caused and increased by pain, ischemia, muscle tension, apprehension, and so forth, interruption of this pain cycle can reduce the spasm. Once the spasm is diminished, the part (such as the low back) can be treated more easily with massage, exercise, or other modalities.
4. *Reduction of spasticity.* In patients with upper motor neuron lesions such as strokes or spinal cord injuries, spasticity can greatly limit function and progress in rehabilitation. The application of cold to a spastic muscle group may reduce the spasticity for as long as 90 minutes.[1] Once the spasticity has been reduced, the involved muscles can be passively stretched to prevent or alleviate contractures. The antagonist muscle groups can be exercised actively, and the patient can perhaps learn to use the limb in a more normal, functional manner.
5. *Facilitation of motor responses.* Techniques such as quick icing can be used on patients with neurologic involvement or patients after orthopedic surgery when the involved muscles need reeducation.
6. Treatment of acute burns. The application of ice-water compresses or immersion of the part in ice water can greatly reduce the pain of burns and the subsequent blistering.[1]
7. Treatment in conjunction with (a) joint mobilization to reduce the possibility of pain and swelling, (b) deep friction massage before and after the massage to reduce pain and irritation, (c) high-volt galvanic or other electro-stimulation to help alleviate swelling, (d) strenuous workouts or competitive events to avoid residual swelling, and (e) rest, compression, and elevation to alleviate increased bleeding and swelling.

Contraindications

1. If a patient has ever had frostbite in the area to be treated, another modality must be chosen.
2. If a patient has Raynaud's disease, severe pain may develop, especially if the hands or feet or nearby areas are treated.
3. If the circulation to a part being treated is compromised, the normal vascular responses to cold application may not take place and frostbite might occur.
4. If a patient is very old or very young, the thermoregulatory responses may not function adequately.
5. If a patient is extremely sensitive or allergic to cold, he or she may not tolerate any cold treatments and another modality must be chosen.

SPECIAL CONSIDERATIONS

The physical therapist must be aware that the application of cold can lead to a reduced speed of muscle contraction because of a slower nerve conduction velocity. Therefore, asking a patient to perform rapid exercises immediately after a cold application could be counterproductive (see, also, Chapter 10).[14] Increased viscosity of joints, tendons, and ligaments may decrease the patient's ability to perform quick movements. The therapist should be aware that the application of cold before exercise remains a controversial issue. The therapist also must keep in mind that cold reduces the ability of collagen tissues to elongate. If the tissue is anesthetized, stretching procedures may tear muscle, tendon, or joint fibers. Therefore, if stretching is prescribed, it must be done with great care and ease.

Some people are extremely sensitive to cold and may develop a rapid drop in blood pressure as a result of a cold application. Others may develop severe itching and erythema. Still others may suffer from Raynaud's phenomenon, which leads to sudden spasm of the small arteries of the feet, hands, and fingers, which can become extremely painful, pale, then blue followed by red. Before treating a patient with ice, the therapist must test a small area of the patient's body to note the response. Patients who lack sensation to temperature must be monitored very carefully to note any of the changes mentioned above. To avoid reactions (eg, frostbite or edema) ice packs used in treatment for pain and acute injuries should be applied intermittently (ie, after a 15–20-min. treatment, remove for the same length of time and then reapply) (see Chap. 9).

As is the case with many other physical agents used in physical therapy, more experimental work must be done with cold to validate what clinicians see as results of a treatment.

■ **KEY TERMS**

cryotherapy	**ice packs**
ice massage	**Cryo/Temp**
chemical cold packs	**vapocoolant spray**
Hydrocollator cold packs	**quick icing**
Col-Pack cold packs	**RICE therapy**
ice towels	

■ **REVIEW QUESTIONS**

1. A 25-year-old runner has just sprained his ankle in the marathon. What type of cold application would you give him if you had the choice of any of the cold modalities described in this chapter? Explain your answer.

2. A 40-year-old woman comes to you with a spasm in her left posterior cervical musculature. You know that cold is a good choice because it reduces pain and spasm. What would you do before choosing a cold modality? Why would you do this?

3. A patient with chronic spasm of the upper trapezius muscles is no longer covered by insurance. Yet you believe that cold, in addition to gentle stretching, is the best way to rid her of her spasm and pain. You have written out a home exercise program for her. What type of cold would you tell her to use at home? Why?

4. A patient comes to the physical therapy area with a severely swollen lower extremity on which there appears to be a diabetic ulcer. Would you use the Cryo/Temp? Why?

5. One of your patients has had a stroke, and now his left bicep brachii are spastic. What could you do for this patient in addition to or before therapeutic exercise?

6. Name two contraindications to ice massage on the foot or hand.
7. How does Fluori-Methane spray cool the skin?

REFERENCES

1. Lehmann JF, ed: *Therapeutic Heat and Cold,* 3rd ed. Baltimore, MD: Williams & Wilkins; 1982.
2. McMaster WC: Cryotherapy. *Physician Sports Med.* 1982; 10(11):113–119.
3. Fox RH: Local cooling in man. *Br Med Bull.* 1961; 17(1):14–18.
4. Goodgold J, Eberstein A: *Electrodiagnosis of Neuromuscular Disorders,* 3rd ed. Baltimore, MD: Williams & Wilkins; 1983.
5. McMaster N, Liddle S, Waugh T: Laboratory evaluation of various cold modalities. *Am J Sports Med.* 1978; 6:291–294.
6. DonTigny RL, Sheldon K: Simultaneous use of heat and cold in treatment of muscle spasm. *Arch Phys Med Rehabil.* 1962; 43:235–237.
7. Weisberg J: Influence of icing and brushing on the achilles tendon reflex in human subjects. *Physiother* (Can). 1976;28(1):21–23.
8. Lowdon BJ, Moore RJ: Determinants and nature of intramuscular temperature changes during cold therapy. *J Phys Med.* 1975; 54:223–233.
9. Travell J, Simons D: *Myofascial Pain and Dysfunction: The Trigger Point Manual.* Baltimore, MD: Williams & Wilkins; 1983.
10. Melzack R, Jeans M, Stratford J, et al: Ice massage and transcutaneous electrical stimulation: comparison of treatment for low back pain. *Pain.* 1980; 9:209–217.
11. Simons D, Travell J: Myofascial trigger points: a possible explanation. *Pain.* 1981; 10:106–109.
12. Travell J, Koprowska I, Hirsch BB, et al: Effect of ethyl chloride spray on thermal burns. *Pharmacol Exp Ther.* 1951; 101:36.
13. Rinzler SH, Stein I, Bakst H, et al: Blocking effect of ethylchloride spray of cardiac pain induced by ergonovine. *Proc Soc Bio and Med.* 1954;85:329–333.
14. Chatfield PO: Hypothermia and its effects on sensory and peripheral motor systems. *Ann NY Acad Sci.* 1959; 80:445–448.

15

Considerations for All Thermal Treatments

Bernadette Hecox, PT, MA

T he previous chapters in this section have shown that the application of thermal modalities can produce systemic as well as local responses. Both ambient conditions and the patient's activity level can augment or diminish these systemic responses. For example, an extremely warm day or swimming rather than just soaking in a heated pool can place greater demands on body systems that are affected by temperature changes. Although healthy adults can usually tolerate these demands, they may be excessive for many patients seen in physical therapy: ie, young children, the elderly, or the debilitated. Therefore, the physical therapist must constantly be alert to the reactions that may occur in these patients.

This chapter briefly discusses the monitoring of signs and symptoms that may indicate overstressed systems. It also reviews ambient conditions that may place extra stress on patients but are unlikely to affect a healthy working therapist. Finally, heat-related problems, their causes, related signs and symptoms, and treatments are discussed.

MONITORING OF SIGNS AND SYMPTOMS

Observing the condition of the patient's skin as well as being aware of the status of all vital signs is essential when applying thermal modalities. In simple cases, when the patient has no systemic involvement, visual observation is sufficient.

The skin reveals changes in blood flow, body temperature, the patient's general health, and the autonomic nervous system's reactions to pain or to emotions such as fear. The general condition and color of the skin must always be observed and any abnormalities noted in the patient's chart.

Depending on the dosage (intensity, duration, and area of the body to which the modality is applied), changes in vital signs may occur. Therapists should know what changes in vital signs to expect and recognize which are within the normal range for the amount of stress produced by the specific treatment. For example, with a 20-minute, very warm Hubbard tank treatment, a rise in core temperature of 2° F is expected, as are temporary fluctuations in blood pressure and pulse rate (see Chapter 9).

Therapists may be treating people who already have raised body temperature (hyperpyrexia), rapid or slow heart rate (tachycardia or bradycardia), high or low blood pressure (hypertension or hypotension), or a combination of symptoms. In many physical therapy departments, such as those in acute care hospitals and nursing homes, a high percentage of patients may have some form of heart disease. When treating patients with these problems, the therapist should do the following:

- Consult with a physician if cardiac or other problems are such that they might be exacerbated by a thermal treatment.
- Proceed cautiously with or discontinue treatment if the patient complains or shows signs of general discomfort, displays a notable increase in respiration, or has a marked increase or decrease in pulse rate.
- Always take the pulse rate before a vigorous or prolonged heat treatment and do so often during the treatment.

Because debilitated patients can experience cardiac stress from thermal treatments, safety guidelines adapted from those prescribed for exercise and for cardiac rehabilitation are presented here.[1–5]

During any normal 20–30 minute heat treatment, the therapist should discontinue the treatment and make a note in the patient's chart if any of the following signs are observed:

- If the pulse rate of a young adult approaches double the resting rate. For deconditioned people, use the age-rate formula: ie, subtract the patient's age from 220; the pulse rate should not exceed 50% of that number.

$$\text{Pulse rate limit} = (220 - \text{age}) \times 0.5$$

- If the strength of the patient's pulse diminishes.
- If the patient's blood pressure changes from pretreatment resting levels, according to the following guidelines: (1) if a non-well adult's systolic pressure declines more than 15–20 mm Hg or increases more than 30 mm Hg; the decrease in systolic pressure is a **major sign of danger,** (2) if the diastolic pressure increases more than 20 mm Hg or goes above 130 mm Hg or if it decreases more than 20 mm Hg, (3) if extreme increases in systolic and diastolic pressures are accompanied by headache or blurred vision, (4) if the systolic pressure and the pulse rate **decrease** progressively **stop treatment immediately and summon a physician.**

Vigorous generalized heat treatments should not be given if the patient's systolic pressure is less than 90 mm Hg. Cardiologists commonly advise patients with ischemic heart disease to avoid extremes in ambient temperature, either hot or cold.

EFFECTS OF AMBIENT CONDITIONS

When considering the physiological changes that occur with application of heat or cold, the therapist should pay attention to the ambient conditions in which the thermal treatments are given. Although wind velocity and atmospheric pressure are important ambient factors, the discussion is limited to ambient temperature and humidity in this text.

In general, healthy people who are accustomed to living in any given climate function well and maintain a constant internal temperature despite day-to-day changes in the weather. Whenever such changes cause the body temperature to deviate even slightly, most people maintain thermal homeostasis by adjusting their behavior—by changing their activity level and the amount of clothing worn and by appropriate alterations in the physiological effector responses such as shivering or sweating.[6] However, if a person is suddenly exposed to different climatic conditions, although the usual effector responses may operate, they may be inadequate for safe and comfortable thermoregulation.

We have all experienced or observed the behavioral and physiological reactions occurring after a flight to a climate that differs from the climate to which we are accustomed. For example, if a New Yorker flies to Florida on a February day that is 25° F in New York and 88° F and humid in Florida, he feels hot and sweaty even though he puts on summer clothes and moves slowly when outdoors. Meanwhile, Floridians are comfortably engaging in their normal activities.

A few days later, a Texan leaves home, where the temperature is 88° F, and arrives in New York City, where the temperature is 50° F, an unusually mild February day. Despite putting on two pairs of warm-up pants and a sweater under her coat, she is extremely uncomfortable, shivering, complaining about the cold, and preferring to stay indoors. Meanwhile, New Yorkers are out strolling, opening their coats and enjoying the unseasonably warm day.

In both cases, the traveler's behavioral responses are appropriate. Because their physiological systems are not "set" to maintain homeostasis in the new environment, the adaptations in their clothing, shelter requirements, and activities protect them from excessive shivering or sweating until their systems are "reset." Each day they become less uncomfortable as physiological changes occur during the process of acclimatization.

Acclimatization can be defined as the means by which humans, when placed in a different climatic environment, gradually make physiologic adjustments that enable them to function comfortably and maintain homeostasis.[7] The terms "artificial acclimatization" and "acclimation" are often used to describe adjustments that occur under laboratory conditions where an artificial change in climate has been created.[8,9] However, all three terms are frequently used interchangeably.

During the process of acclimatization, the activities of the thermoregulatory systems of the body adjust to cope with the new environment. These adjustments occur only if exposure to the changed climatic conditions is sufficient to place a stress on these systems. Such stress is referred to as "heat stress" or "cold stress".[7]

Unfortunately, heat and cold stress can overload the thermoregulatory systems of many patients seen in physical therapy unless the patients are carefully monitored. Patients who are susceptible to systemic breakdowns include those who have recently arrived from other climates, those who are debilitated and attempt therapeutic exercise at the onset of unexpected seasonal changes such as a sudden heat wave, and those who receive prolonged or intense heat treatments to large areas of the body. It has been reported that people with borderline heart conditions may experience severe heart failure in hot weather because the increase in blood flow in the skin necessary for cooling puts an extra load on the heart. When the weather cools again, the cardiac condition reverts to its borderline status.[10] Children also are at high risk for heat-related illnesses. Physiologically, their thermoregulatory systems are less well controlled than are adult systems, and their capacity to sweat and convect heat from core to body surface is not as great. Morphologically, the ratio of their surface area per volume is greater than that of adults; thus, heat is transferred more easily from the environment to their bodies.[11]

In many treatment situations, especially home care, minimally endowed nursing homes, and heated pool areas, therapists are concerned about reactions caused by an increase rather than a decrease in ambient temperature. Therefore this discussion of heat acclimatization is limited to the major points that may help clinicians gauge the intensity of the treatments given when patients are suddenly exposed to hot ambient conditions.

In the past, the ability to function well in specific climates was attributed to racial differences—that is, natural selection favored some individuals. Tolerance for certain climates was attributed to physiologic and anatomic factors inherent to the peoples who had survived in those climates. Although racial factors have not been ruled out, the results of several studies indicate that peoples other than natives can achieve much the same tolerance because humans have the ability to make appropriate acculturational and physiologic adjustments when placed in a different climate.[12–14]

The findings of studies in which young healthy men who were adjusted to working in temperate climates were required to do moderate exercise under hot climatic conditions illustrate the acclimatization process.[15,16] On Day 1 their heart rates increased markedly while stroke volume decreased; thus, their cardiac output remained about the same as it was in temperate conditions. Although the men sweated profusely, their rectal temperature rose, on the average, 2° F higher than it was when they performed the same work in temperate conditions. Over a period of days, adjustments occurred. The men's sweat volume increased, whereas the concentration of sodium in the sweat decreased. Their heat rate and rectal temperature declined to levels similar to those when they were doing equal work in the temperate conditions.

In general, studies have shown that adequate adjustment occurs in 4 to 7 days and acclimatization is nearly complete in 12 to 14 days.[17,18] These physiological adaptations can occur with as little as 1 hour per day of "heat stress," but a greater adaptation occurs if one is stressed for approximately 2 hours. A single 100-minute period of work in heat is shown to be more effective than two 50-minute periods.[15] For children, the rate of acclimatization is slower than that for adults.[11]

Although passive acclimatization has some benefits,[12] in general, investigators agree that a person who is sedentary during the acclimatization period is only adjusted to sedentary conditions in this hot climate.[19] In a hot climate, one must do sufficient work to cause heat-work stress during the acclimatization period. Thus, if a soccer team from Chicago plans to play safely and efficiently in tropical West Africa, the players should not only live in that West African climate for at least 5 days but also practice to the point of stress each day. Adjustments to heat are relative to the amount of stress experienced. Because each person will display individual reactions throughout the adjustment period, heart rate, temperature, and sweat volume must be carefully monitored.[20]

How long acclimatization will be maintained once a person is removed from the heat stress situation has not been determined as yet. Some investigators believe that the physiological adjustments will be maintained for 2 weeks or more,[21] whereas others believe that some decline occurs even over a weekend without heat-work stress.[22] Other adaptations that occur when people live in a hot climate for an extended period need not be addressed in the context of this text.

When one experiences a sudden increase in ambient temperature, the behavioral adjustments, apparently made to alleviate discomfort, are in fact extremely important for maintaining homeostasis. Because the cardiovascular and sudomotor systems are not yet "set," one may sweat a great deal but the sudomotor system is not prepared to provide enough sweat to maintain thermal homeostasis for the hotter conditions. If this loss of fluid continues, with the usual salt concentration, dehydration and a great electrolyte imbalance could result. Much of the fluid required for sweat is furnished by blood plasma. Thus, when the cardiovascular system acts to cool (by dilation of peripheral vessels and increased heart rate, which send more blood to the periphery), it not only brings internal heat to the surface for radiation, it provides fluid for sweat as well. If cardiac output remains constant but the peripheral blood flow increases, blood must be shunted from visceral systems such as the renal system. If this situation continues, vital organs will be deprived of their blood supply. The increased heart rate that occurs can fatigue heart muscles that have not been trained for such activity.

Fortunately, within a few days, the following adjustment mechanisms occur. Total plasma volume increases. There is an increase in blood flow to the skin, which allows more heat dissipation, and to muscles, which increases their ability to do work. The adrenal system adjusts to allow more sweating, which enables more cooling by evaporation. With these increases in cooling mechanisms, vital signs stabilize. The salt concentration in sweat decreases; thus, the electrolyte balance is maintained.

CONSIDERATIONS FOR PHYSICAL THERAPISTS

The information given in this section can have direct application to clinical situations.

1. Patients who are suddenly exposed to a hotter or more humid environment should do some exercise daily with careful monitoring of vital signs and other symptoms of distress. The patient cannot be expected to rest for 5 days, and then be adjusted for normal activities.
2. The therapist must consider the status of each patient because of individual differences in physiologic responses.
3. The therapist should consider a modality other than heat rather than superimpose hot weather, a heat modality, and therapeutic exercise on a patient.
4. The therapist must be aware that patients with cardiac problems are unable to tolerate new cardiovascular demands and that patients with Addison's disease or other adrenal problems are unable to tolerate excessive sweating.
5. The therapist must be aware that children, debilitated people, and elderly people, if unable to tolerate the overload of heat, may have a breakdown in one or more of the many systems involved in thermoregulation and can experience a "heat accident," as described later in this chapter.

REACTIONS CAUSED BY EXCESSIVE EXPOSURE TO HEAT OR COLD

Excessive ambient heat does not "burn up" a body. Rather it causes system "burn out" as a result of overload: in other words, the heat loss mechanisms cannot work hard enough to balance the heat gain. With excessive cold, the body's attempt to increase heat production through shivering and exercise may lead to exhaustion.

Cardiovascular Reactions

If the heart rate, stroke volume, or both, are unable to increase sufficiently to maintain cardiac output, the blood pressure will drop, which in turn may increase the amount of blood pooling in the veins. People who stand in one position in hot weather frequently become faint because blood has pooled in their legs, thus depriving the brain of its supply.[5,19] Increased venous pooling also decreases cardiac filling. When less blood reaches the heart, the ultimate result is less blood for cardiac emptying, which causes a further drop in blood pressure.[23] The heart strives to rectify the situation by increasing the pulse rate, which results in an additional decrease in stroke volume. In turn, the heart rate increases even more in a greater attempt to rectify the decrease in blood pressure. This vicious cycle continues until the attempts of the heart are beyond its capability. If the heart rate increases beyond 140–200 beats per minute, depending on the individual, the time for cardiac filling is insufficient, even in healthy individuals.[24] The result may be cardiac arrest.

Sudomotor Reactions

Because evaporation of sweat is the primary means by which the body loses heat in hot weather, the importance of an intact sudomotor system in maintaining thermal homeostasis cannot be overemphasized. If people are acclimatized to the heat conditions they are exposed to, the adrenal and endocrine systems can usually regulate the fluid-electrolyte balance provided that the body maintains ample fluids and electrolytes to meet the demand. The output of sweat must be balanced by the intake of fluid and food. However, when a nonacclimatized person is exposed to high temperatures for prolonged periods, the demands on the systems that regulate fluids and pH balance may be too great. Excessive sweating without changes in the concentrations of salt and other electrolytes can lead to serious heat-related problems ranging from heat cramps to heat stroke. These problems are discussed later in this chapter.

Metabolic Reactions

Because the metabolic rate is temperature related, excessive heating may increase the rate to the point that the other systems cannot clear metabolic wastes adequately. Consequently, the normal pH balance is disturbed. If an excessive amount of acid escapes with sweat and the blood alkaline level increases, the systems usually react by periodical reversing of the pH in the sweat and blood fluids. However, with extreme demands, the systems may become deregulated.

The metabolic response to a decrease in the temperature of local tissues differs from the response to general body cooling. When the temperature of local tissues drops, the metabolic rate of those tissues decreases. However, if the central thermoregulating areas receive information that the internal temperature of the body is decreasing, the metabolic rate will increase. Although this increased rate is chemically induced in part, it is primarily the result of shivering and the movements one makes to keep warm. But both the movements and shivering, if prolonged, may lead to physical exhaustion.

Fig. 15–1 illustrates which thermoregulatory system is primarily responsible for maintaining thermal homeostasis when a person is exposed to different ambient temperatures. Physical therapists can use this information to make decisions about treating people with borderline systemic problems. The temperatures given are approximate, and the reactions are relative to the severity and duration of the exposure.

An ambient temperature ranging from approximately 71.6° F to 86° F (22° to 30° C) is considered to be the *zone of thermal neutrality*. This is the range in which vasomotor regulation provides sufficient heat loss to balance the metabolic heat

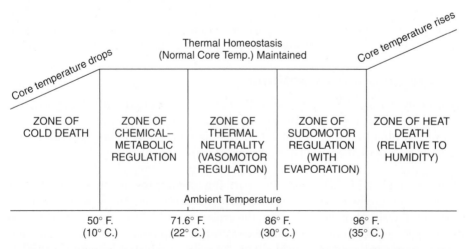

Fig. 15–1. Systems maintaining thermal homeostasis in various ambient temperatures denoted by zones. Relative to the duration of exposure, humans cannot maintain a normal internal (core) temperature if the ambient temperature is lower than 50° F or higher than 96° F relative to the humidity.

gain. The range for a nude resting man is 82.4° F to 86° F (28° to 30° C); if the man is wearing light clothes, doing mild exercise, or both, the range may be lowered to between 71.6° F and 75.2° F (22° and 24° C).[9] When the temperature exceeds this range, the vasomotor activity will increase but the system will be incapable of maintaining a constant core temperature because the effectiveness of radiation diminishes as the temperature gradient between the environment and skin decreases. Thus, the sudomotor system must act to maintain homeostasis. Even when resting, a man's sensible sweating begins when the ambient temperature rises to about 85° F (29° C) and a woman's sensible sweating begins when the temperature reaches approximately 89.6° F (32° C). Sweating increases as the temperature increases. When the ambient temperature equals or is higher than the body surface temperature (approximately 96° F) (35.5° C), radiation ceases or reverses direction.

The temperature range above approximately 86° F (30° C) is considered to be the *zone of sudomotor regulation.* Because the vaporization process is what cools the body, the environment must allow this sweat to evaporate. If the temperature-humidity index is high, evaporation cannot occur and the core temperature and metabolic rate will increase. Thus, the *apparent temperature,* which is based on the relationship between temperature and humidity rather than temperature alone, provides a better description of ambient conditions. Table 15–1 illustrates the differences. If the ambient temperature is 90° F and the humidity is only 20%, the apparent temperature is 87° F. If the humidity is 60%, however, the apparent temperature is 100° F. If the temperature is 85° F but the humidity is 90%, the apparent temperature is 102° F, but if the humidity is 40%, the apparent temperature is 86° F.

In general, disabled people can exercise safely when the ambient temperature is 80° F if the humidity is 40% (apparent temperature 79° F). However, exercise is unsafe if the humidity is 70% (apparent temperature 85° F).[25] Because of the humidity, apparent temperatures are commonly within the range where caution should be used in hydrotherapy areas.

With continued increased in ambient temperature, the danger of system breakdowns increases. Neither the vasomotor nor sudomotor system is capable of functioning adequately to maintain thermal equilibrium. Excessive increases in body temperature and metabolic rate can cause serious problems or death. If the body temperature is higher than about 106° F (41.1° C) long enough, brain damage occurs. If the body temperature is higher than about 110° F for even brief periods, the result may be death. If the increase in metabolic rate is excessive, severe disturbances in pH balance can lead to tetany or death.[8,9]

The range of ambient temperature from approximately 71.6° F to 50° F (22° to 10° C) is considered to be the *zone of chemical-metabolic regulation.* The first systemic reactions that occur to preserve the constant internal temperature are cutaneous vasoconstriction and pilo erections. Although some production of chemical-metabolic heat may begin at ambient temperatures 86° F to 77° F (30° C to 25° C), it increases markedly at temperatures below 68° F (20° C). These chemical-metabolic reactions are the shivering and nonshivering thermogenesis mentioned in the section in Chapter 9 devoted to systemic responses to cold.[26]

TABLE 15–1. EXAMPLES OF APPARENT TEMPERATURES

Ambient Temperature	Relative Humidity	Apparent Temperature
90° F	60%	100° F
90° F	20%	87° F
85° F	90%	102° F
85° F	40%	86° F
80° F	70%	85° F
80° F	40%	79 ° F

*Adapted from a table compiled by the National Weather Service. *Utica Observer Dispatch,* August 4, 1988.

PATHOLOGICAL PROBLEMS CAUSED BY OVEREXPOSURE TO HEAT

Exposure to excessive heat can cause a variety of problems. Dermatologic problems such as prickly heat (miliaria) or temporary dehydration are minor problems, but they can lead to more serious disorders, or heat accidents: ie, heat cramps, heat exhaustion, and heat stroke. Because many patients seen in physical therapy are susceptible to these problems and require precautionary measures, each problem is briefly discussed below. (Many studies and in-depth reports are available.[27-32])

Prickly Heat

Prickly heat is a minor skin infection caused by obstructions in the ducts of the active sweat glands. It is seen in areas of the body that remain moist because of sweating and a lack of exposure to air: for example, in areas that are constantly covered by hot compresses, clothes, or diapers. This infection is characterized by pinpoint-sized lesions and "prickly"-type itching sensations.[33] To prevent prickly heat from developing, the therapist should always allow the patient's skin to dry completely after removing a modality that produces sweating. Knochel[31] reported that any form of sweat gland malfunction or entrapment, including prickly heat, renders people with diseases such as scleroderma or cystic fibrosis more susceptible to heat stroke.

Dehydration

Dehydration is a net decrease in body fluids that occurs when fluid intake is insufficient to compensate for fluids lost normally through sweat, respiration, urine, and feces. In general, the fluid lost per day can be replaced by consuming about 2 quarts of fluids in drink and food each day.[34] The amount of fluid intake required increases, depending on the amount of heating and the activity level. During the Persian Gulf war of 1991, the American military personnel, if active, were instructed to drink six or more gallons of water per day.[35] Vomiting, diarrhea, or intestinal drainage—conditions often experienced by patients seen in physical therapy—can result in a greater loss of both fluid and electrolytes.[36] Such patients can be encouraged to sip fluids during or soon after exercise periods. If the therapist suspects that a patient's electrolyte balance is in jeopardy, however, he or she should consult the physician. Although temporary dehydration is not a serious problem, it may precipitate a more serious heat-related disorder. Ranging from least to most severe, these heat accidents are heat cramps, heat exhaustion, and heat stroke.

Although these heat accidents are discussed separately, more than one component of the thermoregulatory system often breaks down, and early symptoms of heat distress may include characteristics of each component. Thus, the symptoms of these conditions are not as clear cut as the discussions indicate.

Heat Cramps

Heat cramps are believed to result from either an imbalance of electrolytes, primarily reduced salt in muscles, or water depletion.[29,33] The precise cause is not completely understood. The imbalance of electrolytes can occur in hot weather and is the result of either insufficient salt intake or excessive salt output. Insufficient salt intake can occur if a person drinks an excessive amount of nonsalty fluids such as plain water, thus disturbing the fluid or salt balance or if the person's diet provides an insufficient amount of salt. Excessive salt output can occur when a normal output of sweat contains a high salt concentration or when the salt concentration is normal but sweating is excessive.

Laborers and athletes who sweat profusely and replace the water but not the salt often experience heat cramps. The primary symptoms are severe cramps in the extremities, the abdomen, or both areas. Vital signs are usually unchanged with heat cramps.

Treatment includes rest and immediate but gradual replacement of fluid balance by drinking fluids, which perhaps contain a small amount of salt, and by increasing the amount of salt in the diet. The type of fluid that should be ingested, especially its salt and sugar content, is subject to much debate. Some researchers have shown that increasing the amount of salt in the diet is sufficient to balance the amount lost in fluids.[37] Other studies have shown that hypertonic drinks may be more effective in maintaining normal plasma volume and electrolyte balance.[17,38] Since plasma supplies fluid for sweat, a decreased volume of plasma will reduce the rate of sweating. In general, the subjects in these studies were healthy young adults or animals, not debilitated or elderly people; thus, extrapolating the results to patients may be questionable. Salt tablets are not recommended "since their hypertonicity may cause fluid shift into the G.I. tract."[28] According to the current definition of heat cramps, findings or symptoms other than muscular cramps automatically categorize the problem as some form of heat exhaustion.[31]

Heat Exhaustion

Heat exhaustion occurs when a person is exposed to more heat than the thermoregulatory mechanisms are capable of controlling. Although heat exhaustion rarely occurs in pure form, in order to differentiate the causes, it can be categorized as exercise-induced heat exhaustion (heat syncopy), water-depletion heat exhaustion and salt-depletion heat exhaustion.[7]

A form of heat exhaustion called *heat syncopy* is characterized by fainting or collapse when standing or exercising in extreme heat. The peripheral dilation and tachycardia resulting from the heat, the exercise, or both can cause an increase in venous pooling, which in turn results in hypotension, a loss of blood flow to the brain, and fainting.

Water-depletion heat exhaustion may occur in people who do hard work in a temperate climate or moderate work in a hot climate, in children, and in feeble adults who are unable to ask for or obtain water—for example, in residents of marginally staffed nursing homes. Early symptoms include intense thirst, fatigue, weakness, discomfort, anxiety, or impaired judgment. The body temperature is elevated slightly.[28] If the condition is not treated, more serious symptoms or heat stroke can develop.

Salt-depletion heat exhaustion usually afflicts nonacclimatized people who have a high concentration of salt in sweat or who sweat excessively. The symptoms may differ from those resulting in water depletion. The victims do not complain of thirst; they are likely to complain of a headaches or nausea and may experience giddiness, vomiting, or diarrhea. The skin will be pale and clammy. The body temperature may be normal or subnormal. The major symptoms are hypotension and tachycardia.[28]

Although heat exhaustion caused by water and salt depletion have been differentiated, the causes and symptoms frequently overlap. The symptoms of heat exhaustion may actually indicate the early stage of heat stroke.[32]

Treatment includes cooling the patient gradually, positioning the patient's head level with or lower than the trunk to encourage blood flow to the brain, and elevating the patient's legs to encourage venous return from the lower extremities. Massaging the lower extremities also reduces venous pooling. The lost fluid or salt should be replaced **gradually.**

Heat Stroke

Heat stroke, the most dangerous of all heat accidents, may result in coma or death if not treated immediately. Heat strokes occur most commonly during hot humid weather, when sweat does not evaporate, and during exposure to excessive, uninterrupted heat—eg, during a heat wave without cooling periods at night. The body temperature increases, and the cardiovascular system responds excessively in an attempt to bring more blood to the periphery.[31]

Three factors that predispose a person to heat stroke are dehydration, lack of acclimatization to a hot humid environment, and poor physical fitness. Healthy adults who work hard for prolonged periods in heat (eg, road workers laying tar in extremely hot humid weather), the elderly, and the debilitated are susceptible to heat stroke. In addition, people who suffer from malnutrition, diabetes mellitus, or cardiac problems are vulnerable.[30] Finally, drugs such as benztropine mesylate, atropine, and other anticholinergics; phenothiazine; and antihistamines may increase vulnerability.[31]

Heat waves in the United States, even in recent years, have caused many heat stroke-related deaths among elderly people who did not have air conditioners or adequate cooling devices. Because some physical therapy departments and home care settings are not air conditioned, therapists must be aware of their susceptible patients, those who are elderly or have cardiac problems especially if doing exercise.

Although a variety of factors are involved in the etiology of heat stroke, the three prevalent ones are elevated body temperature, metabolic acidosis, and hypoxia. Victims of heat stroke usually have body temperatures higher than 107° F (41.6° C), but if temperatures as low as 104° F (40° C) are maintained long enough, heat stroke can result.[2,39] Heat strokes can occur even in young adults who are experiencing intense heat and in people who are experiencing great heat stress without physical exertion: for example, while in a sauna or a Turkish bath.[32]

Time is of the essence when treating heat strokes. Unless the body temperature is lowered quickly, metabolic acidosis and tissue hypoxia develop.[30] Early symptoms may be similar to those related to heat exhaustion and may or may not include headache, lightheadedness, vertigo, and abdominal distress. However, the major sign is a rapid increase in body temperature, which may lead to delirium, coma, brain damage, or death. The pulse will be fast—130–160 beats per minute—and breathing will be rapid. The skin will be hot but not necessarily dry. The common belief that the major symptom of heat stroke is cessation of sweating is misleading because many victims maintain the sweating function.

Treatment begins by using any possible, even drastic, means of cooling the body in an attempt to lower the body temperature rapidly. Move the person out of the sun, expose the person's entire body to a cool breeze, and elevate the person's head to avoid increased blood flow to the brain. Use whatever means of cooling are available: eg, immerse the body in cool water or wrap it in cold wet towels. Some authors recommend that the rectal temperature should be reduced 0.54° F (0.3° C) every 5 minutes for the first 30 minutes.[30] Cooling the body at a rate faster or slower than this reduces the chance of survival. Cooling should continue until the person's temperature has been reduced to 102° F (38.9° C).

Table 15–2 includes the major causes, symptoms, and immediate treatments for the three major types of heat accidents. Any person who treats or cares for elderly or disabled people or treats patients with heat or exercise, especially in a hot environment, should be familiar with the information given in the table.

SUMMARY

This chapter has discussed factors that should be considered concerning the general condition of patients when being treated with thermal modalities and also precautionary measures that should be taken to avoid problems that can occur. The differences between the ability of healthy adults and many physical therapy patients to tolerate stress on body systems were noted. Such patients include young children and elderly or debilitated individuals. The importance of monitoring a patient's skin and vital signs was emphasized, and various ambient conditions that

TABLE 15–2. FACTORS ASSOCIATED WITH HEAT ACCIDENTS

Factor	Heat Cramps	Heat Exhaustion			Heat Stroke
		Exercise Induced Exhaustion Syncopy	Water Depletion Exhaustion	Salt Depletion	
Etiology	Electrolyte imbalance Negative salt balance in muscles. Caused by drinking excessive amounts of non-salt fluids or food, excessive sweating with normal salt content, or normal sweating with high salt content.	Peripheral vascular dilatation, tachycardia, or both causing venous pooling.	Insufficient water intake for amount of exercise per temperature-humidity performed.	Insufficient salt intake to replenish (1) excessive salt in normal amount of sweat or (2) excessive sweat.	Exposure to excessive heat/humidity, usually for prolonged periods or for short periods of strenuous exercise.
Those susceptible in excessive heat	The very active and the ill or debilitated.	People doing excessive exercise or prolonged standing.	Healthy adults doing prolonged or strenuous exercise in heat without replenishing water; children; nonexercising feeble adults unable to obtain water.	Nonacclimatized people.	People in poor physical condition; those suffering from conditions such as cardiac problems, diabetes mellitus, malnutrition, and healthy people doing strenous exercise.
Symptoms	If active, severe cramps in extremities or abdomen. If ill, minor discomfort and muscle weakness. No change in vital signs.	Fainting or collapse.	Thirst, fatigue, weakness, discomfort, anxiety, impaired judgment. Temperature may be slightly elevated.	Headache, giddiness, nausea, vomiting, pale and clammy skin. Temmperature may be normal or subnormal. Hypotension, tachycardia.	In early stages, may be similar to heat exhaustion. EXTREMELY HIGH TEMPERATURE: 102–107° F or more. Rapid pulse and respiration; skin hot; cessation of sweating (usually but not always).
Treatment	Rest; immediate but gradual replacement of salt intake in fluids and in diet.	Rest. Cooling the patient. Place head level with or lower than trunk. Elevate and massage legs. Begin gradual replacement of fluids or salt in drinks and food. The heat exhaustion problems may overlap.			Keep head elevated. Begin cooling immediately by using cool towel wraps, immersing in cool water, ice massage, or whatever means available. Reduce rectal temperature approximately 0.54° F (0.3° C) every 5 min until 102° F.

affect patients receiving thermal treatments were pointed out. Finally, the causes and signs and symptoms of heat-related problems and basic treatments were discussed.

■ KEY TERMS

acclimatization	heat cramps
zone of thermal neutrality	heat exhaustion
zone of sudomotor regulation	heat syncopy
apparent temperature	water depletion heat exhaustion
zone of chemical-metabolic regulation	salt depletion heat exhaustion
prickly heat	heat stroke
dehydration	

■ REVIEW QUESTIONS

1. What precautionary steps should a physical therapist take when treating a patient who has a cardiac problem?
2. How does the therapist determine the pulse rate limit of a deconditioned 35-year-old man during a 30-minute heat treatment? What should the therapist do if his pulse rate exceeds that limit?
3. What changes in blood pressure should cause a physical therapist to discontinue a heat treatment? What changes in blood pressure are extremely dangerous?
4. What temperature range defines the zone of thermal neutrality?
5. If a physical therapist is treating a disabled 55-year-old woman with heat modalities and the ambient temperature is 80° F (26° C) and the humidity is 40%, is it safe to proceed? Why?
6. While visiting Miami, where the temperature is 88° F, a healthy woman from Montana sprains her ankle and needs physical therapy. Is it safe to use heat modalities? Why?
7. Three months after a back injury, a football player returns to football practice on a hot humid August day. How long should he practice on Day 1?
8. After 2 hours of practice on Day 2, the football player complains of nausea, his pulse rate is fast, and his blood pressure has dropped. How should the physical therapist begin treatment?

REFERENCES

1. Amundsen L, ed. *Cardiac Rehabilitation*. New York: Churchill, Livingstone: 1981.
2. Blair S, Gibbons L, Painter P, et al. *Guidelines for Exercise Testing and Prescription*. 3rd ed. *Amer Col of Sports Med*. Philadelphia, PA: Lea & Febiger; 1986:8–21.
3. Ellestad M. *Stress Testing*. 3rd ed. Philadelphia, PA: FA Davis; 1986; 31:116–118.
4. Irwin S. *Cardiopulmonary Physical Therapy*. St. Louis, MO: CV Mosby; 1985:51.
5. Pollock M, Wilmore J, Fox S. *Exercise in Health and Disease*. Philadelphia, PA: WB Saunders; 1984:315.
6. Hensel H. *Thermoreception and Temperature Regulation*. New York: Academic Press; 1981:199.
7. Leithead C, Lind A. *Heat Stress and Heat Disorders*. Philadelphia, PA: FA Davis; 1964; 16:20–21.
8. Clark R, Edholm O. *Man and His Thermal Environment*. London, UK: Edward Arnold; 1985:136, 155.
9. Houdas Y, Ring E. *Human Body Temperature: Its Measurement and Regulation*. New York: Plenum Press; 1982:59, 97, 108–109, 112, 118, 179–181.
10. Guyton A. *Textbook of Medical Physiology*. 6th ed. Philadelphia, PA: WB Saunders; 1981:353, 623, 894.
11. American Academy of Pediatrics. Climatic heat stress and the exercising child. *Physician and Sports Med*. 1983; 11(8):155–159.
12. Fox R, Budd G, Woodward P, et al. A study of temperature regulation in New Guinea people. *Phil Trans Roy Soc London*. 1974; 268:375–391.
13. Hammel H. Effect of race on response to cold. *Fed Proc*. 1963; 22:795–800.
14. Strydom N, Wyndham C. Natural state of heat acclimatization of different ethnic groups. *Fed Proc*. 1963; 22:801–809.
15. Lind A, Bass D. Optimal exposure time for development of acclimatization to heat. *Fed Proc*. 1963; 22:704.
16. Senay L, Mitchell D, Wyndham C. Acclimatization in a hot, humid environment: body fluid adjustment. *J Appl Physiol*. 1976; 40:786–796.
17. Greenleaf J, Brock P. Na$^+$ and Ca^{++} ingestion: plasma volume-electrolyte distribution at rest and exercise. *J Appl Physiol*. 1980; 48:838–847.
18. Pichan G, Sridharan K, Swamy Y, et al. Physiological acclimatization to heat after a cold conditioning in tropical subjects. *Aviat Space Environ Med*. 1985; 56:436–440.

19. Rowell L. Human cardiovascular adjustments to exercise and thermal stress. *Physiol Rev.* 1974; 54(1):75–159.

20. McArdle W, Katch F, Katch V. *Exercise Physiology.* 2nd ed. Philadelphia, PA: Lea & Febiger; 1986; 448–449.

21. Nadel E, Pandolf K, Roberts M, et al. Mechanisms of thermal acclimation to exercise and heat. *J Appl Physiol.* 1974; 37:515–520.

22. Wyndam C, Jacobs G. Loss of acclimatization after six days of work in cool conditions on the surface of a mine. *J Appl Physiol.* 1957; 11:197–198.

23. Nielson B, Rowell L, Bonde-Petersen F. Heat stress during exercise in water and in air. In: Hales J, ed. *Thermal Physiology.* New York: Raven Press; 1984:395–398.

24. Caldroney R. Heat induced illness. *J Kentucky Med Assoc.* 1982; 80:671–674.

25. National Weather Service table. *Utica Observer Dispatch,* August 4, 1988.

26. Stanier M, Mount L, Bligh. *Energy Balance and Temperature Regulation.* Cambridge, UK: Cambridge University Press; 1984.

27. Borrell R, Parker R, Henley E, et al. Comparison of in vivo temperatures produced by hydrotherapy, paraffin wax treatment, & fluidotherapy. *Phys Ther.* 1980; 60(10):1273–1276.

28. Gollehon D, Drez D. Heat syndromes: a review. *J Louisiana State Med Soc.* 1982; 134(6):9–11.

29. Johnson L. Preventing heat stroke. *Am Fam Physician.* 1982; 26(7):137–140.

30. Khogali M, Mustafa M. Physiology of heat stroke: a review. In: Hales J, ed. *Thermal Physiology.* New York: Raven Press; 1984:503–510.

31. Knochel J. Environmental heat illness. *Arch Intern Med.* 1974; 133:841–864.

32. Shibolet S, Lancaster M, Danon Y. Heat stroke: a review. *Aviat Space Environ Med.* 1976; 47:280–301.

33. Wyngaarden J, Smith L Jr, eds. *Cecil's Textbook of Medicine.* 17th ed. Philadelphia, PA: WB Saunders; 1985:358, 2229, 2304–2306.

34. Guyton A. *Human Physiology and Mechanisms of Disease.* 4th ed. Philadelphia, PA: WB Saunders; 1987:130, 190.

35. Environment adds to challenge facing Desert Shield physicians. *JAMA.* 1991; 265:435, 439–440. Medical News and Perspectives.

36. Anthony C, Thibodeau G. *Textbook of Anatomy and Physiology.* 11th ed. St. Louis, MO: CV Mosby; 1983:567.

37. Costill D, Cote R, Miller E, et al. Water and electrolyte replacement during repeated days of work in heat. *Aviat Space Environ Med.* 1975; 46:795–800.

38. Fox R, Woodward P, Exton-Smith A, et al. Body temperatures in the elderly: a national study of physiological, social, and environmental conditions. *Br Med J.* 1973; 1:200–206.

39. Assia E, Yoram E, Shapiro Y. Fatal heat stroke after short march at night: a case report. *Aviat Space Environ Med.* 1985; 56:441–442.

SECTION 3
HYDROTHERAPY

Historically, people have considered "soaking in water" one of the most common "cures" for human ailments. The popularity of bathing at beaches and pools, as well as other means of "soaking" such as in hot tubs and jacuzzis, attests to the benefits people seek or believe that they gain from some mode of getting into the water. Regardless of whether the benefits are in the body or the mind, if one feels better this use of water has merit. Therapeutically, we recognize that immersion modalities are extremely valuable both physiologically and psychologically.

This section focuses on immersion in water treatments, whirlpools, Hubbard tanks, therapeutic pools, and contrast baths. Most of the other hydrotherapy modalities commonly used in the United States are discussed in Section II, Thermal Agents. This section concludes with a brief discussion of several additional hydrotherapy modalities that are used less often in the United States than they are elsewhere.

Hydrotherapy

Bernadette Hecox, PT, MA

W hen water is used as a treatment for physical or psychological problems, it is termed *hydrotherapy.* Medical hydrotherapy can be defined as the internal or external use of water in any of its three forms, solid, liquid, or vapor, to treat disease or traumas. "Internal use" refers to treatments such as drinking mineral waters, administering enemas, or douching. In the United States, the word internal can be omitted from a physical therapy definition because physical therapists do not treat internally. According to this definition, hot and cold packs, ice modalities, and moist air cabinets are all considered hydrotherapy modalities. Many people also include melted paraffin because it is fluid, and some even include sauna baths in the hydrotherapy category. In essence, however, the medium for hydrotherapy is water.

Water has unique physical properties, including buoyancy, hydrostatic pressure, surface tension, cohesion, adhesion, and fluidity in addition to its well-recognized thermal properties. By immersing the patient's body or part of the body in water, therapists use these properties when performing many therapeutic procedures. Table 16–1 outlines the primary treatment procedures for which immersion in water is useful and the specific properties of water that warrant its use. Because all the properties listed are inherent in water, all act on a person simultaneously. However, each will be discussed individually.

TABLE 16–1. PURPOSES OF IMMERSION HYDROTHERAPY AND THE PROPERTIES OF WATER THAT WARRANT ITS USE

Purpose	Property of Water
Hot or cold treatment modality	Thermal properties
Environment for performing therapeutic exercise procedures (muscle strengthening, balance, ambulation, and range of motion)	Buoyancy, hydrostatic pressure, surface tension, cohesion, and turbulence used for resistance/assistance.
Environment in which to improve circulation, reduce edema, or both	Thermal properties and hydrostatic pressure
Treatment of skin problems and open wounds; debridement; removal of dressings; application of topical medications in solution; skin lubricant	All pressure factors and fluidity and turbulence
Psychological	Any and all properties

IMMERSION HYDROTHERAPY—USES AND RELATED PHYSICAL PROPERTIES

Thermal Effects

Hydrotherapy modalities are considered to be superficial thermal modalities because only the body surface contacts the water and the skin is virtually waterproof. However, when the body is immersed in water, physiologic changes may occur that are different than with the other superficial thermal modalities.

Immersion factors. When the body or body part is immersed in water, the entire circumference of the immersed part is treated simultaneously. Nonfluid superficial modalities may be applied to only one surface of the body. The melted paraffin-mineral oil bath and Fluidotherapy also are immersion modalities, but their thermal properties differ from those of water.

Thermal properties of water. In comparison to the thermal properties of the paraffin mixture, water has higher specific heat and thermal conductivity values thus it contains more heat per temperature and conducts heat more rapidly (see Table 7–3). Because of these thermal properties, water is a good means of heating or cooling the body rapidly.

Heat transfer with immersion. The primary means of heat transfer between skin and water is convection. However, assuming that the immersed body part remains completely still, a limited amount of heat gain or loss may occur via conduction between the skin and water molecules immediately adjacent to the skin. This adjacent water layer may act as a "sealer," deferring further conduction. Everyone has experienced this sealer effect. If one sits still in a tub of very warm water, the water next to the skin soon begins to feel cooler, but as one swishes the water a little or moves a little in it, the cooler water is pushed aside and the warmer water comes close to the skin. The water then feels warmer again. The diver's wet suit exemplifies the use of this sealer effect as a means of insulation. In therapy, agitators are placed in whirlpools primarily to move the water and prevent this sealer effect.

Actually, even if one could remain completely still, some convection would occur. The heat transfer by conduction between the skin and adjacent water molecules results in a temperature of the adjacent water that differs from the rest of the water in the tub. This temperature gradient sets up convection currents, and heat transfer by convection begins (see Chapter 7). The convection power of water is 25 times greater than that of air.[1] Swimming increases the convection as the body moves through the water; agitators do the same because the water is forced to move across the body.

Physiologic effects of immersion. The physiologic and therapeutic effects resulting from the thermal properties of water are similar to those attributed to any heat or cold modality discussed in Section II. However, the tissues affected may be different than those affected by other superficial modalities. Because the body part is surrounded by water, both agonist and antagonist muscle groups are affected simultaneously. When the entire body segment is surrounded by a substance containing much heat, there is less opportunity for normal local heat-loss mechanisms to be effective; therefore, heat may conduct to deeper tissues than is the case with other superficial modalities.[2,3] If so, it may be possible to effect the healing of slightly deeper tissues more than is possible with other superficial heat modalities and to elongate (stretch) deeper tissues such as tendons and capsules more effectively. It has been shown that nonelastic tissues can best be lengthened while heated, but with many heat modalities, the stretching procedures must wait until the heat has been removed. The precise mechanisms for heat transfer from water to the body core are not clearly understood. Nadel points out that the thickness of the subcutaneous fat layer is inversely proportional to changes in internal temperature. Whether this is simply because of the fact that fat, a thermal insulator, influences the conduction of heat or whether other thermal regulatory mechanisms are involved is unclear.[4]

Systemic physiologic changes in water, including changes in all vital signs, (core temperature, blood pressure, pulse rate, and respiration), may be much greater than with other superficial heat modalities because the body's means of heat loss are much less. For example, if the total body is immersed as with a Hubbard tank treatment and the water temperature is greater than the skin temperature, there is virtually no way for sweat to evaporate or for surface heat to radiate to a cooler environment. The ambient temperature in which the patient is existing while in the water is the water temperature, not the room temperature that the therapist is experiencing, and the humidity of the patient's environment is 100%.

The room temperature and humidity also must be considered. If the air in the room is extremely humid—and it may well be because there is so much water in the area—some heat loss may occur through radiation but there is little chance for heat loss through the evaporation of sweat. This is significant not only for patients but for everyone else in the hydrotherapy area as well. Changes in vital signs, fainting, or both may be experienced by anyone in the area. Thus, it is important to keep the room as well ventilated as possible. The temperature of the room should be cool enough to allow some heat to escape but warm enough to avoid chilling the patient when he or she leaves the water. A room temperature of 78° F (25.5° C) with a relative humidity of 50% is suggested.[5] Although Campion[6] suggested an air temperature of at least 86° F (30° C) for pediatric hydrotherapy areas, she stated that it must be lower than the water temperature. To avoid chilling, the patient is always wrapped in dry towels or cotton blankets after coming out of the water.

Aquatic Therapeutic Exercise

Exercising in water is extremely useful. Patients with poor standing balance can stand without fear of falling, patients unable to bear weight on joints in the lower extremities can walk, patients with weak muscles can move body parts, and peripheral and cardiac muscles can be strengthened. Since exercising in water can be so useful, the related properties of water and general concepts of how they are applied in therapeutic exercise will be discussed. Specific hydrotherapeutic exercise programs are beyond the scope of this book, but can be found in the literature.[6–12]

Buoyancy

Buoyancy is defined as the upward thrust of water acting on a body that creates an apparent decrease in the weight of a body while immersed. The Archimedes' Principle tells us that the upward thrust that a fully or partially immersed body experiences is equal to the weight of the water that it displaces. The amount of water displaced depends on the density (mass/unit volume) of the immersed body relative to the density of water (see Chapter 7).

Water density does not always remain constant. It varies with temperature and atmospheric pressure. The density of salt water is greater than that of fresh water; thus, one floats more easily in the ocean than in a fresh-water lake. The density of any volume of water is proportional to its depth. Because deeper water supports the water above, its density is greater.

The densities of various substances, measured in g/cm^3, are described by a pure number value called *specific gravity* (SG) that is given to each substance. The SG value for pure water at $4°$ C is 1.0. Whether another substance will float or sink in water can be determined by comparing its SG value to that of pure water. Specific gravity values for substances relevant to this discussion are given in Table 16–2.[7,9,13–16]

An object whose SG, thus its density, is equal to pure water (1.0) will float submerged just below the surface of the water. If the SG of the object is **greater** than 1.0, the object will sink at a rate that depends on the difference in SGs. For example, aluminum (SG = 2.7) will sink, but it will do so more slowly than iron (SG = 7.8). If the SG of the object is **less** than 1.0, the object will displace a proportional amount of water. For example, the SG of ice is approximately 0.92; thus, 92% is in the water and 8% is floating above. What one sees floating in Arctic waters is indeed just the tip of the iceberg.

Air is far less dense than water (SG = 1.21×10^{-3}), so air-filled pillows, toys, and even surgical gloves blown up like balloons can be used to support body parts and increase a patient's ability to float. Because the SGs of oak and pine woods are less than 0.1, they can be useful as floats if dry. Even wooden seats or crutches can be used to help support a body part or prevent a patient from sinking. Floats also can be used for resistance exercises to increase the resistance encountered when pushing down into the water against buoyancy.

The SG of the average human body with air in the lungs is approximately 0.974, slightly less than water; thus, one floats nearly submerged but 2.6% of the body is fortunately above water. If the floating is prolonged, one hopes this will be the face. Because air is considerably less dense than water, if one inhales deeply, more of the body will be above water, but if one exhales completely, the body may sink because the SG of a body without air is approximately 1.1.

The differences in people's sizes and shapes and the differences in the SG values of various tissues can explain why some people float more easily than others. On the average, approximately 60% of an adult's body is water, which tends to equalize the body's SG with that of the surrounding water. The SG of fat is lower than water, which tends to let the body float, but the SG of some bone may be greater than water, which tends to let the body sink. Therefore, a person with dense bones and little fat will have more difficulty floating than one who has more fat and less dense bones. Conversely, if two people's arms are of equal length and

TABLE 16–2. SPECIFIC GRAVITY OF DIFFERENT SUBSTANCES*

Substance	Specific Gravity Value
Pure water	1.0
Salt water	1.024
Ice	0.917
Air	1.21×10^{-3}
Average human body with air in lungs	0.97
Average human body without air in lungs	1.1
Fat (subcutaneous)	0.85
Bone (varies with density)	
Femur	1.85 (approx)
Vertebral body	0.47 (approx)
Substances used for hydrotherapy equipment	
Wood	
Oak	0.72
Pine	0.42
Aluminum	2.7
Iron	7.8

*From Skinner A, Thomson A,[7] Lehmann J,[15] and McCordle W, Katch F, Katch V.[16]

bone structure but one person is obese and the other is thin and both are standing neck high in water, the obese person will have more difficulty adducting the arms down under the water.

Because buoyancy counteracts weight, when ambulation is desired to maintain a patient's muscle strength, function, or both but weight bearing is contraindicated—for example, after surgery or an injury to a lower extremity—the patient can walk safely in water that is up to the neck. As the patient improves, the water level can be lowered gradually, decreasing the apparent weightlessness. Dancers, runners, and other athletes commonly use this technique to keep in shape while recovering from injuries that necessitate non-weight bearing.

If a body segment is relaxed, weak, or paralyzed, by allowing buoyancy to lift the part, the segment can move upwards toward the water surface. Resistive exercises can be performed by downward movements against this upward thrust. By positioning the body correctly, all joint movements can be performed either with or against buoyance. Just as gravity assists with downward movements out of the water, buoyancy assists with upward movements in the water. Therefore, positions for resistance or assistance exercises are always the opposite when in water than when out of water.

Kinesiological rules for torque (the moment of a force) are as useful when planning hydrotherapy exercises as when planning exercises out of water. The torque (τ) is equal to the rotary force (F) times the lever arm distance (L); thus

$$\tau = F \times L.$$

The rotary component of a force is at a right angle to the moving segment. (For more complete information regarding torque, the reader is referred to kinesiology or biomechanics texts.[17,18,19]

When performing movements out of water, the effect of gravity (a vertical downward force) on the rotary movement of a body segment is greatest when the segment is horizontal (ie, at a 90° angle from the vertical) and the rotational component of this gravitational force decreases as the segment moves toward the vertical (ie, the angle changes from 90°). Similarly, when movements are performed in water, the effect of buoyancy (a vertical upward force) is greatest when the segment is horizontal and diminishes as the segment approaches the vertical (see Fig. 16–1).

Just as the center of gravity (COG) is used as a reference point when analyzing the effect of gravity at a given angle when a movement is performed out of water, the center of buoyancy (CB) of a body segment is the reference point used to analyze the effect of buoyancy on movements at a given angle, performed in water. The CB pertains only to the center of the part of the body that is immersed in the water.

Both the COG and the CB can be used to measure the lever arm distance of a rotating segment. The farther either the COG or CB is located from the axis of rotation, the longer the lever arm distance, thus the greater its effect on the torque produced. The COG or CB can be changed by adding external objects. Adding weights to the distal end of an extremity places the COG more distally; similarly, holding a balloon or float at the hand or foot places the CB more distally, increasing the lever arm distance for the torque produced upward by buoyancy (Fig. 16–2A and B). Thus, a balloon placed in a hand in water adds resistance to an arm pushing down into the water, but assists in allowing an arm positioned nearly vertical in the water to rise (Fig. 16–2 C and D). Bending a knee or elbow moves the COG or CB proximally, thus shortening the lever arm and reducing the torque resulting from either gravity or buoyancy (Fig. 16–2E, F, and G).

When horizontal movements are performed out of water, the effect of gravity is neutralized. Similarly, the influence of buoyancy is neutralized when performing horizontal movements in water. However, buoyancy will give an upward support to a body segment performing such movements.

Because gravity and buoyancy are counteracting forces, the body is stable

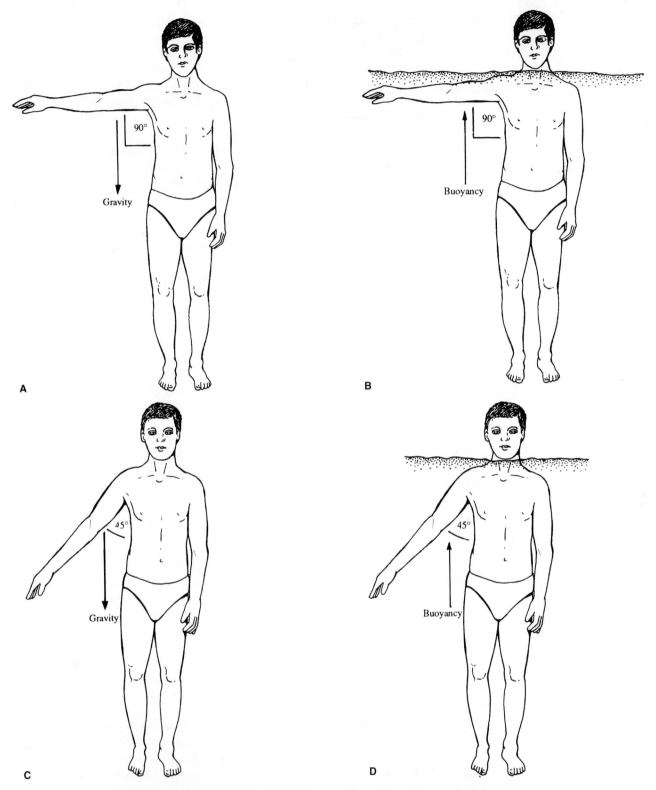

Figure 16–1. Rotary components of gravitational and buoyancy forces on an arm at various angles. F_t = total force and F_r = rotary component of the total force. In the horizontal position, ie, at a 90° angle between the arm and the vertical (the trunk), the total forces of both gravity and buoyancy are rotary forces ($F_t = F_r$). At a 45° angle, the F_t of both gravity and buoyancy must be resolved into rotary components and either a compression or a distraction component; thus, the F_r is less than the F_t. (**A**) When the arm is held at a 90° angle, gravity is a downward vertical force. (**B**) When the arm is held at a 90° angle in water, buoyancy is an upward vertical force. (**C**) With the arm at a 45° angle, the F_t of gravity is resolved into rotary and distraction components, and the F_r is less than the F_t. (**D**) With the arm at a 45° angle in water, the F_t of buoyancy is resolved into rotary and compression components, and the F_r is less than the F_t.

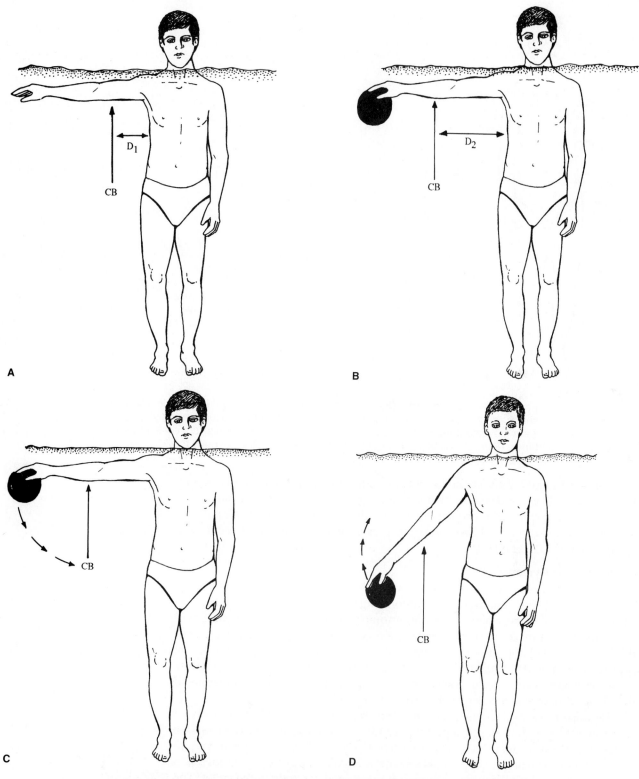

Figure 16–2. Illustrations of different ways of changing the center of buoyancy (CB) of an extremity, thus changing the lever arm distance and the resulting torque. This can increase the resistance or assistance that buoyancy produces to movements in water. (**A**) The lever arm distance (D_1) to the CB of an arm in water is shown. (**B**) An inflated balloon is held in the hand. This moves the CB distally, lengthening the lever arm distance (D_2), thus increasing the torque resulting from buoyancy. (**C**) The balloon adds resistance to downward movements, thus opposing buoyancy. (**D**) The balloon assists buoyancy with upward movements.

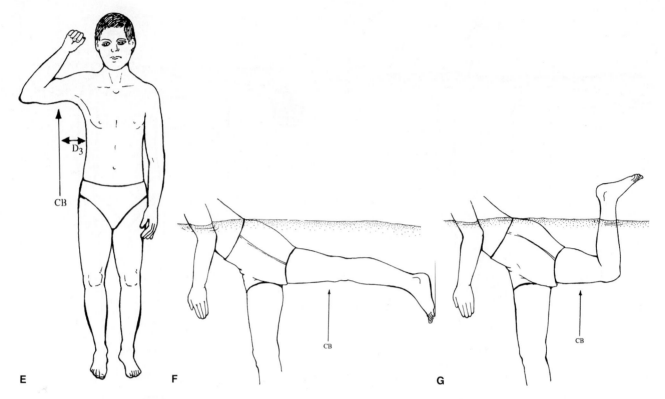

Figure 16–2 (continued). (E) Bending an elbow moves the CB proximally, thus shortening the lever arm distance and decreasing the torque. Consequently, a downward movement meets less resistance, and upward movements receive less assistance. **(F and G)** Similarly, bending the knee alters the effect of buoyancy.

when the COG and CB are aligned vertically. If they are not, rotation occurs (Fig. 16–3A and B). This can be helpful when planning exercises to improve balance or the ability to recover to the vertical after being tipped off balance. Weak patients must be guarded carefully, however, because they can easily be tipped over by the rotation (Fig. 16–3C and D).

Hydrostatic Pressure

Hydrostatic pressure is the pressure exerted by the water on the immersed body. Water surrounds the immersed part, conforming to and enclosing any shape. According to Pascal's law, when a body part immersed in fluid is at rest, the fluid will exert equal pressure on all surface areas at a given depth (Fig. 16–4). The effect of this pressure is significant when treating patients with respiratory problems. The pressure can be used as a resistance when doing exercises to improve lung expansion. However, patients with serious respiratory problems may have difficulty breathing if their lungs cannot expand adequately against so much external pressure.

Because pressure increases with the density of the fluid and the density of water increases with its depth, a pressure gradient is established between surface water and deeper water (22.4 mm Hg for each 30.5 cm).[20] Thus, standing and walking in water can be helpful to patients who have circulatory problems or edema in the legs or feet if the edematous body part is positioned correctly in the water. The distal part, if deeper in the water, will be subject to more pressure. This pressure gradient encourages return flow of fluids in a proximal direction from the extremity (Fig. 16–5).

The combined effects of buoyancy and hydrostatic pressure can be helpful when a patient is practicing standing balance. The pressure provides some support all around the body to an equal degree, and if the patient should fall a little off the vertical when immersed while standing, buoyancy can help him or her regain the vertical position(Fig. 16–6).

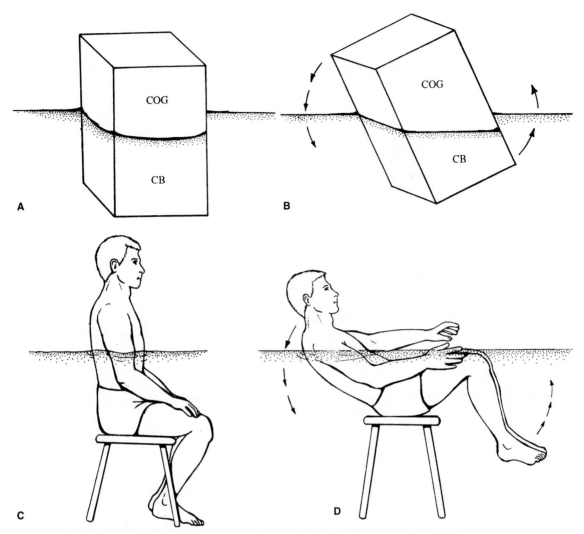

Figure 16–3. When the center of gravity (COG) of a portion of an object that is out of water is in vertical alignment with the center of buoyancy (CB), the object is stable. When it is not in vertical alignment, the object rotates. (**A**) Because the COG and the CB are vertically aligned, the box is stable. (**B**) Because the COG and the CB are not vertically aligned, the box rotates. (**C**) A person sitting partially immersed in water with the COG and the CB in vertical alignment is in a stable position. (**D**) If the COG of the portion of the sitting person that is out of the water is not vertically aligned with the CB of the portion in the water, the person tips over.

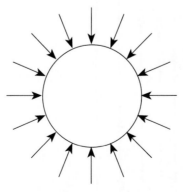

Figure 16–4. Equal hydrostatic pressure at any given depth.

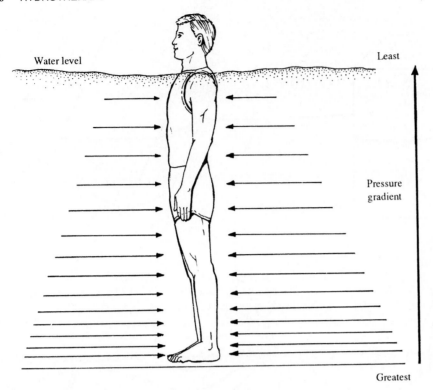

Water level   Least

Pressure
gradient

Greatest

Figure 16–5. The effects of hydrostatic pressure when a patient is standing in water. Density increases with depth increasing the pressure.

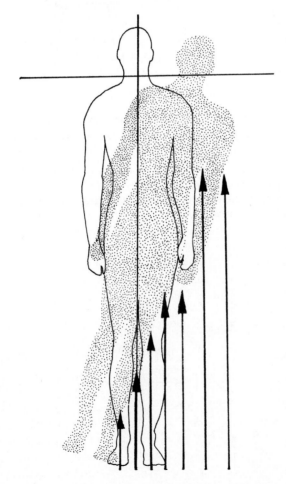

Figure 16–6. Temporary displacement of a vertical body. Buoyancy assists recovery.

When explaining differences in the effect of water on a stationary body versus a moving one, Kolb's differentiation of hydrostatic and *hydrodynamic pressure* is useful. Kolb categorizes both buoyancy and the equal pressure that still water exerts on a static object as hydrostatic pressures and categorizes the pressures caused by movement of either the object or the water as hydrodynamic pressures.[21]

When walking in water, one will encounter the pressures inherent in the fluid. To move the water in the path as one moves forward, one must push against the pressure the water is exerting. The faster one walks, the more resistance is encountered and the more demands are made on the walking muscles. Conversely, in the "wake" of a body moving in water (ie, immediately behind), there is much less pressure. If a patient is extremely weak, the therapist might walk in front of the patient. If the patient is close behind in the therapist's wake, he or she will not encounter the pressure. Baby ducks swimming in line behind their mother exemplify this situation.

Other Properties

Other properties of water to be considered in relation to hydrotherapy exercises are (1) surface tension, (2) cohesion, (3) adhesion, and (4) turbulence.

Surface tension. Water molecules on the surface have a greater tendency to hold together, thus resistance is slightly greater on the surface. Any diver who does a belly flop experiences that tension. Therapeutically, this increased resistance is usually insignificant, but if someone is extremely weak, horizontal movements may be performed more easily in the water just beneath the surface rather than at the surface.

Cohesion is the tendency of water molecules to adhere to each other. The greater the cohesion, the greater the viscosity. This cohesion contributes to the resistance encountered while moving through water because some force is required to separate the water molecules.

Adhesion is the tendency of water molecules to adhere to molecules of other substances. This property is observed daily. Water drops cling to one's body or to the sides of a glass. A damp sponge cleans dirt off a surface better than a dry sponge. It is this adhesion to the sides of therapeutic tanks that requires that they be wiped dry after cleaning. This property of water has no significant influence on movements in water. However, it is a factor when doing volumetric measuring because water drops adhering to the sides of a container are not measured in overflow volume.[22]

Turbulence. Webster's defines a turbulent fluid flow as one in which "the velocity at a given point varies erratically in magnitude and direction." This is in contrast to a smooth "streamline" flow, in which the direction is unchanged.

The movement of objects in water can cause the water to move in circular patterns, creating small whirlpools or eddy currents—turbulence. Moving a body segment through water creates some turbulence. Obviously, a body encounters greater resistance moving through turbulent water or against the current than through calm water or with the current. The faster the movement, the greater the turbulence created which puts more demand on muscles to move the segment. Skinner and Thomson[7] stated that "the quicker the movement, the greater the turbulence and therefore an exercise may be progressed by increasing the speed at which it is taken."

Many studies have been carried out to determine the effects of static immersion or exercise in water. Johnson et al[11] compared identical upper and lower extremity exercises performed by healthy young adults on land and in water and found that both heart rate and oxygen consumption were greater when exercises were performed in water. These investigators suggested that "the metabolic requirement of exercise performed in water is greater than when the same exercise is done on land" and they note that the cardiac recovery cost was reduced.[11] More recently, Kirby et al[23] studied the oxygen consumption of healthy young adults exercising while immersed in a pool heated to 96.8° F (36° C), with a pool area temperature of 77° F (25° C) and a relative humidity of 53%. Interestingly, they found no significant difference in oxygen consumption when a subject sat quietly in the pool, neck high in water, than when resting on land. Exercise ranging from light (walking in the pool) to heavy (running in place) produced proportional increases in oxygen consumption and a gradual increase in aerobic demands. Kirby et al concluded that the higher-intensity exercise appeared to "be within range that is likely to induce aerobic training"—that such exercises might be beneficial for some patients. However, they warned that the exercises should be used with caution because they could "represent a risk to patients with unstable cardiac disease."

It should be noted that few published studies can be found which show the benefits of aquatic vs. land therapeutic exercise. A 1990 unpublished study[24] did compare the effects of an exercise program on land vs. water on subjects with arthritic knees. The results showed a *significantly greater increase* in knee joint range of motion (ROM) and *decrease* in perception of pain for the aquatic group than the land group. Although the study was well executed, the population was small; a duplication of the study with more subjects would be useful.

Peripheral Circulation and Edema Problems

Heat is indicated to hasten healing through increased metabolism and increased blood flow to an area. However, heat applications also may cause edema or venous pooling (see Chapter 2 and 3, Table 3–1). The rationale for the use of compression to reduce edema and increase venous return is cited in Chapters 3 and 28. When a body part is immersed, the tissues are compressed by the hydrostatic pressure of the surrounding water.

If the distal part of an extremity is lowest in the water, the pressure gradient between the surface and deeper water favors reduced accumulation of fluid in distal parts. Although fluid accumulation is common in distal parts while "dangling" extremities out of water, in water, the effect of gravity is counteracted by the effect of buoyancy.[20,25] On the basis of the effects of water pressure, full body (head out) immersion is currently recommended as a treatment for "diuretic-resistant" edema in patients with cirrhosis and nephrosis.[26,27] One might also assume that in water, relative to out of water, the probability of edema or venous pooling at any given temperature also is diminished. Studies of head-out immersion in thermoneutral water at 95° F (35° C) indicate that there is an increase in venous return from the periphery to the central body and a shift of fluid from the interstitial space to the capillary. These changes have been attributed to the hydrostatic pressure.[28,29]

Traditionally, in physical therapy, whirlpool treatments are used for problems involving the extremities, both for their thermal effects and for hydro exercise. However, the effect of whirlpool treatments on edema is debatable. Magness et al,[30] using both healthy adults and patients with rheumatoid arthritis, lymphedema, and hemiplegia as subjects, showed that when an upper extremity was passively immersed in water at various temperatures 92–112° F (33.3° – 44.4° C), edema in both the healthy and patient populations did increase; the increase was proportional to the increase in water temperature. The authors suggest that the *heat* produced the edema and that if the extremity had been active while immersed, the effect might have been ameliorated.

Walsh's[31] reports of studies yet unpublished indicate that swelling occurs with or without exercise in water. The temperatures of the water used in these studies were about 98.6° F (37.6° C) and 104° F (40° C).

The meager evidence available suggests that the effect of heat may be confused with that of immersion. One should not necessarily throw out the bath water with the baby (the heat). In conditions where edema is of great concern, exercise in thermoneutral water might be advised, taking advantage of the hydro pressure to decrease edema. Research is needed to determine the effect of water at such temperatures on edema. In other conditions, the use of hydrotherapy for heat as well as other benefits should be continued until more conclusive evidence is available.

Skin Problems and Open Wounds

The fluidity properties of water enable water to be a useful substance for treating skin problems and open wounds. Fluidity means the rate of flow of a substance. For example, catsup is not as fluid as water. Every liquid has a certain viscosity—ie, a certain amount of friction between the molecules of that substance—that causes resistance. The amount of resistance determines the rate of flow of that liquid, its fluidity. The fluidity of water enables it to get into all crevices quickly and reaching all skin and surface openings regardless of position or shape. The cleansing effect of water, sometimes referred to as the *lavage effect*, is the result of this fluidity. It is useful in therapy for lubricating dry areas, for removing dressings painlessly, and for debridement of dead tissues from ulcers or burns or after cast removal.

Because many chemicals can dissolve in water, a topical medication in solution with water or lubricating oils can be transported to any or all surface areas. Oils, of course, float on top of the water.

When an external force causes water to move more rapidly, the water can exert greater pressure on the body. The massage showerhead currently sold commercially exemplifies this. In therapy, whirlpool agitators with the force directed toward the body are used to create a massage effect, enhance the lavage cleansing effect, or assist in removing dressings and dead tissues. In cases when only a slight increase in pressure is required and the amount of pressure must be well controlled, a dental water irrigating device may be used. A study of normal adults comparing 20–30 minute soaks, agitation, and brief sprays showed that agitation followed by spraying was "significantly better than any single technique in removing bacteria."[32]

Psychological Effects

Most healthy people feel invigorated after taking a bath or shower and enjoy some relief from daily anxieties. Changes in patients' attitudes, the improvements observed during treatments, and patients' reports of feeling good after a tank or pool treatment may be the result of the psychological effects of immersion in water as much as or more than the physiologic effects.

Psychology offers various reasons for these emotional and behavioral changes. People often identify bathing with a leisure-time activity. This identification encourages relaxation. In water, one can be surrounded by a neutral-to-warm environment that also is physically supportive because of the buoyancy and pressure properties of water. Receiving this external comfort and support can be emotionally supportive and help relieve anxiety.

In psychiatric settings, with the increased use of pharmacotherapies and psychotherapies, the use of physical therapies has declined considerably.[33] However, hydrotherapy treatments are still being used in selected cases to alleviate the symptoms of neurotic and psychotic patients.[34]

It is natural for a patient with a physical problem to have accompanying psychological problems. Although the hydrotherapy treatment is given for physically beneficial reasons, psychological problems may be relieved as well.[35]

In this section we have attempted to acquaint the reader with various factors that make hydrotherapy an important physical therapy modality. However, despite the popularity of this modality and the belief in its usefulness, its effects in a disabled population is meager. Most hydrotherapy study populations are made up of healthy young adults. Few studies that compared the effectiveness of water immersion with that of other modalities could be found in the recent literature. Whether physiologic effects of hydrotherapy are the result of the thermal or the other properties of water needs more investigation.

Hydrotherapy does have certain advantages over other modalities: for example, water is readily available and easy to use. Although hydrotherapy treatment may appear to be relatively inexpensive, this is not necessarily true. The cost of buying, maintaining, and cleaning hydrotherapy equipment such as whirlpools and Hubbard tanks, not to mention the municipal charges for water and the energy to heat it, may make these treatments expensive. This cost is ultimately absorbed by patients. For cost reasons, such treatments should not be given capriciously, but neither should they be avoided when they are the treatment of choice. If the therapist regards holistic treatments as most useful, tank or pool treatments are frequently the optimal ones available because both the mind and the body may benefit.

WATER IMMERSION MODALITIES

Whirlpool and Hubbard Tanks

The two most common modalities used in clinics for immersion in water are whirlpool tanks and *Hubbard tanks*; the two share much in common. Their common features are discussed first, then specific information pertaining to each is provided.

Both types of tank can be used as hot or cold thermal modalities, and both transfer heat primarily by convection. Both utilize the properties of water for the therapeutic purposes shown in Tables 16–1 and 16–2.

Equipment
Both whirlpool and Hubbard tanks are made of stainless steel or plastic, which can be easily cleaned. If cared for properly, these tanks will last for decades. The water is supplied by plumbing similar to that for a bathtub. The tanks include the following:

- hot and cold water mixing valves,
- a temperature gauge which indicates the temperature of the water flowing into the tank,
- a water thermometer attached to the inside of the tank to indicate tank water temperature,
- an agitator (a turbine ejector aerator),
- a seat, and
- a gravity drain.

The agitator in the tank mixes the water so that all water in the tank has approximately the same temperature. Agitators are designed so that they can be raised, lowered, and pivoted to direct their force at various levels and angles. Some agitators also are movable. They are attached to a rail on the outside of the tank and the top edge and can slide to any position along the tank. The agitator forces air through openings that **must be immersed** in the water; this force increases the rate of water flow. The amount of force produced by the agitator can be varied manually by ejector controls located out of the water. If the force is trained directly toward one part of the body, it can have a stimulating effect, that is sometimes called a micromassage effect. Patients with low back pain, for example, often enjoy the agitation force directed toward the painful area. This added force and the increased water flow can also assist in both removal of dressings and debridement.

Precautions regarding agitators. Although the agitator has no exposed moving parts that might injure the patient, care must be taken not to allow a finger, toe, or loose bandage to plug the openings. Because the agitator is motorized, attached to an electric source, and used in water, great care must be taken that there are no breaks in the wiring or insulation. Even a minor problem in any part of the electrical mechanism can cause serious electric shock, or even electrocution.[36] The motor must be securely fastened outside of the tanks. **ALL PERSONNEL MUST BE AWARE THAT IF A LIVE MOTOR OF ANY SORT FALLS INTO WATER, ANYONE IN THAT WATER CAN BE ELECTROCUTED.**[31] This equipment must contain hospital-grade plugs, and the receptacles must be fail-safe hospital grade.

New equipment must be provided with ground fault interrupters, (GFI). All hydro equipment must be checked for current leakage at least every 6 months. **NEVER ALLOW THE PERSON IN THE WATER TO SWITCH THE AGITATOR OFF OR ON.**

Additives

Opinions vary concerning the need for and effectiveness of solutions added to the water, but no conclusive evidence supports any opinions. Providone-iodine,[37] saline solutions, or bactericidal agents, including sodium hypochlorite (household bleach), can be added for the treatment of open wounds. An article by Richard[38] provides much information to guide the therapist when using these additives. Mc-Guckin et al[39] reported an outbreak of wound infections caused by *Pseudomonas aeruginosa* that coincided with the discontinuance of the use of sodium hypochlorite (Clorox) in Hubbard tank treatments and ceased when the use of the disinfectant resumed. Steve et al[40] studied the effects of chloramine-t with burn patients, and showed that this additive was effective relative to the concentration: 200 parts per million (ppm) was far more effective than 100 ppm. For recommended concentrations of agents sold for medical use, consult the manufacturer's label on the container. For patients with dry skin, (eg, after cast removal) or for those receiving many water treatments, bath oil can be added. A 4% solution of lidocaine has been suggested to reduce pain during debridement.[41] Adding a scented, colored water softener or foaming solution can be a pleasant bonus for the patient. Care must be taken to insure that patients have no allergic reactions to any solutions used.

General Considerations

Preparation of Tanks

Tanks must be thoroughly clean before water is added. Cleaning procedures are discussed later in this section. Tanks should be filled and ready for patients just before the time of treatment. Although there is much heat in the volume of water contained in these tanks, the water will cool down. Thus, the temperature should be checked at the time of treatment to ensure that it is correct. Allow 10 to 15 minutes for complete filling of the tanks.

General Indications and Contraindications

The effects of the properties of water on an immersed body or body part have been discussed earlier in this section. Tables 16–3 and 16–4 list common indications and relative contraindications for hydrotherapy as related to the effects of the properties of water. Physical therapists must always be alert to factors that contraindicate hydrotherapy for patients who otherwise might benefit from this modality. For example, in cases where there is a danger of cross-contamination or if hydration might exacerbate a skin condition.[42]

General Precautions

Any part of the body that is immersed in water loses its means of heat escape; the heat cannot radiate from that part of the body and the sweat cannot evaporate. When a substantial part of the body is in very warm water, the body temperature may increase, and systemic mechanisms that increase heat loss, heart rate, blood pressure, and respiration may change greatly in an effort to maintain thermal homeostasis. **VITAL SIGNS MUST BE MONITORED.** The patient's oral temperature should be monitored whenever the water temperature is higher than 100° F (37.8° C).

Patients may faint or experience heat distress. Therefore, **THE PATIENT MUST NEVER BE LEFT ALONE DURING OR AFTER A HYDROTHERAPY TREATMENT.**

Opinions vary concerning the amount of activity and the temperature of water that will maintain normal core temperature. Houdas and Ring[1] reported that if a healthy adult is resting immersed in water at a temperature of approximately

TABLE 16–3. GENERAL INDICATIONS FOR WARM AND HOT IMMERSION THERAPY

Indication	Therapeutic Effect	Property of Water
Subacute and chronic soft tissue injuries such as joint strains, sprains, or low-back problems	Decreases swelling (edema)	Pressure
	Hastens healing	Thermal
	Decreases pain/spasms	Thermal
	Increase range of motion	Buoyancy and thermal
	Increases strength	Buoyancy and pressures as resistance
Shortened tissues contractures, scars	Relaxation	Thermal and psychological
	Increases extensibility of nonelastic tissues	Thermal
	Softens scar tissue	Fluidity and thermal
	Assists active motion	Buoyancy
Arthritis: osteo and subacute, chronic rheumatoid	Increases joint mobility	
	Decrease pain	Thermal and buoyancy
	Increase range of motion	
Postfractures	Remove dry scaly skin	Fluidity and pressure
	Increase range of motion	Thermal and buoyancy
	Increase strength	Antibuoyancy pressure
Open wounds, burns, decubitii	Cleanses debrides, Increases circulation	Fluidity and pressure
Partially healed wounds or burns	Softens scar tissue	Thermal and
	Prevents contractures	Buoyancy
Muscle spasms	Increases circulation	Fluidily (turbulence forced pressure)
	Decreases pain	Thermal
Muscle weakness caused by central or peripheral nervous system involvement or by disuse	Increases range of motion	Buoyancy and
	Increases strength	Antibuoyancy pressure
Tension, anxiety, or other emotional or psychological problems	Relief of symptoms	Thermal and Hydrostatic Pressure

TABLE 16–4. GENERAL CONTRAINDICATIONS FOR IMMERSION HYDROTHERAPY*

Contraindication	Rationale
Cardiac dysfunctions	Heart cannot adapt to changes needed for thermal homeostasis adjustment.
Respiratory dysfunctions	Inability to resist hydrostatic pressure, tolerate heat, or both.
Decreased thermal sensation	Inability to report overheating or overcooling. Avoid hot or cold water; recommend cool through warm range (approx. 80° F–98° F) (26.7°–36.7° C)
Severe peripheral vascular disease (diabetes, arterial sclerosis)[†]	Contraindication for heat.
Danger of bleeding or hemorrhage[*]	Contraindication for heat.
Acute rheumatoid arthritis[‡]	Contraindication for heat.
Surface infections (including all fungus infections)[†]	Infection may spread to other areas or cross-contaminate via water.
Uncontrolled bowels (if pelvic area is in water)	Contamination is avoided.
Some dermatological conditions (atopic eczema; Senile or winterpruritus and ichthyosis)	Skin hydration may exacerbate some dermatologic conditions. Water removes natural skin moisture.

*These contraindications are relative to the intensity of the heat and the amount of body immersed.

[†]Avoid water temperatures higher than about 95° F.

[‡]Always add a bactericidal agent to the water.

91° F (33°–34° C), thermal neutrality is maintained: that is, the vasomotor activity will maintain stable core temperature. If the person is exercising strenuously, at three times the resting metabolic rate, a water temperature as low as 79° F (26° C) will maintain thermal neutrality. McCardle and colleagues,[16] also referring to healthy adults, reported that the optimal water temperature for swimming is 82°–86° F (27.8°–30° C). This temperature-activity information may serve as a guideline for treating orthopedic patients who are otherwise healthy. However, temperature ranges must be modified for more seriously debilitated people.

Bierman and Licht[43] reported 3° F (1.7° C) core temperature elevation when subjects stood in 104° F (40° C) water for 10 minutes. Interestingly, the study reported by Kirby et al[23] found no significant change in oral temperature while the subjects were immersed in 96.8° F (36° C) water, regardless of the intensity of their activity. However, the duration of immersion was not reported.

Frequently, patients are apprehensive about hydrotherapy tank treatments and the difficulty of getting into the tanks, especially if lifts are required for safe transfers. Being transported on the lifts can be frightening. Therapists must realize this, reassure the patient, and handle all aspects of the treatment with skill to gain the patient's confidence.

Pre- and Posttreatment Precautions

Before the treatment, the therapist must check patients' records for any problems that would contraindicate an immersion hydrotherapy and use the records as a guide regarding how closely the patients' vital signs must be monitored. When patients come out of the water, they may be chilled. Therefore, they should be dried immediately and covered with cotton blankets or towels to keep warm until they become adjusted to the air temperature.

Considerations Specific to Whirlpool Treatments

Whirlpool tanks are available in various sizes: from a size just large enough for a hand or foot to a size large enough for an adult to be able to sit comfortably (Fig. 16–7). Low Boys, which are similar to bathtubs, allow legs to be extended in a horizontal position. A common size found in clinics is large enough to immerse an entire extremity and allow free movements of the joints of arms or ankles and feet. However, it is difficult to immerse a shoulder joint comfortably. Larger tanks can be equipped with a seat so that an adult can sit with much of the body immersed in the water. A seat, usually made of stainless steel or plastic, can be adjusted to various depths in the water and can easily be removed when not needed (Fig. 16–8A).

A high chair is often placed outside of the tank. This enables patients to sit outside of the tank and immerse much of their lower extremity into the water. The chair also can be used to facilitate lowering patients into a "sitting tank." They first sit on the chair outside of the tank, place their legs into the tank, then lower themselves onto the tank seat. Many patients need one or two people to help them with this transfer (Fig. 16–8B).

Hard rubber hand grips, similar to those used on crutches, are usually placed on either side of the rim of the tank. These can be used to improve the patients' grip while they lower themselves into the tank, or they can be positioned to reduce pressure on vessels and nerves in popliteal or axilla areas if these areas are pressing on the rim of the tank. Motorized lifts also are available and are especially useful for transferring patients into a Low Boy (Fig. 16–8C).

Dosage

Water temperature. Depending on the size of the body area immersed and the patient's physical status, an effective hot or very hot whirlpool may range from 103° F to 115° F (39.9° – 46.1° C).[42] If the patient is sitting waist or chest high in water, the temperature should be at the lower end of the range to avoid great increases in core temperature. If only one extremity is immersed, the upper range can be used, provided the patient is otherwise healthy. The temperature should

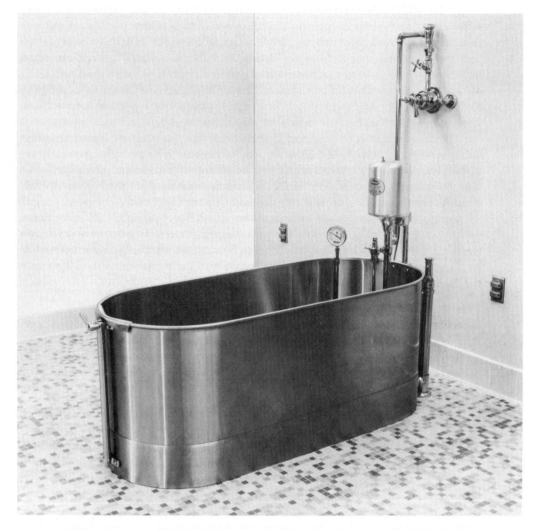

Figure 16–7. A "sit in" sized whirlpool tank, or low boy, with (1) a hot and cold water mixing valve, (2) a water thermometer, (3) an agitator (aerator), and (4) a gravity drain. (*Reproduced with permission from Whitehall Electro Medical Co., Inc. Hackensack, NJ.*)

never be so high that the patient is uncomfortable and the therapist must be alert to changes in vital signs and observable signs of distress.

Duration of treatment. The usual duration of an effective treatment is approximately 20 minutes. If R.O.M. or therapeutic exercises are also done in the tank, the time may be extended.[44]

Treatment Procedures

1. Remove the patient's clothes from area to be treated.
2. Inspect the skin for conditions that may invite cross-contamination or may be exacerbated by moisture.
3. Test for thermal sensitivity.
4. Drape the patient properly. Use towels to protect clothes on other areas of the body from getting wet.
5. Help the patient immerse his or her body or body parts, having second person help if necessary.
6. Place a towel roll over the hand grip under the axilla or knee to avoid pressure on nerves or blood vessels if only the extremity is immersed and the patient leans against the edge of the tank.
7. Advise the patient against getting fingers or toes near the opening in the agitators and against turning agitators off or on.
8. Loosen the bolts and rotate and adjust the height of the agitator to the de-

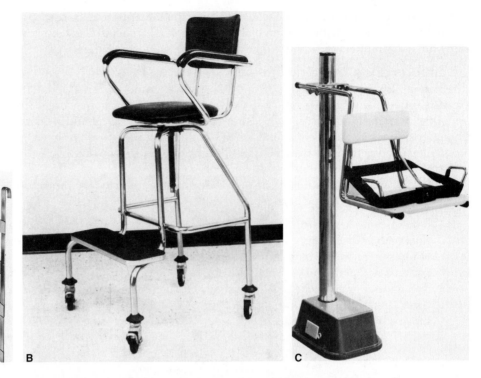

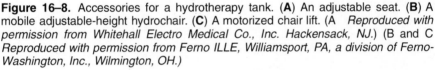

Figure 16–8. Accessories for a hydrotherapy tank. (**A**) An adjustable seat. (**B**) A mobile adjustable-height hydrochair. (**C**) A motorized chair lift. (A *Reproduced with permission from Whitehall Electro Medical Co., Inc. Hackensack, NJ.*) (B and C *Reproduced with permission from Ferno ILLE, Williamsport, PA, a division of Ferno-Washington, Inc., Wilmington, OH.*)

sired position. Tighten the bolts securely. Be careful that the agitator does not rise quickly (buoyancy) and hit you in the face while adjusting. Do **not** adjust the agitator while the motor is on.

9. Turn on the agitator.
10. Reassure and remind the patient that someone will always be in the area.
11. Monitor vital signs as necessary.

Note: If the patient is to sit in the water, advise to urinate before beginning treatment.

Posttreatment Procedures

1. Remove body part from water.
2. Dry thoroughly.
3. Check skin condition and check for unusual changes in vital signs.
4. Avoid chilling by keeping body covered or wrapped.
5. Assist patient in dressing if necessary.

Frequently, the whirlpool treatment is followed immediately by ultrasound (underwater method) while the patient is still in the tank. Berger[45] stressed the importance of therapists wearing rubber gloves during these treatments. He advised that all equipment should be plugged in to ground fault interrupters. Obviously, the agitator should be off not only for safety but to prevent ultrasound from diverging flow.

Considerations Specific to Hubbard Tank Treatments

The Hubbard tank, named after the engineer who designed it, is a large tank with a shape that resembles a keyhole. These tanks, too, are available in various sizes. Generally, the tank is approximately 8 feet long. The width is approximately 6 feet near one end, which enables a supine person to fully abduct the arms, and is approximately 4 feet wide near the other end, which allow the legs to abduct. At mid-side, the width narrows to 36 inches, enabling the therapist to get closer to the patient than is possible with a rectangular-shaped tank. The tank is deep enough to allow full body immersion while sitting or lying on a stretcher (Fig. 16–9).

Indications and Contraindications

Hubbard tanks are usually used for wound care, range of motion, and therapeutic exercise, for people who need full-body treatments for conditions such as generalized arthritis or multiple burns. They also are used for those who should remain in a lying position: for example, patients who have spinal cord injuries; or have had hip surgery or fractures, or patients with back, shoulder or neck problems that warrant hydrotherapy.

The contraindications to Hubbard tank treatments are listed in Table 16–4. Special considerations should be given regarding

- patients with severe cardiac or respiratory problems because they may be unable to adjust to any excessive external pressure caused by the water or to temperatures that may strain the cardiorespiratory systems,
- patients with loose bowels, and
- pregnant women in the first trimester if the heat is sufficient to raise the core temperature greater than 102° F (38.9° C) for 20 minutes because this may be harmful to the fetus.[46]

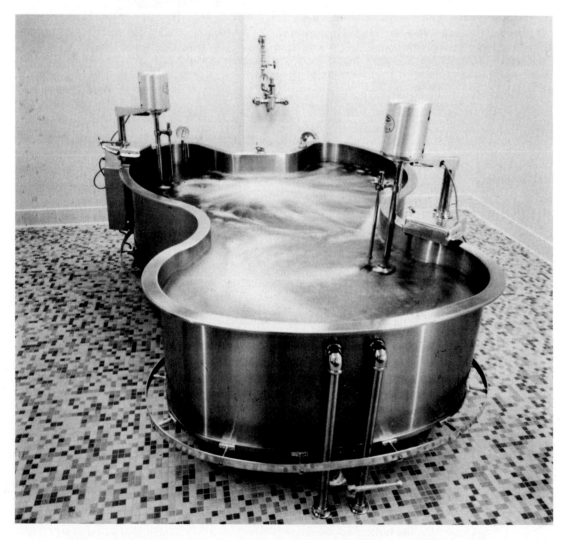

Figure 16–9. A Hubbard tank. (*Reproduced with permission from Whitehall Electro Medical Co., Inc. Hackensack, NJ.*)

Exposure to heat in the form of hot tub, sauna, or fever in the first trimester of pregnancy has been shown to be associated with an increased risk of neural tube defects such as spina bifida. The hot tub appeared to have the strongest effect of any single heat exposure.[47]

Dosage

Water temperature. The water temperature range is 90°–102° F (32.2°–38.8° C). Frequently, the temperature of water used in clinics is about 97°–100° F (36.1°–38.8° C). This temperature may be pleasurable and have a sedative effect, but one must realize that most of the body is immersed in this heat. Whenever ambient temperature is in this range, vital signs, including the core temperature, will change over time. Thus, temperatures in the lower part of the range may be required for patients who cannot tolerate these changes—those with cardiac or respiratory problems or preexisting fevers or those who will be exercising in the water.

Duration of treatment. The usual duration is 20 minutes.[44] If other treatments will be done while in the tank, the time can be extended to 30 minutes.

Treatment Procedures

Patients should wear a bathing suit or light-textured clothing that will not feel uncomfortable when wet and can be removed easily. Hospital gowns or proper draping are acceptable. Disposable paper swim clothes manufactured especially for these treatments are available commercially. Some patients like to wear a cap to keep their hair dry. Patients should be advised to urinate before beginning treatment.

The following steps should be carried out during the treatment:

1. Position the patient usually supine on a stretcher designed specifically for use in water (Fig. 16–10).
2. Secure the patient to the stretcher with straps to keep any body parts from floating off the stretcher.
3. Secure an air-filled pillow or towel roll to the stretcher and place it under the patient's head.
4. Position extremely weak or debilitated patients on the stretcher outside of the tank and use a motorized or hydraulic lift to suspend the stretcher, which then rotates or slides on a track to transport the patient over the tank. Then lower the stretcher into the tank. To ensure safety with these transfers, two people should assist the patient. The stretcher must be steadied and the head end must not be allowed to drop during transfer.
5. Lower the stretcher just to the water line so that the patient can become accustomed to the feeling of the water before being completely immersed.
6. Secure the head portion of the stretcher to the hooks in the tank so that the patient's head is elevated appropriately.
7. Immerse the patient to the depth necessary, keeping the head elevated.
8. Fasten the stretcher securely.
9. Place agitators in the appropriate positions and turn them on.
10. **DURING TREATMENT, MONITOR THE PATIENT'S VITAL SIGNS AND DO NOT LEAVE THE PATIENT UNATTENDED.**

As a responsible physical therapist, ensure that motorized equipment (agitators and lifts) are maintained in good working order and are checked periodically for both electrical and mechanical safety.

Posttreatment Procedures

As soon as the treatment is completed proceed as follows:

1. Lift the patient and stretcher to just above the water line and cover the patient immediately with cotton blankets or dry towels. Let the stretcher drip water into the tank before moving it over dry floor.
2. Remove the patient's wet clothes and dry the patient thoroughly, always keeping the patient covered for modesty and warmth.

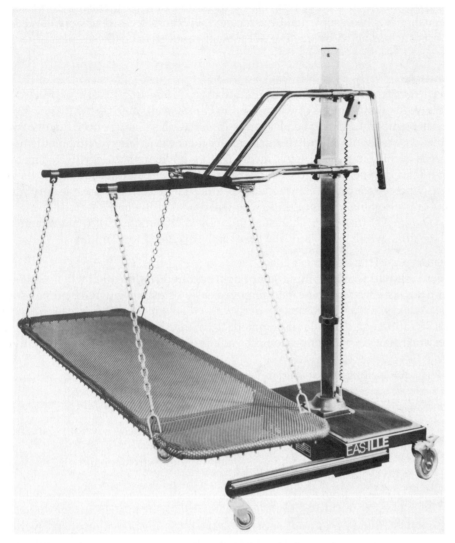

Figure 16–10. A hydrostretcher on an electric lift. (*Reproduced with permission from Whitehall Electro Medical Co., Inc. Hackensack, NJ.*)

3. Return the stretcher to an adjacent area and lower it onto a table or plinth.
4. Help the patient dress, always making certain that the patient is not chilled.

Walking Tanks

Hubbard tanks may have an additional "walking trough," which is approximately 32" deep, below the floor of the regular tank. It may be countersunk into the floor. In some models, the center part of the floor of the basic tank acts as a cover for the trough that can be lifted out when the trough is needed. When the trough is not needed, the cover keeps the trough area dry (Fig. 16–11).

Walking tank treatments are indicated for any patients who require non-weight-bearing standing or ambulation activities (eg, during early recovery from some injuries of the lower extremity or surgical procedures) and for neurological patients who require practice in sitting or standing balance or ambulation.

The trough is equipped with parallel bars and a chair or stool at each end. Patients can practice walking and all forms of hydrotherapeutic exercises in the water. The water level can be altered to meet each patient's needs: for example, it can be shoulder high for non-weightbearing standing or ambulation and be lowered gradually as the patient is able to bear more weight.

Some patients need to be transferred into the water by a sling halter or a chair

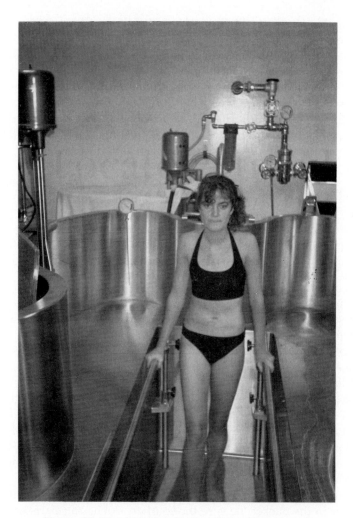

Figure 16–11. A Hubbard tank with a walking trough.

lift. As with stretcher transfers, two people are needed for this transfer. For safety and to reduce the patient's anxiety, the therapist should be in the water before the patient and be ready to assist as the patient is lowered into the water.

Cleaning and Maintenance of Tanks

It is important to keep all hydrotherapy equipment clean and in good condition. In each clinical setting, the procedures used are recorded and must always be followed. In hospital facilities, any laxity in the care and cleaning of equipment may lead to the department's failure to pass the periodic inspections of the American Hospital Association and the American Medical Association as well as endanger the patient or damage equipment.

All physical therapists, physical therapy assistants, and aides should be capable of cleaning tanks thoroughly and efficiently. Although hydrotherapy aides usually clean the tanks, the therapist is responsible for the proper instruction of the aides and for strict adherence to the cleaning protocol.

The cleaning procedures may vary to some extent in each setting, but they are basically the same. The procedures presented here were taken from those used in three large rehabilitation centers, although each center's protocol had slight variations.

Equipment. The equipment required includes disinfectant solutions, protective gloves, brushes with handles that enable all crevices to be scrubbed, buckets, many clean dry towels, and a water hose. Special hoses are available that can select and spray either the disinfectant or clean water, making this task much easier. In some clinics, disposable plastic liners are used for all patients. Cleaning is still required, but it takes less time.

At present, there is no conclusive evidence to recommend any one disinfectant.[48] Studies and reported observations suggest that sodium hypochlorite (5.25%) as contained in household laundry bleach is an effective and inexpensive disinfectant.[39,49] However, Turner et al[50] pointed out that, over time, chlorine corrodes the surface of stainless steel tanks. Their investigation showed that manual scrubbing with a standard germicidal detergent was effective in reducing bacterial contamination, except for drains and bottoms of tanks, which could not be adequately scrubbed.

General procedures. Tanks must be cleaned before and after each patient. They also must be cleaned before water cultures are taken. **EVERYONE MUST BE CAREFUL NOT TO SPLASH THE DISINFECTANT SOLUTION ON ANYONE'S SKIN. SHOULD THIS OCCUR, RINSE THE AREA IMMEDIATELY AND THOROUGHLY WITH COOL WATER.**

The procedure for cleaning the tanks is as follows:

1. Put on protective gloves.
2. Drain all the used water completely.
3. Rinse the entire tank and all equipment used for treatments, being sure all openings in agitators and all drains are included.
4. Wipe out thoroughly all surfaces that touched the water, using a clean towel. (Some clinics put alcohol on the towel.)
5. Spray and wash the entire inside of the tank, including the drains, and the outside of the agitators with lukewarm (not hot) water and the disinfectant delivered through the special hose attached to the tank. The disinfectant is delivered through the hose by depressing the small lever under the nozzle head. Release it to stop the flow of the disinfectant. If this hose is not available, mix the disinfectant with water in a bucket and pour it on all surfaces, then rinse with water using a regular hose. Follow each manufacturer's directions regarding the percentage of disinfectant and water in the bucket. Be sure the solution reaches all parts of any equipment, agitators, and water thermometers that were in the treatment water. Usually, disinfectant is left on approximately 1 minute.
6. Lower the agitators into the disinfectant solution in the bucket, being sure that all openings are in the solution. Turn on the motors for approximately 20 seconds. Turn off the motors. Remove the agitator from the bucket.
7. Rinse the entire tank with water delivered through the hose until all residue is drained. Include all equipment in this rinse.
8. Rinse a final time with water at approximately 115° F to hasten drying.
9. Post a "READY" sign on tank.
10. Wipe both the inside and the outside dry after the final use for the day. Be sure clean towels are used for the inside.
11. Clean the outside of the tank once a week with a stainless steel cleanser, usually a cream or powder. Remove any mineral deposits or discoloration from the inside of the tank with chlorine cleanser.

Some tanks are designed to reduce contamination by eliminating the crevices at the intersection between the floor and the walls. The interior surface is curved and seamless, resembling the design of most bath tubs.[51,52]

Procedures for isolation patients. Isolation patients include those with burns or other acute infectious lesions, surface ulcers, decubitus ulcers, and AIDS-related eruptions. For these patients, tank treatments are useful for cleansing the wounds, changing dressings, applying medication in solution, and debriding dead tissues. Therapists should not treat such patients unless well trained in all techniques to avoid cross-contamination or endangerment of the patient in any way. The specialized treatment procedures are beyond the scope of this book. Currently, tank treatments for isolation patients are being replaced by sprays, showers and topical medications.

Note that when a patient's burns have healed sufficiently, a tank is useful for preventing contractures in scarred areas and for increasing range of motion. At this stage, when the patient is no longer considered an isolation patient, only normal precautions need be taken.

Tanks cannot be completely sterile because the drain must ultimately be connected to a sewer system.[48,53] However, every effort should be made to treat patients in as sterile an environment as possible. Sterilized plastic tank liners are used in an attempt to decrease contamination. Additional cleaning procedures may be required when preparing tanks for and after treating isolation patients. These procedures are as follows:

1. Follow the usual cleaning procedures up to Step 7.
2. Refill the tank with a solution of hot water (approximately 115° F, 46° C) and disinfectant.
3. Allow the solution to stand for approximately 5 minutes. (Some clinics use the agitator during this period.)
4. Drain thoroughly.
5. Rinse thoroughly.
6. Proceed with Step 8 of the usual cleaning procedures.

Tanks must be cleaned immediately after each isolation patient and, in some clinics, again before the next patient uses the tank.

Therapeutic Pools

Although pools are an expensive addition to a physical therapy department, they are extremely valuable for patients in the rehabilitation stage of disability. The primary purpose of pools is therapeutic exercise. Pools are equipped with ramps, stairs, and lifts to help patients get in and out and with parallel bars and attachments for stretchers or chairs that are immersed. The floor of the tank is graded to vary the depth of the water. For rehabilitation purposes, in addition to the properties of water that can facilitate rehabilitation, creative therapists can devise methods of doing exercises that can be fun. All pools should have an assortment of floats, beach balls, and inflatable toys to be used during the exercises. Pools in pediatric rehabilitation centers are extremely popular because swimming, water games, and fun exercises motivate the children to carry out the necessary therapy. Campion's text presents many creative hydrotherapy ideas.[6] Pools are recommended for athletes and dancers who are recovering from injuries to maintain their general strength, flexibility, and function while remaining nonweight bearing. A modified pool that is approximately 4 feet deep and 12 feet wide (Swimex) has recently been introduced for hydrotherapy. It is designed so that a one-directional flow of current can be activated in the water in the upper region. The rate of flow can vary, enabling patients to exercise against a current "set" for an appropriate amount of resistance.

Generally, the temperature of the water in therapeutic pools is warmer than in a regular indoor pool. Temperatures of approximately 90°–100° F (32°–38° C), usually between 94°–98° F (34.4°–36.7° C) are recommended. As was mentioned previously, Kirby et al[24] found no change in the oral temperature of healthy subjects regardless of the intensity of activity at 96.8° F (36° C), but Houdas[1] believed that the temperature at which thermal neutrality is maintained at rest in water is slightly lower than 94° F. Houdas also stated that healthy people who are exercising at three times the resting metabolic rate can maintain thermal neutrality in a water temperature as low as 79° F (26° C); in the rehabilitation setting, however, such a low temperature is not advised.

One must be aware that the amount of exercise one does may determine the optimal temperature. Sagawas et al[54] showed that, in cool water, exercise rather than resting is more advantageous for maintaining core temperature, but if the water temperature is approximately 77° F (25° C), an ordinary man cannot generate enough heat through exercise to maintain his core temperature. Conversely, if the pool temperature is in the higher range, 98° F (36.7° C), exercise must be limited.

The advantages of initially practicing walking, standing, and therapeutic exercise in water were discussed earlier in this chapter. However, there may not be a direct carryover to standing and walking out of water. Both patient and therapist must be prepared for a transition period when progressing to functions out of water. Contraindications and cross-contamination precautions are similar to those given for Hubbard tank treatments.

Contrast Baths

Treatment with *contrast baths* involves placing one or more extremities alternately in very hot and very cold water. Clinically, whirlpool tanks are usually used; for home treatments, patients can use pails or tubs.

Because superficial blood vessels constrict while in the cold water and dilate while in the hot water, contrast baths are considered to be a "vascular exercise." This procedure can increase superficial blood flow in the extremities to a remarkable degree, and it is believed to hasten healing.

An early study, Moor et al[55] reported that a 30-minute contrast bath produced a 95% increase in local blood flow when one lower extremity alone was immersed. When all four extremities were immersed, there was a 100% increase in blood flow in the upper extremities and a 70% increase in the lower extremities. The current literature contains a dearth of studies about the effects attained with contrast baths: for example, changes in muscle strength and in recovery time from fatigue. These studies are not in agreement and are inconclusive.

Dosage. The recommended water temperatures for the cold bath range from 59° to 68° F (15°–20° C). Those for the hot bath should range from 105° to 110° F (40.6°–43.3° C).[56] There are several variations in the timing used. One example is 3–4 minutes in the hot water, followed by 30–60 seconds in the cold water.

Treatment procedures. It is usual to begin with the hot bath and continue alternating for approximately 30 minutes, with the final immersion in the cold. Keep in mind, however, that for vascular exercise, the contrast in temperature is more important than the sequence in which it is applied. It may be advisable, especially for the first treatment, to begin both hot and cold at the more moderate ends of the temperature range, then gradually move toward the extreme ends of the ranges within the patient's tolerance.

Indications and Contraindications

Contrast baths are most commonly used for athletic injuries. This modality is also used for leg ulcers or for orthopedic problems, ie. arm or leg joint strains or sprains. However, these indications are valid only if the patient is otherwise in good health because patients experience extreme thermal shocks with each change in temperature.

The contraindications are similar to those for other thermal modalities (see Chapter 10): cardiovascular problems, peripheral vascular diseases (especially arterial sclerosis), a tendency toward hemorrhage, loss of sensation, pregnancy, and hypersensitivity to temperature.

Precautions. Autonomic fight-or-flight reactions should be expected because substantial alteration and fluctuation in pulse and blood pressure will occur during the treatment. Consequently, therapists must be alert for any signs of distress. The patient's pulse should be monitored frequently throughout the treatment.

If the volume of water is not great, the water temperatures may change markedly during a treatment. Thus, water thermometers should be monitored to ensure that the contrast in temperature remains consistent throughout the treatment. If necessary, more ice can be added to the cold water or more hot water can be added to the hot bath. Be careful when adding the hot water if the body part is already immersed.

OTHER MODALITIES

Although currently not used extensively in the United States, many other forms of hydrotherapy can be useful. Because they are popular in other countries and are occasionally used in the United States, they are discussed briefly here. More complete descriptions for their treatment procedures can be found in other texts.[9,44,55-58]

Moist air cabinets. Approximately one-half of the patient's body can be placed in a cabinet. The patient is usually supine but can be prone or side-lying. Water is heated to 103°–113° F (40°–45° C), and air is forced past the water absorbing much of the moisture; thus, the humidity in the air is extremely high. The air then circulates throughout the cabinet. During a 15–20 minute treatment, the patients' core temperature usually increases 3° F. The high humidity prevents evaporation of sweat in the areas of the body that are in the cabinet. The patient will sweat profusely after treatment to cool down. Patients with chronic low back and arthritis pain report relief, are able to move with greater ease, and exhibit increased range of motion after these treatments.

Sitz baths. In a sitz bath, the water covers the pelvic region. There are tubs specially constructed so that just the pelvic and peroneum areas are in the water. Portable units designed to fit over toilets and maintain the desired temperature are available for home use. However, as a home treatment, patients often sit in bathtubs with water covering that area.

Hot sitz baths require a temperature of 105°–115° F (40.5°–46° C). The duration can range from 2 to 10 minutes. This treatment is intended to reduce pain, increase circulation in the pelvic area, and enhance tissue healing. Dodi and Bogoni[59] showed that at a water temperature of 104° F (40° C), internal anal pressure decreased significantly, whereas this did not occur with water temperature at either 41° F (5° C) or 73.4° F (23° C). They suggested that the pressure change reduces pain. The indications for hot sitz baths are for women after a birth or a hysterectomy, for patients after a hemorrhoidectomy, and for patients with prostatitis, cystitis, or chronic pelvic inflammatory diseases.

Cold sitz baths require a temperature of 35°–75° F (1.7°–24° C). The duration can range from 2 to 10 minutes. This treatment is intended to increase the tone of smooth muscles (atonic constipation) and to reduce uterine bleeding. Although urologists and gynecologists prescribe sitz baths, more investigation is needed to determine the benefits.

Scotch douche. In the Scotch douche, a shower spray of alternating hot (100°–110° F, 37.8° – 43.3° C) and cold (80° – 60°F, 26.7° – 15.5° C) water is passed over the body. First, the hot spray is passed up and down the back of the person standing in a shower stall, followed by a cold spray. This procedure, alternating hot and cold, continues for several minutes. The same procedure is carried out on the front of the body. This treatment is invigorating and also is used with patients who have emotional or psychiatric problems.

Peloids (mineral mud) and fango (moor peat). These substances are heated and applied to the body in a manner similar to the way hot packs are applied. Many people believe that the mineral content of these muds enhances the benefits received from a heat modality.

Wet sheets. Wet sheets are used in some psychiatric settings. The patient is completely wrapped in wet sheets at 60°–70° F (15°–21° C). While wrapped in the sheets, the patient experiences three changes in sensation of temperature: cool, neutral, and then very hot, during which profuse sweating occurs. This treatment is said to reduce anxiety states to a great degree.

Sauna baths. Sauna baths are popular in the general population in both the United States and Europe. First, one rests in a room that has walls, floor, and benches made entirely of wood. The air is extremely dry (low humidity). Stones or bricks are heated so that the air in the room is 140°–176° F (60° – 80° C) or higher.[10] The person sweats profusely, and, because the air is dry, the sweat easily evaporates, cooling the body. Thus, the high temperature can be tolerated but only for brief periods. The next procedure is to take a brief cold shower (or roll in snow), then return to the sauna. The two procedures can be repeated. One must note that although some people enjoy this activity and the feeling of well being it provides, sauna baths place a great strain on all the heat loss mechanisms and may lead to cardiac or heat accidents. Sauna baths are **contraindicated** for cardiac patients, the elderly, and women in the first trimester of pregnancy. Members of many ethnic groups do take sauna baths throughout life and claim no ill effects. Perhaps they become conditioned and therefore don't experience or notice greater reactions with increasing age.

Spas. Areas of effervescent, sparkling water (ie, carbon dioxide springs) can be found throughout the world. Many people strongly believe that these springs have great healing power and report some rejuvenation of health and spirits after spending time at these spas. These spas are often considered to be resorts. Saratoga Springs in New York State and Nauheim and Mannheim in Germany are examples of these spas. At these resorts, massage and other hydro facilities such as saunas, steam baths, and mud baths are usually available.

■ KEY TERMS

hydrotherapy	lavage effect
buoyancy	Hubbard tank
specific gravity	walking tank
hydrostatic pressure	contrast baths
hydrodynamic pressure	moist air cabinets
surface tension	sitz baths
cohesion	Scotch douche
adhesion	peloids
turbulence	fango

CASE DISCUSSIONS

The actual case studies are presented here to (1) demonstrate the complexity of hydrotherapy (or any other treatment), (2) prepare students for the positive and negative holistic effects that may occur, and (3) stimulate class discussion.

CASE STUDY 1

Betsy D, age 19, is a college sophomore. She has had severe rheumatoid arthritis since age 11. Many tendon releases have been performed, but she still has markedly limited range of motion of both hips, knees, shoulders, and elbow joints. She is wheelchair bound but can stand and take a few steps in a walker. She is currently a patient in a rehabilitation center, where she receives Hubbard tank treatments daily for ambulation training and range of motion. Last week, she asked if something else could be substituted for the tank treatments because she hated what her hair always looked like after treatments when visitors came and she felt like "a prune." The staff decided that hot packs applied to all eight joints and tank treatments could be given on alternate days. Would you agree with this decision? Discuss the advantages and disadvantages of each.

Hot Packs

Advantages. There is no need to prepare tanks and all bathing preparations and follow up for the patient. Heat and moisture would be applied only to the involved joints and thus not spoil her hairstyle or skin. They could be applied in positions that would encourage a sustained stretch of (joint) soft tissues while heat is being applied.

Disadvantages. No movement can be performed during the heat treatment. In addition, using eight packs for one patient may deplete the department's supply for approximately 1 hour, considering the treatment time and the time to reheat the packs, thus depriving other patients.

Hubbard Tank Advantages. The entire body is heated, and the patient can move the joints while in the heat, taking advantage of both the heat and hydrotherapeutic properties to increase range and function. The tank may encourage standing and walking in a more erect position.

Disadvantages. The tank increases the expense and time required to give a treatment. In addition, the patient did not want the treatment.

Similarities

Eight hot packs at approximately 104° F applied simultaneously may supply sufficient heat to produce systemic changes and relaxation that are equal to or greater than the Hubbard tank treatment. Can you think of more similarities?

CASE STUDY 2

Mrs. J is hospitalized for the third time with a frozen shoulder. Her range of motion (active and passive) for shoulder flexion and abduction is approximately 0–40°. The cause is undetermined. Because malignancy has not been ruled out, deep heat modalities are not used. The following treatments were tried repeatedly without noted improvement: hot packs applied in a position that would encourage a sustained stretch, cold packs followed by active and passive range of motion, sustained stretch procedures, mobilization, (Codman's pendulum) wall climbing, and proprioceptive neuromuscular facilitation exercises.

Results of Hubbard Tank Treatment

Finally, she was given a Hubbard tank treatment. Within 2 minutes after being completely immersed in 100° F water, lying supine on a stretcher, she said, "Oh, this feels good," and simultaneously abducted both arms as if stretching. Her right shoulder abducted to approximately 110°. Can you explain this?

Discussion

There is a possibility that because abduction was performed in the supine position, the effects of buoyancy and gravity were neutralized and the buoyancy supported the arm so that it floated during the movement. The temperature of the water may have encouraged relaxation. However, the rehabilitation staff believed that the cause of the patient's shoulder problem was psychological.

REFERENCES

1. Houdas Y, Ring F. *Human Body Temperature.* New York: Plenum Press; 1982:69, 192.
2. Clarke R, Hellon F, Lind A. The duration of sustained contractions of the human forearm at different muscle temperatures. *J Physiol.* 1958; 143:454–473.
3. Abramson D, Mitchell R, Tuck S. Changes in blood flow, oxygen uptake and tissue temperature produced by the topical application of wet heat. *Arch Phys Med Rehabil.* 1961; 42:305.

4. Nadel E. *Problems with Temperature Regulation During Exercise.* New York: Academic Press; 1977:91–120.

5. Atkinson G, Harrison A. Implications of the health and safety at work act in relation to hydrotherapy departments. *Physiotherapy.* 1981; 67:263–265.

6. Campion M. *Hydrotherapy in Pediatrics.* Rockville, CO: Aspen Pub; 1985.

7. Skinner A, Thomson A, eds. *Duffield's Exercise in Water.* 3rd ed. London, UK: Baillière-Tindall; 1983:20.

8. Forster A, Palastanga N. *Clayton's Electrotherapy: Theory & Practice.* 8th ed. Philadelphia, PA: WB Saunders; 1981.

9. Licht S, ed. *Medical Hydrology.* New Haven, CT: Elizabeth Licht; 1963:181, 196, 207, 247, 291–299.

10. Golland A. Basic hydrotherapy. *Physiotherapy.* 1981; 67:258.

11. Johnson B, Stromme S, Adamczykj J, et al. Comparison of oxygen uptake and heart rate during exercise on land and in water. *Phys Ther.* 1977; 57:273–278.

12. Davis B, Harris R. *Hydrotherapy in Practice.* London, UK: Churchill Livingstone; 1988.

13. Lehmann J. *Therapeutic Heat and Cold.* 4th ed. Baltimore, MD: Williams & Wilkins; 1990.

14. Halliday D, Resnick R. *Fundamentals of Physics.* Extended 3rd ed. New York: John Wiley & Sons; 1988.

15. McArdle W, Katch F, Katch V. *Exercise Physiology.* Philadelphia, PA: Lea & Febiger; 1986:162, 491–494.

16. Evans F. *Mechanical Properties of Bone.* Springfield, IL: Charles C Thomas; 1973:166.

17. Lehmkuhl D, Smith L. *Brunnstrom's Clinical Kinesiology.* Philadelphia, PA: FA Davis; 1983.

18. Norkin C, Levangie P. *Joint Structure and Function.* Philadelphia, PA: FA Davis; 1983.

19. Enoka R. *Neuromechanical Basis of Kinesiology.* Champaign, IL: Human Kinetics Books; 1988.

20. Greenleaf J. Physiological responses to prolonged bed rest and fluid immersion in humans. *J App Physiol Environ Exer Physiol.* 1984; 57:619.

21. Kolb M. Principles of underwater exercise. *Phys Ther Rev.* 1957; 37:361–365.

22. Beach R. Measurement of extremity volume by water displacement. *Phys Ther.* 1977; 57:286–287.

23. Kirby RL, Sacamno JT, Balch DE, et al. Oxygen consumption during exercise in a heated pool. *Arch Phys Med Rehabil.* 1984; 65:275–278.

24. Douros M. *Comparison of the Effects of Aquatic Therapy vs. Therapeutic (land) Exercise on the Increase of the Range of Motion of the Osteoarthritic Knee.* New York: Program in Physical Therapy, Columbia University; 1990. Master's thesis.

25. Physiologic response to water immersion in man—a compendium of research. Washington, DC: NASA Technical Memo X–3308.

26. Bank N. *N Engl J Med.* 1980; 302:969. Letter to the editor.

27. Brown CD, et al. Water immersion induced diuresis in the nephrotic syndrome—secondary ref. Presented at American Society of Nephrology, Nov, 1979.

28. Epstein M. Renal effects of head-out water immersion in man: implications for an understanding of volume homeostasis. *Physiol Rev.* 1978; 58:529–581.

29. O'Hare J, Heywood A, Dodds P. Water immersion in rheumatoid arthritis. *Bri J Rheumatol.* 1984; 23:117–118.

30. Magness J. Swelling of the upper extremity during whirlpool baths. *Arch Phys Med Rehabil.* 1970; 51:297.

31. Walsh M. Hydrotherapy. In: Michlovitz S, ed. *Thermal Agents in Rehabilitation.* 2nd ed. Philadelphia, PA: FA Davis Co; 1990:76, 119–120.

32. Niederhuber S, Stribley R, Koepke G. Reduction of skin bacterial load with use of the therapeutic whirlpool. *Phys Ther.* 1975; 55:482–486.

33. Kolb LC, Brodie HK. *Modern Clinical Psychiatry.* Philadelphia, PA: WB Saunders; 1982.

34. Singh H. Treating a severely disturbed self-destructive adolescent with cold wet sheet packs. *Hosp Commun Psychiat.* 1986; 37:287–288.

35. Tarnowski KJ, Rasnake KL, Drabman RS. Behavioral assessment and treatment of pediatric burn injuries: a review. *Behavior-Ther.* 1987; 18:417–441.

36. Arledge R. Prevention of electric shock hazards. *Phys Ther.* 1978; 58:1216.

37. Smith P, ed. *Infection Control in Long Term Care Facilities.* New York: John Wiley & Sons; 1984:133.

38. Richard R. The use of chlorine bleach as a disinfectant and antiseptic in whirlpools. *Phys Ther Forum.* August 29, 1988:7–8.

39. McGuckin M, Thorpe R, Abrutyn E. Hydrotherapy: an outbreak of *Pseudomonas aer-*

uginosa wound infections related to Hubbard tank treatments. *Arch Phys Med Rehabil.* 1981; 62:283–285.

40. Steve L, Goodhart P, Alexander J. Hydrotherapy burn treatment: use of chloramine-T against resistant microorganisms. *Arch Phys Med Rehabil.* 1984; 65:301–303.

41. Every inch & 1/2. Suggestions from a reader. Publication of The Jobst Institute, Toledo, OH; undated.

42. Sauer G. *Manual of Skin Diseases.* Philadelphia, PA: Lippincott; 1985:76, 101.

43. Bierman W, Licht S. *Physical Medicine in General Practice.* New York: Paul Holber; 1952: chap 2.

44. Hayes K. *Manual for Physical Agents.* 3rd ed. Chicago: Northwestern University, Program in Physical Therapy; 1984.

45. Berger W. Electrical shock hazards in the physical therapy department. *Clin Management.* 1985; 5:30.

46. Smith D, Clarran S, Harvey M. Hyperthermia as a possible teratogenic agent. *J Pediatr.* 1978; 92:878–883.

47. Milunsky A, Ulcickas M, Rothman K, et al. Maternal heat exposure and neural tube defects. *JAMA* 1992; 268:882–885.

48. Mansell R, Borchardt K. Disinfecting hydrotherapy equipment. *Arch Phys Med Rehabil.* 1974; 55:318–320.

49. Miller J, LaForest N, Hedberg M, et al. Surveillance and control of Hubbard tank bacterial contaminants. *Phys Ther.* 1970; 50:1482–1486.

50. Turner A, Higgins M, Craddock JC. Disinfection of immersion tanks (Hubbard) in a hospital burn unit. *Arch Environ Health.* 1974; 28:101–104.

51. Lawn G, Bohannon R. *Clin Management.* 1984; 4:6. Our readers comment.

52. Bohannon R. *Clin Management.* 1983; 3:50–51. Practice Tips.

53. McMillan J, Hargiss G, Nourse A, et al. Procedure for decontamination of hydrotherapy equipment. *Phys Ther.* 1976; 56:567–570.

54. Sagawas S, Shiraku, Yousef M, et al. Water temperature and intensity of exercise in maintenance of thermal equilibrium. *J App Physiol.* 1988; 65:2413–2419.

55. Moor F, et al. *Manual of Hydrotherapy & Massage.* Mountain View, CA: Pacific Press; 1964.

56. Kottke F, Lehmann J, ed. *Krusen's Handbook of Physical Medicine and Rehabilitation.* 4th ed. Philadelphia, PA: WB Saunders; 1990.

57. Finnerty G, Corbitt T. *Hydrotherapy.* New York: Ungar; 1960.

58. Downer A. *Physical Therapy Procedures.* Springfield, IL: Charles C Thomas; 1975.

59. Dodi G, Bogoni F, Infantino A, et al. Hot and cold in anal pain. *Dis Colon & Rectum.* 1986; 29:248–251.

SECTION 4
ELECTROTHERAPY

The use of electrotherapy can be traced back to ancient times. Its application has passed through periods of popularity and controversy. A few important historical milestones follow. A detailed account of this interesting history can be found in *Therapeutic Electricity and Ultraviolet Radiation* (GK Stillwell, ed. Baltimore, MD: Williams & Wilkins; 1983).

In 48 AD, Scribonius Largus, a Roman physician, used shock from torpedo fish to treat chronic headache and gout. In 1791 Luigi Galvani stimulated frog nerves and muscles with electrical charges from lightning and reported that the animals spontaneously developed electricity. In 1796 Alessandro Volta proved that the electrical charges in Galvani's experiment were the result of current between two dissimilar metals that were in contact with each other and not spontaneously produced by the animals.

Throughout the 19th century, a variety of medical conditions were routinely treated with electrical stimulation: for example, hemiplegia, epilepsy, kidney stones, sciatica, gout, rheumatism, and angina pectoris. In 1849 Guillaume B. Duchenne used "induced current" to treat atrophy and paralysis. He reported that he could apply this current to a patient in a less painful manner by using moistened surface electrodes and concluded that induced current was better than galvanic current. In 1870 L. Erb recommended the use of both induced and galvanic currents to stimulate nerve and muscles in the belief that these currents stimulated nutrition to atrophied muscles. During the polio epidemic of 1920, electrical stimulation was routinely used to treat paralysis. Some of the basic techniques used today were developed during that time. In subsequent years, electrotherapy went through periods of rising and declining interest.

At present, there is a renewed interest in the use of therapeutic electricity to stimulate nerve and muscle tissues. In addition, its application has been extended to the treatment of pain, the healing of wounds and fractured bones, and the introduction of ions to tissue. Electrical stimulation also is used as an evaluative tool.

Numerous electrotherapeutic devices are available today that offer a wide range of choice with respect to current type, frequency, mode, and ease of application. The selection of an electrotherapeutic device with the appropriate type of current, voltage, frequency and intensity for effective use is a difficult task. To simplify this task and to use this physical agent appropriately, physical therapists must have a good understanding of basic electricity and its effect on the body and be thoroughly familiar with the devices. Furthermore, therapists should remember that the treatment goal is the most important guide to the choice of electrical device and its appropriate setup.

The electrotherapy and electrophysiologic testing section of this text consists of seven chapters. Chapter 17 covers basic electricity and some of the background information necessary to understand the topic. Chapters 18 and 19 discuss the effects of electrical stimulation on the body and the clinical application of this physical agent. Chapters 20 and 21 describe the application of iontophoresis and transcutaneous electrical nerve stimulation (TENS) for the treatment of pain, and Chapter 22 reviews the point locator and stimulator, which is used to find trigger or acupuncture points, then stimulate them. Chapter 23 addresses the topics of electrophysiologic tests, nerve conduction velocity and electromyography.

17

Therapeutic Electricity

Tsega Andemicael Mehreteab, PT, MS

E lectrical stimulation is used to assess and treat nerve and muscle tissues and to manage different neuromuscular conditions. For example, it is used to evaluate the integrity of neuromuscular tissues with tests such as nerve conduction velocity, electromyography, and the strength-duration test. Electrical stimulation is commonly used in physical therapy to treat neuromuscular conditions, enhance local circulation and tissue healing, decrease pain, and increase range of motion. This chapter looks at the basic physical concepts of electric current, voltage, resistance, and waveforms. It also applies these concepts to the various types of electrical stimulators available and presents the body's response to electrical stimulation. Later chapters will look in more detail at different uses of electrical stimulation in normal and pathological conditions.

ATOMIC STRUCTURE

The atom is primarily composed of electrons, protons, and neutrons. The *electron* has a negative charge (–), the *proton* has a positive charge (+), and the *neutron* has no charge. The amount of positive charge carried by the proton is equal to the amount of negative charge carried by the electron. A neutral atom has an equal number of electrons and protons. If an atom gains or loses an electron, it is no longer neutral and is referred to as an *ion*. When an atom gains an electron, the number of its electrons becomes greater than the number of its protons, and the atom becomes a negatively charged ion. Conversely, if an atom loses an electron, the number of its electrons will be less than the number of its protons and it becomes a positively charged ion. Superscripts (–) and (+) are used to designate the charge of the ion. When more than one electron is transferred to or from an atom, a number next to the + or – signs is used to indicate the number of electrons transferred. For example, Cu^{2+} indicates the loss of two electrons from copper. SO_4^{-2} indicates the gain of two electrons by sulfate. The amount of charge carried by any substance is proportional to the number of charged individual atoms or molecules. For example, Cu^{+2} or SO_4^{-2} has twice as much charge as Cu^+ or NO_3^-, respectively. Similarly, a substance containing eight ions of Cu^+ has twice the amount of charge as the same amount of substance containing only four ions of Cu^+. The unit used for charge is the coulomb. The *coulomb* (C) is equivalent to the combined charge of 6.29×10^{18} electrons.

ELECTRICITY

The movement or flow of charged particles such as electrons or ions from one place to another constitutes an *electric current*. In metals, electricity is conducted by the flow of electrons; in solutions, electricity is conducted by the flow of ions. The amount of electrical current depends on the number of electrons or ions passing a given point per unit of time. The unit of current is an *ampere* (A). One ampere represents particles with a total charge of 1 C flowing every second through a given point. Thus 1 A = 1 C per second. Smaller units are the milliampere (mA) = 10^{-3} A and the microampere (μA) = 10^{-6} A.[1] To demonstrate the role of ions and electrons in the generation of electricity, the electrolytic cell is discussed below.

Electrolytic Cell

Fig. 17–1 represents an example of an electrolytic cell, a simple circuit containing a solution of copper chloride ($CuCl_2$) and water (H_2O), two metallic rods known as *electrodes*, and a battery. Each electrode is connected with a wire to the battery on one end and is immersed in the electrolytic solution on the other end. The positively and negatively charged ions in solution that conduct current are called *elec-*

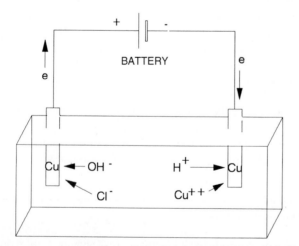

Figure 17–1. An electrolytic cell containing a solution of copper chloride ($CuCl_2$) in water (H_2O), two electrodes, and a battery. The two copper electrodes are connected to the battery with wire. As the battery is turned on, the negatively charged ions, OH^- and Cl^-, are attracted toward the anode (+ charged electrode) and the positively charged ions (anions), H^+ and Cu^{2+}, are attracted toward the cathode (– charged electrode). The electrolytes in this solution are OH^-, Cl^-, H^+, and Cu^{2+}. The battery is represented by ⊣⊢.

trolytes. In this circuit, the electrolytes are copper (Cu^{2+}), chloride (Cl^-), hydronium (H^+), and hydroxide (OH^-) ions.

The electrode attached to the positive side of the cell is called the *anode,* and the electrode attached to the negative side of the cell is called the *cathode.* Thus the cathode (–) is electron rich and the anode (+) is electron deficient. The positive (+) and the negative (–) signs are used to designate the anode and the cathode, respectively. In this circuit, the ions (Cu^+, H^+, Cl^-, and OH^-) are responsible for carrying the electrical charges through the solution. However, the electrical current flowing through the electrodes and through any wires used in the circuit is the result of the flow of electrons.

At the metal-solution interface (see Fig. 17–1), electrons are exchanged between the electrodes and the ions in the solution. The negatively charged ions are attracted and flow toward the anode. These ions are called *anions.* At the anode, the anions give up their excess electrons to the electron-deficient electrode. At the same time, electrons are leaving the negative side of the battery and flowing toward the cathode. In solution, the positively charged ions, called *cations,* are attracted to and flow toward the cathode, where they pick up excess electrons.

Electricity passes through the solution circuit as long as the excess of electrons in the cathode and deficiency of electrons in the anode are maintained. That is, a *difference in potential* between the two ends of the circuit exists. In an electrolytic solution, the ions migrate in two opposite directions: cations (+) toward the cathode and anions (–) toward the anode. A two-way migration of ions in solution is known as *convection current.*[2] Because body fluids contain electrolytes, electrical current through tissue fluids not only is conducted but also involves convection current.

Fig. 17–2 represents a typical electrical circuit; it is a diagrammatic representation of the basic components for electrical current flow. The circuit must be completed: that is, a continuous loop is required for charges to flow. In such a circuit, the electric current continues until the battery is no longer charged or the electrolytes in the solution are depleted. In other words, all the cations are reduced or pick up electrons ($Cu^{++} + 2e \text{-------} > Cu$) or all the anions are oxidized or lose their excess electrons ($2Cl^- \text{-------} > Cl_2 + 2e$). Note that electrons flow from the negative electrode (cathode) to the positive electrode (anode). However, by arbitrary convention, the direction of current was historically designated to be from the positive to the negative electrode.

Body fluids such as blood, sweat, interstitial fluid, and urine all contain electrolytes such as potassium (K^+), sodium (Na^+), calcium (Ca^{2+}), chloride (Cl^-), and sulfate (SO_4^{2-}). As electrical current pass through such electrolytic solutions, a number of chemical reactions can occur. The magnitude of these electrochemical

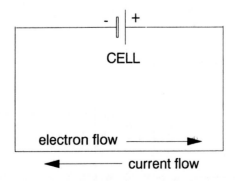

Figure 17–2. A schematic representation of a complete electrical circuit. The arrows depict the direction of electron and current flow. Electrons flow from the cathode (–) toward the anode (+), but, by arbitrary convention, the direction of current is designated to be from the positive electrode (anode) toward the negative electrode (cathode). Current continues to flow until the battery is turned off or the electrolytes are depleted. The battery is represented by ┤├ .

reactions depends on how long the current is applied and on the current density. *Current density* is the amount of current per unit of electrode area and is proportional to the current amplitude (intensity). Current amplitude, electrode size, and current duration are important factors in the safe application of electrical stimulation.

Types of Current Used in Physical Therapy

The two types of electrical current available for therapeutic purposes are direct current and alternating current. Direct current (DC) is the constant unidirectional flow of electricity. For example, the electrons flow continuously in one direction from the isoelectric point. The isoelectric point is a standard reference point used to describe the direction of electrical flow (Fig. 17–3). In DC circuits, the electrodes maintain their positive or negative polarity; therefore, when these electrodes are used to stimulate tissues, positive and negative fields will be established and maintained under the positive and the negative electrodes, respectively.

Direct current can induce chemical reactions in body tissues. For example, at the anode, oxidation of the anions results in *acidic reactions,* whereas at the cathode, reduction of the cations results in *alkaline reactions.* These electrochemical reactions are referred to as *polar reactions* and are outlined in Table 17–1. The extent of such reactions depends on the duration and intensity of the current applied. Different chemical reactions occur at the positive and negative electrodes. The direct current output can be modified to deliver either a continuous or interrupted direct current mode. Therapeutically, continuous direct current is mainly used to induce chemical reactions and to transfer ions, a method called iontophoresis. (see Chapter 20).

Interrupted direct current is used to stimulate motor, sensory, and autonomic nerves and muscle tissues. An interrupted direct current, which has a monophasic pulse of long duration can be produced easily by manually interrupting the direct current circuit with a "make or break" key. Interrupted direct current produced mechanically by the device at a preset rate may have an extremely brief duration.

Some electrical stimulators such as the so-called high-voltage pulse stimulator, deliver unidirectional, monophasic waveforms. The duration of each pulse is less than 100 microseconds, which is too short to induce a significant chemical reaction or to stimulate denervated muscle tissues. But such stimulators are used to stimulate intact neuromuscular tissue and other soft tissues.

Alternating current (AC) is a current that changes its direction of flow periodically; thus, its electrodes change polarity alternately. For example, A and B in Fig. 17–4A represent two ends of the circuit; the current moves from A to B; then, as the polarities of A and B change, current moves in the opposite direction: ie, from B to A. Unlike direct current, a positive and a negative field under each electrode are not maintained. Instead, the electrical fields change polarity (alternate) and the current rises to peak amplitude in the positive phase, falls back to the **isoelectric point,**

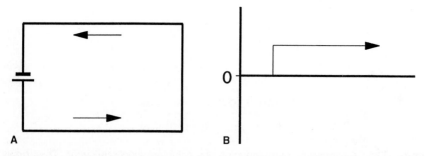

Figure 17–3. (A) A schematic representation of a direct current circuit, where the current flows in only one direction and the two ends of the circuit maintain their positive or negative charges. **(B)** The line with an arrow represents a continuous flow of direct current beginning at the isoelectric line. Current flows continuously until the circuit is disconnected or the battery is turned off. The battery is represented by ┤├ .

TABLE 17–1. POLAR REACTIONS UNDER EACH ELECTRODE

Anode (+)	Cathode (−)
Attraction of anion (−ions)	Attraction of cations (+ions)
Acidic reactions	Alkaline reactions
Example: formation of HCl	Example: formation of NaOH
Solidification of protein	Liquification of protein
Hardening of tissue	Softening of tissue
Hyperpolarization	Hypopolarization
Increased nerve excitability	Increased nerve excitability

(Davis, RB (ed). *Pediatric Neurology for the Clinician.* Norwalk, Conn.: Appleton & Lange; 1992, with permission).

and rises to the negative peak field before returning to the isoelectric point. An isoelectric point is the zero point on the graphic representation of a given stimulus (Fig. 17–4B).

Biphasic waveform and bidirectional current are two other names used for alternating current. The electrodes used to deliver such current to the body tissue change their polarity with each change in the direction of the current. Any chemical reaction that may have occurred during one half-cycle, or phase, of the output is neutralized by the subsequent phase, which is opposite in direction and similar in magnitude. Therefore, with this type of stimulation, no net polar (chemical) reaction occurs.

CHARACTERISTICS OF AN ELECTRICAL CIRCUIT

An electrical circuit is a pathway through which electrons or other charged particles move. Fig. 17–1 represents a circuit made up of electrodes, electolytic solution and battery. For a current to exist, all components of the circuit (eg, battery, electrodes, switches) must be in physical contact so that electrons or other charged particles can move from one area to another. The flow of electrons or charged ions is called *current*.

Electromotive Force

To have a continuous flow of charges, or current, in a circuit, a driving force is required. This driving force is essentially a difference in potential between two ends or points of the circuit and is often called an *electromotive force* (EMF). However, this term is misleading because EMF is a measure of the maximum work per unit charge rather than a measure of force. A difference in potential is established when the amount of charges at one end of the circuit is greater than that at the other end or between any two points of the circuit. This difference in potential can

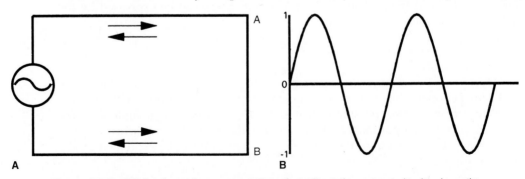

Figure 17–4. (A) A schematic representation of an alternating current circuit, where the current changes direction. This occurs as the polarity (field charge) of the two ends of the circuit, A and B, changes from positive to negative. **(B)** Each cycle of the current is graphically represented by a sine waveform. One complete cycle contains both positive and negative phases. The source of the alternating current is represented by ⊖ .

be established by a motor or a battery. For example, the cathode end of a battery supplies excess electrons (–), whereas the anode end is deficient of electrons; therefore, if the two ends of the battery are connected, electrons will flow from the cathode to the anode and an electrical current will be established in the circuit. The electrons or other charged particles will continue to flow as long as the difference in potential is maintained and the circuit is completed. The difference in potential is expressed in *volts* (V); smaller units are expressed in millivolts (mV, 10^{-3} V) and microvolts (μV, 10^{-6} V).

Resistance

When electrons or ions flow through the circuit, they encounter *resistance* (R) by the medium through which they are made to flow. The unit used for resistance is the ohm (Ω); larger units are the kilo-ohm (10^3 Ω) and mega ohm (10^6 Ω). Materials that offer less resistance and readily allow electric current to pass through them are called *conductors*. For example, copper, silver, and tap water are good conductors. Materials that offer high resistance and impede the passage of current are called *insulators*. For example, glass, rubber, paraffin, and distilled water are good insulators. Materials that are neither good conductors nor insulators are called *semiconductors*. For example, silicon and germanium, which are used in solid-state circuits, are good semiconductors.

The resistance encountered in a circuit depends on the following factors: the type, size, shape, and composition of the conductor material. In addition, other factors such as temperature may influence the resistance of a circuit. For example, increasing the temperature of a metal may decrease its conductivity, whereas increasing the temperature of a tissue may improve its electrical conduction because of an increase in body fluids (eg, blood or sweat) in the area. A moist piece of gauze or paper is used as a conductive medium between the skin and the electrode in transcutaneous electrical stimulation.

The type of conductor material determines the level of resistance to the current. For example, metals have less resistance than do nonmetals. Silver and copper have the least resistance among the metals; thus they are good conductors. Copper wires are commonly used for house current. Nonmetals such as rubber, formica, and various other plastics have high resistance and are used to insulate electrical circuits. Even among good conductors and good insulators differences in the degree of resistance are encountered. In liquids, the degree of resistance in the system is determined by the composition of the solution: ie, the materials that make up the medium through which current is passing. Solutions such as salt water, which have many electrolytes, offer less resistance than do solutions such as tap water, which have few or no electrolytes. Body fluids such as blood, sweat, and interstitial fluid contain many electrolytes and therefore are good conductors.

The length (L), the cross-sectional area (A), and the *resistivity* (ρ) of the conductor also determine the resistance (R) of a circuit. These can be expressed by the following equation:

$$R = \frac{\rho L}{A}$$

For example, a thin copper wire offers higher resistance than a thick copper wire and a long copper wire offers greater resistance than a short copper wire. As electrical current encounters resistance, heat is generated. According to Joules law, the heat produced is proportional to the resistance, the intensity and the duration of the current. The electrical-to-thermal energy conversion can be expressed by the following equation:

$$H = 0.24 \times I^2 \times R \times t$$

where 0.24 is a constant, H is heat in joules (gram- calories), I is current intensity in amperes, R is resistance in ohms and t is time in seconds. To avoid hazardous consequences, the appropriate type and size of wiring should be used in electrical de-

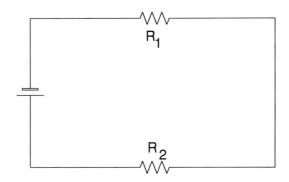

Figure 17–5. Electrical circuit with resistance. This schematic diagram illustrates an electrical circuit with two resistors, R₁ and R₂. The symbol ⎓ᴧᴧᴧ⎓ represents the resistors and ⊣⊢ represents the battery, the electromotive force, or the voltage.

vices. Otherwise, heat buildup may lead to breakage of machinery and even electrical fire.

Electrical circuits are represented in Fig. 17–5. The resistance of the system is represented by a resistor whose symbol is (⎓ᴧᴧᴧ⎓). These resistors are physical elements that are placed in the circuit or may represent hindrance offered by various components of the circuit. The two resistors are represented by R_1 and R_2, and the driving force, or voltage, is represented by the symbol for battery (⊣⊢). The amount of electrical current, or intensity (I), through the circuit depends on the voltage or potential difference usually symbolized by E or V and the resistance (R). The greater the voltage (difference in potential), the higher the intensity. On the other hand, for a given voltage, the greater the resistance, the lower rate of electrical flow. This relationship is shown by the following equation called *Ohm's law:*

$$I = \tfrac{E}{R} \text{ or } E = IR,$$

where I is the current intensity in amperes, E is the potential difference in volts, and R is the resistance in ohms.[3]

If any two of the above electrical quantities are known, the third can be calculated. For example, in a circuit with a 10 Ω resistor and a 45 V potential difference, what is the amount of electric current flowing through the circuit? The answer is

$$I = \tfrac{E}{R} = \tfrac{45}{10} = 4.5 \text{ A.}$$

Arrangement

The components of an electrical circuit can be arranged in series or parallel to each other. Most electrical circuits consist of a combination of series and parallel components.

Series circuits. When several resistors, such as R_1, R_2, and R_3 in Fig. 17–6 are arranged so that the same current flows through each of them, they are said to be in series with each other. When electrical stimulation is administered transcutaneously (that is, through the skin), the skin and fat layers can be considered to be in series. The total resistance (R_T) is the arithmetic sum of the resistors in series: that is,

$$R_T = (R_1 + R_2 + R_3 \ldots \ldots R_n.)$$

The same amount of current (I_T) flows through each resistor; thus,

$$I_T = I_1 = I_2 = I_3$$

From Ohm's law,

$$I_T = E/R_T.$$

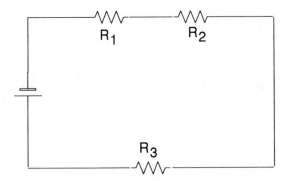

Figure 17–6. Resistors in series. This schematic diagram illustrates a circuit with three resistors, R_1, R_2, and R_3, in series. The ⌇ represents a resistor and ⊣⊢ represents the battery, the electromotive force, or the voltage.

Note that voltage (E) must be sufficient to overcome the total resistance (R) for current (I) to exist. For example, in the series circuit above, if $R_1 = 100\ \Omega$, $R_2 = 200\ \Omega$, and $R_3 = 300\ \Omega$, and the voltage = 60, what is the intensity through this circuit?

$$R_T = 100\ \Omega + 200\ \Omega + 300\ \Omega = 600\ \Omega$$
$$I_T = E/R_T = 60V\ /\ 600\ \Omega = 0.1\ A$$

Parallel circuits. In Fig. 17–7, resistors R_4, R_5, and R_6 are arranged so that the current has multiple alternative pathways. This circuit is said to be arranged in parallel. In a parallel circuit, the reciprocal of the total resistance $1/R_T$ is equal to the sum of the reciprocals of each resistor in parallel: that is,

$$1/R_T = (1/R_4 + 1/R_5 + 1/R_6 + \ldots \ldots\ 1/R_n)$$

For example, in the above parallel circuit, if $R_4 = 100\ \Omega$, $R_5 = 200\ \Omega$, and $R_6 = 200\ \Omega$, then the total resistance (R_T) can be calculated as follows:

$$\frac{1}{RT} = \frac{1}{R4} + \frac{1}{R5} + \frac{1}{R6} = \frac{1}{100}\Omega + \frac{1}{200}\Omega + \frac{1}{200}\Omega = \frac{1}{50}\Omega$$
$$R_T = 50\ \Omega$$

Therefore, R_T is equal to 50 Ω. With a voltage of 250 across the resistors, the total current, I_T, across all the resistors can be calculated as follows:

$$I_T = \frac{E}{R_T} = 250V/50\Omega = 5\ A$$

In a parallel circuit, the voltage across each resistor is the same. Because current takes the path of least resistance, the current (*I*) through each resistor in parallel is inversely proportional to their resistance. The current across the individual resistors is calculated as follows:

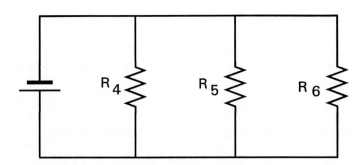

Figure 17–7. Resistors in parallel. This schematic diagram illustrates a circuit with three resistors, R_4, R_5, and R_6, in parallel. The ⌇ represents the resistors and ⊣⊢ represents the battery, the electromotive force, or the voltage.

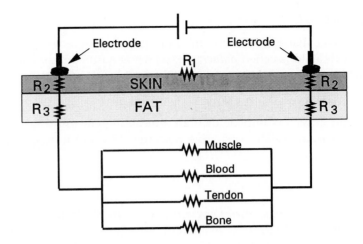

Figure 17–8. Resistive components of tissue. This schematic diagram represents the flow of current through a biologic tissue. The resistive components representing the skin and fat are arranged in series, and muscle, blood, tendon, and bone are arranged in parallel. Muscle tissue and blood offer less resistance to current than do skin and fat. R_1 = resistance along skin. R_2 = resistance through skin. R_3 = resistance through fat.

$$I_1 = \frac{250}{100} = 2.50A$$
$$I_2 = \frac{250}{200} = 1.25A$$
$$I_3 = \frac{250}{200} = 1.25A$$

Therefore,

$$I_T = I_1 + I_2 + I_3 = 2.5 \text{ A} + 1.25 \text{ A} + 1.25 \text{ A} = 5 \text{ A},$$

the same answer as that obtained by first calculating the total resistance (R_T) in the above example.

Note that for a parallel circuit, the resistance is effectively reduced. In fact, the total resistance ($R_T = 50 \, \Omega$) of the circuit is less than the resistor which offers the least resistance ($R_4 = 100 \, \Omega$). The circuit also can be arranged with a mixture of series and parallel components. In such an arrangement, the components must first be resolved segment by segment before the values of the total circuit can be calculated.[1] In the body, the resistive components are arranged in series and in parallel. As shown in Fig. 17–8, skin and fat are arranged in series. In the deeper tissues, the electrical current takes the path of least resistance; thus muscle, blood, tendon, and bone can be considered to be resistors in a parallel circuit.

In addition to the above circuit arrangement, other physical characteristics of a circuit influence the pattern and magnitude of current flow. Three such characteristics are capacitance, inductance, and impedance.

Capacitance

The characteristic that enables a device or circuit to store electrical charges in an electrostatic field is called *capacitance,* which is based on the voltage of the circuit. Capacitance is measured in units of *farads (F).* One farad is the amount of capacitance of 1 C of charges stored in a circuit with difference in potential of 1 V (F = C/V). Because a farad is an enormously large unit, capacitance is measured in microfarads (10^{-6} F) and picofarads (10^{-12} F). An electronic device called a capacitor is used to store electrical charges and release them at a later time. It is made up of two conductors with a dielectric (insulating) material in between. A capacitor does not allow direct current to pass through it, whereas it does allow alternating current to pass.

Inductance

The characteristic that enables a circuit or device to store electrical energy in an electromagnetic field is called *inductance,* which is a function of current intensity. Inductance is measured in *henries (H).* Smaller units are the millihenry (mH, 10^{-3}H) and microhenry (μH, 10^{-6}H). The symbol for inductance is *L.* An *inductor* is a device that stores electrical energy in an electromagnetic field. Both capacitors and inductors impede or limit alternating current flow in a circuit. These hindrances are called capacitive reactance (X_c) and inductive reactance (X_L), respectively.

Impedance

Similar to the resistance in a direct current circuit, the hindrance to current flow encountered in an alternating current circuit is call *impedance* (Z), which is measured in units of ohms. Biological tissues, because of their complex composition, present various factors and interactions that limit current flow. The hindrance to current flow caused by body tissues is called impedance. Body tissue such as muscle, nerve, fat, and skin offer various degrees of impedance to electrical current passed through them. Impedance is composed of resistance (*R*), Capacitive reactance (X_C) and inductive reactance (X_L) and is expressed by the following equation:

$$Z = \sqrt{R^2 + (X_L - X_c)^2}$$

Where R^2, X_L and X_C are static resistance, inductive reactance, and capacitive reactance, respectively.

As shown in the following equation, capacitive reactance (X_C) is inversely proportional to the frequency of the alternating current. In general, the higher the frequency of the stimulating current, the lower the impedance of the tissue:

$$X_C = \frac{1}{2\pi f C}$$

Where π = 3.14, *f* is the frequency of applied voltage in hertz (cycles per second) and *C* is capacitance in farads. For a more detailed review of concepts presented above, the reader should consult a general physics text.[4] Skin contains keratin and offers the highest impedance to electrical current. If the skin is slightly abraded, the impedance decreases by 50–100% Although necessary for accurate electrical testing, abrading the skin is not usually necessary for routine electrical stimulation. Removing dirt, oil, and dead skin with alcohol or soap and water is usually sufficient for this procedure. In addition, the clinician should note that the tissue impedance may decrease as stimulation time progresses. Therefore, clinically, the body part should be stimulated a few times before setting up the final amplitude. Furthermore, the amplitude should be checked frequently during the first few minutes of stimulation.

Other factors that influence the effectiveness of electrical stimulation are current density and the composition and volume of the tissue stimulated. Current density (current/unit area) depends on the intensity, the size of the electrodes, and the site of the tissue stimulated. For example, the subcutaneous fat in obese people presents high resistance. Therefore, effective stimulation of the nerve or muscle requires an extremely high intensity, which the person may not tolerate. In addition, the body acts as a volume conductor: ie, the current spreads in all directions in the immediate vicinity of the electrode. This may reduce the effective density of the stimulating current. In general, the more fluid and the greater the electrolyte content, the greater the conductivity of the tissue. The percentage of water content in the various body tissues can be used as a guide for the relative conductivity. For example, muscle contains 72–75% water, whereas fat contains 14–15% water.[5]

CLASSIFICATION OF ELECTRICAL STIMULATORS

General Characteristics of the Stimulus Output

Numerous electrical devices can be used to achieve physical therapy treatment goals. The different designs of available electrical devices make it difficult to select the appropriate device for a desired objective. To simplify this task, the most common electrical stimulators can be classified according to the general characteristics of their stimulus output: namely, the waveform, duration, and frequency of the output. In addition, electrical stimulators have been classified according to their frequency and voltage. For example, low versus medium frequency and low versus high voltage are terms sometimes used to refer to a particular type of electrical device.

Waveforms

Waveform is the geometric representation of an electrical wave or stimulus. The shape of the wave depicts the amplitude and pulse duration of each stimulus. Electrical stimulators may offer a choice of waveforms or may operate on only one preset waveform. The main variables of a waveform are the amplitude, duration, and rise and decay times. Some typical waveforms available in electrotherapeutic devices are shown in Fig. 17–9. Note that the monophasic waveforms do not transverse the *isoelectric line,* the line that crosses the zero point on the representative graph of the waveform. The waveforms above or below the isoelectric line are in the positive or negative phase, respectively. The *phase* is the flow of charges in one direction for a finite period of time. Waveforms representing direct current can be in either the positive or negative phase and are called *monophasic.*

Waveforms representing alternating current cross the isoelectric line, contain a negative and a positive phase, and are called *biphasic.* Biphasic waveforms are symmetrical if the shape and area under the positive and negative phases are equal. Some biphasic waveforms are asymmetrical: ie, shape and area under the positive and negative phases are not equal. The area under a phase represents a phase charge. In an asymmetrical biphasic waveform, the phase charge can be balanced or unbalanced. In a balanced asymmetrical biphasic waveform, the net positive and negative phase charges are equal and the output is electrically neutral. On the other hand, in an unbalanced asymmetrical biphasic waveform, the net positive and negative phase charges are unequal and the output is not electrically neutral. Typical names used to refer to waveforms are faradic, sine, rectangular

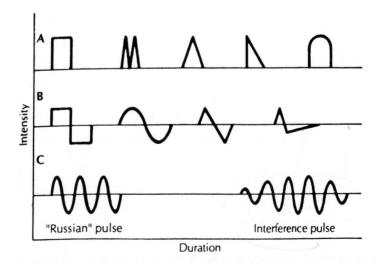

Figure 17–9. Basic waveforms. **(A)** monophasic, **(B)** biphasic, and **(C)** polyphasic. (*Reproduced with permission from* Clinical Electrotherapy. *RM Nelson, DP Currier. 1987, Appleton & Lange.*)

biphasic, and asymmetrical biphasic. A single waveform representing a stimulus output is called a pulse. The *pulse duration* represents the time elapsed from the beginning to the end of the waveform and is given in units ranging from microseconds to seconds. The *interpulse interval* represents the time between two successive pulses. The rate at which these pulses occur in a second is the pulse rate or frequency and is given in pulses per second (pps).

The amount of current used can be expressed as peak current amplitude, average current, or current density. *Peak current amplitude* is the maximum amplitude of the waveform. For some waveforms, such as the twin peak waveform of the high-voltage pulsed current stimulator, the peak current amplitude can be reached only for a brief period. *Average current* (the total current per unit of time), on the other hand, is the current amplitude averaged over the total duration of the waveform. This is determined by dividing the area under the waveform by the duration of the waveform. Another way of expressing current amplitude is the mathematically derived root mean square (RMS). The current amplitude depends on the shape of the waveform (see Fig. 17–10). For example, the RMS of a sinusoidal waveform is 0.70 of the peak amplitude, whereas the average current is 0.64 of the peak amplitude.[6] For electrical stimulators, the stimulus intensity or amplitude is usually given in units of milliamperes or microamperes.

Other characteristics of a waveform are its rise and decay times. The *rise time* (speed of rise) represents the time required to reach peak amplitude. Some waveforms, such as the square waveform, almost immediately rise to peak amplitude, whereas others, such as the triangular or saw tooth waveforms, have a slower rise time. The rise time may affect the response of tissues to the stimuli. For example, nerve tissue fails to respond to a slowly rising pulse, whereas a denervated muscle tissue does not. The reason is that nerve tissue accommodates to the stimuli and muscle tissue does not. *Decay time* represents the amount of time the pulse takes to go from peak to zero amplitude. This also may affect the response of tissue to the stimuli. The frequency and duration of the waveform or pulse also can be modified to produce a variety of stimulus outputs.

Waveform Modulations

The stimulus output, the waveform, can be modified to alter the quality of the response to the stimulation. This modification is called output modulation, which can be achieved in many ways. The most common modulations are phase duration modulation, phase amplitude modulation, and pulse rate modulation. The duration, amplitude, or frequency of the waveform is modified to increase and decrease gradually. The quality of the response changes as the basic characteristics of the stimulus output change (see Fig. 17–11).

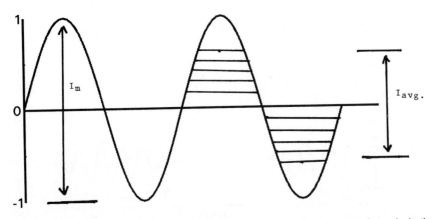

Figure 17–10. Peak and average current amplitude of a sinusoidal waveform. I_m is the peak current amplitude measured from the isoelectric point to the peak of the current waveform. I_{avg} is the amplitude of current averaged over the duration (t) of the waveform. $I_{avg} = 0.64 \times I_m$.

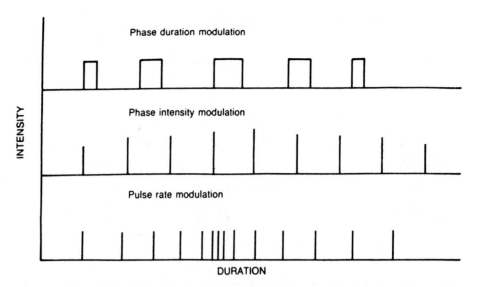

Figure 17–11. Dynamic modulations of pulse characteristics. Modulation of phase duration, intensity, pulse rate and duration, and combined amplitude. (*Reproduced with permission from* Clinical Electrotherapy. *RM Nelson, DP Currier. 1987, Appleton & Lange.*)

Surged modulation is produced when the individual pulses within a series or train of pulses are programmed so that the peak amplitude of each sequential pulse is either gradually or abruptly increased to peak amplitude and is gradually or abruptly decreased to zero amplitude. The time required to reach a maximum amplitude of the surged mode is called *ramp time*. A train of pulses can be ramped up or down. The pulse duration also can be modulated by increasing or decreasing the duration of successive pulses. Because of the gradual recruitment of motor units, surged modulations elicit a muscle contraction that builds up gradually. The increasing intensity, or duration, recruits motor units with increasing stimulus thresholds. The surged mode rate is expressed in surges per minute. The gradual increase and fall in stimulus intensity may be better tolerated. Note that some authors use rise time and ramp time interchangeably. For the sake of clarity, the term ramp time is used for surged pulses and the term rise time is used for a single waveform or pulse.

In addition to the amplitude, duration, and frequency modulation, the stimulus output can be delivered continuously or interrupted periodically. A continuos mode or pattern is an ongoing, nonmodified series or train of pulses. When the series of pulses commence and cease at regular intervals, an interrupted or *burst mode* is produced. The rate of bursts or interruptions per second determines the quality of muscle contraction. For example, an interruption rate of 10 pulses per second produces a twitch contraction, whereas an interruption of 50 pulses per second produces tetanic contractions. For example, the so-called "Russian" electrical stimulator delivers polyphasic waveforms at 2500 Hz. These pulses are patterned to deliver bursts of pulses 50 times per second, with each burst or envelope of pulses lasting 10 milliseconds (see Fig. 17–12).

Duty Cycle

In addition to the surged modulation, the pulse output can be modified by selecting patterns with different total on-versus-off periods of the output. This is referred to as the *duty cycle*. The duty cycle is the ratio of the on-time of the trains of pulses to the total period. It relates the net on-time of the stimuli to the total time period (on + off) of the stimuli. The duty cycle is usually expressed as the percentage of on-time to the total period (on + off). For example, when a train of stimuli is on for 10 seconds and off for 30 seconds, the duty cycle is 25% (10 ms/40 ms × 100%), or a ratio of 1 to 3. The longer the on-time of a given duty cycle, the greater the possibility that the stimulated muscles will become fatigued.

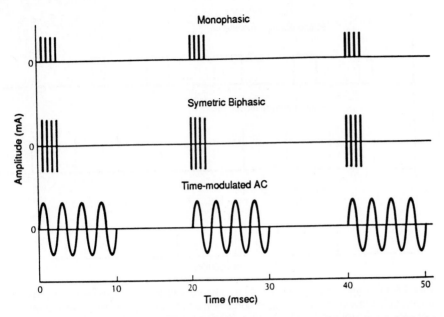

Figure 17–12. Burst modulation of various pulses. The stimulus output is modulated so that the pulses last for only a brief period. Monophasic pulsed bursts usually last only 1 millisecond, whereas biphasic bursts last 10 milliseconds. (*Reproduced with permission from* Clinical Electrotherapy. *RM Nelson, DP Currier. 1987, Appleton & Lange.*)

Frequency

The classification of therapeutic electrical devices can be based on the frequency of the stimuli output or the "carrier" frequency used. This classification includes devices that deliver low-frequency output (1–1000 Hz), medium-frequency output (1000–10,000 Hz), and high-frequency output (10,000 Hz or more). Devices with low-voltage direct and alternating current and those with high-voltage pulsed current are examples of low-frequency units.

The interferential current stimulators use two medium-frequency circuits in the range of 4000–5000 Hz. One circuit delivers a preset frequency of 4000 Hz; the second circuit delivers a variable frequency of 4001–4150 Hz (Fig. 17–13). The tissue is apparently stimulated by a net frequency of 1–150 Hz.[7]

The designation high frequency is reserved for electrical devices that use extremely high-frequency currents. Such high frequencies do not stimulate muscle or nerve tissues and are used for therapeutic heating of tissue. Examples of this category of treatment are the shortwave and microwave diathermies. Note that frequency as a basis for classification of electrical stimulators tends to be confusing because the terms low frequency and medium frequency are so relative.

In addition to waveform and frequency, the type of current and the voltage are sometimes used to classify electrical stimulators. Type of current refers to direct current or alternating current (biphasic waveform), and voltage refers to the low-voltage versus the so-called high-voltage designations of electrical stimulators. The low-voltage stimulating devices use approximately 0–150 volts, and their stimulus amplitude or intensity is measured in terms of milliamperes. The stimulus output is displayed in current intensity rather than the actual voltage used to deliver such current. The so-called high-voltage pulsed current stimulator, on the other hand, displays voltages as high as 500 to deliver limited average current of 1.0–1.5 milliamps. The stimulus amplitude in such devices is given in terms of volts, as displayed on the voltmeter. The terms low voltage and high voltage are relative and should only be used to distinguish between these two types of clinical devices. The term "high voltage" used in the nontherapeutic sense represents devices carrying at least 2500 V. Relative to such devices, the clinical high-voltage pulsed-current units can be considered in the low volt range.

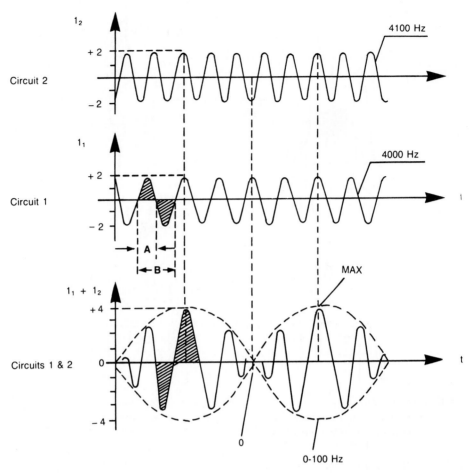

Figure 17–13. Generation of interference current. A = phase duration, B = pulse duration. Note that when the two circuits are in phase, the amplitude of the envelope is twice as high, thus providing an intensity that is adequate for excitation. (*Reproduced with permission from* Clinical Electrotherapy. *RM Nelson, DP Currier. 1987, Appleton & Lange.*)

Constant Current and Constant Voltage Stimulators

The stimulus output used to stimulate tissues encounters an ever-changing environment because of changes in the impedance of electrodes, skin, and other tissue. To deliver a constant stimulus output, electrical devices are designed either as constant voltage or constant current units. This adjustment occurs in the output amplifier section of an electrical device and is a response to changing load: that is, the total impedance encountered by the stimulus output. Constant voltage generators are designed to adjust current flow so that the voltage of the stimulus output is maintained within a set amount. Constant current generators are designed to adjust the voltage so that the current amplitude is maintained within the set amount. In addition, such devices limit the voltage changes within set ranges to prevent skin burns when the load suddenly increases, as in the case of a dry electrode. (A more detailed discussion of this concept can be found elsewhere.[8])

PLACEMENT OF ELECTRODES

In general, for a given current amplitude, the smaller the electrode, the higher the current density and the stronger the stimulus. Current density, the amount of current concentrated under an electrode, is expressed in milliamperes per unit of area (mA/sq cm). For example, for an electrode of 2 cm^2 that is delivering 10 mA, the

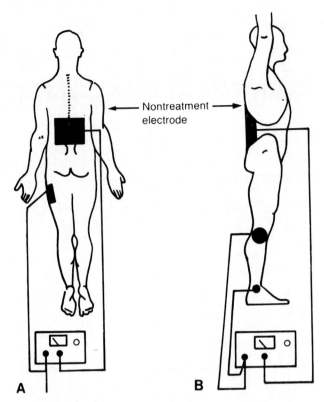

Figure 17–14. Monopolar technique of placing electrodes. **(A)** The simple method, **(B)** The method with a bifurcated lead so that both knee and ankle can be treated simultaneously. (*Reproduced with permission from* Clinical Electrotherapy. *RM Nelson, DP Currier. 1987, Appleton & Lange.*)

current density directly under the electrode is 10 mA/2 sq cm or 5 mA/sq cm. Current density is considered when choosing the appropriately sized electrode for stimulating or for current dispersion. In therapeutic electrical stimulation, the smaller electrode delivering higher current density is referred to as the active or stimulating electrode and the larger electrode, which is mainly used to complete the circuit, is referred to as the dispersive electrode.

For any electrical stimulation to be effective, the circuit must be completed: that is, the two leads with at least two electrodes must be secured to the body part to be stimulated. Because the body is a good conductor, placing these electrodes on any part of the body would complete the circuit. For effective stimulation of the target tissue, however, the electrodes should be placed selectively. For the purposes of electrophysiologic testing and therapeutic application, electrodes of the same circuit are placed on the target area either in a *monopolar* or a *bipolar* arrangement. The designation monopolar or bipolar is based on the relative size and location of the electrodes used for stimulation.

Monopolar placement. In a monopolar placement, a single small electrode (the active or stimulating electrode) is placed on the target area to be stimulated—the area where the greatest effect is desired, eg, the motor point. The second, larger electrode (the dispersive or reference electrode) is placed on the same side of the body and away from the target area. In this arrangement, the current density under the smaller electrode is higher than it is under the larger dispersive electrode (see Fig. 17–14).

Bipolar placement. In a bipolar placement, two electrodes of the same size are placed on the target area in such a way that the electrical current of the circuit efficiently stimulates the target tissues. In this arrangement, the electrical current is concentrated in the target area (see Fig. 17–15). Note that more than two electrodes in a circuit (channel) can be used by bifurcating the leads of the circuit. The total electrode area is determined by adding the areas of all electrodes used in each lead

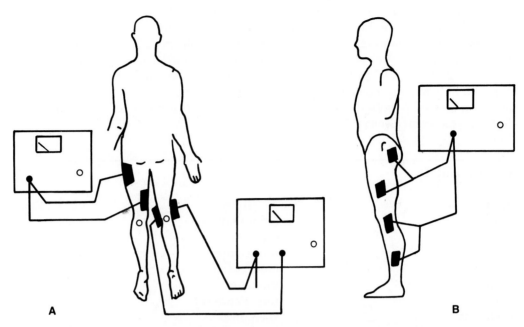

Figure 17–15. Bipolar technique of placing electrodes. **(A)** The simple method over a joint or muscle, **(B)** The bifurcated method along the dermatomal distribution. (*Reproduced with permission from* Clinical Electrotherapy. *RM Nelson, DP Currier. 1987, Appleton & Lange.*)

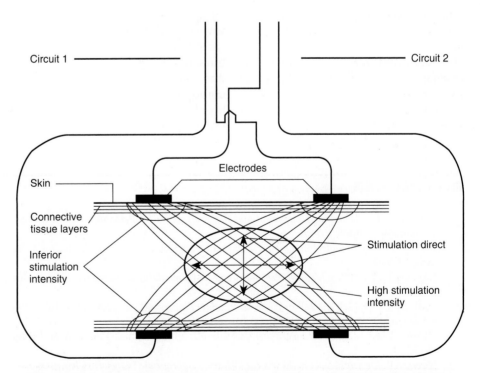

Figure 17–16. Quadripolar technique of placing electrodes. Electrodes of Circuit 1 are placed in a crossed pattern with the electrodes of Circuit 2. The maximum interference of current of the two circuits occur where they cross. In this area, the modulated amplitude of the stimulus output is higher than it is under either electrode. (*Adapted with permission from Traditional and Modern Aspects of Electrotherapy. A Hansjorgens, HU May, 1982.*)

of the circuit. More than one channel can be used to stimulate a large area of the body. Different areas of the body also can be stimulated at the same time using different channels. For example, two channels with four electrodes can be used to stimulate a large area such as the back—an arrangement referred to as a quadripolar electrode placement The electrode of each channel can be oriented parallel to (adjacent) or in a crossed pattern to each other. The interferential current stimulator uses a crossed pattern of electrode placement referred to as the quadripolar electrode placement (See Fig. 17–16).

■ KEY TERMS

electron	resistivity
proton	Ohm's law
neutron	capacitance
ion	inductance
coulomb (C)	henries (H)
electric current	inductor
ampere (A)	impedance (Z)
electrodes	waveform
electrolytes	isoelectric line
anode	phase
cathode	monophasic
anions	biphasic
cations	pulse duration
difference in potential	interpulse interval
convection current	peak current amplitude
current density	average current
acidic reactions	rise time
alkaline reactions	decay time
polar reactions	surged modulation
current	ramp time
electromotive force	burst mode
resistance	duty cycle
conductors	monopolar
insulators	bipolar
semiconductors	impedance

REFERENCES

1. Tammes AR. *Electronics for Medical and Biology Laboratory Personnel.* Baltimore, MD: Williams & Wilkins; 1971:8.
2. Scott PM. *Clayton's Electrotherapy and Actinotherapy.* Baltimore, MD: Williams & Wilkins; 1975:42.
3. Karselis T. *Descriptive Medical Electronics and Instrumentation.* Thorofare, NJ: Charles B Black; 1973:12.
4. Halliday D, Resnick R, Walker J. *Fundamentals of Physics.* 4th ed. New York: John Wiley & Sons; 1993.
5. Shriber WA. *Manual of Electrotherapy.* 4th ed. Philadelphia, PA: Lea & Febiger; 1975:120.
6. Newton R. *Electrotherapeutic Treatment: Selecting Appropriate Waveform Characteristics.* A Preston; 1984:5–6.
7. Savage B. *Interferential Therapy.* Boston: Faber & Faber; 1984:19.
8. Stillwell K. *Therapeutic Electricity and Ultraviolet Radiation.* 3rd ed. Rehabilitation Medicine Library Baltimore, MD: Williams & Wilkins; 1983:91.

18

Effect of Electrical Stimulation on Nerve and Muscle Tissues

Tsega Andemicael Mehreteab, PT, MS

Physiological Responses

   Action Potential

   Impulse Propagation

   Effectiveness of Electrical Stimuli

Electrophysiologic Tests

Strength-Duration Test

Chronaxie Test

Reaction of Degeneration Test

Key Terms

B oth nerve and muscle cells are excitable. For example, electrical stimulation of a normal peripheral motor nerve elicits a muscle contraction. This chapter reviews the normal physiologic responses of nerve and muscle tissue to electrical stimulation and discusses the use of electrophysiologic tests to determine the integrity of nerve and muscle tissue.

PHYSIOLOGICAL RESPONSES

Action Potential

Electrical stimulation of a normal peripheral motor nerve elicits a muscle contraction. This response involves the excitation and conduction of a nerve impulse. *Excitation* refers to the events leading to the generation of an action potential, and *conduction* refers to the transmission or propagation of the action potential away from the site of stimulation.[1] Both nerve and muscle cells respond to different kinds of stimuli, such as electrical, thermal, mechanical, and chemical stimuli. This excitability of nerve and muscle cells is caused by a change in their transmembrane potential, which is established by the unequal distribution of charged ions between the inside and outside of the semipermeable membrane. The resting potential or the voltage difference between the inside and outside of nerve or skeletal muscle fibers (cells) at rest is between 60 mV and 90 mV, the inside being more negative. Adequate stimulation of a nerve axon or a muscle cell causes an abrupt change of the resting membrane potential, leading to the development of an *action potential* (excitation of the cell).[2]

The action potential depicted in Fig. 18–1 is made up of sequential events. A stimulus initiates a *depolarization phase,* or a reduction of its negative charges, which also represents a reduction of the membrane potential of the cell. When the depolarization or excitation of the membrane reaches its peak, it is followed by a

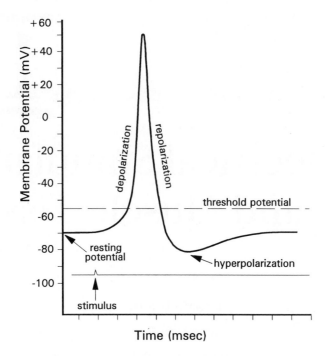

Figure 18–1. Changes in membrane potential during an action potential. A stimulus causes a cell membrane to undergo an action potential. The transmembrane potential is rapidly depolarized. When it reaches its maximum intensity, it dips below the resting potential and becomes even more negative, or hyperpolarized, then returns to its resting potential.

repolarization phase that reestablishes the resting potential. The nerve axon requires sufficient time to recover after one stimulus and before another stimulus can be effective. The repolarization phase includes a *refractory period*, during which the nerve axon either fails to respond to a (absolute refractory period) or requires more intensity (relative refractory period) to respond to a subsequent stimulus. This rest period may range from 0.5 – 1 millisecond.[1] When a nerve-muscle complex is electrically stimulated, the rest period should be at least equal to the refractory period of the nerve so that a subsequent stimuli can be just as effective.

Impulse Propagation

The action potential, or impulse, self-propagates from the site of stimulation in all directions. For example, electrical stimulation of a peripheral motor axon causes the conduction of a nerve impulse from the point of stimulation toward the neuromuscular junction. There, the impulse causes the release of neurochemical transmitters that generate a muscle action potential and elicit muscle contraction. Orthodromic conduction and antidromic conduction are terms used to describe the direction of impulse conduction. When an impulse travels along its normal or physiologic direction, the conduction is referred to as *orthodromic conduction:* for example, a motor axon conducting an impulse from a proximal site of stimulation toward its neuromuscular junction. *Antidromic conduction* occurs when the impulse is conducted in the opposite direction of its normal or physiologic direction: for example, a motor axon conducting an impulse from a distal (peripheral) site of stimulation toward the cell body (proximally).

Effectiveness of Electrical Stimuli

The effectiveness of an electrical stimulus depends on its intensity (amplitude), duration, and speed of rise (rise time).

Intensity. The intensity of a stimulus that is just sufficient to depolarize the cell membrane and cause an action potential is called a *threshold stimulus.* An intensity lower than threshold is called a subliminal or *subthreshold stimulus.* The subthreshold stimulus may cause some changes in the immediate environment of the tissue stimulated, but it does not depolarize the membrane sufficiently to trigger an action potential. Conversely, increasing the amplitude, duration, or both, higher than threshold does not increase the magnitude of the action potential; thus, generation of an action potential follows the "all or none" principle of excitation. Because nerves usually contain many axons with different excitation threshold, thus increasing the stimulus amplitude, they excite the axons with high stimulus threshold in addition to those with low threshold, resulting in a stronger response. Such a response is caused by the recruitment of more axons rather than by an increase in the magnitude of any individual action potentials.

Stimulus duration. In addition to the stimulus amplitude, the duration of the stimulus must be long enough to excite the tissue. The minimum stimulus duration required by a tissue depends on the characteristics of the tissue. For example, nerve tissue is more excitable than muscle tissue and thus requires a shorter duration stimulus than does muscle tissue. Other factors such as the temperature and general condition of the tissue may influence the minimum duration required to excite the tissue. For example, increasing the temperature and local circulation of the tissue may decrease its resistance and thus require a shorter stimulus duration and less intensity.

The quality of neuromuscular response to electrical stimulation also depends on the rate, or frequency, of the stimuli. For example, a low frequency of 1 or 2 stimuli per second will produce a single response referred to as a *twitch contraction.* This is followed by complete relaxation of the contractile elements of the muscle. At higher frequencies, eg, 15 pulses per second, there is not enough time for relaxation and the action potentials begin to summate, giving rise to a partial or incomplete contraction called an unfused tetanus. A *tetanus* is a sustained muscle contraction caused by a rapid succession of stimuli. As shown in Fig. 18–2, at progressively higher frequencies—greater than 30 stimuli per second, for exam-

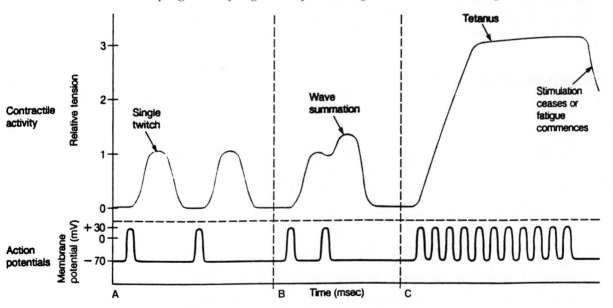

Figure 18–2. Wave summation and tetanus: twitch, partial tetanus, and fused tetanus. **(A)** If a muscle fiber is restimulated after it has relaxed completely, the second twitch is the same magnitude as the first twitch. **(B)** If a muscle fiber is restimulated before it has relaxed completely, the second twitch is added on to the first twitch, resulting in a wave summation and a partially fused muscle contraction or an incomplete tetanus. **(C)** If a muscle fiber is stimulated so rapidly that it has no opportunity to relax between stimuli, a maximal sustained contraction called tetanus occurs. *(Reproduced with permission from* Human Physiology: From Cells to Systems. *Sherwood L. 1989: West Publishing Co.)*

ple—summation of the action potentials is more complete and produces a fused tetanus. It should be noted that higher stimulus frequencies, which produce tetanic muscle contraction and duty cycles with short rest periods, promote muscle fatigue. Therefore, to avoid fatigue, sufficient rest between stimuli should be provided.[3]

Rise time. The third criterion that a stimulus must meet to be effective is a sufficient rise time. Rise time is the time required for the stimulus to reach its maximum intensity or peak amplitude. This characteristic is dependent on the waveform of the stimulus. The rise time of a square waveform is virtually immediate compared with that of an exponential waveform. If the stimulus reaches peak amplitude slowly, nerve tissue accommodates to the passage of such current and fails to respond to it. Accommodation is the rise in the excitation threshold of nerve tissue resulting from a gradually increasing stimulus intensity. Clinically, the phenomenon of accommodation occurs only in nerve tissue, not in muscle tissues.

The three parameters—stimulus amplitude (intensity), duration, and rise time—can be used to measure the response of the tissue to a given stimulus and are useful measurements in electrophysiologic tests. The results of these tests compared with the results from the normal contralateral side may indicate whether the nerve axon is intact or whether the muscle is partially innervated or completely denervated.

ELECTROPHYSIOLOGIC TESTS

Nerve tissue is more excitable than muscle tissue. Thus, normal nerve tissue has a lower threshold than muscle tissue and is expected to respond to stimuli with a lower intensity and shorter duration than is required by muscle tissue. A number of electrophysiologic tests based on this inherent difference in excitability help determine the excitability of nerve and muscle tissues. The following are the most common tests: (1) strength- duration (SD), (2) chronaxie, (3) reaction of degeneration (RD), nerve conduction velocity (NCV), and electromyography (EMG) tests. The nerve conduction velocity and electromyography tests are described in Chapter 20.

Strength Duration Test

The intensity and duration of a stimulus are inversely related. In general, the shorter the duration, the higher the intensity required for excitation. The relationship of intensity and duration is a quantitative measure of the excitability of muscle and nerve tissues. This relationship is demonstrated by the intensity-duration curve, commonly referred to as the *strength-duration* (SD) curve (Fig. 18–3). This curve is obtained by plotting on a graph the stimulus amplitude required to produce a minimally visible contraction of a muscle as the stimulus duration is varied. It should be noted that there is a minimum stimulus duration below which the tissue ceases to respond regardless of the intensity available. Similarly, there is a minimum intensity below which the tissue ceases to respond regardless of the duration available.

In addition to the relative position of the curve, two points on the SD curve, chronaxie and rheobase, should be noted. *Rheobase* is the minimum intensity required to elicit a minimally visible contraction when the duration is infinite. Clinically, duration of 100–300 milliseconds is used. *Chronaxie* is the duration required for a stimulus with twice the rheobase intensity to elicit a minimally visible contraction.

The SD test is a quantitative test because the intensity required to produce minimally visible contractions in response to a stimulus of a given duration is measured and is compared with the intensity on the normal contralateral side. The intensity values obtained for different durations are then plotted on a graph with duration and intensity coordinates (see Fig. 18–3). For example, nerve tissue has a

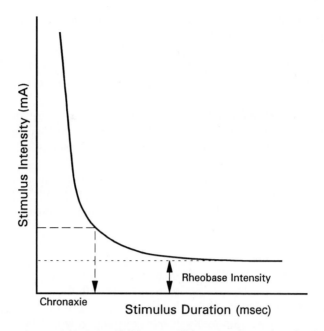

Figure 18–3. Strength/duration (S/D) curve. This curve shows the stimulus amplitude (intensity) required to produce a minimally visible contraction (response) of a muscle as the duration of the stimulus is varied. There is a minimum duration below which the tissue does not respond regardless of the intensity of the stimulus. The rheobase is the minimal intensity of infinite duration that is required to elicit a response. The chronaxie is the duration of a stimulus that is twice the intensity of the rheobase and is required to elicit a response.

considerably lower chronaxie (approximately 0.03 millisecond) than a denervated muscle tissue (approximately 10 milliseconds). A chronaxie greater than 1 millisecond is considered to be abnormal for a nerve and may indicate muscle denervation. The excitatory response of nerve fibers depends on the inherent impedance of the tissue. The large-diameter nerve fibers such as the A and C fibers are excited sooner than smaller-diameter fibers that transmit sensory or noxious stimuli.[4]

Procedure

To conduct the SD test, a direct-current generator with a square waveform and a variable duration (300–0.01 millisecond) is used. An ammeter is used to measure the required intensity. For the test results to be accurate, the test conditions must remain as constant as possible. The body part should be positioned appropriately, and there should be proper lighting so that any changes in response can be observed easily and accurately. The position of the electrode on a given motor point should not be changed as the test proceeds. Ideally, an assistant should be present to record the results. It should be noted that the test has some inconsistencies regarding contractions and possibly some experimental inconsistencies. Such limitations can be minimized by having the same person conduct the tests on the same patient.

The steps listed below should be followed when conducting the SD test:

1. Explain the test and what to expect to the patient. Position the patient in a comfortable position and prepare an SD or chronaximeter for testing.
2. The body part to be tested should be supported in a semistretched position. The area should be well lit so that any response can be seen easily.
3. Set the instrument on automatic interruption mode so that stimulation occurs every 0.5 to 2 seconds.
4. Set the duration on 100–300 milliseconds. 100 msec may be more comfortable for some patients.
5. For the active, stimulating electrode, use a handheld stimulator with an

extremely small electrode tip. Place a dispersive pad on an appropriate area proximal to the area to be stimulated.

6. Locate a motor point of a muscle innervated by the peripheral nerve to be tested. At least one proximal and one distal muscle innervated by that nerve should be tested and compared with the normal contralateral side, established normal values, or both.

7. To insure consistent results after locating the motor point, decrease the intensity until observable contractions disappear and then increase the intensity gradually until a minimally visible contraction is noted. Record the intensity used.

8. Sequentially decrease the duration from 100 to 0.01 millisecond. For example, set the duration at 100, 50, 30, 20, 10, 5, 3, 2, 1, 0.5, 0.2, 0.1, 0.05, and .01 milliseconds. For each duration, record the intensity used to produce the minimally visible contraction.

9. On a special SD log paper, plot the intensity versus the duration used. Connect the points on the graph to form a curve.

10. Compare the results of proximal versus distal muscles innervated by the peripheral nerve. Also, compare the results with those of the normal side.

11. On the SD curve, identify the rheobase: the minimum stimulus amplitude required to elicit a minimally visible contraction when the stimulus duration is infinite (100–300 milliseconds).

12. On the SD curve, identify the chronaxie: the stimulus duration required to produce the minimally visible contraction when the stimulus intensity is twice that of the rheobase.

Interpretation

As shown in Fig. 18–4, the SD curve of a denervated muscle requires a higher intensity for a given duration than does an innervated muscle. Therefore, the SD curve of a denervated muscle is shifted up and to the right on the SD coordinate. The relative position of the SD curve of the tested nerve and the progress or lack of

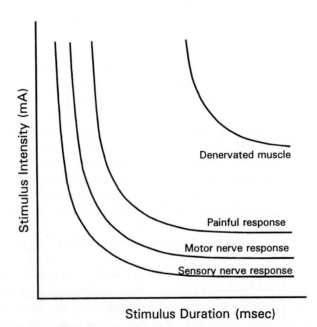

Figure 18–4. Strength/duration (S/D) curves comparing the intensity and duration of stimuli necessary to elicit a response from different tissues. The relative position of the curves indicates that a normal sensory nerve responds more quickly than a motor nerve does and requires a lower stimulus amplitude and duration. Sensory nerve fibers that transmit pain or noxious stimuli require a higher amplitude and a longer duration. Denervated muscle, although an excitable tissue, requires a stimulus of higher amplitude and longer duration than does a normally innervated muscle.

progress in subsequent tests are useful to document the status of the nerve-muscle complex and to arrive at a prognosis for a given condition. In addition, the shape of the SD curve may indicate partial denervation or partial innervation in subsequent tests. For example, such curves may be discontinuous or have a bend or kink on them.

Chronaxie Test

The chronaxie test is a quick means of obtaining a chronaxie value without having to test for every duration and plot a complete graph. Note that the procedures for setting up the test are the same as those for SD test:

1. Explain the test and what to expect to the patient. Position patient in a comfortable position. Prepare an SD or chronaximeter for testing.
2. The body part to be tested should be supported in a semistretched position. The area should be well lit so that any response can be seen easily.
3. Set the instrument on automatic interruption mode so that stimulation occurs every 0.5 to 2 seconds.
4. Set the duration on 100–300 milliseconds; 100 milliseconds may be more comfortable for some patients.
5. For the active, stimulating electrode, use a handheld stimulator with an extremely small electrode tip. Place a dispersive pad on an appropriate area proximal to the area to be stimulated.
6. Locate a motor point of a muscle innervated by the peripheral nerve to be tested. At least one proximal and one distal muscle innervated by that nerve should be tested and compared with the normal contralateral side, established normal values, or both.
7. To insure consistent results after locating the motor point, decrease the intensity until observable contractions disappear, then increase the intensity gradually until a minimally visible contraction is noted. Record the intensity used.
8. Record the rheobase and turn the duration to zero.
9. Set the instrument at double (2x) the rheobase intensity.
10. Gradually increase the duration until the minimally visible contraction is reproduced. This duration at double the rheobase intensity is the chronaxie value.
11. Compare the obtained value with normal established chronaxie values or with the chronaxie of the normal contralateral side.

Reaction of Degeneration Test

The reaction of degeneration test is a qualitative test based on a characteristic difference between the response of nerve and muscle tissues to a long-or short-duration electrical stimulus. This test is also called the faradic/galvanic test. To conduct the test, an electric generator that can produce both monophasic long-duration and biphasic short-duration pulses is used. To minimize the spread of current through the area through volume conduction, a handheld electrode with a small area of stimulation is used. For long-duration stimuli, the test uses interrupted monophasic pulses with pulse durations of 100 milliseconds that are repeated approximately once a second. For short-duration stimuli, the test uses biphasic pulses with a duration of less than 1 millisecond that are applied at a frequency higher than 120 Hz. Such stimuli will elicit a tetanic contraction of a normally innervated muscle. The quality of muscle contraction in response to the short-versus long-duration stimuli is used to characterize the response as twitch versus tetanic, brisk versus sluggish, or diminished contractions. The presence or absence of a response also is indicative of the condition of the tissue. Table 18–1 depicts the possible responses to short- versus long-duration stimuli. The possible results of a RD test are normal reaction, partial reaction, complete reaction, or absolute reaction.

TABLE 18–1. REACTION OF DEGENERATION TEST

Reaction	Stimuli of Short Duration	Stimuli of Long Duration
Normal		
Nerve	Tetanic contraction	Brisk twitch contraction
Muscle	Tetanic contraction	Brisk twitch contraction
Partial		
Nerve	Diminished or partial	Diminished or partial individual contraction
Muscle	tetanic contraction	Sluggish contraction
Full		
Nerve	No contraction	No contraction
Muscle	No contraction	Sluggish contraction
Absolute		
Nerve	No contraction	No contraction
Muscle	No contraction	No contraction

Procedure

Locate a motor point of a muscle innervated by the peripheral nerve to be tested. At least one proximal and one distal muscle innervated by that nerve should be tested and compared with the normal contralateral side. Begin the test on the normal side to establish a baseline.

Test for response to pulses of short duration. The steps listed below should be followed when conducting this test:

1. Explain the test and what to expect to the patient. Position the patient in a comfortable position.
2. The body part to be tested should be supported in a semistretched position. The area should be well lit so that any response can be seen easily.
3. Select an electric generator that can produce both monophasic long-duration and biphasic short-duration pulses.
4. Test with the short-duration stimuli first. Set the generator on tetanizing current: that is, at a stimulus frequency higher than 120 Hz and a stimulus duration less than 1 millisecond.
5. Place a dispersive electrode over an appropriate area proximal to the area to be stimulated. A large smooth area such as the upper back or shoulder for the upper extremity tests and the lower back or buttocks area for the lower extremity test is recommended. Place the electrodes on the same side of the body to avoid stimulation across the heart.
6. For the active, stimulating electrode, use a handheld electrode equipped with an extremely small tip equipped with a "make-or-break" switch for manual interruption of the stimulus output.
7. Locate and stimulate the motor point of the muscle to be tested. If the muscle responds, increase the intensity to obtain a strong contraction.
8. Note and record the quality of the muscle contraction in response to the short-duration tetanizing current. Short-duration tetanizing stimuli elicit a tetanic contraction of a normally innervated muscle. Decrease the intensity back to zero.
9. **Do not remove** the stimulating electrode from the motor point. For consistent results, the same motor point should be used for the next segment of the test.

Test for response to pulses of long duration. The steps listed below should be followed when conducting this test.

1. Maintain the same position of the stimulating electrode over the motor point tested above.
2. Change to the long-duration stimulus current of the generator. Set the duration on 500 milliseconds. Set the instrument on the automatic interrup-

tion mode so that the stimulus output occurs once each second. If an automatic setting is not available, interrupt the current manually every 500 milliseconds with the "make-or-break" switch on the stimulating electrode.

3. Select the cathode for the stimulating (active) electrode and the anode for the dispersive electrode.
4. Stimulate the motor point of the muscle to be tested, and if the muscle responds, increase the intensity to get a strong brisk twitch contraction.
5. Note and record the quality of the muscle contraction in response to the long-duration stimulus. If the muscle is normally innervated, a brisk twitch contraction is elicited. Any variation of the observed response should be noted and compared with those in Table 18–1.
6. Decrease the stimulus output to zero intensity.
7. Repeat these procedures on the involved side.

■ KEY TERMS

excitation	threshold stimulus
conduction	subthreshold stimulus
action potential	twitch contraction
depolarization phase	tetanus
repolarization phase	strength/duration (S/D) curve
refractory period	rheobase
orthodromic conduction	chronaxie
antidromic conduction	

REFERENCES

1. Sherwood LL: *Human Physiology from Cells to Systems.* St. Paul, MN: West Publishing; 1989.
2. Nelson RM, Currier DP: *Clinical Electrotherapy.* Norwalk, CT: Appleton & Lange; 1991.
3. Benton LA, Baker LL, Bocoman BR, et al: *Functional Electrical Stimulation: A Practical Guide.* Downey, CA: Rancho Los Amigos Rehab Engineering Center, Rancho Los Amigos Hospital; 1981.
4. Li CL, Bak A: Excitability characteristics of the A- and C-fibers in peripheral nerve. *Exp Neural.* 1976; 50:67.

19

Clinical Uses of Electrical Stimulation

Tsega Andemicael Mehreteab, PT, MS

Muscle Reeducation and Facilitation

Maintenance of Muscle Integrity

Spasticity

  Direct Stimulation of Spastic Muscles

  Stimulation of Antagonistic Muscles

  Reciprocal Stimulation of Spastic and Antagonistic Muscles

Muscle Holding or Spasm

  Intermittent Stimulation

  High-Frequency Stimulation

Denervated Muscles

Edema

Tissue Repair (Wound Healing)

  Low-Amplitude Continuous Unidirectional Stimulation

  Monophasic Short-Duration Stimulation with High-Voltage Pulsed Current

Electrical stimulation is used as an adjunct in the management of many disorders, including neuromuscular, musculoskeletal, vascular, and soft-tissue injuries. This chapter reviews the use of therapeutic electricity to reeducate and facilitate muscles, such as in idiopathic scoliosis; maintain muscle integrity; reduce spasticity, muscle holding, and edema; and heal tissue and bone. The use of therapeutic electricity for these disorders is based on empirical and limited scientific research.

MUSCLE REEDUCATION AND FACILITATION

Neuromuscular electrical stimulation of an area with deficits increases a patient's awareness of contractile motions by providing proprioceptive, kinesthetic, and sensory input. This modality can be used in the management of upper motor neuron dysfunctions such as spasticity, peripheral nervous system injuries such as Bell's palsy, muscle imbalance such as in idiopathic scoliosis; and other conditions that cause pain, weakness, and immobility. The goals of treatment are to reeducate a muscle toward normal function and to facilitate motion. A number of studies have demonstrated that electrical stimulation can be used to facilitate muscle action during functional training involving gait and the upper extremities.[1-3] Others have used electrical stimulation in conjunction with biofeedback and report that it is an effective modality in training paretic muscle.[4-6]

In reeducation and facilitation of muscles, electrical stimulation is used as a guide to improve the patient's proprioceptive and visual sense of the motions and activities being facilitated. Because this requires concentration and effort, prolonged sessions and overstimulation should be avoided to prevent either mental or physical fatigue. Patients should be encouraged to coordinate their efforts for voluntary movements with the stimuli. As soon as progress is noted, electrical stimulation should be gradually withdrawn.

Before initiating the treatment:

1. Explain to the patient the procedure to be performed.
2. Place the patient in a comfortable position.
3. Clean all body parts to be treated with soap and water or alcohol to reduce skin impedance.
4. Place the muscle or muscle groups in a supported position.
5. Use the gravity assisted or eliminated position.

Then place bipolar electrodes of one or more channels over the large muscles or muscle groups, and select the following stimulus parameters:

• Waveform: symmetrical or asymmetrical biphasic pulses with a duration of 200–500 microseconds.
• Pulse rate: greater than 60 pps biphasic pulses to produce tetanic muscle contractions.
• Stimulus amplitude: amplitude adjusted to maximum tolerable contraction.
• Duty cycle: a 1:1 cycle to produce rhythmical muscle contractions.
• Duration of treatment: approximately 15 minutes (the time may vary, depending on the patient's tolerance and the effectiveness of the session).

In the treatment of idiopathic scoliosis, the procedure for facilitation and strengthening of weak muscles by electrical stimulation differs from those stated above. Electrical stimulation is used to stimulate the overstretched, weakened muscles on the convex side of the curve.[7-9] Electrodes are placed over the muscles at the apex of the curve, and the muscles are stimulated for 7–8 hours during sleep. According to Eckerson and Axelgaard,[10] candidates for this procedure are carefully screened using the following selection criteria: (1) the idiopathic curve must measure anywhere from 20° to 40° using the Cobb method, (2) the child must have at least one more year of spinal growth, and (3) the child must be a compliant, cooperative individual with a stable personality who can tolerate electrical stimulation. The specific procedure listed below is based on the protocol developed by Eckerson and Axelgaard.[10]

Before initiating the treatment:

1. Explain to the patient the procedure to be performed, and instruct a family member to help patient with the daily application of the treatment at home.
2. Position the patient in a comfortable position.
3. Clean the body part to be treated with soap and water or alcohol.

Then place bipolar or quadripolar electrodes over the overstretched and weakened muscles on the concave side of the curve, and select the following stimulus parameters:

• Waveform: rectangular monophasic waveform with 220-microsecond output from a portable batter-operated dual-channel stimulator.
• Pulse rate: 25 pps
• Stimulus amplitude: 50 to 70 mA.

- Duty cycle: a 1:1 ratio: for example, a cycle with 6 seconds on and 6 seconds off.
- Duration of treatment: gradually increased until patient tolerates 8 hours of stimulation.

MAINTENANCE OF MUSCLE INTEGRITY

Studies of healthy subjects indicate that electrical stimulation increases muscle strength; however, electrical stimulation does not appear to be superior to voluntary training.[11–15] On the basis of these and other studies, electrical stimulation is used when peripheral nerve innervation is intact but normal voluntary motion is weak or lacking as a result of atrophy after prolonged casting, pain, or surgery.

Well-documented clinical studies demonstrate that electrical stimulation is effective in retarding disuse atrophy, as measured by limb girth measurements and the maximum voluntary isometric torque. Electrical stimulation promotes early active range of motion in postsurgical and cast-immobilized limbs.[16–19] For example, Morrissey et al.[20] compared the use of electrical stimulation of the quadriceps of immobilized patients following anterior cruciate ligament reconstruction with unexercised patients. They used 350-microsecond, monophasic pulsed current at 50 pps to stimulate the quadriceps. Their results showed a less pronounced decrease in thigh circumference and maximum voluntary isometric torque in the immobilized group than in the unexercised group. In another study, an alternating current of 2500 Hz, delivering 50 bursts per second, was used to stimulate the quadriceps and hamstrings of patients following anterior cruciate ligament reconstruction. The results indicated increase in the maximum voluntary isometric torque of knee extension and flexion.[21]

For greater effect, the authors recommend that the patient coordinate his or her voluntary activity with the stimulation. The goals of treatment in such cases are to maintain muscle integrity, retard disuse atrophy, and disrupt the "pain-guarding cycle" so that an active exercise and rehabilitation program can begin as early as possible. It should be noted that the parameters used in studies in this area vary significantly. For example, current amplitudes vary from 33% to 80% of the maximum voluntary isometric torque. Pulse duration has varied from 20–300 microseconds, and the treatment has been given 3 to 5 days per week for 3 to 5 weeks. Further clinical research is needed to determine the specific parameters of stimulation.

Before initiating the treatment:

1. Explain to the patient the procedure to be performed,
2. Position the patient in a comfortable position,
3. Clean all body parts to be treated with soap and water or alcohol to decrease skin impedance.
4. Place the muscle or muscle groups in a semistretched and supported position.
5. Use the gravity-assisted or gravity-eliminated position for weak muscles.

Then place the electrodes over the area to be treated: monopolar electrodes for small muscles such as those of the face, hand, and foot; bipolar electrodes over the major muscles or muscle groups involved; or reciprocal stimulation of muscle groups when indicated. Finally, select the following stimulus parameters:

- Waveform: 20–300 microsecond, monophasic or biphasic waveforms or 2500 Hz delivered in 50 bursts per second.
- Pulse rate: greater than 40 pps for monophasic or biphasic pulses to produce tetanic muscle contraction.
- Stimulus amplitude: high enough to produce maximum tolerable muscle contractions.

- Modulation: amplitude or frequency modulated for a gradual and smooth muscle contraction.
- Duty cycle: A 1:5 cycle should be used to allow for sufficient rest between stimulations and avoid muscle fatigue.
- Duration of treatment: can vary in length, depending on the patient's training, activity level, condition, and tolerance.

The patient should be encouraged to perform voluntary contractions of the muscles involved while the stimulus is on.

SPASTICITY

Spasticity resulting from a lesion or dysfunction in the central nervous system is a major concern for the physical therapist. Some studies have indicated that electrical stimulation in conjunction with other exercise and training programs can be an effective treatment tool to overcome spasticity. Short-term effects of treatment and lack of carry-over are common to all such studies. Clinicians who advocate the use of electrical stimulation point out that relief of spasticity, even for a short period, allows the patient to experience a decrease in abnormal tone and possibly an increase in normal volitional movement. Functional training also can be provided during this time.

Varying rationales have been posed to explain the mechanism responsible for reducing spasticity by electrical stimulation. Walker et al.[22] demonstrated that a 20 pps spike waveform stimulation of the radial, median, and saphenous nerves, applied for 1 hour twice a day for 1 week, suppressed clonus via spinal reflexes. The effect was reported to have lasted approximately 3 hours. Stimulation of the spastic muscles resulted in a generalized decrease of abnormal tone and the flexion-reflex response. One possible mechanism involved in reducing spasticity is sensory habituation of cutaneous reflexes. High-frequency stimulation of spastic muscles to produce tetanic muscle contraction and an amplitude adjusted to produce the maximum tolerable contraction has also been shown to reduce spasticity in patients with spinal cord injuries.[23–25] The reduction in tone lasted approximately 30 minutes after stimulation. The two possible rationales for the decrease in tone may be fatigue following the barrage of electrical stimulation of the same motor neurons and antidromic activation of the axon of an alpha motor neuron. In the latter case, the antidromic stimulation of the alpha motor neuron activates the motor unit and, through recurrent collaterals, excites a pool of Renshaw cells. In turn, the Renshaw cells inhibit the alpha motor neurons of the activated pool and the motor neurons of synergistic muscles. An in-depth discussion of motor neurons and the role of Renshaw cells can be found elsewhere.[26]

Electrical stimulation of the antagonist muscle has been associated with concomitant inhibition of the spastic agonist muscle. Baker et al[6] reported a reduction of flexor spasticity in hemiplegic patients following bipolar stimulation of wrist and finger extensors. They used a monophasic stimulus of 200 microseconds duration at a rate of 33 pps, with a 7 seconds on–10 seconds off duty cycle and an amplitude high enough to produce a sustained isotonic muscle contraction through the full range of motion. Alfieri[27] demonstrated a reduction in spasticity lasting from 10–15 minutes to 2 hours in 96 hemiplegic patients when muscles antagonistic to those with spasticity were stimulated.

Electrical stimulation of spastic muscles and their antagonists with a rhythmical reciprocal pattern of stimulation, activating agonist and antagonists alternately, has effectively reduced spasticity. Vodovnic et al[28] reported a reduction in the hypertonicity of knee flexors and extensors of patients with spinal cord injuries following a reciprocal pattern of bipolar stimulation of quadriceps and hamstrings. The stimulus used was asymmetrical biphasic pulses of 300 microseconds duration at a rate of 30 pps and 100 mA current amplitude. Stimulation lasted for 30 minutes.

Three methods of electrical stimulation are used to decrease spasticity: (1) direct stimulation of the spastic muscles, (2) stimulation of muscles antagonistic to the spastic muscles, and (3) reciprocal stimulation of spastic muscles and their antagonists. The following procedures should be used in the initial session, and parameters appropriate to the individual should be adjusted in subsequent sessions:

Direct Stimulation of Spastic Muscles

Before initiating the treatment:

1. Explain to the patient the procedure to be performed.
2. Place the patient in a comfortable position.
3. Clean all body parts to be treated with soap and water or alcohol to decrease skin impedance.
4. Place the muscle or muscle groups in a supported position.
5. Use the gravity-assisted or gravity-eliminated position.

Then place bipolar electrodes of one or more channels over the spastic muscles or muscle groups and select the following stimulus parameters:

- Waveform: symmetrical or asymmetrical biphasic pulses with 200–500 microseconds duration.
- Pulse rate: greater than 60 pps biphasic pulses to produce tetanic muscle contraction.
- Stimulus amplitude: amplitude adjusted to maximum tolerable contraction.
- Duty cycle: a 1:1 cycle to produce rhythmical muscle contraction.
- Duration of treatment: approximately 15 minutes, but this may vary in length depending on the patient's tolerance and the effectiveness of the session.

Stimulation of Antagonistic Muscles

Before initiating the treatment, follow procedures 1 through 5 above. Then place bipolar electrodes of one or more channels on the muscles antagonistic to the spastic muscles and select the following stimulus parameters:

- Waveform: monophasic or biphasic pulses with a 200–500 microsecond duration.
- Pulse rate: 30–50 pps to produce tetanic muscle contraction.
- Stimulus amplitude: amplitude adjusted to produce tolerable muscle contractions.
- Duty cycle: a 1:1 to 1:5 cycle to produce rhythmical muscle contraction.
- Duration of treatment: approximately 15 to 20 minutes. To avoid fatigue, the duration may vary in length, depending on the patient's tolerance and the effectiveness of the session.

Reciprocal Stimulation of Spastic and Antagonistic Muscles

Before initiating the treatment, follow procedures 1–5 above and prepare two circuits for the rhythmical and reciprocal stimulation of the muscle groups involved. Then place bipolar electrodes over the spastic muscles and their corresponding antagonistic muscles and select the following stimulus parameters:

- Waveform: monophasic or biphasic pulses with duration of 300 microseconds.
- Pulse rate: 30 pps to produce tetanic muscle contraction.
- Stimulus amplitude: adjusted to produce tolerable muscle contractions.
- Duty cycle: 5 seconds on and 5 seconds off to produce rhythmical, reciprocal muscle contractions.

- Duration of treatment: approximately 15 to 20 minutes. To avoid fatigue, the duration may vary in length, depending on the patient's tolerance and the effectiveness of the session.

MUSCLE HOLDING OR SPASM

Trauma, pain, and muscle weakness may lead to irritation and pain; this condition is commonly referred to as muscle spasm or muscle-holding state (see Chapter 4). The cause and mechanism of this condition is not clearly understood. The possible causes include microtrauma, accumulation of metabolic irritants, and pain. Anxiety and tension seem to increase the occurrence or severity of this condition. Regardless of the original cause, pain and discomfort result in more pain and protective muscle holding; thus, a vicious cycle of "pain-spasm-pain" is established. Electrical stimulation, by increasing the circulation in large vessels[29,30] and enhancing nutrition, may be an effective means of disrupting this cycle and thus facilitating normal function. The goals of treatment are to relieve pain, promote relaxation of the involved muscles, and restore normal motion to the area of pain.

There are two methods for treating muscle spasm with electrical stimulation: (1) intermittent electrical stimulation and (2) high-frequency stimulation to elicit a sustained and continuous contraction of the muscles in spasm.

Intermittent Stimulation

Intermittent electrical stimulation causes alternating muscle contraction and relaxation. Such rhythmic activation of the muscles causes an increase in the local circulation, helps remove metabolic irritants from the area, and provides a mechanical stimulation to muscle fibers.

Before initiating the treatment:

1. Explain to the patient the procedure to be performed.
2. Place the patient in a comfortable position.
3. Clean all body parts with soap and water or alcohol to reduce skin impedance.
4. Place the muscle or muscle groups in a supported and relaxed position.

Then prepare two circuits for the rhythmical, reciprocal, or intermittent stimulation of the muscle groups involved. Place bipolar electrodes over the muscles in spasm, and select the following stimulus parameters:

- Waveform: biphasic pulses with a duration of 200–300 microseconds.
- Pulse rate: 30–50 pps to produce tetanic muscle contraction.
- Modulation: surged at a moderate rate.
- Stimulus amplitude: high enough to produce a comfortable muscle contraction.
- Duty cycle: a 1:3 cycle with 5 seconds on and 15 seconds off to produce an intermittent muscle contraction.
- Duration of treatment: approximately 15 to 20 minutes. Avoid fatigue. The duration may vary in length, depending on the patient's tolerance and the effectiveness of the session.

High-Frequency Stimulation

High-frequency stimulation is used to elicit sustained and continuous muscle contractions of the muscles in spasm. The goal is to induce fatigue in the muscle in spasm. The patient's tolerance and the predisposition of the muscle to local ischemia should be carefully assessed before this approach is used. Because sustained muscle contractions may impede normal blood flow to the area, lower stimulating frequencies should be used.

Before initiating the treatment, follow procedures 1–4 above. Then place bipolar electrodes over the muscles in spasm (two circuits can be used to stimulate large areas) and select the following stimulus parameters:

- Waveform: monophasic or biphasic pulses with a duration of 200–300 microseconds.
- Pulse rate: greater than 60 pps to produce tetanic muscle contraction.
- Modulation: continuous
- Stimulus amplitude: adjusted to produce maximal, tolerable muscle contractions.
- Duration of treatment: approximately 15 to 20 minutes. (the time may vary, depending on the patient's tolerance and the effectiveness of the session).

DENERVATED MUSCLES

Electrical stimulation with monophasic long-duration pulses such as interrupted direct current may be beneficial by producing muscle contraction and increasing circulation and nutrition to a denervated muscle. These effects may help slow down the changes resulting from the lack of physical activity of the denervated muscles. Studies in animal models have indicated that electrical stimulation of denervated muscles retards atrophy.[31–33] Other studies have shown that electrical stimulation of denervated muscles may actually interfere with peripheral nerve regeneration.[34–36] The controversy over the benefits and disadvantages of this approach are supported by numerous studies. (An in-depth review of this topic appears elsewhere.[37]) In light of the controversial results of the studies in this area and the possible disadvantage of electrical stimulation in denervated muscles, the physical therapist's primary goal of maintaining joint mobility and function in patients with peripheral nerve injury resulting in denervation can be accomplished by other therapeutic approaches such as therapeutic exercise and positioning.

EDEMA

Trauma may cause an excessive amount of body fluids to accumulate in the interstitial spaces. Congestion of body fluids also may occur because of compromised peripheral vascular function such as venous insufficiency. Muscle contractions during routine daily activities such as walking provide pumping action, which aids venous return. Interference with the pumping action of muscles can occur as a result of trauma; decreased activity, as in prolonged bed rest; or weakness, pain, or other neuromuscular problems. Electrical stimulation of these muscles may improve the pumping action and thus improve circulation to the area.

Before initiating the treatment:

1. Explain to the patient the procedure to be performed.
2. Place the patient in a comfortable position.
3. Measure the extent of the edema by taking girth or volumetric measurements before and after treatment to document the progress in reducing the edema.
4. Clean all body parts with soap and water or alcohol to reduce skin impedance.
5. Elevate the body part so that drainage of fluid is aided by gravity.

Then place bipolar electrodes of one or more channels over the major muscle groups for reciprocal contraction and relaxation of the agonist-antagonist muscles in the vicinity of the edema or for intermittent stimulation of muscles proximal and distal to the edematous area. Finally, select the following stimulus parameters:

- Waveform: monophasic high-voltage pulsed current or symmetrical or asymmetrical biphasic pulses with a duration of 200–500 microseconds
- Pulse rate: greater than 60 pps to produce tetanic muscle contraction.
- Modulation: reciprocal or intermittent stimulation of major muscle groups to achieve the desired pumping action,
- Stimulus amplitude: adjusted to produce maximum tolerable contraction.
- Duty cycle: a 1:1 cycle should allow time for adequate ejection and filling of the blood vessels.
- Duration of treatment: approximately 20–30 minutes (this time may vary, depending on the patient's tolerance of the patient and the effectiveness of the session).

TISSUE REPAIR (WOUND HEALING)

Electrical stimulation at a wound site has been claimed to accelerate and enhance healing by retarding bacterial growth, increasing local circulation, or enhancing the natural process of tissue repair. In vitro and in vivo studies have supported the bactericidal effects of electrical stimulation. In vitro electrical stimulation of *Staphylococcus aureus*[38] and *Escherichia coli*[39] with continuous low-intensity direct current have been shown to have bactericidal effect either by retarding or inhibiting bacterial growth. Furthermore, Rowley et al[40] stimulated ischemic skin ulcers of humans with low-intensity direct current (200–1000 uA) using the negative electrode and found that the stimulation retarded the growth of *Pseudomonas aerguinosa*. The bacterial count in their study either decreased or remained stable, whereas the count for the control group increased. Kincaid and Lavoie[41] reported that the growth of three species of bacteria was inhibited by stimulation with high-voltage monophasic pulses.

The precise mechanism for the bactericidal effect is not clearly understood. One plausible rationale is the depletion of substrates as a result of continued cell membrane excitability as the microorganism attempts to maintain homeostasis. Another plausible rationale is that the electrical fields alter the internal processes of the microorganism and thus cause its death.[42] These mechanisms may work together or separately. For the bactericidal effect, a negative electrical field and low-amplitude current are used.

In addition to its bactericidal effect, electrical stimulation may accelerate tissue healing by promoting the natural healing process. This process includes the establishment of a difference in potential between the wound area and the surrounding healthy tissue. The difference in potential at the wound site, commonly called "injury potential" initially becomes positive 24 to 48 hours after the injury and becomes negative 8 or 9 days after the injury. As the wound heals, the difference in potential gradually returns to baseline.[43,44] According to this theory, electrical stimulation with the positive field can be used to enhance the natural process of tissue recovery and to promote tissue healing.

The healing process of wounds also includes the formation and migration of epithelial cells, the activation of phagocytes, an increase in the number of polymorphonuclear leukocytes and lymphocytes, and an increase in the synthesis of fibroblast and collagen. Electrical stimulation, especially at the positive electrode, has been shown to increase the number of polymorphonuclear leukoctyes, increase collagen synthesis, and accelerate wound epithelialization.[45] Clinicians generally agree that the positive electrical field is more effective for tissue healing and that the negative electrical field has a greater bactericidal effect. The average rate of wound healing is approximately 1 mm per day. As indicated in these studies, the polarity of electrodes over the wound site should be changed when the wound-healing plateau is reached.

In addition to the use of continuous unidirectional current, short-duration monophasic pulses, such as the stimulus output of the high-voltage pulsed current, have been shown to promote wound healing in humans.[46] According to the results of these and other similar studies, electrical stimulation can be used as an adjunct in the management of wounds. One should remember, however, that standard parameters and guidelines have not been established for electrical stimulation used for wound healing. Further clinical research is needed to clarify and establish criteria for the treatment of various types of ulcers and wounds.

In the wound healing procedure, the wound is cleaned and debrided, the wound area is packed loosely with sterile saline- saturated gauze, and an electrode is secured over the area. The positive electrode is used for tissue healing. If a bacterial infection is evident, the negative electrode is used first until the infection clears up, then followed by positive electrode stimulation for tissue healing. To avoid spot burns and discomfort, electrode packs should be cut to fit the size and contour of the wound. Two types of stimuli can be used for this procedure: (1) low amplitude continuous unidirectional current and (2) monophasic short-duration pulses of high-voltage pulsed current. In addition, neuromuscular stimulation in the vicinity of the wound may promote healing by enhancing the circulation and nutrition to the area. In this case, the stimulating electrodes should be placed away from the wound site.

Low-Amplitude Continuous Unidirectional Stimulation

Before initiating the treatment:

1. Obtain a recent culture of the wound.
2. Explain to the patient the procedure to be performed.
3. Place the patient in a comfortable position.
4. Measure the size and depth of the wound or photograph the wound site before and periodically after treatment to document progress.
5. Clean and debride the wound site before packing it with sterile saline-saturated gauze.
6. Place the anode over the gauze-packed wound site. If a wound culture indicates bacterial infection, apply the cathode over the wound site until the infection clears up. Continue stimulation with the anode until tissue heals.
7. Clean the dispersive electrode site well with soap and water or alcohol and place a dispersive pad over a convenient, large body surface such as the back or shoulder.

Select the following stimulus parameters:

- Waveform: continuous unidirectional current.
- Stimulus amplitude: low amplitude of 200 to 1000 μA.
- Duration of treatment: 1–2 hours several times a day.

Monophasic Short-Duration Stimulation with High-Voltage Pulsed Current

Before initiating the treatment, follow instructions 1–7 above. Then place the monopolar electrodes of the stimulator over the gauze-packed wound site and place a dispersive pad over a convenient, large body surface such as the back or shoulder. Select the following stimulus parameters:

- Waveform: monophasic
- Phase duration: 20–100 microseconds.
- Pulse rate: 80–105 pps.
- Modulation: continuous pulses
- Stimulus amplitude: subthreshold level of motor stimulation. (If the wound is in a muscular area, increase the amplitude until a minimally visible muscle contraction is elicited, then turn down the amplitude to sub-

threshold level. Note that the wound is devoid of skin and its impedance is lower than the surrounding tissues.)

• Duration of treatment: 30–60 minutes a day until the wound heals.

REFERENCES

1. Uros Bogataj, Nusa Gros, et al: Restoration of gait during two to three weeks of therapy with multi-channel electrical stimulation. *Phys Ther.* 1989; 69:319–327.
2. Crastam B, Larson E, Previc T: Improvement of gait following functional electrical stimulation. *Scand J Rehabil. Med.* 1977; 9:7–13.
3. Parker K, Baumgarten J: Upper extremity control in Rancho Los Amigos Rehab Engineering Downey, Ca *Annual Report of Progress* pg 4, 1981.
4. Winchester P, Montgomery J, et al: Effect of feedback stimulation training and cyclical electrical stimulation on knee extension in hemiplegic patients. *Phys Ther.* 1983; 63:1096–1103.
5. Bowman B, Baker L, Waters R: Positional feedback and electrical stimulation: an automated treatment for the hemiplegic wrist. *Arch Phys Med Rehabil.* 1979; 60:497–502.
6. Baker LL, Yeh C, et al: Electrical stimulation of wrist and fingers for hemiplegic patients. *Phys Ther.* 1979; 59:1495–1499.
7. Freidman HG, et al: Electrical stimulation for scoliosis. *Am Fam Physician.* 1982; 24:155–160.
8. Axelgaard J, Brown JC: Lateral electrical surface stimulation for the treatment of progressive idiopathic scoliosis. *Spine.* 1983; 8:242–260.
9. Grimfby G, Nordwall A, et al: Changes in histochemical profile of muscle after long-term electrical stimulation in patients with idiopathic scoliosis. *Scand J Rehabil Med.* 1985; 17:191–196.
10. Eckerson LF, Axelgaard J: Lateral electrical surface stimulation as an alternative to bracing in the treatment of idiopathic scoliosis. *Phys Ther.* 1984; 64:483–490.
11. Currier DP, Mann R: Muscular strength development by electrical stimulation in healthy individuals. *Phys Ther.* 1983; 63:915–921.
12. Wolf S, Gideon B, et al. The effect of muscle stimulation during resistive training on performance parameters. *Am J Sports Med.* 1986; 14:18–23.
13. Selkowitz DM: Improvement in isometric strength of the quadriceps femoris muscle after training with electrical stimulation. *Phys Ther.* 1985; 65:186–196.
14. Laughmann RK, Youdas JW, Garrett TR: Strength changes in the normal quadriceps femoris muscle as a result of electrical stimulation. *Phys Ther.* 1983; 63:494–499.
15. McMiken DF, Todd-Smith M, Thompson C: Strengthening of human quadriceps muscles by cutaneous electrical stimulation. *Scand J Rehabil Med.* 1983; 15:25–28.
16. Knight KL: Electrical muscle stimulation during immobilization. *Phys Sport ed.* 1980; 8:147.
17. Eriksson E, Haggmark T: Comparison of isometric muscle training in the recovery after major knee ligament surjery. *Am J Sports Med.* 1979; 7:169–171.
18. Godfrey CM, Jayawardena H, et al. Comparison of electro-stimulation and isometric exercise in strengthening the quadriceps muscle. Physiother. Cana. 1979; 31:265–267.
19. Gould N, Donnermeyer D, et al. Transcutaneous muscle stimulation to retard disuse atrophy after open menisectomy. *Clin Orthop Rel Res.* 1983; 178:190–197.
20. Morrissey MC, Brewster CE, et al. The effect of electrical stimulation on the quadriceps during post operative knee immobilization. *Am J Sports Med.* 1985; 13:40–45.
21. Delito A, Rose SJ, et al: Electrical versus voluntary exercise in strengthening the thigh musculature in patients after anterior cruciate ligament surgery. *Phys Ther.* 1988; 68:660–663.
22. Walker JB: Modulation of spasticity a prolonged suppression of spinal reflex by electrical stimulation. *Science.* 1982; 216:203–204.
23. Lee WJ, McGovern JP, Duval EN: Continuous tetanizing currents for relief of spasm. *Arch Phys Med.* 1950; 31:766–771.
24. Bowman B, Bajd T: Influence of electrical stimulation on skeletal muscle spasticity. In: *Proceedings of the International Symposium on External Control of Human Extremities.* Belgrade, Yugoslavia: Committee for Electronics and Automation; 1981: 561–576.
25. Vodovnik L, Bowman BR, Hufford P: Effects of electrical stimulation on spinal spasticity. *Scand J Rehabil Med.* 1984; 16:29.

26. Somjen G: *Neurophysiology: The Essentials.* Baltimore, MD: Williams & Wilkins, 1983.
27. Alfieri V: Electrical treatment of spasticity. *Scand J Rehabil Med.* 1982; 14:177–182.
28. Vodovnic L, Stanic U, et al. Functional electrical stimulation for control of locomotor systems. *Crit Rev Bioeng.* 1981; 6:63–131.
29. Randall BF, Imig CJ, Hines HM: Effect of electrical stimulation upon blood flow and temperature of skeletal muscle. *Am J Phys Med.* 1953; 32:22.
30. Currier D, Petrilli C, Threlkeld J: Effect of medium frequency electrical stimulation on local blood circulation to healthy muscles. *Phys Ther.* 1986; 66:937.
31. Davis H: Is electro-stimulation beneficial to denervated muscles? a review of results from basic research. *Physiother Can.* 1983; 35:306–310.
32. Harada Y, Nakano K, Fujiwara M: Effects of electrical stimulation on the denervated rat muscle. *Acta Med Hypogoensia.* 1979; 4:129.
33. Pachter BR, Eberstein A, Goodgold J: Electrical stimulation effect on denervated skeletal myofibers in rats: a light and electron microscopic study. *Arch Phys Med Rehabil.* 1982; 63:427.
34. Girlanda R, Dattola R, Vita G, et al: Effect of electrotherapy on denervated muscles in rabbits: an electrophysiological and morphological study. *Exp Neurol.* 1982; 77:483.
35. Brown MC, Holland RL, Ironton R: Nodal and terminal sprouting from motor nerves in fast and slow muscles of the mouse. *J Physiol.* 1980; 306:493.
36. Ironton R, Brown MC, Holland RL: Stimuli to intramuscular nerve growth. *Brain Res.* 1978; 156:351.
37. Spielholz N: Electrical stimulation of denervated muscle. In: Nelson R, Currier D, eds. *Clinical Electrotherapy.* 2nd ed. Norwalk, CT: Appleton & Lange; 19:121–142.
38. Barranco S, Berger T: In vitro effect of weak direct current on *Staphylococcus Aureus.* *Clin Orthop* 1974; 100:250–255.
39. Rowley B: Electrical current effects on *E. coli* Growth Rates. *Proc Soc Exp Biol Med.* 1972; 139:929–934.
40. Rowley B, et al: The influence of electrical current on an infecting micro-organism in wounds. *Ann NY Acad Sci.* 1974; 238:543–551.
41. Kincaid C, Lavoie K: Inhibition of bacterial growth in vitro following stimulation with high voltage, monophasic pulse current. *Phys Ther.* 1989; 69:651–655.
42. Wolcott L, et al. An accelerated healing of skin ulcer by electrotherapy: preliminary clinical results. *South Med J.* 1969; 62:795–801.
43. Burr H, et al. An electrometric study of the healing wound in man. *Yale J Biol Med.* 1940; 12:483–485.
44. Becker RO, Murray DG: Method for producing cellular dedifferentiation by means of very small electrical currents. *Trans NY Acad Sci.* 1967; 29:606.
45. Carley P, Wainapel S: Electrotherapy for acceleration of wound healing: low intensity direct current. *Arch Phys Med Rehabil.* 1985; 66:443–446.
46. Kloth LC, Feedar JA. Acceleration of wound healing with high voltage, monophasic, pulsed current. *Phys Ther.* 1988; 68:403.

20

Iontophoresis

Tsega Andemicael Mehreteab, PT, MS

Dosage and Density

Contraindications

Procedure

Clinical Applications

Key Terms

I ontophoresis is the treatment technique in which an electric current is used to drive ions of various substances through the skin and into underlying tissues. Continuous direct current is used to transfer the charged ions into the tissues. The substances must dissociate into their charged ionic form and must be readily available for transfer into the skin under the electrode. Although some studies are available on the use and effect of some therapeutic ions, there is a dearth of standard clinical procedures for application and of published studies supporting the efficacy of iontophoresis. This chapter presents general guidelines and procedures for application as well as a chart listing sample ions with their sources, therapeutic effects, recommended dosages, and references that will provide additional information.

Continuously flowing direct current from an electric generator that provides constant current is used to drive ions into the skin and other tissues. The ions are delivered to the tissue as they are repelled by an electrode with the same polarity. Therefore, the polarity of the ion must be known before the appropriate polarity of the active electrode can be determined. For example, a positively charged ion such as zinc (Zn^{2+}) is applied under the positive electrode (the anode), and chloride ion (Cl^-) is applied under the negative electrode. In other words, matching the ion and the appropriate electrode is an extremely important step in the procedure. To determine the polarity of the ion, consult a pharmacist, refer to established literature, or use the periodic table of elements found in most chemistry books. In cases of ionic compounds composed of two elements, the first element is positively charged and the second is negatively charged. For example, in sodium chloride (NaCl), sodium is positive and chloride is negative.

DOSAGE AND DENSITY

The ion to be applied must be available in its charged form and should be soluble in both water and lipids. For example, the ion can be prepared in water or be suspended in an inert base (ointment). Because the concentration of the ions as well as the physical size of each ion may vary, the dosage must be carefully determined before the ion is applied. Dosage for the selected ionic concentration is expressed as a product of the intensity used in milliamperes and the duration of the treatment expressed in minutes. For example, a dosage of 20 mA-minutes may represent a current with an intensity of 4 mA applied for 5 minutes or an intensity of 2 mA applied for 10 minutes.

For safety, the density of the current should be considered. *Current density* is determined by dividing the current amplitude by the total area of the electrode. The range of density used for iontophoresis is between 0.1 and 0.5 mA per cm sq.[1] The maximum safe current density is approximately 1 mA per square inch. One must exercise caution to avoid an allergic reaction to the direct current, commonly referred to as a *galvanic rash.* This reaction is usually the result of hypersensitivity to a direct current. A galvanic rash may develop within 5 minutes of electrical stimulation. In addition, possible allergies or sensitivities to the substances used for iontophoresis should be carefully and thoroughly investigated before they are applied.

A commercially prepared electrode with a direct-current generator is also available for iontophoresis. This type of unit contains an electrode unit with a cavity for the ionic solution, a portal for filling the cavity with the solution, a semipermeable membrane that is placed directly over the skin, and a lead that connects the electrode unit to the current generator. A second lead and a dispersive electrode complete the circuit.

The net amount of ions deposited in the tissue can be affected by a variety of factors. For example, the local circulation may move ions away from the local area of application, or other ions in the area with a similar charge may compete with the ions to be applied. In addition, the higher the concentration of ions, the lower the uptake by the tissue. This has been shown by the uptake of different concentrations of radioactive phosphorus by iontophoresis.[1]

CONTRAINDICATIONS

Thoroughly investigate for possible allergies or sensitivities to the substances and direct current to be applied. The skin offers a significant impedance to current flow. Area devoid of its skin covering lacks this natural protection. In addition, current tends to concentrate in areas of least resistance; therefore, avoid current application over areas with broken skin, cuts, or bruises. Iontophoresis is contraindicated when there is acute injury and bleeding in the area to be treated.

In addition, iontophoresis is contraindicated in the following conditions: recent scars or new skin in the area to be treated; lack of sensation; metallic implants, wire or staples in the immediate vicinity of the area to be treated; patients with pacemakers; and conditions where electrical stimulation is contraindicated.

PROCEDURE

The following are the basic procedures for setting up an iontophoresis treatment.

1. Clean the skin and inspect it for cuts or bruises; check for sensation.
2. Explain to the patient the procedure and what to expect from the treatment.
3. Position the patient and the area to be treated appropriately.
4. Use a direct current generator with constant current output and well-calibrated controls (the ammeter should indicate the exact intensity delivered in milliamperes).
5. Follow the manufacturer's suggested procedures if using the commercially prepared electrode and a direct-current generator. The electrode comes with a cavity and portal system; the premeasured medication is directly injected into this cavity.
6. Use two electrodes (if the electrodes are self-prepared), an active electrode with the same polarity as the ion to be applied, and a larger, dispersive electrode. The dispersive electrode should be at least four times the size of the active electrode and should be placed on a distant area. Electrodes should be made of a flexible metal such as tin, cooper, aluminum, or aluminum foil that is cut to the appropriate size. Flexible electrodes conform easily to the body's contours and provide better contact.

7. Secure several layers of gauze or sponge saturated with the solution containing the ion over the area to be treated. Place the flexible metal electrode over it. If the ion is in a topical form, spread a thin layer of the ointment over the area to be treated and apply several layers of gauze moistened with distilled water over the ointment. To keep the metal from contacting the skin, the size of the electrode should be slightly smaller than the gauze preparation and the other side of the electrode should be covered with insulating material.

8. Use electrode leads, alligator clips, and clamps to connect the electrodes to the current generator. Apply the electrode evenly and avoid air bubbles.

9. Use nonmetallic straps or weights to ensure firm and even contact of the electrode with the body part.

10. Determine the dosage by taking the area of the active electrode into consideration—the maximum safety limit is 1 mA per square inch. The dosage should be increased gradually over time and must be consistent with the results of the treatment. When the current is turned on or off, the intensity should be gradually increased or decreased to avoid a twitch response.

11. Pay special attention when the cathode (−) is used as the active electrode. The chemical or polar effects of the cathode include alkaline reactions that affect the epidermis and further decrease skin resistance. This may cause a burn, commonly referred to as a "negative electrode burn."

12. Turn the current intensity up or down gradually to avoid an abrupt interruption of the direct current.

13. Observe the skin every 3–5 minutes during treatment for any adverse reactions such as a galvanic rash or burn. Also observe the skin after treatment and instruct the patient to observe and report any adverse reactions.

14. Ensure that the antidote ion or substance is readily available.

The ions available for clinical use may vary in concentration and in the type of carrier used: an aqueous solution or an ointment base. To prevent undesirable ions of the same charge from being delivered, the aqueous solution or the ointment carrier should not contain competing ions. The carrier substance should be chemically stable. There are recommended concentrations for various ions; however, a standard guide for concentration and dosage is lacking. (See Table 20–1 for recommended dosages for some ions used in physical therapy.)

TABLE 20–1. SAMPLE IONS AND THEIR CLINICAL USES

Ion/Charge/ Electrode	Main Source	Therapeutic Use	Recommended Dosage	References
Acetate/ (−) cathode	Acetic acid, 2% solution	Calcified tendonitis; decreases calcium deposits	3–5 mA for 10–20 min.	2,3
Copper / (+) Anode	Copper Sulfate 1% solution	Fungicidal; athlete's foot	10 mA for 15 min for 2 weeks. Bath method.	4
Dexamethasone and xylocane/ (+) Anode	Decadron ointment	Anti-inflammatory; arthritis, bursitis, tendonitis	1–5 mA for 15–20 min.	5–7
Hyoluronidase / (+) Anode	150 USP units in 250 cc of 0.1 M acetate buffer solution at 5.4 pH Wydase	Reduce edema	1–2 mA per 2.5 sq cm electrode for 20–40 min.	8, 9
Lidocaine / (+) Anode	Lidocaine Hydrochloride	Analgesia; bursitis, neuritis	2 mA for 1 min. and 4 mA for 5 min. Current density < 0.65 mA/sq cm.	10
Salicylate / (−) Cathode	1% sodium salicylate 2% sodium salicylate	Analgesia; myalgia Plantar warts	4–5 mA for 45 min 10 mA for min.1/wk.	11, 12
Tap water / (+) or (−) Anode or cathode	Tap water	Hyperhidrosis of palms or feet	15–29 mA for 10–15 min, 2–3 wk.	13, 14
Zinc / (+) Anode	01. M zinc oxide ointment	Bactericidal; ischemic ulcer	4–5 mA for 15 min, 2×/day.	15

CLINICAL APPLICATIONS

Table 20–1 lists the applications of sample ions and their clinical use. The names and charges of the ions are listed in Column 1, the main sources of the ions and the concentration of the desired substances are listed in Column 2, the therapeutic uses and effects, the recommended dosages, and references are listed in Columns 3, 4, and 5, respectively. (The references provide additional information on these ions).

■ **KEY TERMS**

current density   galvanic rash

REFERENCES

1. O'Malley EP, Oester YT: Influence of some physical chemical factors on iontophoresis using radio-isotopes. *Arch Phys Med Rehabil.* 1955; 36:310–316.
2. Psaki C, et al: Acetic acid ionization: a study to determine the absorptive effects upon calcified tendonitis of the shoulder. *Phys Ther Rev.* 1955; 35:84.
3. Khan J: Acetic acid iontophoresis for calcium deposits. *Phys Ther.* 1977; 57(6):658–659.
4. Haggard H, et al: Fungous infections of hand and feet treated by copper iontophoresis. *JAMA.* 1939; 112:1229.
5. Glass J, et al: The quantity and distribution of radio labeled depamethasone delivered to tissues by iontophoresis. *Int J Dermatol.* 1980; 19:519.
6. Harris PR: Iontophoresis: clinical research in musculo-skeletal inflammatory conditions. *J Orthop Sports Phys Ther.* 1982; 4:109.
7. Bertolucci L: Introduction of anti-inflammatory drugs by iontophoresis: double blind study. *J Orthop Sports Phys Ther.* 1982; 4:103.
8. Shwarth M: Hyaluronidase by iontophoresis in the treatment of lymphodema. *Arch Intern Med.* 1955; 95:662.
9. Russo J, et al: Lidocaine anesthesia: comparison of iontophoresis, injection, and swabbing. *Am J Hosp Pharm.* 1980; 37:843–847.
10. Magistro C: Hyaluronidase by iontophoresis. *Phys Ther.* 1964; 44:169.
11. Garzione J. Salicylate iontophoresis as an alternative treatment for persistent thigh pain following hip surgery. *Phys Ther.* 1978; 58:570.
12. Gordon A, Weinstein M: Sodium salicylate iontophoresis in the treatment of plantar warts. *Phys Ther.* 1969; 49:869–870.
13. Levit F: Simple device for treatment of hyperhidrosis by iontophoresis. *Arch Dermatol.* 1968; 98:505.
14. Shrivastava S, Sing G: Tap water iontophoresis in palm and plantar hyperhidrosis. *Br J Dermatol.* 1977; 96:189.
15. Cornwall M: Zinc iontophoresis to treat ischemic ulcers. *Phys Ther.* 1981; 61:359.

21

Transcutaneous Electrical Nerve Stimulation

Joseph Weisberg, PT, PhD

Transcutaneous electrical nerve stimulation (TENS) can be defined as the procedure of applying controlled, low-voltage electrical pulses to the nervous system by passing electricity through the skin via electrodes placed on the skin.[1] The popularity of treating pain with electricity increased with the development of TENS. Originally, TENS was developed as a by-product of the Dorsal Column Electrical Stimulator, which was made to stimulate the nerves in the dorsal column directly as a means of controlling pain. Because this device had to be surgically implanted, finding a way to test the effects of such stimulation before implantation became important. Consequently, TENS was developed as a noninvasive technique based on the same principle as the Dorsal Column Electrical Stimulator. However, once TENS was used to screen patients for this stimulator, it was realized that, in many cases, treatment with TENS was sufficient to reduce the pain and the surgical procedure could be avoided. During the 1970s, the therapeutic use of TENS was refined and became a convenient and effective method of treating pain.

TENS currently has many applications. Because it is a safe and effective method of treating pain and has survived the scrutiny of the Food and Drug Administration (FDA), TENS is used after many surgical procedures,[2-8] in obstetrics,[9,10] and for acute and chronic pain caused by many different conditions.[11-18] According to the FDA's medical device regulations, TENS is considered to be a Class II device—its distribution and application to patients must be prescribed by a licensed physician.

PAIN THEORIES

Several theories have been postulated to explain why TENS changes the perception of pain. The first theory, and the one responsible for the development of TENS, is the Gate-Control Theory, which states that stimulation of non-nociceptors or their axons can interfere with the relay of sensation from nociceptors to higher centers in the brain where pain is perceived.[19] According to the theory, TENS stimulates sensory A fibers with high-frequency stimulation. The impulses of this stimulation flood the pathway to the brain and close the "gate" to transmission of pain. This type of stimulation seems to manage the pain threshold.[20]

The second theory is based on the existence of natural opiates (pain suppressors) in the body. These opiates are produced by the pituitary gland (beta-endorphins) and in the spinal cord (enkephalins). Stimulation of sensory nerves with low-frequency TENS stimulates the release of these opiates, thus affecting the perception of pain.[21]

A third theory relates to the findings by Leandri et al[22] that TENS stimulation induces local vasodilation in patients with myofascial symptoms. They postulated that the induced local vasodilation affects pain that is caused by trigger points. Fassbender[23] demonstrated that the trigger points are related to ischemic areas in connective tissue or in muscle. The vasodilation produced by the TENS treatment possibly alters the ischemic area, thus affecting the pain.

A fourth theory relates to acupuncture. It is not within the scope of this book to discuss acupuncture. Briefly, however, acupuncture is based on energy lines (meridians) and entry points (acupuncture points). The theory is that TENS can be used to stimulate acupuncture points that affect the flow of energy, thus altering the condition that causes the pain. Recent studies indicate that stimulating acupuncture points as a treatment for pain may be as effective or even more effective[24,25] than using TENS on other somatic points.

Treating pain with TENS is not a simple matter because patients are not alike and their conditions are different. Furthermore, each practitioner claims success with different treatment protocols. Therefore, the therapist must realize that the key to clinical success lies in understanding the modality and its limitations, not in relying on a specific formula that seemed to work for someone else.

Although the literature on how TENS works is controversial, the view that TENS is an effective treatment for pain is widely accepted.

INDICATIONS AND CONTRAINDICATIONS

The indications for TENS treatment are pain syndromes such as acute pain, chronic pain, phantom limb pain, postoperative pain, obstetric pain, cardiopulmonary pain, and neurological pain (shingles). It also is indicated before potentially painful treatments (such as stretching a contracture or debridement) to elevate the patient's pain threshold .

TENS is contraindicated for some patients. For example, it may cause interference if a patient has a demand-type pacemaker. If applied over the carotid sinus, it might cause a hypotensive response. Because its effects on the embryo are unknown, TENS should not be used on a pregnant patient during the first trimester.

The following precautions should be adhered to:

- Anterior neck area. Stimulating the area close to the carotid sinus should be avoided.
- Cardiac disease. Stimulation across the chest should be avoided.
- Epilepsy. TENS should be avoided over the head and neck of epileptic patients.
- Over the eyes. The effects are unknown.

- Mucosal surfaces. TENS is not used to treat over such surfaces.
- Cerebrovascular accident patients and other central nervous system disorders. The effects of stimulation to the head in patients with such disorders are not known.
- Incompetent patients. Some patients may not be able to manage the device. Also, the device should be kept out of the hands of children.
- Dependency on the device. Due to the effect of the opiate released, some patients may become dependent on the device.
- Breaks in the skin.

In general, TENS is a safe modality. The only adverse reaction reported is skin irritation, which might be an allergic reaction to the gel or adhesive, poor application technique (eg, lack of gel, inadequate cleansing of skin, or uneven electrode contact), excessive treatment time, or rough removal of the electrodes.

EQUIPMENT

Although many different TENS units are available, most have the following:

- Solid-state generators for durability.
- A rechargeable battery for convenience and economy.
- Single, dual, or multiple-channels (for multiple sites).
- An intensity control: Large myelinated fibers require less current than the small unmyelinated fibers. Some therapists favor minimal intensity for an optimal effect, relying on the Arndt-Schultz law for support.
- A pulse rate control: Large myelinated fibers respond effectively to a high rate (more than 100 Hz), whereas small unmyelinated fibers respond more effectively to a low rate (less than 100 Hz).
- A pulse width control: Large myelinated fibers respond effectively to impulses with a narrow width (50 ms), whereas small myelinated fibers respond to impulses with a wide width (200 milliseconds).
- Wave characteristics that are either biphasic, with a negative spike component, or monophasic, with a positive rectangular component only.
- A modulation control, which allows the therapist to vary the current characteristics by at least 10%, usually the frequency or pulse width, to delay accommodation of the nervous system to the TENS.
- Electrodes (the most commonly used types are discussed later).

In addition, most TENS units are portable; that is, they are designed to be worn by the patient for convenience.

PROCEDURE

Initial Evaluation

A complete evaluation of the patient's pain symptoms should include a medical history, the etiology and duration of pain, previous treatments, current pain medication, pending litigation that is related to the pain, employment status, as specific a description of the pain as possible (quality, location, frequency), and a physical examination. In addition, the therapist should monitor the patient's vital signs for any changes resulting from the treatment.

Approach to the Patient

After deciding that TENS is the appropriate treatment, the therapist should explain the procedure to the patient to allay any anxiety he or she may have concerning electrical modalities. The therapist also should describe the type of sensation that is usually associated with such a treatment and the fact that the patient controls the intensity and can terminate the treatment at any time.

Furthermore, the therapist should emphasize the fact that TENS will not cure the underlying problem. It is a useful tool that, with persistence, could help relieve the pain. When TENS is used for postsurgical pain relief, the therapist should explain the procedure to the patient before the surgery. After the surgery, the therapist must make certain that the patient fully comprehends the instructions; this usually takes two to four visits. The patient should then be permitted to take the TENS unit home.

Modes of Application

There are four commonly used modes of application: conventional, acupuncture-like, bursts of pulse trains, and brief and intense.

Conventional. Conventional TENS is the most commonly used type. It primarily affects the large afferent (A) fibers, thus affecting the transmission of pain (according to the Gate theory). In our opinion, for optimal results the rate should be high (60–80 pulses per second, pps) and the width should be narrow (50–100 microseconds). The patient should experience a comfortable tingling sensation with no muscle contraction. Treatment time is usually 30 minutes. The treatment can then be repeated.

Acupuncturelike. Acupuncturelike TENS is directed toward the small-diameter (C) fibers. The stimulation characteristics are low rate (2–4 Hz) and wide width (200 microseconds). The intensity can be as high as the patient can tolerate and usually causes visible contractions. This type of stimulation may affect the secretion of endorphins, which would explain the relatively longer relief the patient experiences: ie, several hours and, at times, days.

Bursts of pulse trains. TENS applied in this mode involves high-rate (100 pps) stimulating current administered in bursts at a low rate (1–4 pps). This type of stimulation also causes visible muscle contractions. The effects of the initial treatment may last as long as 4 hours, probably as a result of the secretion of endorphins.

Brief and intense. This technique involves brief and intense high-rate (above 100 pps) and high-width (above 200 microseconds) current at an intensity as high as the patient can tolerate. This produces a tetanic contraction and results in surface analgesia for 5 to 10 minutes. Brief and intense TENS is a noxious stimulus and is used before painful procedures such as burn debridement, passive stretching, or minor surgery.

Because the literature is unclear regarding which mode is more effective and for which patients and regarding what conditions respond better to which mode and with what parameters, the therapist should be flexible. One approach is to begin with conventional TENS because it is the mode that patients can tolerate most easily. If the patient's initial response is poor, the therapist can try varying the placement of the electrodes first, then manipulate the parameters. Only when all else fails should the therapist try other modes. The patient should be told in advance that it may be necessary to change the parameters to achieve maximum results.

Selection of the TENS Unit

Many TENS devices are available on the market and most permit the manipulation of three variables: (1) the amplitude (or intensity) of the stimulus, (2) the pulse frequency (rate), and (3) the pulse duration (width).

Once the patient understands and can follow treatment protocols, the therapist must select the appropriate unit for that patient. The following questions should be answered before deciding which device the patient should buy.

- Did the patient respond well to treatment with a particular unit?
- Do the characteristics of the unit encompass all that is required for effective treatment?
- Is the unit easy to operate, especially by patients with poor dexterity?

- Is the unit durable and serviceable? (These units are expensive and therefore should serve the therapist or patient for many years.)
- Are rental units available for patients who need the units for a relatively brief period?
- Is the unit small enough to be carried in a pocket or be clipped to an article of clothing such as a belt?

Selection of the Electrodes

Many different types of electrodes are available, and most are effective. The advantages of some electrodes are their disposability and ease of application; the advantage of others is that they are reusable and more economical.

Three types of electrodes are commonly used. The first type is the fabric-covered orthopedic felt electrode that is soaked in tap water. It causes the least amount of skin irritation, but it must be rewet every 2–3 hours. The second type is the carbon-impregnated rubber electrode, which requires the application of a gel and can be left in place for 24 hours or more. This electrode is used more often than the fabric-covered electrode. A third type is the carbon-filled silicone electrode.

When selecting electrodes, the therapist should consider the relative size of the electrodes because the size determines the relative current density. The larger the electrode, the lower the current density. In most situations, the size of the two electrodes should be equal to permit equal current density under both. Furthermore, the therapist also should consider the patient's mental ability, dexterity, financial condition, and the location of the sites to be stimulated.

Placement of the Electrodes

There is no optimal electrode placement that is applicable for all patients, even for those who have a similar syndrome. Whenever possible, however, the electrode should be placed on a body part the patient can reach. The electrode is usually placed directly over the painful area. For most modes of application, the stimulation sites are (1) skin overlying the painful region, (2) the superficial point of the peripheral nerve, (3) the dermatome distribution of the nerve involved, (4) trigger points or acupuncture points, (5) segmentally-related myotomes, and (6) motor points (points on the skin where the least amount of current activates the muscle).

Selecting the site depends on the etiology, location, and character of the pain as well as on the patient's response to the selected site. If the desired results are not achieved by the initial placement, another site should be tried.

When the electrode placement is changed, the intensity of the current that the patient can tolerate also may change, especially if the distance between the electrodes is changed. Remember that skin resistance to the flow of current varies directly with the distance between the electrodes. Therefore, the closer the electrodes, the more superficial and concentrated the stimulus. Accordingly, to avoid blistering or burning, electrodes should not be placed closer than 1 cm from each other.

Electrodes can be placed unilaterally or bilaterally and can be bracketed or crossed. The electrodes can be placed along a peripheral nerve or along a dermatome. They also can be placed transcranially unless contraindicated.

The stimulation sites for acupuncturelike TENS are restricted to (1) acupuncture points, (2) superficial aspects of peripheral nerves, and (3) segmentally-related myotomes.

Application of the Electrodes

After the appropriate electrode sites have been selected, the conducting gel should be applied uniformly on the electrodes. Each electrode should be secured to the skin to ensure total contact. Poor skin contact may cause burning in the area surrounding the electrode rather than the desired paresthesia (tingling or numbness).

Remember that the adverse effect reported from TENS is skin irritation, which can be minimized by following these suggestions:

- Keep the skin and the electrodes clean. The skin can be cleaned with alcohol.
- Alternate the coupling media at the first sign of irritation.
- Place the electrodes on alternate sites.
- Avoid placing the electrodes too close together.
- Minimize the number of times the electrodes are removed from the skin.

Some patients are allergic to commercially available electrode gels or to adhesive tape when used over a long period and may develop contact dermatitis. This skin condition usually disappears within 3 days after the use of the gel or adhesive tape is discontinued. Treatment is discontinued only rarely because of skin irritation.

Adjustment of the Stimulation Parameters

Adjustment of the stimulating parameters depends on the patient's pathology, the mode being used, and the patient's tolerance. The following sequence of adjustments has proved to be effective for conventional TENS:

1. Preset the width (low) and the rate (high).
2. Turn on the unit and increase the amplitude until the patient reports the desired tingling sensation.
3. Readjust the width and rate within the above-cited range relating to the specific modes within the patient's tolerance. Achieve the visible contraction (tetanic contraction with brief intensity) within the patient's tolerance.
4. Readjust the amplitude (intensity). The intensity may need to be readjusted within the first 5–10 minutes because patients often report a change in sensation, which may be a result of changes in resistance caused by the passage of the current through the skin.

Treatment time can range from minutes to hours. Usually, the treatment is given daily for about a week before the results are evaluated. If the results are positive, as determined by the patient's subjective response, the patient is asked to rent the device on a 30-day trial basis to evaluate its long-term effectiveness.

Posttreatment Evaluation

To evaluate the effectiveness of the treatment properly, the patient must demonstrate an understanding of the procedure before taking the TENS unit home. In addition, the patient should be followed for 30 days to insure that he or she is adhering to the procedure.

The evaluation is difficult and imprecise because of the subjecting nature of pain. Nonetheless, a clinician can assess the effectiveness of the treatment in the following ways (see, also, Chapter 4):

- By using a descriptive pain scale ranging from no pain through mild, moderate, severe, and very severe pain.
- By using a pain rating index from 1 to 10, where 1 equals no pain and 10 equals excruciating pain.
- By using the patient's verbal description of the pain experience.
- By using a combination of any of the above.
- By using objective improvement of function (eg, increased range of motion, increased tolerance to an activity).

NEED FOR FUTURE RESEARCH

As with any other therapeutic method, the placebo effect may be responsible, in part, for the positive effect of TENS on pain. To exclude the placebo effect, a double-blind experimental study should be conducted with the device.

The effects of TENS need to be investigated further. A comparison of different techniques used for the same condition would be extremely helpful as we seek ways to improve treatment. These studies should consider the type of stimulator used, the type of stimulation, the specific parameters used (pulse width, pulse rate), the placement of electrodes, the type of electrode, the duration of treatment, and the frequency of treatment.

REFERENCES

1. Mannheimer JS, Lampe GN. *Clinical Transcutaneous Electrical Stimulation.* Philadelphia, PA: FA Davis; 1984.
2. Klin B, Uretzky G, Magora F. Transcutaneous electrical nerve stimulation (TENS) after open heart surgery. *J Cardiovasc Surg.* September-October 1984; 25:445–448.
3. Lagas H, Zuurmond W, Rietschoten W, et al. Transcutaneous nerve stimulation for the treatment of post-operative pain. *Acta Anesthsiol Belg.* 1984; 35:253–257.
4. Navarathnam R, Wang Y, Thomas D, et al. Evaluation of the transcutaneous electrical nerve stimulator for post-operative analgesia following cardiac surgery. *Anaesth Intensive Care.* 1984; 12:345–350.
5. Ticho U, Olshwang D, Magora F. Relief of pain by subcutaneous electrical stimulation after ocular surgery. *Am J Ophthal.* 1980; 89:803–808.
6. Arvidsson I, Eriksson E. Post-operative TENS pain relief after knee surgery. Objective evaluation. *Orthopedics.* 1986; 9:1346–1351.
7. Jensen JE, Conn RR, Hazelrigg G, et al. The use of transcutaneous neural stimulation and isokinetics testing in arthroscopic knee surgery. *Am J Sports Med.* 1985; 13:27–33.
8. Smith MJ, Hutchins RC, Hehenberger D. Transcutaneous neural stimulation used in post-operative knee rehabilitation. *Am J Sports Med.* 1983; 11:75–82.
9. Evron S, Schenker J, Olshwang D, et al. Post operative analgesia by percutaneous electrical stimulation in gynecology and obstetrics. *Eur J Obstet Gynecol.* 1981; 12:305–313.
10. Hollinger J. Transcutaneous electrical nerve stimulation after cesarean birth. *Phys Ther.* 1986; 66:36–38.
11. Bauer W. Electrical treatment of severe head and neck cancer pain. *Arch Otolaryngol.* 1983; 109:382–383.
12. Magora F, Aladjemoff L, Tannenbaum J, et al. Treatment of pain by transcutaneous electrical stimulation. *Acta Anaesth Scand.* 1978; 22:2–8.
13. Olahgang D, Aladjemoff L, Magora A. Five years experience with transcutaneous electrical stimulation (TES) in a pain clinic. Jerusalem, Israel: Department of Anesthesiology, Hadassah University Hospital; 1978:227–231.
14. Peled I, Wexler M, Rousso M, et al. Electrical stimulation in the treatment of the painful hand. *Ann Plast Surg.* 1982; 8:434–437.
15. Schuster G, Marsden B. Treatment of pain with TENS: a clinical evaluation of 61 patients. *J Neurol Orthop Surg.* 1980; 1:137–141.
16. Thurin E, Meehan P, Gilbert B. Treatment of pain by transcutaneous electric nerve stimulation in general practice. *Med J Aus.* 1980; 1:70–71.
17. Bending J. TENS in a pain clinic. *Physiotherapy.* 1989; 75:292–294.
18. Longobardi AG, Clelland JA, Knowles CJ, et al. Effects of auricular transcutaneous electrical nerve stimulation: a pilot study. *Phys Ther.* 1989; 69:10–17.
19. Melzack, Wall PD. Pain mechanisms: a new theory. *Science.* 1965; 150:971–977.
20. Singer K, D'Ambrosia R, Graf B, et al. Electrical modalities. In: Drez P Jr, ed. *Therapeutic Modalities For Sports Injuries.* Chicago, IL: Yearbook Medical Publishers;1989.
21. Salar G, Job I, Mingrino S, et al. Effect of transcutaneous electrotherapy on CSF beta-endorphin content in patients without pain problems. *Pain.* 1984; 10:169–172.
22. Leandri M, Brunetti O, Parodi CI. Telethermographic findings after transcutaneous electrical nerve stimulation. *Phys Ther.* 1986; 66:210–213.

23. Fassbender HG. Non-articular rheumatism. In: Fassbender HE, ed. *Pathology of Rheumatic Diseases*. New York: Springer-Verlag; 1975:313–314.

24. Lein DH Jr, Clelland JA, Knowles CJ, et al. Comparison of effects of transcutaneous electrical nerve stimulation of auricular, somatic and the combination of auricular somatic acupuncture points on experimental pain threshold. *Phys Ther*. 1989; 69:671–678.

25. Noling LB, Clelland JA, Jackson Jr, et al. Effect of transcutaneous electrical nerve stimulation at auricular points on experimental cutaneous pain threshold. *Phys Ther*. 1988; 68:328–332.

22

Point Locator/Stimulator

Joseph Weisberg, PT, PhD

Sites of Trigger and Acupuncture Points

Stimulation of Trigger and Acupuncture Points

Treatment Technique

Key Terms

A *point locator/stimulator* is a device that finds trigger or acupuncture points and is then used to stimulate the points for treatment purposes. Trigger points and acupuncture points are often associated with myofascial and visceral pain and dysfunction. Many clinical approaches have been developed to treat pain and dysfunction, one of which is stimulating these points either electrically or with a cold-laser beam. The effectiveness of electrical stimulation or cold-laser stimulation of trigger or acupuncture points is not well established, and a great need exists for more scientific investigation in this area.[1]

A *trigger point* can be defined as a small area on the body that is tender when palpated and one over which deep palpation elicits referred pain. The impedance of the skin over this point is lower than most of the surrounding skin.[2] Stimulating the trigger point reduces its sensitivity and reduces the referred pain.

An *acupuncture point* is a point located on a meridian (a line of energy described in Chinese medicine). Acupuncture points are considered to be the entry points into the body's energy system. They are usually tender to palpation in the presence of pathology or dysfunction ("disharmony"). Stimulating these points helps to "rebalance" the disharmony in the body's energy system, thus reducing the "pathology of the dysfunction." The skin impedance of the acupuncture points is also lower than the impedance of the surrounding skin.[3,4] Stimulating either a trigger point or an acupuncture point causes the impedance of these points to increase temporarily to the level of the surrounding tissue.[5]

SITES OF TRIGGER AND ACUPUNCTURE POINTS

The sites of the trigger and acupuncture points have been mapped; thus, the clinician can consult textbooks, articles, and poster charts for the specific site of each point. From an anatomic viewpoint, these points are nebulous because they cannot be identified in the body; no one has been able to dissect them. Historically, the sites of trigger points and acupuncture points were established at different times and with different philosophical understanding. However, the sites of the two types of points correlate to a great extent. For example, a correspondence of 71% was found between the sites of trigger and acupuncture points in relation to pain.[6]

Finding a trigger point manually involves palpation and location of the most tender spot in the area involved. The therapist can be confident that a trigger point has been found when the response to pressure applied over it results in local or referred pain. To find an acupuncture point manually, one must first refer to an anatomical chart of acupuncture points. This chart enables the therapist to find the approximate site of the point. The therapist then finds the point by searching for a sensitive spot on the skin overlying the specific anatomic landmark such as a crease, a bony prominence, a hairline, or a depression in the underlying bone.[7] This spot is the acupuncture point. A therapist must be experienced and skilled to find a trigger or acupuncture point manually. However, with a point finding instrument that is sensitive to skin impedance, even an inexperienced therapist can locate these points with confidence.

STIMULATION OF TRIGGER AND ACUPUNCTURE POINTS

Skin impedance varies significantly among individuals. Moreover, skin impedance in one person varies from area to area. For example, the impedance of the skin in the palm of the hand is much less than it is in the dorsal aspect of the hand.[8] In addition, the impedance of the skin at any site may change over time as conditions affecting the physiology of the skin change. For example, pathology—especially hypothyroidism or hyperthyroidism,[8] sympathetic hyperactivity or sympathetic hypoactivity,[9,10] and mental state[8]—can cause physiologic changes in the skin that can affect its impedance.

As was mentioned earlier, acupuncture and trigger points have lower impedance values relative to their surrounding tissue; the lower impedance value at these points is constant.[2,11,12] However, once these points are stimulated, eg, with a cold-laser beam, the skin impedance may increase to the level of the surrounding tissue. This change in impedance may be associated with improvement in a patient's symptoms.[2]

The point locator part of a point locator/stimulator produces extremely low-voltage current, which is enough to flow only through points of low impedance. When this current flows, it activates visual signals, auditory signals, or both in the unit, thereby indicating the sites of the points. Some units are investigative units—they use the cold-laser beam to stimulate the trigger or acupuncture points. Most of the other types of units are currently accepted as therapeutic modalities, and their mode of stimulation is electrical current. Clinicians who use these devices claim clinical success. However, 5% of patients report an increased sensitivity to pain after the initial stimulation; this sensitivity then subsides after the second or third treatment.[13]

TREATMENT TECHNIQUE

When treating patients, the therapist carries out the following steps:

1. Cleanse the skin in the suspected area, preferably with 70% isopropyl alcohol to reduce the impedance of the skin.
2. Place a hand-held electrode in the patient's hand to complete the electrical circuit.
3. Palpate for the pain-sensitive area and identify the general location of the trigger or acupuncture point.
4. Turn on the point locator of the unit and adjust the sensitivity knob.
5. Move the probe tip over the area to pinpoint the spot and apply just enough pressure to ensure good contact. When the probe tip is immediately over the point, the therapist will hear a signal or see a display of lights or a moving needle, depending on the type of unit. This indicates

that the impedance of the spot the probe is touching is lower than the surrounding tissue.

6. Stimulate the spot with electrical stimulation. The probe should remain in contact with the skin over the spot while the therapist switches the control from the point locator to the point stimulator and increase the current to the highest level the patient can tolerate. If a cold-laser beam is used, it is best to pull the probe away from the skin about 1 mm and focus the beam at the site of low impedance.[14] For both electrical and laser stimulation, the duration of stimulation is 15–60 seconds per site.

For indications and contraindications to these modalities, see the indications and contraindications for TENS and laser treatments in Chapters 21 and 26. In addition, the therapist is advised to consult the manufacturer of the unit for more specific information.

■ KEY TERMS

point locator/stimulator   acupuncture point
trigger point

REFERENCES

1. Paris DL, Baynes F, Gucker B. Effects of neuroprobe in the treatment of second degree ankle inversion sprain. *Phys Ther*. 1983; 63:35–40.
2. Snyder-Mackler L, Bork C, Bourbon B, et al. Effect of helium-neon laser on musculoskeletal trigger points. *Phys Ther*. 1986; 66:1087–1090.
3. Hyrarinen J, Karisson M. Low-resistance skin points that may coincide with acupuncture loci. *Med Biol*. 1977; 55:88–94.
4. Reichmanis M, Marino AA, Becker RO. Electrical correlates of acupuncture points. *IEEE Trans Biomed Eng*. 1975; 22:533–535.
5. Brown ML, Ulett GA, Stern JA. Acupuncture loci: techniques for location. *Am J Clin Med*. 1974; 2:67–74.
6. Melzack B, Stillwell DM, Fox E. Trigger points and acupuncture points for pain: correlations and implications. *Pain*. 1977; 3:3023.
7. Kaptchuk TJ. *The Web That Has No Weaver*. New York: Congdon & Weed; 1983:78–80.
8. Richter CP. Physiological factors involved in the electrical resistance of the skin. *Am J Physiol*. 1929; 88:596–615.
9. Van Metre TE Jr. Low electrical skin resistance in the region of pain in painful acute sinusitis. *Bull Johns Hopkins Hosp*. 1949; 85:409–415.
10. Riley LH, Richter CP. Uses of electrical skin resistance method in the study of patients with neck and upper extremity pain. *Johns Hopkins Med*. 1975; 137:69.
11. Hyrarinen J, Karisson M. Low-resistance skin points that may coincide with acupuncture loci. *Med Biol*. 1977; 55:88–94.
12. Reichmanis M, Marino AA, Becker RO. Electrical correlates of acupuncture points. *IEEE Trans Biomed Eng*. 1975; 22:533–535.
13. Roy Steven R, Richard I. *Sports Medicine: Prevention, Evaluation and Rehabilitation*. Englewood, NJ: Prentice-Hall; 1983:103.
14. Kahn J. *Low Volt Technique (Clinical Electrotherapy)*. 4th ed. Syosset, NY: Joseph Kahn; 1985:2.

23

Clinical Electroneuromyography

Arthur Nelson, Jr., PT, PhD

INTRODUCTION

The comprehensive evaluation of the patient referred for physical therapy services should include clinical *electroneuromyography* (ENMG) when a patient presents with flaccid paralysis, atrophy of muscles, and sensory loss or pain radiating to limbs. Any pattern of progressive weakness also may serve as the motivation to perform an ENMG examination. The ENMG exam is used to differentiate between disorders of the central nervous system (CNS) and peripheral nervous system. It also is regularly used in the comprehensive evaluation of people with cervical and lumbar pain syndromes to search for evidence of nerve root compromise. Serial studies also may be used to identify progression or regression of a neuropathy, myopathy, or a neuromuscular junction. The ENMG also may be used to predict the time of recovery of function in selected patients.

The ENMG examination typically consists of two components: (1) nerve conduction studies, or evoked response component, and (2) electromyographic examination of the muscles, or the electromyography (EMG) component. A *nerve conduction* study entails electrical stimulation of a peripheral nerve at a number of sites along its course. This involves the selective stimulation of motor or sensory components of the peripheral nerve. *Electromyography* involves the insertion of needle electrodes in a muscle to identify the nature of the electrical discharges when the electrode is inserted, when the muscle is at rest, and when it contracts with various intensities.

This chapter is divided into three sections. The first section provides information about the ENMG examination that is required before embarking on discussions about *nerve conduction* studies and the EMG examination. Before conducting the actual ENMG examination, the examiner must review the patient's medical history, carry out a clarifying neurologic assessment, and inspect the patient's skin, nails, and hair distribution. The patient's medical history includes pertinent medical information, medications taken over the past several months, laboratory data, radiologic and other reports, and a detailed description of the onset of symptoms, their duration and constancy, their intensity, and the factors that alter those symptoms. A summary of this history is typically contained in the ENMG report.

On the basis of the findings of the medical history and the patient's complaints, further clarification would be obtained by assessing the sensory system, manual muscle testing, reflex responsiveness at selected areas, and other procedures appropriate to the patient's history and complaints. It is useful for the examiner to have disposable pins, cotton wads, and a tendon hammer for this clarifying assessment.

The purpose of evaluating the sensory system is to uncover a pattern of loss or distortion that conforms to some recognizable distribution that would be ultimately compared to the findings of the ENMG examination. It might be surprising to uncover sensory loss in the area where a person is experiencing pain. Patients often cannot discern sensory loss until the examiner pinches them. Many times patients will say a limb is "numb" when in actuality they are describing a sensory dysesthesia of "pins and needles," not hypoesthesia or loss of sensation. The distribution of sensory change may help distinguish between a nerve root, a peripheral nerve, or another pattern. This will be used later to correlate with the ENMG findings.

The manual muscle test used differs from the conventional one in that it is frequently performed bilaterally to assess differences from side to side. In some instances, one must perform a definitive muscle test on individual muscles, but, generally, this assessment is to obtain an overview of groups of muscles. During this testing, the examiner observes for atrophy, wasting, or trophic changes in the skin. These are noted in the report along with muscle test findings.

Deep-tendon jerk responses are elicited at the major sites associated with the suspected problem of the patient. These would be recorded as absent, brisk, or exaggerated, using a definition of numerical scale on the report form. Any other responses such as the plantar (Babinski) reflex should be reported as well. Some examiners use tuning forks to assess response to vibratory stimuli. The special tests for vision, hearing, taste, smell, and equilibrium (caloric test) may not be conducted unless they are pertinent or are absent from the patient's records.

The purpose of the clarifying examination is to provide the examiner with a clearly focused direction for the testing. It may be advantageous to examine the part that exhibits the clinical findings. This may provide more information than would initiating a set procedure and having the patient abort the test prior to getting to the most essential area.

THE ELECTRONEUROMYOGRAPHIC EXAMINATION

Purpose

The ENMG examination can be viewed as an extension of the manual muscle test that permits a more detailed look at the internal electrical state of the muscle during varying states of activity and the responsiveness of nerves to stimuli at various sites along the nerve path. When a person has a peculiar feeling of heaviness but does not exhibit gross loss of strength, it may be possible to uncover changes within the muscle that are not visible without the EMG. Similarly, total paralysis from a nerve injury may reveal early, subtle changes that signal the return of innervation.

The ENMG examination is helpful in distinguishing between CNS disorders and peripheral disorders. For instance, a patient suffering from sensory disturbances in one leg and one arm can be evaluated to determine if this indicates a problem in the cerebral hemisphere or a cervical or lumbar nerve root disorder.

Identifying the severity of a lesion is an important goal of this test, and serial studies can be used to form a prognosis for recovery. The monitoring of progressive disorders such as muscular dystrophy may help primary caregivers determine the rate of progression and its distribution. This information would contribute to program planning and the appropriateness of surgical intervention or the use of orthoses, and to other critical decision making.

It is also necessary to determine if a more acute disturbance has been superimposed on a chronic one: for example, if someone with a chronic cervical radiculopathy has had another injury to the neck and is now complaining of additional symptoms. How much acute change versus the chronic findings has occurred? The answer can have important legal or liability implications.

The ENMG findings may provide information regarding the optimal time to begin treatment. A study by Brown & Ironton[1] suggests that if initiated too early after denervation, electrical stimulation may retard reinnvervation; therefore, it is probably wise to wait until a significant reduction in fibrillation within the muscle has occurred. Similarly, the effectiveness of treatment can be monitored with ENMG to determine if there is objective evidence of improvement.

The ultimate purpose of the ENMG examination is to identify what the problem actually is, what structures are involved, and to what extent.

Some typical problems confronting the physical therapist include weakness, numbness and tingling, pain, dizziness or light-headedness, loss of equilibrium, fatigue, inability to perform tasks previously accomplished, and loss of skill. These complaints are reviewed in the context of the patient's history, laboratory findings, the clarifying neurological assessment, and other pertinent information to form a statement of the problem. Patients often tell examiners what the problem is, but the examiners have already made up their mind and do not listen with an open mind.

Suppose the patient complains of dizziness. Where does one begin? The history should be reviewed to determine when the dizziness occurs: upon first arising in the morning or after straining to have a bowel movement? Has the patient had a significant cardiac or respiratory problem? Has there been a history of middle ear infections? Do other family members have similar problems? What does the person do to alleviate the symptoms? Does activity improve or worsen the problem? What happens to the person's blood pressure when he or she rises from a sitting position? If you find that none of the previous questions provides any clues, then perform a sensory examination. If you find that there is a stockinglike loss of sensation from midcalf to the toes to stimulation with a wisp of cotton, you know the direction the ENMG examination should take. The problem now becomes one of looking for changes compatible with peripheral neuropathy, caudae equinae lesions, or compromise of the lumbosacral nerve roots.

A peripheral neuropathic disorder results in changes that are generally correlated anatomically with it. Does the person have peculiar, unexplained sensations in the feet and lower legs? Does the person experience more dizziness when in a dark room? Have the toe nails changed? Do the feet "go to sleep" easily? Do the legs tire more easily than they used to? Is there significant back pain? Does the patient have radiation of pain to the legs? Does the patient have "pins and needles" in the lower legs and feet? Lumbosacral nerve root compression can produce numbness of legs and weakness of selected lower extremity muscles.

The examiner then conducts a neuromuscular evaluation to delineate what nerves and muscles will be examined and in what order. If the neuromuscular examination reveals sluggish jerk responses in the Achilles tendon and a loss of response to light touch with a wisp of cotton in a stockinglike distribution of both legs, the impression of peripheral neuropathy is supported. However, these findings may be caused by lumbosacral nerve root or plexus compression, or a caudae equinae lesion. With these alternative conditions in mind, the examiner conducts the ENMC to delineate and thereby rule-out two of the four possibilities.

Therefore, the structure of the ENMG examination will include study of the peripheral nerves of the lower legs and feet. The study of a peripheral nerve involves stimulating the nerve at two sites and measuring the velocity with which it conducts the stimuli. A distal muscle is used to determine the response of the nerve to stimuli. The magnitude of its response, known as the amplitude, also is an important bit of information. The distal portion of the conduction also is helpful. This examination process then continues to the other major nerve in each leg to provide a basis of comparison to the nerve in question and to normal values. Special studies of the proximal segment of the nerve are conducted to determine its status and thereby assess the lumbosacral plexus and the nerve roots. Electromyography follows a similar line of reasoning: evaluating the distal musculature of a given peripheral nerve, looking at a proximal muscle of that nerve, then examining muscles that are innervated by nerve roots or components of the lumbosacral plexus. For instance, the paralumbar muscles can be examined to reveal a more proximal problem such as a lumbar or sacral nerve root compression.

Principles

Some of the principles involved in conducting a proper ENMG examination include the following:

1. Examine both a distal and a proximal muscle in a given peripheral nerve. A distal and a proximal muscle innervated by a particular nerve root also should be examined to delineate the lesion. This principle is known as the proximal and distal rule.
2. Examine muscles that are innervated by the same nerve roots but different peripheral nerves to localize the changes to one or the other.
3. Keep examining muscles until normal values are uncovered because it is impossible to delineate the level of involvement until the findings are within normal limits.

In summary, the first principle is proximal versus distal, the second is nerve root versus peripheral nerve, and the third is to keep going until normal values are found.

To understand the findings obtained in an ENMG examination, it is imperative to explore some anatomic and physiologic correlates such as the motor unit, the fascicular organization of nerve and muscle, the resting membrane potential, the junctional potentials, the action potential, neuromuscular transmission, and electromechanical coupling. For a more complete treatment of these subjects, consult a neurophysiology text.

Anatomic Correlates

The motor unit is the most fundamental element of neuromuscular control. A motor unit consists of the motor neuron and its axon, which extends from the anterior horn region of the spinal cord to the muscle fibers innervated by that axon. The ratio of muscle fibers innervated by a single axon has been identified by Weddell, et al[2] as ranging from as few as 7–9 muscle fibers per axon in extraocular muscles to as many as 1400 muscle fibers per axon in the medial gastrocnemius muscle. Obviously, the lower the ratio, the greater the control of that muscle. The muscle fibers innervated by an axon are distributed throughout a fascicle in a checkerboardlike configuration. This ensures that the tension of the motor unit will be evenly distributed throughout the muscle-tendon unit. Buchthal[3] estimated that the motor unit detected by an electrode will occupy between 5 and 15 sq mm of a muscle and will be mixed with three to six other motor units. If the tip of the exploring electrode can effectively determine 2 to 3 sq mm, it is clear that this electrode must be shifted to a number of sites within the muscle to survey adequately the motor units within the muscle in question.

The axons are collected into bundles, and those bundles are collected into larger bundles that finally accumulate in the nerve trunk. Each collection of bundles has a sheath of connective tissue with the nerve trunk having a covering of perineural connective tissue that encloses the entire structure. It also should be noted that these fascicles are not found in a parallel arrangement but in a loose type of braid within the nerve trunk. For this reason, stimulation applied to the nerve trunk must be of sufficient intensity to ensure that 100% of the axons are stimulated; a lesser stimulus may not stimulate the same fibers at another level of the nerve. This intense stimulus is known as a *supramaximal stimulus.*

Physiologic Correlates

The cell membrane of nerve as well as muscle possesses an electrical charge known as the *resting membrane potential.* If a micropipette electrode is inserted into this membrane and connected to a voltmeter, it will register a negative charge of 70–90 mV. The membrane in a resting state acts as a type of storehouse of electrical charge, much like a battery. This resting charge requires an ionic imbalance of excess sodium on the outside of the membrane and excess potassium on the inside of the membrane. In addition, a metabolic pump must maintain this imbalance using an adenosine triphosphate (ATP) energy source. The membrane is thereby relatively impermeable to sodium and less so to potassium. The resting membrane potential is close to the equilibrium potential of potassium.

When an electrical stimulus is delivered to a nerve membrane, it apparently discharges the capacitance of that portion of the membrane, resulting in a dramatic change in the permeability of the membrane to sodium. This leads to a dramatic reversal of the membrane potential so that the inside of the membrane becomes positive. This reversal of the potential is called a *depolarization.* Because this depolarization occurs three-dimensionally in a progression from the point of stimulation, it is called the wave of depolarization. Once this depolarization reaches its peak, the sodium egress is maximal while potassium also has been exiting the membrane at a slower rate. A repolarization then takes place with the membrane potential returning to a negative value. The actual value reached is more negative than the resting potential. This overshoot is called *hyperpolarization.* This hyperpolarization makes the membrane refractory to stimuli at this instant. This ensures a set frequency of discharge of nerve and muscle membrane so that the motor neurons designed for high-frequency firing will have short afterhyperpolarization periods and low-frequency firing motor neurons will have shorter ones.

If an electric current is applied with an extremely slow increase of intensity, there may be no change in the resting membrane potential, which is termed *accommodation.* However, if, after the slow increase in current has resulted in no response, the sudden cessation of the current will result in a change in the resting membrane potential. Therefore a response may be elicited by turning the current off.

It is clear that proper electrolyte balance will be necessary for the optimal function of these reversal depolarization and repolarization potentials. Moderate increases in extracellular potassium reduces the concentration gradient and lowers the resting potential of the nerve and muscle membranes. Small increases in extracellular potassium produces partial depolarization, and the cell will fire easily and sometimes spontaneously. This is recognized as an abnormality on the ENMG examination of a muscle. Large increases in potassium concentration can produce a depolarization block, resulting in profound paralysis and the danger of cardiac failure. These electrolyte imbalances may be encountered in kidney disease and in hyperkalemic periodic paralysis. Anoxia and hypoxia resulting in a decreased oxygen concentration produces an accumulation of potassium extracellularly. This results in transient signs and symptoms. These symptoms may be reflected in the sensory system as tingling, loss of vision, or "seeing stars." In the motor system, it may be manifested as loss of strength, twitching of muscles, or lack of endurance.

If sodium conductance is interfered with, eg, in tetrodotoxin poisoning, the wave of depolarization, the *action potential,* will be blocked. Structural changes in the nerve membrane brought on by disease, injury, or ischemia may lead to a leakage of sodium, which could increase excitability or, if extreme, a complete block in conduction. An increase in extracellular sodium will increase the amplitude and the rise time of the action potential will be faster. Conversely, a decrease in sodium outside the membrane results in a reduced action potential amplitude and a slower rise time of the action potential. If the decrease of sodium is severe, it may block the action potential formation entirely.

Calcium ions act as a membrane stabilizer, and if they are absent, the result is a decreased concentration gradient of sodium and potassium. For example hypocalcemia will reduce the resting membrane potential, resulting in increased excitability seen on the EMG as spontaneous firing of motor units called fasciculations. The most common symptoms of hypocalcemia will be twitching, tingling, or both. It also is likely that synaptic transmission will be interfered with, which would result in weakness. Excess calcium tends to reduce the action potential and enhance synaptic transmission but is difficult to determine clinically.

Drugs (eg, cocaine) that interfere with sodium conductance in the axon membrane will block the action potential, starting with the thinnest fibers first; hence its value for blocking pain conduction. Vincristine affects the neurotubule system and therefore results in deterioration of the delivery of substances such as transmitters to the terminal axon. This may result in a deterioration of the distal axon known as a dying-back neuropathy.

When nerves have been injured and the axons have degenerated, a supersensitivity of the postsynaptic terminus of those axons will develop. In the case of muscle fibers innervated by a degenerated axon, the muscle fibers will become supersensitive to acetylcholine, and if any of this transmitter is near those fibers, they will spontaneously fire. The muscle fibers will be irritated by mechanical stimulation such as the insertion of the needle electrode during the ENMG examination. The irritability can then be represented as increased insertional activity, fibrillation potentials at rest, or positive sharp waves while the muscle is at rest.

Variables influencing conduction velocity of nerve. The velocity of nerve conduction is proportional to the diameter of the axons within the nerve trunk and to the degree of myelinization around each axon. The amount of myelin is significant because it enhances the conduction seven times more than would occur without myelin sheathing. Therefore, if demyelination occurs, it will severely reduce conduction velocity. The thickest axons and the most richly myelinated ones are the primary afferents derived from the muscle spindles that are responsible for the tendon jerk response. Because thick axons are more vulnerable to compressive lesions, the tendon jerk will be among the first deficits observed.

Conduction of evoked stimuli in the nerve trunk. When short duration pulses of current (0.1–0.2 milliseconds) are delivered to a nerve trunk, more and more axons are added to those thickest fibers that respond earliest. Electrical stimulation elicits responses in the thickest axons first and then, as the intensity increases, smaller and smaller diameter fibers are brought in. Because all the pulses of current are arriving simultaneously in all the axons, the result is a compilation of all the individual motor units firing in a confined period of time. The result is a single response known as a *motor action potential* (MAP). To be certain that all the axons are responding and none are left out, the response is observed on the oscilloscope screen while the intensity of the pulses of stimuli is slowly increased until there is no further increase in the amplitude of the MAP. This is then referred to as a *supramaximal stimulus* because no further increase in amplitude has taken place despite the 10% increase in the intensity of the stimuli (Fig. 23–1).

Voluntary recruitment of motor units. The final determiner of whether muscular action will occur is the excitation of the anterior horn cell, also known as the alpha

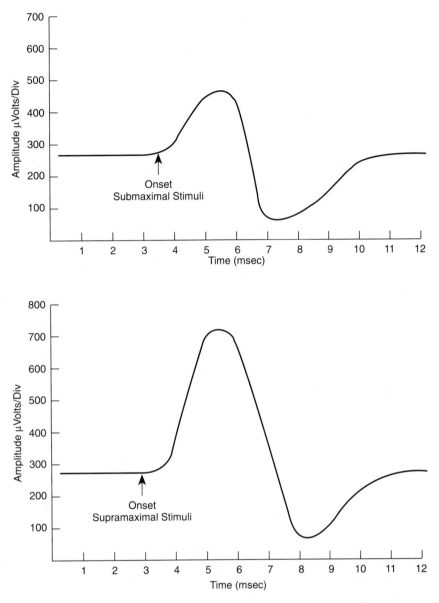

Figure 23–1. Influence of supramaximal stimuli on latency. The latency is 2.7 milliseconds with supramaximal stimuli and 3.4 milliseconds with submaximal stimuli.

motor neuron. Once the anterior horn cell is activated at the axon hillock, the action potential is conducted at either maximum amplitude or not at all throughout its course. This property is known as the all-or-none law, which ensures that whatever firing frequency is established in the anterior horn cell will be the frequency that is applied to the neuromuscular junction and subsequently to the muscle membrane, assuming no disorder of the neuromuscular junction or muscle membrane. This means all muscle fibers supplied by each axon, which can be as high as 1400 muscle fibers in the medial head of the gastrocnemius or as few as 5 or 6 in the extraocular muscles. Because these individual muscle fibers are spread through the fascicle, the needle electrode of the EMG will act as a type of averager and there will be an amalgamation of the individual action potentials from the many muscle fibers into a *compound motor unit potential* (cMUP) (Fig. 23–2).

Duration of the motor unit potential. The duration of the compound motor unit potential (cMUP) is determined by the spread of the end-plate zone in relation to the total length of the muscle fibers. For example, the abductor pollicus brevis muscle has an end-plate zone that is 50% of the total length of the fibers of the muscle. Conversely, the biceps brachii has an end-plate zone that is only 10% of the

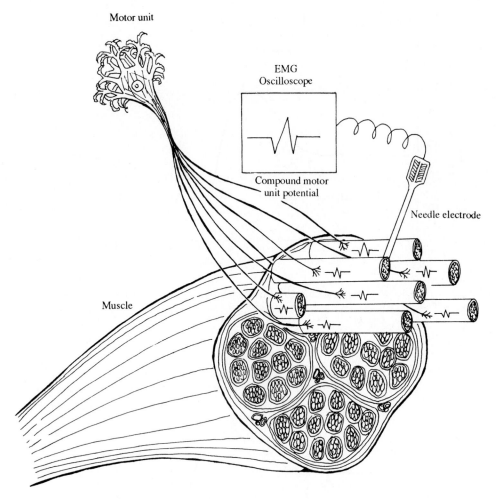

Motor unit

EMG
Oscilloscope

Compound motor
unit potential

Needle electrode

Muscle

Figure 23–2. Formulation of a compound motor unit potential. The action potentials from each muscle fiber are amalgamated into an averaged potential.

total length of the muscle fibers. This results in a longer duration of the cMUP of the abductor pollicis brevis muscle than the biceps brachii muscle.

Amplitude of the motor unit potential. The size or amplitude of the cMUP is determined by the circumference of the muscle fibers with respect to the total cross-section of the muscle. Therefore, larger diameter fibers in a relatively small muscle will result in a higher amplitude cMUP in that muscle when sampled with EMG. For example, the abductor pollicis brevis will have a higher amplitude MUP than does the biceps brachii. As noted previously, the extracellular sodium can influence the amplitude of the cMUP as well.

Recruitment of motor units. During voluntary contraction or reflex activation of muscle, the smallest motor units with the lowest amount of tension will be recruited first. They will increase their frequency of firing from 5 per second to 12 or 15 per second. As the smaller motor unit (MU) reaches its plateau of frequency, it is supplemented with a larger motor unit, which begins at a higher frequency and eventually may achieve maximum frequency of firing of 50 per second in an extremely strong contraction. This orderly *recruitment* from small to larger motor units is known as the size-order principle of recruitment attributed to Hennemann et al.[4] During an EMG, it is instructive to observe the increased rate of firing of motor units. If a person has few motor units, the units will fire more frequently when the person is trying to contract the muscle more forcefully. If the person is feigning weakness, the frequency remains unchanged. Clinicians can use confusion movements to outwit the patient into a better recruitment pattern than the patient may want to convey.

Neuromuscular transmission. The axon does not conduct the action potential directly to the muscle fibers but must release chemical transmitters at the neuromuscular junction. The wave of depolarization releases calcium from the neuroplastic reticulum. In the presence of calmodulin, the calcium ruptures the vesicles containing acetylcholine, which spills out into the synaptic cleft between the nerve and the muscle membrane. The acetylcholine molecules bind to the receptor sites on the muscle membrane, thus changing the permeability of the membrane to sodium and potassium. The change in permeability leads to an increase in the positive charge on the inside of the membrane that is proportional to the number of activated gates. The new potential is referred to as a *graded junctional potential or an end plate potential* because it is proportional to the amount of acetylcholine binding to the membrane. Once that graded potential reaches threshold, an action potential is formed on the muscle membrane which is subsequently conducted along the surface of the muscle membrane at a rate of 3 to 5 meters per second.

Electromechanical coupling. Once the muscle action potential reaches the openings of the transverse tubule system, it enters the depths of the muscle fiber. There, the action potential activates calcium in the sarcoplasmic reticulum in the presence of calmodulin. The released calcium bonds to troponin, which is wrapped around the actin molecules and bound to tropomyosin, which is released by the calcium binding to troponin. When this occurs, an electrostatic inhibition between actin and myosin is released, permitting actin and myosin to bind. The hinge of the myosin molecule bends, thereby exerting tension when this actin-myosin binding takes place. This tension is exerted by a new molecule called myosin-actin-ATPase. The energy is provided by the breakdown of adenosine triphosphate for the formulation of the bond. To release the bond, energy is also required through the breaking down of ATP in the presence of magnesium. This is accompanied by an active pumping of calcium back into the sarcoplasmic reticulum. If calcium remains in the region of the actin and troponin, the bond will not release and a rigor will remain within the sarcomere that does not require an action potential. Thus, it is possible, under this special circumstance, to have contraction of a muscle without EMG potentials being in evidence.

All electroneuromyographs used in clinical investigations have two basic components: the nerve conduction mode and the electromyography mode. The two components are contained within a single unit called an electromyograph (EMG). The essential elements of the EMG consist of the oscilloscope; the stimulate mode; the EMG mode, the manual modes and gain-and-sweep speed controls; and a printer mode with buffer. Attendant to this EMG are a preamplifier with a long cable and a stimulator with another cable attached to the body of the stimulate mode. An essential element within the EMG is the *differential amplifier,* which is essential to distinguish extremely small voltages from larger ones that surround us in every environment. The electrodes are attached to the preamplifier to complete the circuit.

The examiner's choice of the proper electrodes to bring the small signals from the patient's body to the EMG is a crucial one. The current recommendation is to use disposable needle electrodes for EMG, metal disk electrodes for motor nerve conduction studies, and ring or clip electrodes for sensory nerve conduction studies. The electrodes are the most critical link in the entire system and also are subject to many sources of error. The electrodes are used to transfer the essential physiologic information from the subject to the EMG preamplifier and the differential amplifier, which expands the information and displays it on an *oscilloscope* and also converts it to sound that can be heard on speakers. The interaction of metal needles with the biologic tissue is a complex one and varies in many circumstances, producing distortions of the tiny electrical signals.

If one considers the tiny contact of a needle electrode within a muscle, which moves and twists the electrode during contraction, one begins to sense the larger problem of obtaining reliable information from the electrode. The purpose of the electrode within the muscle is to pick up the microvolt potentials while there are much larger electrical influences in the adjacent area such as electric power wiring, appliances, and lighting. The trick is to distinguish between the tiny biologic signals within the body and the rather large electrical signals surrounding the body. Most electrical interference is handled by applying an appropriate ground that effectively nullifies the larger currents or isolates the biologic signals from the larger ones. It is helpful to disconnect all equipment that may be plugged into the wall socket in the vicinity of the EMG. The design of the amplifier is an important factor in providing a dependable signal-to-noise (information-versus-error) ratio.

The electrodes and the ground plate are connected to the preamplifier, a box-like structure with pin receptacles labeled for the input of cathode, anode, and ground. The purpose of the preamplifier is to increase the magnitude of the signals taken from the electrodes without requiring long leads (wires) from them. In place of long unshielded wires or leads, the preamplifier has a shielded cable of sufficient length to reach the subject being tested and not incur the distortions of long leads and the influences of surrounding currents that would distort the signals. A good preamplifier must have low electronic noise levels and it should have high input impedance and differential amplification with high *common mode rejection*. The latter will be discussed later.

Electronic noise (unwanted electrical messages) is always a part of any instrument, and it does not contribute to the identification of useful biologic data. Electronic noise may develop from within the instrument, and the better the design of the amplifier, the less noise there will be. External sources of noise are called interference or artifacts. These may arise from fluorescent lighting, wall power outlets, dimmer switches, poor grounding within the electrical circuits in the building, and broadcast radio signals within range of the patient. When internal noise is smaller than the biologic signal, the distortion may not prevent accurate recognition of the biologic EMG signal. This becomes critical when the signal is extremely small: eg, a sensory evoked response, which will be less than 10 μV. The internal electronic noise may be 20 μV, thereby overshadowing the sensory response and making it invisible. A technique known as averaging is used to record only the signal that is always taking place at the same time and rejecting the signals that are occurring

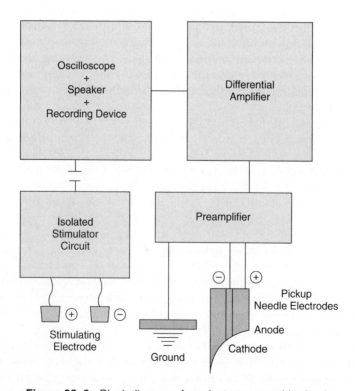

Figure 23–3. Block diagram of an electromyographic circuit.

randomly. Once the small signals leave the electrodes and are conducted to the amplifier, their power and size is such that the smaller internal noise is no longer a major source of distortion. Thus, the electrodes used and the quality of the preamplifier are the most important factors for minimizing the distortion of the biologic signal.

Another important property of the preamplifier is the proper match between the impedance of the electrode system and the impedance of the preamplifier. *Impedance* is defined as the combined effect of resistance capacitance, and inductance of any circuit. It is desirable for the electrodes to have low impedance at the site of the signal pickup; however, at the terminals of the preamplifier, it is essential to have an extremely high impedance. In simpler words, the signal should be conducted, unhampered, from the source to the amplifier, where it should not be conducted but, in actuality, stopped from conduction. It also is important for the impedance of the two terminals to be well matched. If there is a mismatch, the current will move into the terminal of lower impedance and thereby create a drop in voltage. Because voltage or electromotive pressure is the signal being measured, any drop will distort the signal markedly.

When dealing with biologic signals, one is frequently looking at alternating voltages and currents. This means that the EMG circuit must deal with Ohm's law, where current is equal to voltage divided by impedance. The formula would be stated as

$$I = E/Z,$$

where the letter Z is impedance. Because the frequency also changes, the factor of inductance must also be accounted for. The ideal preamplifier should have high input impedance to have the least amount of distortion and loss of amplitude, which would be the voltage of the signal. High impedance is defined as high resistance and small capacitance.

Differential amplification is the capacity of the preamplifier to amplify selectively the signals that are confined to the input exploring and reference electrodes as they relate to the ground plate. Because differential amplification concerns the response to minute voltage differences between the two points noted previously, the resistance, size, and interface of the exploring and reference electrodes should be as similar as possible to the tissue being explored. Because voltage can be likened to pressure and current can be likened to the flow of water, it is evident that restricting the flow of water increases the pressure. Conversely, opening the restriction reduces the pressure quickly. The latter is referred to as a voltage drop and results in large distortions of the biologic signal being measured.

Differential amplification occurs when voltage signals affect the exploring electrode differently from the reference electrode as each of these relate to the ground. Much larger voltages, such as those found in house current, will not be amplified because they affect both exploring electrode and reference electrode simultaneously with the same amount of voltage despite the fact that the voltage is thousands of times higher. This results in high common mode rejection.

A *calibration signal* is usually available that will display a known signal, which can be used as a reference to measure the biologic signals against. This is crucial for reliable and consistent measurements of these tiny biologic signals.

The amplifier receives the preamplified signal, which the examiner can increase or decrease according to the needs of the particular study being conducted. The control on the face of the ENMG usually is termed sensitivity, voltage, or gain control. The EMG signals are measured in microvolts; therefore, one would select a gain or sensitivity setting for EMG at 100 μV. In a motor nerve conduction study, one might set the gain at 5000 μV. In conducting a sensory evoked test, a typical gain or sensitivity setting would be 10 μV.

In an effort to reduce distortion, the *frequency bandwidth* or cycles per second (Hz) over which the amplifier must operate varies for particular studies. If one is conducting sensory studies of conduction, it is unnecessary to extend the frequency band too far in the high range, whereas EMG requires a low-frequency as well as a high-frequency range to detect the wide range of signals being generated in normal and pathologic states. Electronic filters are often used to remove some characteristically annoying signals such as 60 cycle or 60 Hz wall currents.

The amplified display on the cathode–ray oscilloscope is then filtered sufficiently to avoid distorting the display or reducing its amplitude so that it is possible to measure critical components of the waveforms displayed. The displayed signal can then be transferred to a printer for a paper display that can be stored as a permanent record.

In an effort to eliminate 60-cycle interference (found commonly from house current), inexpensive EMG feedback devices limit the low frequencies to no lower than 100 Hz. Consequently, this results in cutting out all of the MUPs less than 100 Hz, which includes the small motor units that fire from 5 to 15 Hz.

Amplification of the signal will decrease for alternating current test signals at frequencies above and below the frequency bandwidth of the instrument. The bandwidth limit consists of the frequencies that reduce or attenuate the amplitude 30% or more from that encountered in the midband region. Similarly, the amplifier should have a sufficiently rapid rise time of 20 microseconds and a much slower decay time of at least 8 milliseconds.

Amplifier noise can become extremely troublesome when conducting a sensory study, which requires high amplification. The electronic noise usually present in newer models of EMG, when shorting out the input terminals, is between 4 to 7 μV. This amplifier noise will increase geometrically with the frequency bandwidth. Thus, restricting the frequency bandwidth will reduce the amplifier noise, permitting better identification of the evoked sensory response. Another factor that increases noise is the electrical resistance in the electrode circuit connecting the patient to the preamplifier. This underscores the need to reduce skin resistance and to use relatively short wire leads to connect the active biologic signal source to the preamplifier. Because this biologic signal is an alternating one, the conducting leads must not offer excessive impedance: ie, the combined effect of capacitance and inductance plus the electrical resistance of the patient circuit. It is essential to have low-impedance conducting signals from the patient through the leads to the amplifier, after which the amplifier circuit should offer high input impedance so that the voltage will not drop asymmetrically and thereby distort the biologic signal. If electrode paste accidentally enters one terminal but not the other, the terminals would not be matched for impedance. Therefore, the difference between the terminals would be amplified, resulting in an error signal on the oscilloscope. This distortion, known as a voltage drop, attenuates (reduces) the rapid parts of the waveform and leaves the slower components unchanged. The result is a major waveform distortion.

Time is a critical variable to measure in an ENMG. Therefore, a mechanism of controlling this variable must be used. This setting is regulated by a control usually labeled as "sweep speed" or "time base." The sweep speed is on the X axis and can be compared to the calibration signal placed on the screen when measuring the displayed waveforms. Typical settings for the *sweep speed* would be: EMG at 10–20 ms/cm (X axis), motor nerve conduction at 5 ms/cm, and sensory nerve conduction at 2 ms/cm.

The nerve conduction mode uses a stimulation circuit that is electronically isolated from the differential amplifier. In addition, the nerve conduction velocity mode is synchronized so that the sweep is initiated at the left-hand margin of the screen. This provides for a consistent location of the stimulus and the evoked responses. Without this synchronization, it would be necessary to measure each distance and anticipate where the response will appear on the screen. Its appearance would not be consistently at the same place on the screen as it is currently with the synchronized *isolated circuits.*

Modern ENMG devices have *storage oscilloscopes* that can "freeze" the waveform on the screen for detailed study. Generally, both EMG and nerve conduction velocity tracings can be stored and, in turn, printed on paper for permanent records.

Another technological advance that is incorporated in the ENMG is the *averager.* This device only amplifies signals that arrive within a given time period, which the examiner selects to approximate the time frame in which the signal is expected to arrive. Only signals that appear regularly in that window (time frame) are amplified. This makes it possible to identify extremely small potentials even though much larger potentials are present but fall outside of this time window.

The following are common sources of distortion of electrical signals from the patient to the apparatus:

- Lead wire of an electrode is partially broken
- Lead wire moves during recordings
- Wrong electrodes are connected to the amplifier input
- Stimulator electrodes are near or on the recording electrodes
- The ground electrode is loose
- Dried electrode paste is on the surface electrode
- Too much electrode paste is creating a bridge between poles
- Power cords are plugged into a receptacle near the patient
- Fluorescent lighting is in the testing area
- Electronic dimmers are nearby or on same circuit
- Audio that is too high is causing feedback
- Citizen-band radio or taxi broadcaster is nearby
- Radio or television transmitter is nearby
- Diathermy or other electronic equipment is nearby
- Wall receptacle is poorly grounded
- Examining table is metal or a wheelchair is ungrounded

It is important to avoid having patients come into contact with the casing of the ENMG because there may be small *leakage currents* coming from the case. The ENMG has the power cord attached at the rear of the unit, which reduces the possibility of contact with the patient considerably. The shock from this source, although small, could be serious if the patient's cardiac status is unstable or if the patient has an implanted pacemaker.

Stimulators should always have the intensity control returned to zero so that a large stimulus will not be delivered to the patient inadvertently. When stimulating, the intensity should be gradually advanced to avoid an excessive amount of stimulation. Care should be exercised so that the limb to be stimulated is not on a metal or conductive surface because this may lead to unpredictable effects on the patient.

The final common pathway is the anterior horn cell and its axon and all the muscle fibers attendant to it. The all-or-none law assures that once the anterior horn cell is activated by threshold stimuli, the axon also will be fired with the same all-or-none response, and, presuming there is no neuromuscular junction deficit, the action potential will be transmitted to the muscle membrane, resulting in the activation of all (8–1400) muscle fibers of that particular motor unit. The spread of the end-plate zones on the skeletal muscles will be varied and, in some muscles, will represent a wide distribution when comparing the end-plate zone to the total length of the muscle fibers. When an EMG electrode is inserted within a muscle and it detects action potential sweeping along the course of the muscle membranes, it actually blends the individual action potentials together and forms a type of average called the *motor unit potential* (MUP). The duration of the MUP is determined by the spread of the end-plate zone in relation to the total length of the muscle fiber. For example, the abductor pollicis brevis muscle has an end-plate zone that is 50% of the total length of the fibers of that muscle. Conversely, the biceps brachii has an end-plate zone that is only 10% of the total length of the muscle fibers, which results in a shorter duration of the MUP than in the abductor pollicis brevis muscle (Fig. 23–4).

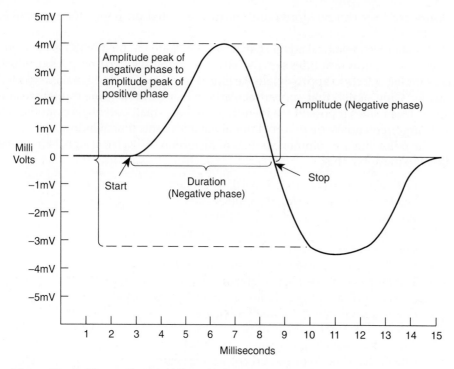

Figure 23–4. Motor unit potential; evoked response. Determination of amplitude and duration as seen on the oscilloscope.

The amplitude or size of the MUP is determined by the circumference of the muscle fibers with respect to the cross section of the total muscle. Therefore, larger diameter fibers in a small muscle will result in a higher amplitude MAP in that muscle when sampled electromyographically.

During voluntary contraction of a muscle, the small motor units within the muscle are activated first and will increase their frequency of firing from approximately 5 per second to 10 or 15 per second. As the smaller unit increases its rate of firing and more force is being called for, larger and larger motor units are then added, and they in turn increase their rate of firing. This process is referred to as the size principle of motor unit recruitment, as identified by Hennemann et al.[4] By observing the increased rate of firing, one can estimate the degree of effort. If a person has only a few motor units available to fire actively, and they are "asked" to contract the muscle with greater and greater force, the frequency of firing will increase in those available motor units. But if a person is feigning weakness, the rate of firing remains stable. Confusing the person with reciprocating motions usually reveals increased rates of firing in the muscle in question. DeLuca et al believed that the highest rate of firing of motor unit potentials would range from 35 to 45 per second, during maximal effort.[5]

If short-duration pulses (0.1–0.2 milliseconds) of direct current are delivered to a nerve trunk, more and more axons are activated, beginning with the larger diameter fibers first, as the intensity of the stimulus becomes stronger. When the nerve fibers are fired simultaneously, an action potential that is an amalgamation of all active units within the muscle is formed and is therefore a *compound action potential* (CAP). As was noted previously, a greater-than-maximal, or a supramaximal, stimulus is used to assure that all nerve fibers are activated, thereby providing a basis for later comparison of the active fibers within a given nerve trunk.

Instrumentation

All electromyographs used in clinical investigations have two basic components: the nerve conduction mode and the electromyography mode. One crucial element in the EMG is the differential amplifier, which enables the detection of extremely small voltages within the muscle. The most important fact to grasp is that the differential amplifier discriminates differences in voltage between two points. Because it is concerned with response to minute differences in voltage between two points in the muscle, its input terminals are designed to have an extremely high impedance to the flow of current. Because voltage is likened to pressure and current is likened to the flow of water, it is evident that restricting the flow of water will increase the pressure and, conversely, removing the restriction would reduce the pressure quickly. The latter is referred to as a voltage drop and should be avoided during electrical measurement because it distorts the signal.

Another aspect of differential amplification is that the small voltages within tissue can be identified even in the midst of much higher voltages (eg, wall outlets, lights, diathermy units and other electrical devices). The reason the small voltages can still be detected rather than be drowned out by the larger wall currents is that the differential amplifier compares both the active electrode and the dispersive electrode to ground and thus can ignore the larger voltages that are common to both poles or electrodes as well as the ground. Therefore, voltages common to all three are rejected; this is called common-mode rejection ratio (CMRR). A good EMG should have a CMRR of 1000:1. This will lead to the ability to detect small voltages even in the field of extremely high voltages.

When conducting an EMG, the size and duration of the wave forms or action potentials will be important items. The horizontal axis provides a time base that can be modified by the control on the EMG called the sweep speed or the time base. The vertical axis is used to determine the *amplitude* or size of the action potential. When the sweep speed is on 5, each centimeter on the horizontal axis has 5 milliseconds (or 5/1000 of a second). If the sweep is changed to 10, each centimeter is equal to 10 milliseconds.

The vertical axis is used to determine amplitude and is also called the gain on the EMG. The gain or voltage can be changed. If the gain is set at 5 mV, it means that each vertical centimeter attained by the action potential will be 5000 μV in amplitude. Similarly, if the gain setting is changed to 100, it implies that each vertical centimeter is equivalent to 100 μV. When the gain has a higher number, it is less sensitive, and, when the gain has a lower number, it is more sensitive. If a gain setting of 2000 is used and a CAP attains a height of 2 cm, it is evident that the amplitude is 4000 μV or 4 mV.

The nerve conduction mode uses a stimulation circuit that is electronically isolated from the differential amplifier. In addition, the nerve conduction velocity mode is synchronized so that the sweep is initiated at the left-hand margin of the screen. This provides for a consistent location of the stimulus and the evoked responses. Without this synchronization, one would have to measure each distance and also expect it at different locations.

An essential element of an ENMG is control of the frequency band to which it responds. Action potentials of short duration require a high-frequency response capability. If the frequency capability of the instrument is not high enough, the amplification of high-frequency action potentials will suffer. Conversely, if the low frequencies are cut off, low frequency potentials will be distorted. In an effort to eliminate 60-cycle interference, inexpensive EMG feedback devices limit the low frequencies to more than 100 Hz. This results in cutting out the frequencies that are less than 100 Hz, which includes most, if not all, of the small motor unit discharges at a frequency of 5 to 15 Hz. Amplification will decrease for alternating current test signals at frequencies above and below the range, or band, of the instrument. The bandwidth limit consists of the frequencies that reduce the amplitude 30% of the midband value. Similarly, the amplifier must have a sufficiently rapid rise time of 20 microseconds and a slower decay time of 8 milliseconds.

Another troublesome factor that can lead to difficulty administering an ENMG exam is amplifier noise. This noise may become especially evident when conducting a sensory conduction study because it involves extremely high amplification. The electronic noise that is typically present with the input terminals shorted is between 4 to 7 μV. The noise increases geometrically with the increase in the frequency bandwidth. Therefore, restriction of the bandwidth reduces the noise on the signal. Another factor that increases noise is the electrical resistance in the circuit connecting the patient to the amplifier. This underscores the need to reduce skin resistance and to use relatively short leads to connect the active areas to the amplifier. Because the signal is an alternating one, the conducting leads must not offer excessive impedance, which is the combined effect of capacitance and inductance as well as the electrical resistance of the circuit. It is desirable to have low impedance from the patient through the leads up to the amplifier, after which the amplifier circuit should offer high impedance so that the voltage signal will not be distorted. If electrode paste enters one of the input terminals, it may result in a large shunt capacitance, which would attenuate or reduce the rapid parts of the waveform and leave the slower components unchanged. The result would be a major wave form distortion.

Environmental temperature has a significant influence on nerve conduction values. These temperatures have an even greater influence when circulatory disturbance or paralysis of musculature is present.

The relationship between temperature and conduction velocity is linear for the range between 29 to 38° C. When beyond this range in temperature, the conduction velocity increases 5% per degree increase or decreases the same percentage per degree decrease. For example, in nerve conducting between 40–60 meters per second, if the environmental temperature decreases 1° C, the conduction velocity will decrease 2 to 3 meters per second. The distal latency from wrist to hand muscle will increase by 0.3 millisecond per degree of cooling for both median and ulnar nerves.

The skin temperature is often taken if these changes in conduction velocity would prove to be critical when interpreting the results on a particular patient. If testing is performed in an environment with a variable temperature, the skin temperature, the conduction velocity, and the latency values should be recorded at the same time.

NERVE CONDUCTION STUDIES

Motor Nerve Conduction

To study the conduction of nerve fibers that supply muscle fibers, it is necessary to place surface electrodes over the muscle to pick up the response. The cathode (black) pickup electrode is placed over the center of the belly (motor point) of the muscle selected for study and the anode (red) is placed distally on top of the muscle tendon junction. It is important to clean the skin of any oils or dirt to reduce skin impedance to an acceptable level (usually 5000 Ω or less) under each electrode. A moderate amount of electrode paste is placed on each cathode and anode as well as on the ground plate. Then, the electrodes are secured with enough tape to assure that they will not slip or move during the stimulation (Fig. 23–5). It is best to have patients recline for the test because some may become lightheaded or feel faint if upright. This posture also facilitates relaxation of muscles.

With the pickup electrodes in place and with the ground plate fixed between them and the stimulating electrodes, the nerve conduction mode of the ENMG instrument is chosen. This mode typically provides a gain setting of 2 to 5 mV per centimeter division and a sweep speed of 5 milliseconds per centimeter division. The stimulus frequency most commonly is 1 per second; however, one can activate the stimulus every time one presses on a foot switch. The duration of the stimulus will depend to some extent on the state of conductivity of the nerve: that is, a diseased nerve will require a longer duration than does a healthy nerve. One typically begins with a duration of 0.1 millisecond; if no response is obtained, the duration is increased to 0.2 millisecond.

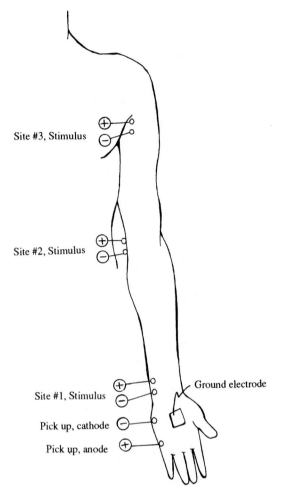

Site #3, Stimulus

Site #2, Stimulus

Site #1, Stimulus

Ground electrode

Pick up, cathode

Pick up, anode

Figure 23–5. Placement of pickup and stimulating electrodes over the ulnar nerve on the left arm (anterior view) at three sites.

A distal point is selected on the nerve to be tested next, and the cathode (black) is placed distal to the anode (red). The stimulator handle contains an intensity control that advances the stimulus gradually while pressing the electrodes firmly into the skin over the nerve. Once a response is obtained, the stimulus intensity is advanced gradually until no further increase in the amplitude of the response wave is noted. When the intensity is then advanced 10% more, the stimulus is termed a supramaximal one. This is done to assure that all conducting fibers are included in the study of that nerve. Once an optimal response is obtained, the response is stored on the screen. Then a marker, called a cursor, is moved out from the left side of the screen to the beginning of the takeoff of the negative (up-going) phase of the response wave. This duration is called the distal latency and is measured in milliseconds: it is the time required for the stimulus to be conducted along the motor nerves to the muscle fibers, from which they are picked up and displayed as the response wave. The *amplitude* of that response is measured from baseline to the peak of the negative phase and is recorded as millivolts (see Fig. 23–1).

Then a second site is chosen on the same peripheral nerve and, again, a *supramaximal stimulation* is conducted and the response wave is stored on the oscilloscope screen. The second, proximal latency is recorded by moving the cursor to the second response wave when it first departs from the baseline in an upward sweep. Similarly, the amplitude is again measured from baseline to the peak of the negative phase (see Fig. 23–1).

A tape measure is used to determine the distance from the distal cathode stimulus site to the proximal cathode site, which is determined in millimeters. The skin temperature is then recorded at a distal site on the limb being tested.

The steps required to test motor nerve conduction can be summarized as follows:

1. Select the instrument component—the nerve Conduction Mode.
2. Use a sensitivity setting of 2–5 mV.
3. Use a sweep speed of 5 ms/division.
4. Use a stimulus rate of 1/s and a duration of 0.1 ms.
5. Position the patient in the supine position with the limb supported.
6. Prepare the skin for recording electrodes over the muscle.
7. Place the cathode (negative) recording electrode over the center of the belly of the muscle.
8. Place the anode (positive) recording electrode over the tendon of the same muscle.
9. Place the ground electrode between the stimulating and recording electrodes.
10. Tape all recording electrodes securely in place.
11. Apply the stimulating electrodes with the cathode (negative) directed distally toward the muscle.
12. Increase the intensity of the stimulus progressively.
13. Continue to increase 10% more once the impulse is maximal to assure that no axons are left out.
14. Record three responses from the distal point.
15. Record three responses from the proximal point.
16. Measure the distance from the proximal to the distal points.
17. Record the proximal and distal latencies and the measurements from the proximal to distal points.
18. Determine the skin temperature over the distal limb and record it.
19. Calculate the conduction velocity of that segment of the nerve.
20. Repeat the previous steps for the next proximal segment of the nerve.

To calculate the conduction velocity of motor components, the distal latency is subtracted from the proximal latency to obtain the time of conduction through that segment of the nerve. This conduction time is then divided into the distance measured (in millimeters) to determine the conduction velocity of that segment of the nerve. That is,

$$\text{Conduction velocity} = \frac{\text{distance (mm)}}{\text{conduction time (ms)}}$$

More than two points can be studied in the same manner if they are accessible to the electrode through the skin. By studying each segment, one can compare different segments to each other to determine if there is relative slowing in one portion versus the other or if there is a drop in amplitude in one area versus another. Each laboratory should conduct tests on a series of normal subjects to determine the normal values for each segment. It also is helpful to print these values on the reporting form. A sample reporting form for nerve conduction is shown in Fig. 23–17 on page 359).

Sensory Nerve Conduction

Because all fibers in a nerve trunk are stimulated simultaneously when electrical pulses of more than threshold are applied, differentiation of motor and sensory components of the peripheral nerve is achieved by placement of the pick-up electrodes. To determine the sensory components of a peripheral nerve, it is customary to place ring electrodes around the fingers for the specific upper extremity nerves to be tested and over skin areas of the feet or toes for selected lower extremity nerves. Obviously, the motor components also are stimulated when the entire nerve trunk is stimulated; however, removing the skin pick-up area from the area of discharge from the muscle provides a distinct signal that represents the sensory or skin innervation for that nerve.

Orthodromic procedure. Sensory axons normally, or orthodromically, conduct impulses from the periphery to the center of the body. Therefore, one can stimulate on the digits and place pick-up electrodes over the nerve trunk at one or more sites to permit determination of sensory conduction velocity (as in motor nerve conduction testing). This orthodromic *sensory nerve action potential* (SNAP) response will be of much lower amplitude than the motor response; therefore, the sensory conduction mode will use 10 to 20 µV gain settings and a sweep speed of 2 milliseconds. Because electronic noise will be close to the signal response, it is helpful to reduce the upper part of the frequency band and compress it between 30 and 200 Hz. This narrow frequency band provides an optimal amplification of the signal.

Antidromic procedure. Sensory studies also can be conducted in an antidromic fashion; that is, against the normal flow of the sensory signal. In this situation, the pick–up electrode is the ring around the finger (cathode proximal and anode distal). The stimulating electrode is the same one used in motor component studies. In both orthodromic and antidromic studies, the amplitude is measured from the takeoff from baseline to the peak of the negative spike. Typical upper extremity amplitudes are 20 to 50 µV, whereas lower extremity values range from 5 to 15 µV.

The *distal latency* is determined in the same manner that it is determined in motor conduction, subtracted from the proximal latency of the sensory response, then divided into the distance measured between the cathode stimulation sources when performed antidromically. If orthodromic, the two times of conduction would be compared to the distance in millimeters from one pickup site to the other. One should expect the amplitudes to be much lower in orthodromic than antidromic sensory studies. For this reason, sensory studies are subject to more interference and technical errors than are the larger amplitude motor studies.

The steps required to test sensory nerve conduction can be summarized as follows:

1. Place the patient in a comfortable supine position.
2. Prepare the skin by cleaning it with alcohol.
3. Place the recording rings or disc electrodes over the cleaned recording and stimulating electrode sites.
4. Place the ground plate between the stimulating and recording electrodes.
5. Follow the orthodromic technique of sensory testing by (1) placing stimulating rings or clips on digits with the cathode (negative) proximal, (2) placing the recording electrodes over the nerve that is being stimulated with the cathode distal, and placing the ground plate between the stimulating and recording electrodes.
6. Follow the antidromic technique of sensory testing by (1) placing the recording electrodes on digits or the distal portion of the nerve being tested with the cathode proximal and the anode distal, (2) placing stimulating electrodes on the distal segment of the nerve with the cathode distal and the anode proximal, and (3) placing the ground between the stimulating and recording electrodes.
7. Select the sensory nerve conduction mode with a 10 µV gain setting and a 2 millisecond sweep speed setting.
8. Stimulate distally and pick–up at the nerve at the two sites on the nerve in the orthodromic technique or stimulate on the nerve and pick-up from the distal site in the antidromic technique.
9. Record three tracings from each site.
10. Record the skin temperature over the distal limb.
11. Measure the distance between the stimulating and proximal recording electrode and the distal recording site (orthodromic technique).
12. The antidromic technique is the same as in motor nerve conduction.
13. Calculate the conduction velocity from the recorded proximal and distal latencies.
14. Record the latencies and the conduction velocity values on a chart for particular nerve in question.

Proximal conduction procedure. Selected peripheral nerves can be stimulated with the cathode directed proximally, the sweep speed reduced to 20 msec/division and the gain increased to 200 µVolts. With this arrangement one can evoke responses in the nerve so as to stimulate axons from distal to proximal. As stimulation of a nerve axon will be conducted in both the proximal and distal directions, the latter will be detected at the distal latency time and will be of large amplitude (eg, 8–12 mV) and is known as an M wave. A proximal conduction observed is an H reflex which is obtained through stimulation of the Posterior Tibial nerve (Fig. 23–6).

The F Wave. The technique for eliciting the F wave response is as follows:

1. Place the patient in a supine, relaxed position.
2. Select the nerve conduction mode on instrument.
3. Use sweep settings of 20 ms/division.
4. Use a gain setting of 200 µV.
5. Use the procedures outlined for motor nerve conduction with regard to skin preparation, electrode placement, and so on.
6. Reverse the position of the stimulating electrode so that the cathode is directed proximally.
7. Advance the stimulation progressively using the same frequency and du-

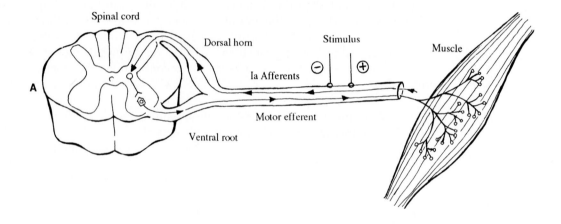

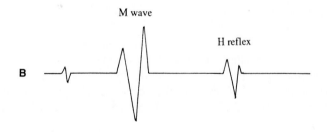

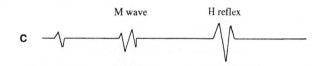

Figure 23–6. **(A)** An idealized H reflex under circumstances of diminishing stimulus intensity. **(B)** Both M and H responses at a threshold stimulus of 0.5 milliseconds duration and a frequency of less than 1 second. **(C)** The M wave decreases as the stimulus decreases. However, the H reflex remains constant in amplitude and duration with a stimulus of 0.5 milliseconds duration, but lower intensity at a frequency of 1 second.

ration as in motor nerve conduction. The M wave will appear at the motor latency on the left of the screen, and after several impulses a much smaller response of 50–150 μV will appear at a much longer latency.

8. Record eight long-latency F waves.
9. Measure the limb length from the seventh cervical vertebrae to the styloid process of the ulna.
10. Compare the proximal conduction to the conduction of the distal segment as a ratio of proximal to distal.
11. Compare the latency of one side to the latency of the other side and if no limb length discrepancy exists, use the longer F wave latency to indicate proximal slowing.

The *F wave latency* is believed to represent a type of echo reaction via the alpha motor neurons that Magladery et al[6] first noted and labeled the F wave. The F wave is called a wave because it does not involve any synaptic transmission. The impulse is believed to travel antidromically proximally in the alpha motor neuron to the cell body, then reflect back again to the motor axon to produce the extremely small and variable response wave in the muscle. If the dorsal roots (carrying sensory axons) are sectioned, the F wave is still readily elicited; therefore, it is assumed that the motor nerves are responsible for its conduction. However, whether the F wave is the product of some other mechanism, perhaps even conduction through other efferents or through afferents that enter the spinal cord through the ventral root is not completely resolved. The F wave latency is variable within a narrow range in normal individuals, and its amplitude also changes in the same individual. These may represent variability in the placement of the stimulating electrode during the test or other technical factors or the F wave could represent some form of multisynaptic transmission.

The F wave is readily obtained by using a supramaximal stimulus on the distal point of most peripheral nerves, and the frequency can be at one per second. This is not found with the H reflex testing, which requires submaximal stimulation at irregular and widely spaced intervals.

Because the F wave is believed to reflect the adequacy of conduction of the axons proximally, it is helpful for the determination of lesions that affect the proximal portion of the axons, such as the Guillain-Barré syndrome and thoracic outlet and nerve root compression lesions. It is helpful to compare the conduction of the distal segment to the proximal segment so that a peripheral (distal) neuropathy does not provide a false positive impression of proximal slowing if one looks only at the F wave conduction.

The H reflex. The H reflex has been studied extensively in clinical and physiologic investigations since it was first identified by Hoffman in 1918.[7] It was not designated the H reflex until the studies of Magladery[6] et al. The H reflex has been the subject of numerous articles over the past 40 years, and Crone, et al[8] and Leonard and Moritani[9] have advocated its use dynamically to determine the neural basis of movement disorders in neurologically impaired individuals. In the typical application in the clinical setting, the H reflex is used to determine the adequacy of the dorsal root containing the Ia afferents from the muscle spindle and to determine the excitability of the Alpha motor neuron pool.[10] Crone and Nielsen[11] found that H-eliciting stimulations that were less than 1 second apart do not allow for the complete recovery of the H reflex to baseline levels. Similarly, the H reflex is stimulated by submaximal stimuli of longer duration (0.5 milliseconds) so that a response is elicited in the thicker afferent (spindle afferents) fibers first and not primarily to elicit motor axons (see Fig. 23–6).

The technique for eliciting the H reflex is as follows:

1. Position the patient prone with the head in the midline.
2. Place the recording electrode (the cathode) over the midpoint between the length of the tibial nerve from the popliteal fossa and medial malleolus, on the medial gastrocnemius, and the anode over the Achilles tendon.

3. Tape the cathode and anode stimulating electrode over the posterior tibial nerve in the popliteal fossa with the cathode directed proximally.
4. Place the ground electrode between the recording and stimulating electrodes.
5. Set the oscilloscope screen to a gain of 500 μV and a sweep speed of 20 milliseconds.
6. Set the stimulus duration for 0.5 milliseconds and the frequency for less than 1 per second or for the best elicitation by the foot switch.
7. Advance the stimuli slowly and to less than maximal so that an M response is evoked. At a latency of nearly 27–32 milliseconds, an H response should be detected.
8. Decrease the intensity after the H response is obtained to the point where the amplitude of the M response declines by 30–40% and the H response remains unchanged.
9. Record the H wave latency and its amplitude from each side.
10. Compare the latencies with each other and with normal values.

Braddom and Johnson[12] found that submaximal stimulation of the posterior tibial nerve in the popliteal fossa in 100 normal subjects with a wide age range had a H reflex latency of 29.8 milliseconds, with an SD of 2.74 milliseconds. The latency is correlated with leg length and with age, so it can be said that H latency is equal to 9.14 + 0.46 leg length in centimeters + 0.1 age in years. When Braddom and Johnson measured the H latencies in 25 subjects of all ages, they noted that there was a mean difference of only 0.3 milliseconds. The standard error of the means from one leg to the other was 0.40 milliseconds. If one uses three standard errors from the mean, it would imply that 1.20 milliseconds would become a significant difference from one limb to the other. It is useful to use this test when compromise of the lumbosacral nerve root is suspected because it reveals S1 nerve root lesion deficits. Obviously, an absence of the response on one side but not on the other also would be indicative of an S1 compromise on that side. Schuchmann[13] conducted H reflex testing of unilateral L5 radiculopathy and found no significant differences in the latencies (see Fig. 23–6).

The H response can be readily obtained from other nerves in addition to the posterior tibial nerve when there is a lesion in the CNS, presumably because the inhibition is removed from the spinal cord circuit.

The blink reflex. Kugelberg[14] described the response of the orbicularis oculi to a stimulus over the brow on the opthalmic branch with an electrode. He noted an early ipsilateral blink reflex response with a latency of 12 milliseconds and a late response bilaterally in the orbicularis oculi muscles of 21 to 40 milliseconds. The blink reflex is currently elicited with an electrical pulse to the opthalmic branch of the trigeminal nerve at the supraorbital foramen; the impulse is then conducted to the anterior hind brain and synaptically transfers the stimulus to the facial nerve, where it is then conducted to the orbicularis oculi muscles for pickup by the electrodes. Kimura et al[15] described a technique in which two channels are used to determine the simultaneous response in both eyes to stimulation on each side independently.

The procedure for eliciting the blink reflex is as follows:

1. Place the patient in the supine position on the examining table.
2. Tape the cathode disk electrode to the outer border of each eye.
3. Tape the reference (anode) electrode to the outer wall of the nostril on each side.
4. Tape the ground electrode to the chin.
5. Select the nerve conduction mode for the oscilloscope.
6. Bring up two channels with the same settings of 200 μV gain and 20 millisecond sweep speed.
7. Stimulate the opthalmic branch at the supraorbital foramen with the cathode while the anode is on the brow.

8. Use a stimulus intensity of 50 V and a duration of 0.1 milliseconds. The ipsilateral response (R1)will be 10.6 milliseconds (SD, 0.82 milliseconds) in normal subjects. The bilateral second response (R2) will be found ipsilaterally at 31.3 milliseconds (SD, 3.3 milliseconds), and the contralateral R2 will be found at 31.6 milliseconds (SD, 3.78 milliseconds).

9. Repeat the stimulation from the opposite supraorbital site to obtain R1 and R2 responses ipsilaterally and contralaterally from that side.

10. Compare both sides for symmetry; a difference of three standard deviations from one side to the other is considered significant.

The *blink reflex* test is useful for testing individuals with facial palsy. This test can activate the proximal portion of the facial nerve, where it is frequently impaired through the facial canal in the temporal bone. A complete loss of conduction leads to an absence of ipsilateral responses but not of the contralateral responses because the trigeminal nerve is unimpaired. If conduction slows, the ipsilateral response will be prolonged, but the latency of the contralateral one will be normal.

The blink reflex also has potential value for testing individuals with blepharospasm or hemifacial spasm. It has been used to document facial and trigeminal involvement in people with acoustic neuromas.[16] Other applications are being investigated for trigeminal neuralgia and migraine headaches.

Repetitive stimulation of the neuromuscular junction. An older method of testing the neuromuscular junction used high-frequency stimulation of more than 50 Hz, which was extremely uncomfortable. The technique has been supplanted by one described by Desmedt, a series of pulses applied at two pulses per second, which results in a significant decrement after the fourth pulse and a return to initial values from the fourth through the tenth pulse. Intercurrent exercise is applied after the first train of 10 pulses. Immediately after the exercise of the muscle being tested, another train of 10 pulses is applied at two per second.[17]

Summary

Nerve conduction studies should always be based on sound clinical judgments, and they are actually an extension of the physical examination of the patient. As Brooke[18] suggested, you should listen to patients because they are trying to tell you what is wrong. The selection of the testing is determined by the review of the patient's history and physical findings. Nerve conduction studies depend on exacting technique and careful recording of data. The quality of the instrumentation is crucial and staff in each laboratory should establish their own normal values.

The interpretation of the results of nerve conduction studies depends on the examiner's knowledge of neurophysiology and neuropathology. For example, a diabetic neuropathy leads to demyelination that results in slowing of conduction, whereas an alcoholic toxic neuropathy leads to degenerative changes in the axon, resulting in a reduction in the amplitude of the evoked responses. Some disorders of the peripheral nerve may not exhibit changes in the periphery if they are found initially in the proximal region of the nerve, such as in the Guillain-Barré syndrome. However, the F wave, the H reflex, or both may be delayed or absent in the same subjects because the ventral roots are implicated in this disease.

Common anatomic variations such as the Martin-Gruber anastomosis between the median and ulnar nerves in the forearm must be considered. Another variation may occur in the peroneal nerve in the lower leg. Sensory symptoms are often inconsistent with textbook configurations, and, because there is much variation in this area, the examiner should not reach the hasty conclusion that the patient is not telling the truth. Also, symptoms such as numbness and hyperesthesia are frequently confusing to the examiner depending on the words a patient uses to describe his or her symptoms.

A neuropractic lesion (one that results in loss of conduction at one location on the nerve) at the elbow, will not reveal any loss of conduction unless one stimulates through that segment. One major deficit in nerve conduction testing is the

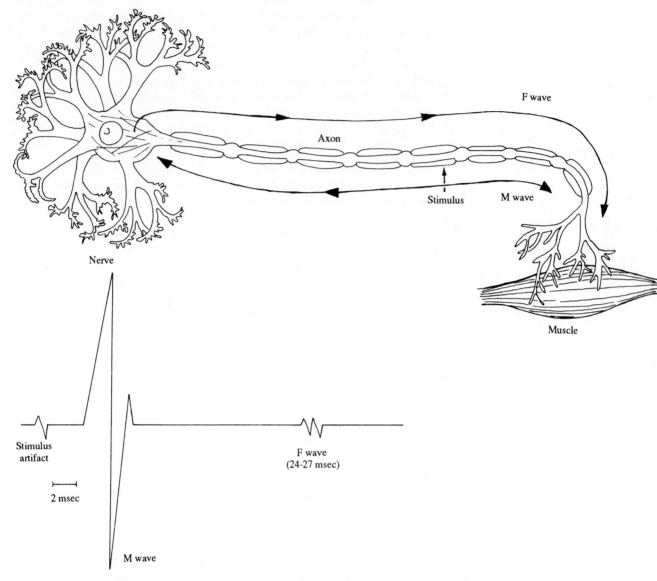

Figure 23–7. Representation of the M wave and F wave in the ulnar nerve of a young adult.

problem of whether the available segments of a given nerve have been studied sufficiently. Although a nerve may be transected completely, it can still conduct impulses for 72 hours after the lesion, but it will not conduct across the site of the transection. Use of statistical comparisons should not replace sound clinical judgment as well as a comparison from one limb to the other and between one nerve and another. Differences in amplitude are unreliable to a degree, but a difference of more than 10% would be of consequence if the study were performed in a standardized manner for each limb. A reduction in amplitude would be found when axons have been eliminated or have stopped conducting because this would result in a loss of many more muscle fibers from the motor unit. In an acute lesion, the loss of one axon would result in 6–700 muscle fibers (motor unit ratio); therefore, 10 axons would result in a loss of 60–7000 muscle fibers. When a lesion has been present for several months, some sprouting of neurons from other healthy ones begin to take over the denervated territory by collateral sprouting, thus reducing the impact on the amplitude to some extent and increasing the numbers of phases producing a SLAP potential (Fig. 23–8).

The duration of the CMAP will be prolonged if the conduction velocity within the nerve trunk is variable. This may be the first sign of axonal degeneration in

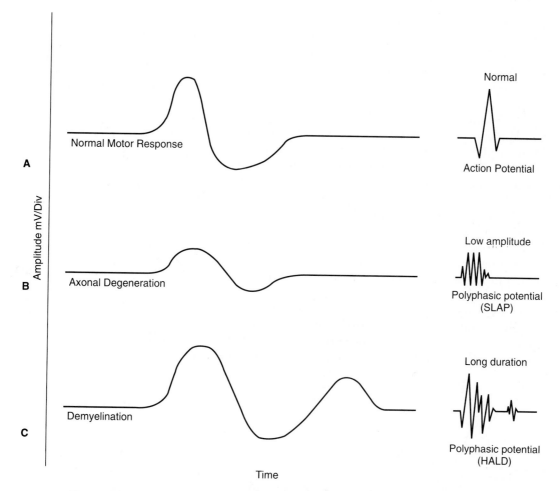

Figure 23–8. Effects of demyelination and axonal degeneration on the evoked motor response and the electromyogram. Axonal degeneration results in reduced amplitude of the evoked response and low amplitude EMG potentials (SLAP), whereas the response from demyelination produces a prolonged duration and a complex EMG potential that also is of longer duration. (**A**) Normal action potential. (**B**) Low short duration amplitude polyphasic potential (SLAP). (**C**) Long high amplitude duration polyphasic potential (HALD).

peripheral nerves affected by Guillain-Barré syndrome or another progressive demyelinating disease of the peripheral nerves. These *demyelinating diseases* also may produce focal slowing of conduction of peripheral nerves; thus, it is important to test more than one segment in nerves that are suspected victims of this type of disorder (see Fig. 23–8).

Prolongation of the distal latency of a nerve may occur with localized compression of that nerve. A common site of compression is the medial nerve through the carpal tunnel or the posterior tibial nerve through the tarsal tunnel. Other disorders will cause the distal portion of the nerve to die back. Sumner[19] implicated distal motor latencies as the most common early sign of toxic dying back of a nerve. They noted the wide variety of toxic agents that are encountered in this modern age, ranging from heavy metal poisoning to volatile industrial toxins; and the list steadily grows longer. These agents should be part of any screening for the etiology of a disturbance that is not readily explained by trauma or other means.

Electrophysiologic studies may uncover changes in conductivity that are not clinically apparent. Thus, it is important to distinguish between a *carpal tunnel syndrome* and a *dying-back neuropathy* caused by an industrial toxin. Clearly, if a nerve is dying back, surgical release of the transverse ligament will not improve nerve function (see Fig. 23–8).

Trauma to a peripheral nerve can result in a loss of conduction called neuropraxia or axonal degeneration; a loss of nerve continuity called axonotmesis; or discontinuity called neurotmesis. In a neuropraxia, the part of the nerve distal to the lesion responds to stimulation normally but will not produce a response distal to the site of neuropraxia when stimulating above it. With axonotmesis and neurotmesis, response distal to the lesion will be good until Wallerian degeneration takes place in the distal segment; then, the response will be nonexistent if the nerve is completely degenerated or partial if the degeneration is incomplete. During regeneration, some rudimentary conduction will take place but it will lag behind changes in the EMG. The EMG will be discussed in a later section (Fig. 23–9).

Failure at the neuromuscular junction results in a progressive declination of the amplitude with repetitive stimulation. When studying patients with an abnormally low amplitude with a single shock, a train of pulses at 2 Hz should be applied, along with intercurrent exercise, to rule out the *Eaton-Lambert phenomenon* or the myesthenic reaction.[20] In addition, other disorders of the neuromuscular junction result in variable amplitudes if the rate is faster than one per second. Whenever variable amplitudes are detected, repetitive stimulation testing should be instituted.

Good technique is the most important factor in avoiding errors in nerve conduction studies. One common source of error is the placement of electrodes and their fixation to the skin. The cathode or negative recording electrode is usually black and should be fixed securely with tape after the skin is cleaned with alcohol

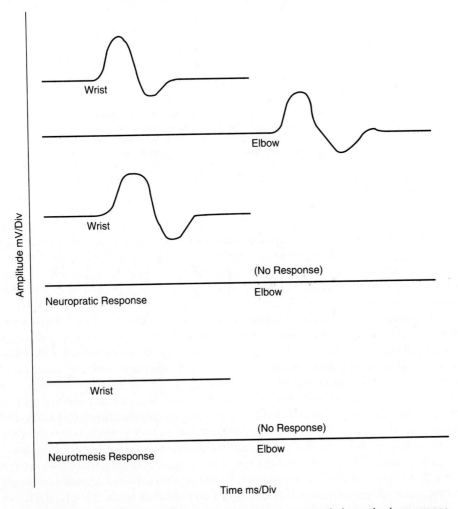

Figure 23–9. Comparison of neuropractic versus neurotmesis in evoked responses of the ulnar nerve at the level of the elbow. (See the normal values on the top tracing.)

to remove any dirt or oils. This electrode should be placed over the center of the belly of the muscle that is customarily the motor point of that muscle. If the active recording electrode is not over the motor point, it may result in an initial positive deflection followed by the negative one. This makes it extremely difficult to determine the precise point of takeoff of the evoked CMAP. The reference electrode is then placed on the musculotendinous junction of that same muscle. Placement of the reference electrode on the tendon junction will provide the best circumstance for reliable amplitude readings. If a person should perspire during the test, the tape may loosen and the amplitude of the recording will become decreased or fragmentary and may even prolong the duration of the CMAP. Similarly, if the electrode paste is bridged from one stimulating electrode to the other, a partial short may occur and cause incomplete stimulation of the nerve under the electrodes.

The use of too much electrode paste, permitting paste to bridge from the active to the reference or recording electrode will result in a distorted signal that is difficult to distinguish from a pathologic entity. Loosening of a ground electrode also will increase electronic noise *(interference)* with a greater distortion of baseline. Before calling the manufacturer's representative, check the electrodes for continuity and good fixation to the body.

Improperly placed stimulating electrodes leads to the need to increase the intensity until the stimulus is extremely painful for the patient. Adequate pressure over the nerve helps to place the electrode as close to the nerve as possible; however, if the pressure displaces the nerve from the vicinity of the stimulus, it decreases the effectiveness of the stimulus. Most studies begin with stimulation of a distal point on the nerve to avoid cross-stimulation from one nerve to another when close together (eg, in the median nerve at the wrist versus in the upper arm). If one is careful to duplicate the response wave at each site along the nerve, you are likely to be stimulating the same nerve throughout. This duplication process also may help when confronted by anomalous innervation such as Martin-Gruber anastomosis of median and ulnar nerves in the forearm or the accessory peroneal nerve, which is found posterior to the lateral malleolus.

Patients with a considerable amount of subcutaneous fat or with a bulky musculature may require longer duration pulses to stimulate the nerve adequately. In a large individual, this may become more evident in the proximal region of the nerve, and an increased pulse width should be used if the response wave changes substantially from the distal one, which involves less tissue. Conversely, if too much stimulation is applied, it may splash to other adjacent nerves, resulting in a confusing pattern of response. When stimulating with high-intensity stimuli, the stimulus might be conducted by volume conduction to the recording electrode which may produce a false signal that would produce a false result. This is most commonly encountered in sensory conduction studies in which the motor nerves are responding and the sensory are not. This results in motor responses that are volume conducted from the muscle to the finger tips, where the recording electrode is located, when recording antidromically.

Measurement is another source of error and should always be taken from pen marks on the skin to avoid errors. The measurements are taken from stimulating cathode to cathode or from stimulating cathode to the recording cathode. The use of calipers have been recommended; however, if metal tape is used carefully, it will result in reproducible results. The measurement should be over the course of the nerve, but this may be difficult to follow in some areas: for example, through the axilla or around the elbow for the ulnar nerve. In the latter, Nelson and Currier[21] recommend flexing the elbow to 90° at the elbow. Whatever position is used, it should be consistent from one test to the next. The shorter the distances, the greater the error. This is most evident in the ulnar nerve at the elbow, where the short distance from above the elbow to below the elbow can be avoided by measuring from above the elbow to the wrist and from below the elbow to the wrist. This will not only produce a less dramatic drop in conduction but also avoid an error of 1 cm resulting in a major error in the determination of conduction velocity.

For instance, an error of 1 cm over 10 cm is a 10% error, but a 1 cm error over 25 cm is a 4% error.

Distal latencies can be standardized to a greater extent through the process of having consistent distances from stimulating cathode to recording cathode. This distance is usually 8 cm for the hand and 14 cm for the foot.

When testing in cold climates, the examiner must allow for warming of limbs and insure that the environmental temperature is adequate to avoid a chill. If necessary, a heating pad or blanket can be applied for 10–15 minutes before testing begins. The recording of skin temperatures is essential in these circumstances to interpret the results in a reasonable fashion.

The patient's age also must be considered because the very young and the very old will have decreased conduction velocity. Other factors that affect conduction, such as peripheral vascular disease, which result in greater cooling of the part, also should be attended to. Determining whether a patient needs vascular surgery when vascular insufficiency and reduced conduction velocity are present is a difficult clinical problem. Paralysis from a cardiovascular accident also may decrease the limb temperature and thereby reduce the conduction velocity of the peripheral nerves within that limb.

During *repetitive stimulation* of a given muscle, unless both the stimulating electrodes and the recording electrodes are taped securely to the patient, any slight movement of either set of electrodes will cause a change in amplitude. Because a change in amplitude of 10% is considered pathologic in the repetitive stimulation technique described earlier, it is crucial to avoid movement of the electrodes during the recording. In addition, the limb should be strapped to a board to insure additional reliability of the measurements.

Nerve Conduction Studies of Specific Nerves

This section outlines the application of the conduction techniques to specific peripheral nerves. The instrument settings are outlined for each nerve, the position of the patient and the placement of electrodes are described, and the stimulation sites are indicated for the major sites used in most clinical situations. The sites of stimulation are labeled S1, S2, S3 and so forth. A more complete description of the conduction velocity procedure will be found elsewhere.

The following technical comments will be helpful to students as they review the procedures for testing specific nerves. When responses are evoked in the facial nerve, the patient may experience a flash of light with each pulse and should be counseled that this is natural, not harmful. The patient also may experience a transient taste of metal in the mouth from slight ionization of metal fillings in the teeth. Again, the patient should be told about this in advance. Only one site is available in the facial nerve; thus, the response to stimuli is recorded as a latency and compared with the opposite side regarding time as well as the amplitude of the CMAP.

Other peripheral nerves are recorded by the nerve and side, and each site of stimulation is labeled with the latencies from each one. As many sites as practical should be used to insure that the lesion is not proximal to the segment studied. The amplitude also is recorded for each site, and some examiners also record the temporal dispersion of the CMAP. In addition, the distance between each site is recorded, and the difference between sites is divided by the time difference between the two stimulus sites to arrive at the conduction velocity, which is also recorded for that segment.

The proximal latencies are recorded on the nerve conduction record for each nerve studied in this way. The H reflex and the amplitudes of the proximal response or reflex also are recorded. Some laboratories conduct an M conduction versus an F conduction to report a ratio of F to M by measuring the length of the limb and calculating a conduction velocity of the proximal latency versus the conduction velocity of the distal segment of the nerve. In this way, one can determine if the distal segment is faster than the proximal segment, which would pervade in a disorder of the proximal components and would be the reverse in the normal situation. All modern ENMG instruments have a variety of printing capabilities, and all the recordings can be displayed on paper with the calculated conduction velocity values, amplitudes, and CMAP waveforms.

Repetitive stimulation studies are reported as amplitude changes as compared with the initial single shock to the muscle being examined. Each series of 2 Hz pulses are calculated and displayed on a paper trace of the responses. The amplitudes that were obtained should be noted after the brief exercise as well.

MEDIAN NERVE (MOTOR)

Electromyograph Instrument Parameters

Filter settings/frequency response: 10,000–10 Hz
Sweep speed: 2–5 ms/division
Sensitivity/gain: 1,000–5,000 µV/division

Patient Position

The patient is positioned supine with the arm abducted approximately 45°. The forearm is fully supinated, and the wrist is in a neutral position.

Electrode Placement

The active recording electrode is positioned directly over the anatomic center of the abductor pollicis brevis muscle. The electrode is placed half the distance between the metacarpophalangeal joint of the thumb and the midpoint of the distal wrist crease.

The reference electrode is positioned **off** the abductor pollicis brevis muscle on the distal phalanx of the thumb over bone or tendon.

The ground electrode is firmly positioned on the dorsum of the hand between the active and stimulating electrodes.

Electrostimulation

Percutaneous electrostimulation is performed at the appropriate anatomic sites in the following order:

S1. Distal stimulation is performed at the wrist between the palmaris longus and flexor carpi radialis tendons. The cathode (negative) pole of the stimulator is placed proximal to the center of the active recording electrode on the abductor pollicis brevis muscle.

S2. Stimulation above the elbow is performed proximal and medial to the antecubital space and proximal to the elbow crease between the belly of the biceps muscle and the medial head of the triceps muscle. The stimulator is positioned just lateral to the brachial artery to minimize the possibility of inadvertent electrostimulation of the ulnar nerve.

S3. Proximal stimulation is performed in the axilla at least 10 cm proximal to the above elbow site and immediately lateral and anterior to the brachial artery.

Technical Comments:

Evoked muscle action potential responses from all three sites should be similar in waveform, amplitude, and duration of response.

Wrist-site stimulation voltage, stimulus pulse duration, or both should be increased gradually and monitored carefully because a high-voltage/long pulse-width stimulation at the wrist may volume conduct to the adjacent ulnar response.

The clinical response should be observed carefully to avoid mistaking an ulnar for a median response. At the wrist, median stimulation elicits thumb palmar abduction and opposition, whereas ulnar stimulation elicits thumb adduction and metacarpal phalangeal flexion. At stimulation sites above the elbow and axilla, median nerve stimulation elicits wrist flexion and radial deviation involving the flexor carpi radialis muscle, whereas ulnar nerve stimulation involves wrist flexion and ulnar deviation by contraction of the flexor carpi ulnaris muscle.

The wrist should be maintained in a neutral position while one measures forearm distance. Wrist flexion decreases and wrist extension increases the distance. All distance measurements should be taken with a metal tape measure. The measurement of distance should approximate the anatomic course of the nerve being tested.

ULNAR NERVE (MOTOR)

Electromyograph Instrument Parameters

Filter settings/frequency response: 10,000–10 Hz
Sweep Speed: 2–5 Ms/division
Sensitivity/Gain: 1,000–5,000 µV/division

Patient Position

The patient is positioned supine with the arm abducted to 90° and externally rotated with the elbow in midflexion at 60°–90°, palm up, and the wrist in a neutral position. When the patient is positioned supine, the palm of the hand faces the ceiling.

Electrode Placement

The active recording electrode is positioned on the ulnar border of the hand directly over the anatomic center of the abductor digiti minimi muscle at the point midway between the distal wrist crease and the crease at the base of the fifth digit at the level of the web space.

The reference electrode is positioned **off** the abductor digiti minimi muscle on the ulnar aspect of the fifth finger at the level of the web space.

The ground electrode is positioned on the dorsum of the hand between the active and stimulation electrodes.

Electrostimulation

Percutaneous electrostimulation is performed at the appropriate anatomic sites in the following order:

S1. Distal stimulation is applied at the wrist, medial **or** lateral to the flexor carpi ulnaris tendon. The cathode (negative) pole of the stimulator is placed proximal to the center of the active recording electrode on the abductor digiti minimi muscle (see Fig. 23–5).

S2. The below-elbow stimulation site is situated just distal to the medial humeral epicondyle in line with the cubital tunnel (a point midway between the medial epicondyle and the olecranon process) of the elbow and the distal wrist stimulation site.

S3. The above-elbow stimulation site is located at least 10 cm proximal to the below-elbow stimulation site in line with the ulnar groove of the elbow and the midportion of the shaft of the humerus in the axilla.

S4. The axilla stimulation site is located at least 10 cm proximal to the above elbow site at the midpoint of the humerus in the axilla.

Technical Comments

Evoked muscle action potential responses from all four sites should be similar in waveform, amplitude, and duration of response.

Wrist stimulation voltage, stimulus pulse duration, or both should be increased gradually and monitored carefully because high-voltage/long pulse-width stimulation at the wrist may volume conduct to the adjacent median nerve at the wrist, eliciting a volume-conducted median nerve response.

The upper extremity should be maintained in the same standard position while the test and measurements of segmental distances are performed.

A major source of error in performing segmental studies is stimulation below the elbow and across the elbow. The below-elbow stimulation site must allow access to the ulnar nerve **before** it enters the flexor carpi ulnaris muscle in the forearm. It is important to select an above-elbow stimulation site at least 10 cm proximal to the below-elbow stimulation site.

The above-elbow stimulation can be accomplished best by positioning the stimulation electrodes at the midhumeral area just posterior to the medial intermuscular septum. Care should be taken not to stimulate too anteriorly (causing contraction of the biceps muscle by direct stimulation or stimulation of the median nerve) or posteriorly (causing contraction of the triceps or failure to stimulate the ulnar nerve).

RADIAL NERVE (MOTOR)

Electromyograph Instrument Parameters

Filter settings/frequency response: 10,000–10 Hz
Sweep speed: 2–5 ms/division
Sensitivity/gain: 1,000–5,000 μV

Patient Position

The patient is positioned supine with the arm abducted approximately 45°. The elbow is slightly flexed and the forearm is fully pronated.

Electrode Placement

The active recording electrode is positioned over the extensor indicis proprius muscle of the dorsal forearm.

The reference surface electrode is positioned away from the extensor indicis proprius muscle on the dorsum of the hand.

The ground electrode is placed between the active and stimulating electrodes on the dorsal surface of the forearm.

Electrostimulation

Percutaneous electrostimulation is performed at the appropriate anatomic sites in the following order:

S1. Distal stimulation is applied at the forearm proximal to the active and ground electrodes. This site is approximately 8–10 cm proximal to the active electrode and just lateral to the extensor carpi ulnaris muscle.

S2. The elbow stimulation site is situated at or about the groove between the brachioradialis muscle and the biceps tendon approximately 6–10 cm proximal to the lateral epicondyle of the humerus.

S3. The axilla stimulation site is situated in the groove between the coracobrachialis muscle and the medial edge of the triceps muscle. (**Note:** The third stimulation is accomplished after the arm is externally rotated and the forearm is supinated.)

Technical Comments

This is a technically difficult test to perform. Surface or needle active (recording) electrodes can be used, but it is crucial in either case to obtain similar evoked responses from all stimulation sites. When using surface electrodes, the response commonly has an initial positive deflection. If so, this should be obtained at all sites for valid calculations. Then, the latency is measured at the same place for all three waveforms.

Any distal extensor muscle of the upper extremity innervated by the radial nerve can be used as a recording site. The extensor indicis proprius is the most distal. To localize this muscle, the examiner should palpate it and evaluate the function during extension of the index finger.

DEEP PERONEAL NERVE (MOTOR)

Electromyograph Instrument Parameters

Filter settings/frequency response: 10,000–10 Hz
Sweep speed: 2–5 ms/division
Sensitivity/gain: 500–2,000 μV/division

Patient Position

The patient is positioned in a comfortable, relaxed side-lying position facing away from the examiner. The hip and knee are slightly flexed, with the ankle positioned in neutral. A single pillow is placed between the patient's knees for comfort and to support the limb being examined.

Electrode Placement

The active recording electrode is positioned over the anatomic center of the extensor digitorum brevis muscle in the anterior, lateral aspect of the proximal midtarsal area of the foot.

The reference electrode is placed on the tendon of the extensor digitorum brevis muscle on the fifth toe.

The ground electrode should be positioned on the lateral or medial malleolus between the active and stimulating electrodes.

Electrostimulation

Percutaneous electrostimulation is performed at the appropriate anatomic sites in the following order:

S1. The nerve is stimulated initially below the head of the fibula and anterior to the neck of the fibula. The stimulator is positioned to approximate the anatomic course of the nerve around the neck of the fibula.

S2. Distal stimulation is applied at the anterior ankle proximal to the center of the active electrode situated on the extensor digitorum brevis muscle. The distal site at the anterior ankle is between the extensor digitorum longus and extensor hallucis longus tendons.

S3. The popliteal space stimulation site is at least 10 cm proximal to the fibular neck site. The peroneal nerve is situated in the lateral border of the popliteal space near the lateral hamstrings.

Technical Comment

Evoked muscle action potential responses from all three sites should be similar in waveform, amplitude, and duration of response.

When applying proximal stimulation in the popliteal fossa, the clinical response in the leg or calf should be monitored to avoid volume-conducted stimulation of the posterior tibial nerve. Ankle eversion ensures that the peroneal nerve is being stimulated, whereas plantar flexion of the ankle indicates stimulation of the tibial nerve.

Distal stimulation is performed approximately halfway between the malleoli, lateral to the extensor hallucis longus tendon, and just proximal to the level of the anterior tarsal tunnel. Occasionally, the response can be improved by stimulating more laterally to the extensor digitorum longus tendon. In obese patients, or in patients with edema or induration, the ankle response may be difficult to elicit. Increasing the stimulus intensity, the pulse duration, or both may overcome this difficulty.

POSTERIOR TIBIAL NERVE (MOTOR)

Electromyograph Instrument Parameters

Filter settings/frequency response: 10,000–10 Hz
Sweep speed: 2–5 ms/division
Sensitivity/gain: 1,000–5,000 μV/division

Patient Position

The patient is positioned prone with a single pillow placed under the ankles to allow slight flexion of the knees.

Electrode Placement

The active recording electrode is positioned over the abductor hallucis muscle, 1 cm inferior (toward the plantar surface) and 1 cm distal (toward the great toe) to the navicular.

The reference electrode is positioned distally on the abductor hallicus muscle tendon on the medial border of the great toe.

The ground electrode is positioned on the medial or lateral malleolus between the active and stimulating electrodes.

Electrostimulation

Percutaneous electrostimulation is performed at the appropriate anatomic sites in the following order:

S1. Stimulation at the ankle is performed at a point halfway between the medial malleolus and the Achilles tendon proximal to the center of the active recording electrode and proximal to the flexor retinaculum.
S2. Proximal stimulation is performed at the popliteal fossa slightly lateral to the midline along the flexor crease of the knee.

Technical Comments

The prone position makes this test more convenient for the examiner. The electrical and clinical responses should be closely monitored, especially during proximal stimulation. Care must be taken to ensure that all evoked muscle action potential responses to ankle and popliteal stimulation have similar waveforms, amplitudes, and durations of response. Plantar flexion ensures that the tibial nerve is being stimulated, whereas ankle eversion indicates peroneal nerve stimulation.

The waveform often exhibits an initial positive deflection. Repositioning of the active electrode on the abductor hallucis muscle minimizes but may not eliminate this problem. If the active electrode is repositioned, the distance to the stimulator must be adjusted to ensure that stimulation is proximal to the flexor retinaculum. In the event that the positive deflection remains after repositioning, accept the waveform and ensure that the waveform at each subsequent stimulation site has the same configuration and that all latencies are marked in a consistent manner.

FEMORAL NERVE (MOTOR)

Electromyograph Instrument Parameters

Filter settings/frequency response: 10,000–10 Hz
Sweep speed: 2–5 ms/division
Sensitivity/gain: 1,000–5,000 µV/division

Patient Position

The patient is positioned supine in a comfortable resting position. The leg is slightly abducted and externally rotated. A pillow can be placed under the knee to maintain this position.

Electrode Placement

The active recording electrode is placed over the center of the vastus medialis oblique muscle.

The reference electrode is placed away from the muscle on the patella or medial joint line.

The ground electrode is placed on the anterior thigh between the stimulating and active electrodes.

Electrostimulation

Percutaneous electrostimulation is performed at the appropriate anatomic sites in the following order:

S1. Distal stimulation is applied at Hunter's canal in the medial aspect of the thigh between the quadriceps and adductor muscles. This site is approximately 8–10 cm proximal to the active electrode.
S2. Surface stimulation is performed below the inguinal ligament and just lateral to the femoral artery.
S3. Surface stimulation is performed above the inguinal ligament and just lateral to the femoral artery.

Technical Comments

For recording, placement of the active electrode over the most prominent portion of the vastus medialis oblique muscle is most useful when recording the maximum motor response.

The inguinal ligament forms an arc, the convexity of which points downward, that extends between the anterior superior iliac spine and the pubic tubercle. Stimulation can be accomplished above and below this ligament approximately 4–8 cm apart.

MEDIAN (ANTIDROMIC) SENSORY NERVE

Electromyograph Instrument Parameters

Filter settings/frequency response: 20,000–20 Hz
Sweep speed: 1–2 ms/division
Sensitivity/gain: 5–20 μV/division

Patient Position

The patient is positioned supine with the arm abducted approximately 45°. The forearm is fully supinated; the wrist is in a neutral position. The fingers may flex slightly when in a "resting" position.

Electrode Placement

The active recording electrode is attached to the index finger at the midpoint of the distance between the phalangeal flexion crease and the web space of the index finger so that a distance of at least 10 cm, but not more than 14 cm, is maintained between the stimulation and active electrodes.

The reference electrode is positioned at or about the distal interphalangeal flexion crease of the index finger so that a distance of at least 3 cm is maintained between the active and reference electrodes.

The ground is positioned on the dorsum of the hand between the active and stimulating electrodes.

Electrostimulation

Percutaneous electrostimulation is performed at the wrist between the palmaris longus and flexor carpi radialis tendons proximal to the transverse carpal ligament.

Technical Comments

Low-intensity stimulation is usually adequate to elicit the antidromic sensory response. Motor response and volume-conduction effects can be reduced by decreasing the electrostimulation intensity, decreasing the pulse width duration of the applied electrostimulation, or both. (**Note:** Motor responses from hand muscles and volume conduction are more of a technical problem when using antidromic techniques than when using orthodromic techniques.)

Special concern. Care must be taken to maintain a separation between the active and reference electrodes on the index finger. Do not allow conducting gel to bridge this interelectrode space.

MEDIAN (ORTHODROMIC) SENSORY NERVE

Electromyograph Instrument Parameters

Filter settings/frequency response: 20,000–20 Hz
Sweep speed: 1–2 ms/division
Sensitivity/gain: 5–10 μV/division

Patient Position

The patient is positioned supine with the arm abducted approximately 45°. The forearm is fully supinated; the wrist is in a neutral position. The fingers may flex slightly when in a "resting" position.

Electrode Placement

The active recording electrode is positioned directly over the cathode (distal) stimulation site used to evoke the median motor response at the wrist.

The reference electrode is positioned 2–3 cm proximal to the active electrode. This electrode is positioned so that it is directly over the anode (proximal) stimulation site used to evoke the median motor response at the wrist.

The ground electrode is positioned on the dorsum of the hand between the active and stimulation electrodes.

Electrostimulation

Percutaneous electrostimulation is applied over the digital nerve through electrodes attached to the index finger. The cathode is positioned at the midpoint of the proximal phalanx of the index finger, and the anode is positioned at or about the distal phalangeal joint line. A distance of no less than 10 cm, but no more than 14 cm, is maintained between the stimulation cathode on the index finger and the active electrode at the wrist.

Technical Comments

A low stimulation intensity is usually adequate to elicit an orthodromic sensory response. The orthodromic technique reduces the possibility of obtaining a spurious motor response.

Motor response and volume conduction effects can be lessened by decreasing the intensity of the electrostimulation, decreasing the pulse-width duration of the applied electrostimulation, or both.

Special concern. Care must be taken to maintain a separation between the stimulation cathode and the anode on the index finger. Do not allow conduction gel to bridge this interelectrode space.

ULNAR (ORTHODROMIC) SENSORY NERVE

Electromyograph Instrument Parameters

Filter settings/frequency response: 20,000–20 Hz
Sweep speed: 1–2 ms/division
Sensitivity/gain: 5–10 µV/division

Patient Position

The patient is positioned supine with the arm abducted to 45°. The forearm is fully supinated, palm up, and the wrist is in a neutral position with the fingers slightly flexed in a "resting" position.

Electrode Placement

The active recording electrodes are positioned directly over the cathode (distal) stimulating site used to evoke the ulnar motor response at the wrist.

The reference electrode is positioned 3 cm proximal to the active electrode. This electrode is positioned directly over the anode (proximal) stimulating site used to evoke the ulnar motor response at the wrist.

The ground electrode should be positioned on the dorsum of the hand between the active and stimulating electrodes.

Electrostimulation

Percutaneous electrostimulation is applied over the digital nerve through electrodes attached to the fifth finger. The cathode is positioned at or about the midpoint of the proximal phalanx of the fifth finger. The anode is positioned at or about the distal interphalangeal joint line of the fifth finger so that a distance of no less than 10 cm, but no more than 14 cm, is maintained between the stimulating cathode on the digit and the active electrode at the wrist.

Technical Comments

A low stimulation intensity is usually adequate to elicit an orthodromic sensory response. The orthodromic technique reduces the possibility of obtaining a spurious motor response.

Motor response and volume conduction effects can be lessened by decreasing the intensity of the electrostimulation, decreasing the pulse-width duration of the applied electrostimulation, or both.

Special concern. Care must be taken to maintain a separation between the stimulation cathode and the anode on the little finger. Do not allow conducting gel to bridge this interelectrode space.

ULNAR (ANTIDROMIC) SENSORY NERVE

Electromyograph Instrument Parameters

Filter settings/frequency response: 20,000–20 Hz
Sweep speed: 1–2 ms/division
Sensitivity/gain: 5–20 μV/division

Patient Position

The patient is positioned supine with the arm abducted approximately 45°. The forearm is supinated, palm up; the wrist is in a neutral position and the fingers are slightly flexed in a "resting" position.

Electrode Placement

The active recording electrode is attached to the fifth finger at the midpoint of the proximal phalanx so that a distance of at least 10 cm, but no more than 14 cm, is maintained between the stimulating electrode and the active electrode. (See Fig. 23–5).

The reference electrode is positioned at or about the distal interphalangeal joint line of the fifth finger so that a distance of at least 3 cm is maintained between the active and reference electrodes.

The ground electrode should be positioned on the dorsum of the hand between the active and stimulating electrodes.

Electrostimulation

Percutaneous electrostimulation is performed at the wrist, medial **or** lateral to the flexor carpi ulnaris tendon.

Technical Comments

The intensity of sensory electrostimulation is usually adequate to elicit the antidromic sensory response. Motor response and volume conduction effects can be lessened by decreasing the intensity of the electrostimulation, decreasing the pulse-width duration of the applied electrostimulation, or both. (**Note:** Motor impulses from hand muscles and volume conduction are more of a technical problem when using antidromic techniques than when using orthodromic techniques.)

Special concern. Care must be taken to maintain a separation between the active and reference electrodes on the fifth finger. Do not allow conducting gel to bridge this interelectrode space.

SUPERFICIAL RADIAL (ANTIDROMIC) SENSORY NERVE

Electromyograph Instrument Parameters

Filter settings/frequency response: 20,000–20 Hz
Sweep speed: 1–2 ms/division
Sensitivity/gain: 5–20 μV/division

Patient Position

The active recording electrode is positioned over the portion of the nerve that can be palpated over an extended extensor pollicis longus tendon at or about the dorsal-radial aspect of the wrist.

The reference electrode is positioned distal to the active electrode in the first web space midway between the first and second metacarpophalangeal joints.

The ground electrode is placed between the active and stimulating electrodes on the dorsal surface of the forearm.

Electrostimulation

Percutaneous electrostimulation is applied along the dorsolateral border of the radius lateral to the cephalic vein at least 10 cm proximal to the active (recording) electrode.

Technical Comments

The extensor pollicis longus tendon forms the medial border of the "snuff box." By running the index fingernail along this tendon distal to the wrist, the examiner can palpate the superficial radial sensory nerve. The active (recording) electrode should be placed at the intersection of the tendon and nerve.

Stimulation of the superficial radial nerve is usually accomplished using a low-voltage, short-duration stimulus. Stronger stimulation may spread to the anterior interosseus branch of the median nerve and produce an unwanted motor response or a volume-conducted artifact. When this occurs, slight flexion of the distal phalanx of the thumb is observed.

The patient may be able to help find the nerve by reporting a "tingling" sensation along the dorsum of the thumb, index, or second finger when a stimulus is delivered.

SURAL (ANTIDROMIC) SENSORY NERVE

Electromyograph Instrument Parameters

Filter settings/frequency response: 20,000–20 Hz
Sweep speed: 1–2 ms/division
Sensitivity/gain: 5–10 μV/division

Patient Position

The patient is positioned in a comfortable, relaxed, side-lying position facing away from the examiner. (The patient also can be positioned supine or prone.) The hip and knee should be slightly flexed with the ankle positioned in neutral. A single pillow can be placed between the patient's knees for comfort and to support the limb being examined.

Electrode Placement

The active recording electrode is positioned inferior to and in line with the lateral malleolus and parallel with the sole of the foot.

The reference electrode is positioned distal to the active electrode along the lateral border of the foot and parallel with the sole of the foot.

The ground electrode is positioned on the medial or lateral malleolus between the active and stimulating electrodes.

Electrostimulation

Percutaneous (antidromic) electrostimulation of the sural nerve is performed 14 cm proximal to the center of the active electrode. Stimulation is performed slightly distal to the lower border of the belly of the gastrocnemius muscle at or about the junction of the gastrocnemius muscle and the Achilles tendon. Stimulation begins 14 cm proximal to the active electrode in the midline of the posterior calf and proceeds laterally (maintaining at least 10 cm but no more than 14 cm distance) until a satisfactory evoked sensory response is obtained.

Technical Comments

The major difficulty encountered when stimulating the sural sensory nerve is finding the nerve in the posterior calf. The patient may be able to help by reporting "tingling" along the posterior or lateral calf or the lateral foot when a stimulus is delivered.

The sensory response is often obscured by a large muscle response. This may be avoided by using a low-voltage stimulus intensity with a short pulse duration.

ELECTROMYOGRAPHY

The electrical characteristics of the normal motor unit are the basis for the EMG. These characteristics are detected by inserting an electrode into the muscle while the muscle is at rest, mildly contracting, and vigorously contracting. The electrical discharges within the muscle are the result of the depolarizations of the active muscle fibers connected to the particular motor unit. If the motor unit has five or six muscle fibers supplied by one axon, all of those fibers will fire at roughly the same time. This results in a synthesis of the firing of each individual muscle fiber into an amalgamated MUP that represents the summation of each individually discharging muscle fiber within the muscle (see Fig. 23–2). The properties of interest to the electromyographer are (1) the duration of the MUP, (2) the amplitude of the MUP, and (3)the number of phases and their configuration.

Normal Muscle

The normal MUP consists of no more than four phases; two or three phases are most typical. (See the normal motor unit tracing in Fig. 23–4). A phase is initiated each time the tracing passes through baseline and is completed when the tracing returns to baseline again. The duration of the MUP is determined by the initial departure from baseline and the return of the potential to baseline again at the end of the entire potential. The amplitude is measured in one of two ways; from baseline to the peak of the negative phase or from the peak of the negative phase to the peak of the positive (downgoing) phase. Obviously, the laboratory must specify how amplitude measurements are taken. The values reported in this chapter are baseline to peak of the negative phase.

Motor unit duration. The normal *MUP duration* is reported as 7 milliseconds (SD, 3.5 milliseconds).[22] The duration of the MUP is determined by the spread of the end-plate zone as it relates to the total length of the muscle. For example, the abductor pollicis brevis has an end-plate zone that occupies 50% of the total length of the muscle, resulting in a duration of the MUP of 8–9 milliseconds. Conversely, the biceps brachii has an end-plate zone that occupies 10% of the total length of the muscle fibers. This results in a duration of 5–6 milliseconds for the MUP (Fig. 23–10).

Motor unit amplitude. The amplitude of the MUP is measured from baseline to peak of the negative (upward) phase, and it varies from 300 to 5000 μV in the normal individual.[22] The amplitude is representative of the size of the active membrane area with respect to the total size of the muscle. Therefore, a small muscle consisting of large individual muscle fibers such as the abductor pollicis brevis will result in a larger amplitude MUP than will the biceps brachii in a sedentary person.

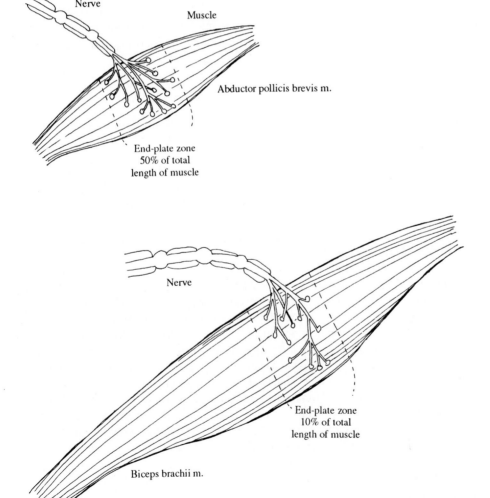

Figure 23–10. Relative spread of the end-plate zone versus the total length of the muscle.

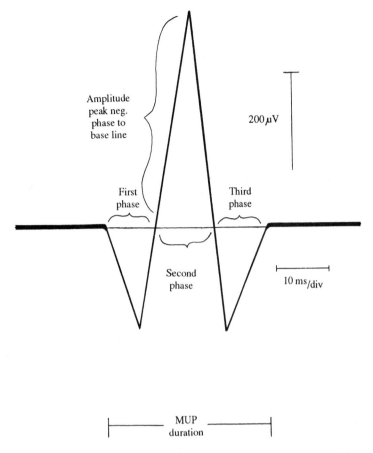

Figure 23–11. A normal motor unit. The motor unit consists of the anterior horn cell, its axon, the neuromuscular junction, and all muscle fibers it innervates. Motor unit potential (MUP) is the synchronous discharge of all muscle fibers innervated by the anterior horn cell. They occur during volitional activity. Initial deflection can be either positive or negative. The amplitude of the motor unit action potential depends on the number of motor unit muscle fibers in close proximity to the recording electrode. The rate of rise time of the motor unit action potential depends on the closeness of the recording electrode to the active muscle fibers. The duration of the action potential of the motor unit depends on the relative density of the muscle fibers in the recording area.

If the muscle fibers are hypertrophied, the amplitudes will increase slightly but will not do so in a predictable manner that is correlated with the hypertrophy. The study of MUP concerns the difference between the MUP obtained from patients and normal values (Fig. 23–11).

Motor unit phases. The number of phases or crossing of the MUP across base-line is determined by the wave of depolarization sweeping along the muscle fibers in a synchronized fashion. If there is a wide spread to the motor end-plate zone, there will be a greater tendency to have more than two or three phases because the summation of the wave of depolarization is not as well synchronized. The minimum number of phases must be two because the wave of depolarization is an alternating wave from negative to positive or vice versa, depending on the position of the recording needle electrode. When the number of phases exceeds four, the MUP is termed a polyphasic MUP. The polyphasic MUP is associated with a MUP that is in the process of reorganization—when the denervated muscle fibers are becoming innervated by collaterals from healthy motor units. This adds many more immature muscle fibers to the original motor unit and spreads the depolarization of these additional fibers over a much larger area. This results in the addition of these multiple phases, forming the *polyphasic MUP* (Fig. 23–12).

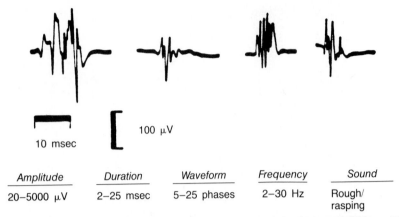

Amplitude	Duration	Waveform	Frequency	Sound
20–5000 μV	2–25 msec	5–25 phases	2–30 Hz	Rough/rasping

Figure 23–12. Complex (polyphasic) action potential of a motor unit with multiple phases. This probably results from asynchronous discharge of muscle fibers in the motor unit. It represents the electrical expression of a motor unit that is undergoing reorganization. Polyphasics are observed in partial compressive neuropathies and in muscular dystrophy. The initial deflection can be either positive or negative. They occur during volitional activity. High-amplitude long-duration (HALD) polyphasic potentials are usually seen in long-standing chronic neuropathies.

Reorganized motor unit. When a motor unit is reorganizing, it also causes the end-plate zone to spread out because the healthy motor unit collaterals reach out to the denervated muscle fibers. Spread of the end-plate zone determines the duration of the MUP, which, in the reorganizing motor unit, will be of longer duration. The duration may exceed 12 milliseconds; some MUPs have been recorded in excess of 20 milliseconds.

Initially, the amplitude of the reorganizing MUP is no larger than the intact MUP, and the amplitudes of some phases will be lower than normal because the previously denervated fibers are atrophic. As the newly innervated fibers increase in diameter, the amplitude of the MUP also increases. A newly organized MUP will produce a relatively short-duration, low-amplitude polyphasic action potential (*SLAP*) (see Fig. 23–8).

A later-stage reorganized MUP will have a polyphasic action potential with a higher amplitude and a longer duration (*HALD*). This type of action potential is encountered in chronic neuropathic lesions in late-stage reorganization of the motor units.

Needle-insertion activity. Inserting a needle into a normal muscle results in a brief burst of electrical activity known as insertional activity. When pierced, the normal muscle liberates electrical discharges that last as long as the actual insertion lasts. If the muscle is denervated—that is, the axons have degenerated after being severed—the denervated muscle fibers revert to a more primitive state that exists in the fetus before motor nerves innervate muscle fibers. When denervated, a skeletal muscle fibrillates: that is, the individual muscle fibers fire spontaneously, producing a small depolarization in all the denervated muscle fibers. Because denervated muscle is extremely sensitive to mechanical irritation, inserting the needle causes a shower of fibrillation potentials in that muscle. The fibrillation potentials are of low amplitude, less than 100 μV and of very short duration, 1–2 msec, with an initial positive deflection followed by a negative phase (Fig. 23–13). The *fibrillation* potential may be confused with end-plate noise, which is of similar amplitude and duration but has an initial negative phase followed by a positive one. The end-plate potential also is associated with considerable discomfort, which can be relieved readily by slight movement of the electrode that pulls the electrode away from the end-plate zone of the nerve. The end-plate potential is normal, not indicative of denervation (Fig. 23–14).

Electrical activity at rest. At rest, a normally innervated muscle exhibits no electrical discharge. The baseline is isoelectrical and no spontaneous discharges are

FIBRILLATION POTENTIALS

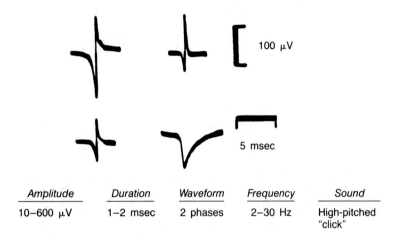

Amplitude	Duration	Waveform	Frequency	Sound
10–600 μV	1–2 msec	2 phases	2–30 Hz	High-pitched "click"

Figure 23–13. Fibrillation potentials representing spontaneous, repetitive discharges of a single muscle fiber. The initial deflection is positive; it indicates altered muscle membrane excitability and an unstable muscle membrane that depolarizes in a variety of circumstances and may be the result of denervation (separation of muscle from nerve), metabolic dysfunction (altered electrolytic states), inflammatory diseases (polymyositis), trauma (injection sites), or lack of trophic influence (stroke or spinal cord injury).

noted. Conversely, denervated muscle has spontaneous discharges of fibrillation while at rest and may have trains of *positive sharp waves* that also discharge while the muscle is at rest (Fig. 23–15).

Electrical activity during mild contraction. With mild contraction of a muscle, the smaller motor units initially discharge, followed by the large and larger motor

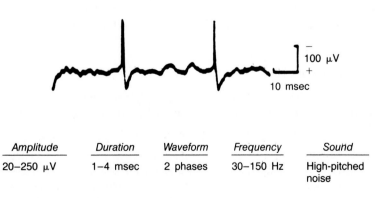

Amplitude	Duration	Waveform	Frequency	Sound
20–250 μV	1–4 msec	2 phases	30–150 Hz	High-pitched noise

Figure 23–14. End-plate potentials. These potentials are produced when the EMG needle electrode comes into contact with nerve fibrils within the muscle. Patients complain of increased pain when these potentials are present. Slight movements of the needle should relieve pain, eliminate the end plate "noise," and clear the screen display of these potential. The initial deflection is negative.

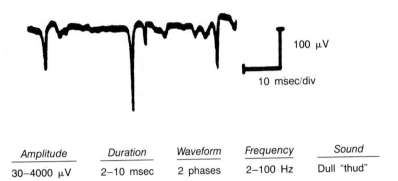

Amplitude	Duration	Waveform	Frequency	Sound
30–4000 μV	2–10 msec	2 phases	2–100 Hz	Dull "thud"

Figure 23–15. Positive sharp waves. These waves may represent asynchronous discharge of a number of denervated muscle fibers. They reflect an alteration in the excitability of the muscle membrane. The initial deflection is positive. Its shape is the most constant of all EMG potentials. Positive sharp waves appear spontaneously at rest and are unpredictable. They are seen in both neuropathies and myopathies.

units as more demand is placed on the muscle for contraction force. This is known as the Henneman size principle of motor unit recruitment. If a muscle is partially denervated, the only motor unit remaining will be the ones the person can activate. If no further motor units can be recruited, the existing motor unit must fire at an increasing rate. If a person is not denervated but the person attempts to imitate this state, only a few motor units will fire. When asked, the person does not increase the rate of firing of those few motor units. This is a helpful method of determining how many motor units are available to a patient and whether the nerve axons are truly partially denervated.

Electrical activity during maximum contraction. When a muscle is required to contract with greater intensity, recruitment of motor units will progress through the small to large motor units and also increase the rate of firing of the motor units recruited. This results in a complete obliteration of the oscilloscope screen with MUPs; this phenomenon is labeled a complete interference pattern and is termed good recruitment. If there are gaps in the recruitment, the recruitment is termed fair and called a partial interference pattern. If even less recruitment occurs and there are discreet MUPs on the screen, the phenomenon is termed a poor recruitment pattern and is called an incomplete interference pattern.

Normal muscle provides good recruitment with a complete obliteration of the baseline on the oscilloscope. This finding is recorded as good recruitment with a complete interference pattern.

Abnormal Muscle

The EMG is particularly helpful for detecting peripheral neuropathies and anterior horn cell disorders and classfiying them regarding the degree of axonal interruption and state of recovery from the denervation.

Characteristics

Insertional activity. Whereas insertion of an electrode into a normal muscle elicits a brief discharge of less than 100 milliseconds, a muscle that is denervated becomes highly responsive to mechanical stimuli, and inserting an electrode into it results in a shower of fibrillation potentials (see Fig. 23–13).

If a muscle is denervated and the muscle membrane is unstable, inserting a needle electrode may give rise to trains of positive sharp waves (see Fig. 23–15). The positive waves may be intermingled with fibrillation potentials. Recall that fibrillation potentials should not be confused with end-plate potentials.

The muscle at rest. A denervated muscle at rest reveals spontaneous discharges without any voluntary effort on the patient's part. These spontaneous discharges may be fibrillation, positive sharp waves, or both. These fibrillation potentials should be stored on the oscilloscope screen and studied carefully to determine that they have an initial positive deflection, followed by a negative deflection, and that they are 1–2 milliseconds in duration and of 50–100 μV in amplitude. The fibrillation potentials have a sound that simulates that of "fat frying in a pan" or "crinkling of cellophane" (see Fig. 23–13). Another spontaneous discharge found in denervated muscle is the positive sharp wave, which begins with an initial and sudden positive (downward) deflection of 50–100 μV and a variable duration of 2–100 milliseconds. The sound is a popping sound and may appear in trains or a series (see Fig. 23–15).

When the anterior horn cells (Alpha motor neurons) are undergoing degeneration or when an inflammatory state is present in that region, the muscles may reveal that fasciculation potentials are spontaneously firing. These fasciculations appear suddenly without any voluntary activation of the muscle. They are either normal bi- or triphasic MUPs, or they may be HALP or SLAP potentials (see Fig. 23–8). It should also be emphasized that these potentials can be found in normally innervated persons who have exercised to fatigue and the motor units are firing spontaneously as a result. These fatigue fasciculations are benign and should not, in themselves, lead to the conclusion that a neuropathy is present. The frequency of firing of benign fasciculations is regular, whereas the frequency of firing of fasciculations associated with anterior horn cell disease are irregular.

Types of Abnormalities

Neurotmesis and axonotmesis. When a muscle is completely denervated, all the axons are completely separated from the muscle. This situation, called a neurotmesis, results in complete loss of voluntary recruitment of MUPs distal to the lesion. With an axonotmesis—incomplete interruption of the axons within a nerve trunk—some surviving axons may be able to fire a few MUPs. This circumstance results in an extremely weak, tremulous contraction. The MUPs elicited will fire at a regular frequency, and, when the patient is asked to contract more vigorously, the frequency of firing of those MUPs will increase. It is impossible for a person with an intact nerve trunk to duplicate this pattern of recruitment because the normally innervated muscles will recruit larger and larger MUPs while increasing the rate of firing of the previous MUPs. Partially denervated patients have no other MUPs to recruit; thus, they fire the available MUPs at a higher frequency.

The *axonotmesis* lesion undergoes a reorganization known as collateral sprouting from healthy axons to supply the muscle fibers that have lost their own supply of axons. When skeletal muscle is denervated, it reverts to a more primitive embryologic state, and its surface membrane, the sarcolemma, becomes supersensitive to acetylcholine. This supersensitivy is associated with the process of attracting healthy axons to the denervated muscle fibers. The healthy motor unit sprouts additional axons, which seek out the denervated fibers, perhaps by specific RNA messengers that have neural attracting agents within them. As these sprouts attach themselves to the now atrophic muscle fibers, the original motor unit expands to include the new muscle fibers. This expands the end-plate zone of the motor unit and increases the duration of the MUP. The newly innervated muscle fibers are atrophic and therefore develop lower amplitude potentials that are separated from the original MUP. This will form the SLAP units noted earlier (see Fig. 23–8).

As a motor unit becomes reinnervated through collateral sprouting, the previously denervated fibers begin to enlarge; therefore, the amplitude of the MUP increases. The end-plate spread caused when the collaterals reach out for the denervated fibers remain spread out. Therefore, the duration of the MUP increases. This results in the HALD unit, which also was noted previously (see Fig. 23–12).

Neuropractic lesions. In a *neuropractic* lesion, which represents a transient loss of conduction in a segment of the nerve, a loss of MUP recruitment will occur distal to the conduction block. Because the neuropractic lesion frequently rectifies itself within hours or several weeks, the recruitment of MUPs will reappear with the ability to conduct impulses in the nerve. It is not uncommon for the nerve to begin conduction after being stimulated electrically above and below the block. However, one cannot always predict when this will occur. The absence of spontaneous discharges at rest is another indication that this is not an *axonotmesis* or *neurotmesis*.

Myoneural function disorders. In myasthenia gravis, the progressive declination of the transmission of the wave of depolarization from the nerve across the myoneural junction may eventually lead to a variable wave of depolarization of the muscle membranes. This will result in a poorly synchronized firing of the MUP that is recognized as variability in the same MUP as it fires repeatedly. The amplitude of the normal MUP, or of even the neuropathic MUP, will not vary during sampling of many motor units. The duration of the MUP also may vary, depending on how many individual myoneural junctions in the motor unit fire synchronously. Because some of these junctions may be less functional than others and the junction is fired at various rates, it is apparent that more and more junctions will fail when the rate of firing increases. The high rate of firing is associated with intense contractions, which will manifest the loss of tension or weakness earliest in the course of the disease.

The Eaton-Lambert phenomenon, the myasthenic reaction, has been linked to toxicity associated with bronchogenic carcinoma of the lung.[20] This disorder is characterized by an extremely low-amplitude response with a single supramaximal stimulus. The amplitude may be only 10% of the normal expected values. When the person produces several voluntary isometric contractions, the amplitude becomes potentiated, sometimes as much as 600%.[23] This would be recognized in EMG discharge as an initial low-amplitude response, followed by the potentiation of the response, then a progressive declination of amplitude when the neuromuscular junction becomes depleted again. A number of other neuromuscular junctional abnormalities, such as botulism intoxication, myotonia, amyotrophic lateral sclerosis, and syringomyelia, also produce EMG evidence of neuromuscular blockage.[24]

Primary muscle disease. If the muscle fiber itself is diseased (eg, in muscular dystrophy), a selective process of degeneration of Type II muscle fibers may result in preservation of the Type I, or slow twitch fibers. As the Type II fibers atrophy, the EMG will reveal low amplitude MUPs in great abundance. Because the axons supplying these atrophic muscle fibers are not lost, the person can recruit them readily. A key difference between normal recruitment and myopathic recruitment is the relative ease with which the patient produces a complete interference pattern with relatively little effort.

An analysis of the MUPs reveals complex units of low amplitude and relatively short duration. The reason for the short duration is that the motor-unit territory shrinks as the total muscle shrinks; therefore, the end-plate spread will be less and result in a decreased duration. As the muscle fibers undergo atrophy, the amplitude is reduced proportionately (see Fig. 23–8).

Some inflammatory muscle diseases, such as *polymyositis*, demonstrate increased irritability to the probe of the needle electrode. The insertional activity is prolonged, and scattered fibrillation may be noted when the muscle is at rest. Contraction of the muscle will result in normal motor unit discharges in the early stages; however, as the inflammatory process produces deterioration, atrophy of fast twitch fibers and a resultant drop in amplitude of the MUP occur. The inflammatory state will not result in abundant recruitment, but, in its place, there will be fair recruitment with partial interference patterns, albeit of lower amplitude.

Congenital or acquired *myotonia* manifests a waxing and waning discharge of MUPs when a needle electrode is inserted into affected muscles. These MUPs have a sound that resembles a dive bomber in a steep dive. The muscles are silent at rest. With moderate contraction, however, the MUPs have a variable amplitude with normal recruitment in the early stages. A distinguishing feature is an inability to terminate muscular contraction, which results in prolonged MUP discharges after a request to relax. This sustained contraction is the most debilitating feature of myotonia because it results in an inability to perform repetitive actions.

The Examination

Following a clarifying assessment of the patient's sensory, motor, and reflex statuses, the affected parts of the body to be examined are outlined. Generally, neuropathic disorders are characterized by a pattern of greater involvement in distal versus proximal muscles, whereas myopathic disease is found more commonly in proximal musculature. The purpose of the sequence of testing selected is to identify changes in muscles that will probably be affected.

If a peripheral neuropathic disorder is suspected, it is appropriate to examine the conduction velocity and distal latencies of lower extremity nerves initially. If the values are less than 40 meters per second in a middle-aged person, further consideration of a peripheral neuropathic disorder is warranted. Similarly, if the distal latencies are prolonged, they would be associated with a dying-back neuropathy.

The next part of the examination is to sample muscles from the distal extreme of the nerve distribution and another muscle at the beginning of the distribution. This procedure is repeated for each lower extremity nerve that exhibits a reduced conduction velocity and a prolonged distal latency. One common pattern would be that the more distal the nerves, the greater the manifestation of denervation. Nerves in the upper extremities would be considerably less affected in peripheral neuropathic disorders. Reduced conduction velocity values, coupled with prolonged distal latencies plus neuropathic EMG findings, would be consistent with a *peripheral neuropathy multiplex.* This designation is given when multiple nerves are involved. If only one peripheral nerve is involved, it is called a mononeuropathy.

A patient who has a long history of low-back pain who was doing spring gardening that involved an excessive amount of stooping and lifting complains of pain radiating to the right leg and describes it as a streak of lightening that extends to the foot. The physical examination reveals hypoesthesia of the dorsolateral lower leg and foot on the right side. The ankle tendon jerk response is depressed on the same side. When testing the peroneal and posterior tibial nerves bilaterally, the conduction velocities are found to be symmetrical and in a range of 45–50 meters per second with distal latencies of less than 4 milliseconds. Would lumbosacral *nerve root compression* result in an increase in nerve conduction velocity? Even if the compression compromised more than 30% of the axons within the nerve root, it would not cause any loss of conduction velocity. However, it would reduce the amplitude on the affected side versus the unaffected side. Because the lesion is found proximally, in the region of the origin of the nerve, the F wave and H reflex latencies would reveal slowing in nerves supplied by the lesioned nerve root or roots. In addition, muscles would be affected in a root distribution pattern versus one that would follow a peripheral nerve distribution. For example, one must select muscles that derive innervation from the same root distribution but are innervated by different peripheral nerves. In this case, one may find neuropathic EMG findings in the tensor fascia latae and in the extensor hallucis longus and extensor digitorum brevis muscles, all of which derive innervation from the fifth lumbar nerve root but are innervated by two separate peripheral nerves. Further investigation of paraspinal musculature in the region of the fifth lumbar vertebrae would place the offending lesion in the nerve root—the common source for this wide range of involvement.

The Report

The reporting of EMG and nerve conduction values or electroneuromyographic findings are usually presented in a tabular form known as the ENMG or EMG report. The report is separated into two major components; the nerve conduction values and the EMG data. In addition to the data presented, the report includes the patient's history and subjective complaints, pertinent clinical findings, and the time of onset and general course of the disorder. A summary of physical findings also are included.

The nerves studied are typically presented in a tabular form, with the proximal and distal latencies of each segment and the distances of those segments of the nerve. The amplitudes for each site of stimulation are presented in millivolts for motor nerves and in microvolts for the sensory components of each nerve. In addition, the proximal latencies; the F wave response and H reflex latencies and their amplitudes are recorded for each nerve on each side (see Fig. 23–6).

The EMG data are presented in the manner in which the information is collected: with insertion of the electrode, with the muscle at rest, with the muscle moderately contracted, and with maximal contractile effort. The needle electrode insertion activity is recorded as brief (which is normal), prolonged, or waxing and waning (as in myotonia). When a muscle is at rest, even when the electrode is in it, the normal muscle will not have any electrical discharges. The denervated muscle will have spontaneous discharges such as fibrillation or positive sharp waves. The fibrillation potential discharge is usually recorded as few and scattered (+1), frequent and found in more than one site (+2), numerous and only a few gaps between them (+3), or abundant and continuous (+4). When positive sharp waves are identified, they are given similar ratings; however, the positive waves typically appear as trains of sharp waves and are ranked according to their duration. The shorter the duration, the lower the numerical rating.

Recording the MUPs during moderate contraction involves the process of analyzing the number of phases, the duration, and the amplitude and frequency of firing with increased demands for more contraction. Some investigators actually store 20 or 30 MUPs and determine the percentage of polyphasic MUPs and note which form they take, SLAP or HALP. Most normal muscles have 10% or less polyphasic MUPs. With increasing age, the percentage of polyphasic MUPs increases, possibly because of remodeling of the end-plate zones. The recording of increased percentages of polyphasic MUPs in a particular nerve root, peripheral nerve, or some other anatomic distribution is helpful, along with other data, to form an impression of the site of the deficit. These percentages of polyphasicity are then listed under the column indicating waveform (see Fig. 23–16).

					Motor Unit Configuration				
Muscle	**S I D E**	**Innervation**	**Insertion**	**At Rest**	**Shape**	**Amplitude**	**Duration**	**Motor Unit Recruitment**	**Comment**

DETAILED ELECTROMYOGRAPHIC FINDINGS

Figure 23–16. An example of an electromyography record, indicating the essential information needed.

Full-effort contractions are recorded when the patient contracts isometrically against the examiner's resistance. The examiner must elicit the patient's maximal effort and judge if there is genuine input to the muscle contraction. One method of assessing this is to track the increase in recruitment and the frequency of firing, as noted in an earlier section. In a normal muscle, recruitment is rated as good and productive of a complete interference pattern. If the recruitment is diminished to a minor degree, it is labeled fair and the interference pattern is labeled as partial. When the recruitment is diminished to a great extent, it is listed as poor and the interference pattern is labeled incomplete. Poor recruitment also may be called discreet MUP recruitment.

Although the reporting forms used are varied, all of them should present complete nerve conduction values and the electromyographic data. That is, the latencies for each site of stimulation and distances between stimulus sites must be listed in a clear manner. The amplitudes of these responses and the latencies

Name _____ Age ___38___ Sex ___M___ Test Date ___3/25/85___

Address _____ , NJ 07094 ___ Status __Priv_____ Case # __0018_____

Chief Complaint ___Low back pain w/ radiation to left leg_____ Onset Date __several months__

Clinical Findings ___Hypesthesia lateral aspect of left foot_____ Referring Dr. _____

— ELECTROMYOGRAPHIC FINDINGS —

MUSCLE AND SIDE		INSERTION	REST	MODERATE	RECRUITMENT	MAXIMUM
Ext. Dig. Brevis	(L)	prolonged	hi-frequency	25% polyphasic	fair	partial
Ext. Hallucis Longus	(L)	prolonged	hi-frequency	25% polyphasic	fair	partial
Medial Gastroc.	(L)	prolonged	hi-frequency	25% polyphasic	fair	partial
Erector Spinae L_5–S_1	(L)	prolonged	hi-frequency	25% polyphasic	fair	partial
Erector Spinae L_5–S_1	(R)	brief	silence	10/15% polyphasic	fair	partial
Erector Spinae $L_{3,4}$	(L&R)	brief	silence	10/15% polyphasic	fair	partial
Medial Gastroc.	(R)	brief	silence	10/15% polyphasic	good	complete
Anterior Tibialis	(L&R)	brief	silence	10/15% polyphasic	good	complete
Vastus Medialis	(L&R)	brief	silence	10/15% polyphasic	good	complete
Ext. Hall. Long	(R)	brief	silence	10/15% polyphasic	good	complete
Ext. Dig. Brevis	(R)	brief	silence	10/15% polyphasic	good	complete
Abductor Hall.	(L&R)	brief	silence	15% polyphasic	fair	partial

— CONDUCTION VELOCITY FINDINGS —

NERVE: Peroneal (L)	NERVE: Tibial (L)	NERVE: Peroneal (R)	NERVE: Tibial (R)
PROX: 10.4 4 mVolts	PROX: 12.2 10 mVolts	PROX: 10.8 7 mVolts	PROX: 10.5 10 mVolts
DISTAL: 4.0 4 mVolts	DISTAL: 4.0 10 mVolts	DISTAL: 4.2 7 mVolts	DISTAL: 4.0 10 mVolts
VEL: 48 M/SEC.	VEL: 45 M/SEC.	VEL: 45 M/SEC.	VEL: 59 M/SEC.
DISTANCE: 31 CM.	DISTANCE: 36 CM.	DISTANCE: 29 CM.	DISTANCE: 36 CM.
F=51.4 msecs	F=49.5 msecs	F=50.2 msecs	F=45.9 msecs
NERVE: Sural (L)	NERVE: L H-Reflex =	NERVE: R H-Reflex =	NERVE: Sural (R)
PROX:	PROX:	PROX:	PROX:
DISTAL: 3.52 10 µVolts	DISTAL: 31.2 msecs 350 µV	DISTAL: 28.9 msecs 500 µV	DISTAL: 3.51 10 µVolts
VEL: M/SEC.	VEL: M/SEC.	VEL: M/SEC.	VEL: M/SEC.
DISTANCE: CM.	DISTANCE: CM.	DISTANCE: CM.	DISTANCE: CM.

IMPRESSION: The EMG findings and prolonged proximal latencies of F waves and H reflex responses on the left side are compatible with an L_5,S_1 radiculitis on the left side.

Figure 23–17. An example of an electrodiagnostic report. Some typical recordings of muscle and nerve conduction values are shown.

also must be juxtaposed. Then, the calculation of the conduction velocity of each segment of the nerve is entered. The EMG data should indicate the name of the muscle studied; its side; the result of needle insertion; the state during rest; the waveforms, amplitude, and duration of the motor units during contraction; and the quality of the recruitment plus the interference pattern produced. (See Fig. 23–17 for an example of a reporting form used in many laboratories.)

Application to Patient Care

Determining the pathophysiologic mechanism that underlies a clinical problem is essential to optimal patient care. A common example is an elderly patient who complains of weakness of both legs. The patient has not been diagnosed as diabetic but has not been tested specifically for diabetes in the past year. What might give rise to this weakness? The sources of weakness might include a CNS lesion, a spinal cord disorder, a peripheral nerve disease, a myoneural junctional disorder, a muscular disease, or psychological factors such as depression, anxiety, or an emotional disorder. The ENMG may delineate whether the weakness derives from the motor neuron, the peripheral nerve or nerves, the myoneural junction, or the muscle itself. The testing of CNS disorders also can be evaluated with cortically evoked studies of the spinal cord, brain stem, or auditory and visual systems. The latter studies are special applications of electrophysiology that is covered in other sources.[25]

Another benefit to the physical therapist is to monitor progress or regression in specific patients. With serial ENMG studies, one can establish realistic goals and expectations. Prediction regarding when these goals can be attained are rendered more precise; therefore, attainment of function can be predicted with more certainty. The therapist must guide the patient who has sustained a foot drop or peroneal palsy regarding the treatment required and whether orthotic support is indicated and what type. If, in the latter case of foot drop, the ENMG reveals axonotmesis at the neck of fibula in the common peroneal nerve, it is known that peripheral axons will regenerate at a rate of approximately 1

TABLE 23–1. NORMAL CONDUCTION VALUES

Nerve	Distance (cm)	Amplitude (using 6 mm disk)	Nerve Conduction Velocity (msec)	Distal Latency (msec)
Ulnar				
Motor (forearm)	6.5	6–16 mV	49–71	≤ 3.5
Sensory (5th digit)	11.0	>10 mV		≤ 3.0
Sensory (palm)	10.0			≤ 2.4
Median				
Motor (forearm)	8.0	4–18 mV	49–70	≤ 4.4
Sensory (index)	13.0	> 15 µV		≤ 3.5
Sensory (palm)	10.0	≥ 30 µV		≤ 2.4
Radial sensory				
Disk electrode	10.0	> 15 µV		≤ 2.5
Peroneal				
Motor (foreleg)	9.0	2–12 mV	43–58	≤ 6.6
Sural sensory				
Behind lateral malleolus	14	5–50 µV		≤ 4.0
Post Tibial Nerve				
Abductor Hallucis Brevis (knee > ankle)	12.9	3–26 mV	41–53	≤ 7.0
Abdi Digiti Minimus	19.0	2–16 mV		≤ 7.3

inch (2.5 cm) per month. If the peroneal nerve is 27 cm long, it is evident that this patient has a recovery period of 2 years and some months. During that 2-year wait, it is essential to avoid stretching paralyzed muscles; thus, the patient must be fitted with an orthosis. The type of orthosis should be one that distorts normal locomotion the least because the patient will be walking with this device for 2 years and habit patterns are established in less time than that (Table 23.1).

Another consideration regarding the patient with a common peroneal palsy is to determine when to begin electrical stimulation, or even whether one should begin electrical stimulation confirmed by the ENMG data. For example, according to Davis,[26] the presence of fibrillation is a contraindication for electrical stimulation of denervated muscle. He suggested that once fibrillation has subsided, it may be more appropriate to stimulate the skeletal muscle. The major question that arises is: If this stimulation is to take place over two or more years, is it reasonable to expect a patient to comply over this period? And if the patient does comply, will it result in improved function of the target muscle? Pachter et al[27] explored some of these issues in animal studies and concluded that stimulation produced some benefits but only for relatively short periods. Kosman[28] cautioned that these studies on denervated animal models are not applicable to the longer durations needed for human regeneration; therefore, he opted against electrical stimulation for such long periods. The electromyographic findings also reveal early reinnervation to determine when it is appropriate to institute muscle reeducation. Obviously, when SLAP discharges are uncovered in a previously denervated muscle, one must actively exercise those muscles to the point of tiredness but not fatigue.[28] The SLAP discharges are only seen on the EMG; they are not visible contractions. Therefore, the EMG is absolutely necessary to identify these early electrophysiologic changes and provide feedback to the patient.

■ KEY TERMS

electroneuromyography	amplitude
nerve conduction	sensory nerve action potential (SNAP)
electromyography	distal latency
supramaximal stimulus	F wave latency
resting membrane potential	H reflex
depolarization	blink reflex
hyperpolarization	demyelinating disease
accommodation	carpal tunnel syndrome
action potential	dying-back neuropathy
motor unit potential (MUP)	Eaton-Lambert phenomenon
recruitment	interference
graded junctional potential	repetitive stimulation
end plate potential	MUP duration
differential amplifier	polyphasic MUP
oscilloscope	SLAP MUP
impedance	HALD MUP
common mode rejection	fibrillation
electronic noise	positive sharp waves
calibration signal	neuropractic
frequency bandwidth	axonotmesis
sweep speed	neurotmesis
isolated circuits	polymyositis
storage oscilloscopes	myotonia
averager	peripheral neuropathy multiplex
leakage currents	nerve root compression

■ REVIEW QUESTIONS

1. An elderly woman who was receiving chemotherapy for a bronchogenic carcinoma is now in remission but is complaining of dizziness. Is this patient a candidate for an ENMG? What would you look for if you knew that chemotherapy produces lesions in peripheral nerves?

2. If the elderly woman's conduction velocity of both peroneal nerves is 36 milliseconds and she is 63 years old, would that conduction velocity be viewed as abnormal?

3. If a response of the ulnar nerve is obtained at the wrist and also at the elbow but no response is obtained above the elbow, what does this indicate?

4. If the distal latency of the median nerve is 4.75 milliseconds and the latency of the ulnar nerve is 2.75 milliseconds, what is the possible significance of these findings?

5. If the F wave latency of the right median nerve is 32 milliseconds, and the F wave latency of the left medial nerve is 29 milliseconds, what is the significance of this difference?

6. In the case described in Question 5, if abundant polyphasic MUPs were found in muscles innervated by the fifth and sixth cervical nerve roots on the right side, would this be compatible with the findings in Question 5?

7. To perform an antidromic test of the sural nerve, where should the recording electrodes be placed?

8. In an individual with legs of equal length, an H reflex latency of 32 milliseconds is found on the left side and a latency of 28 milliseconds is found on the right side. Is this difference within normal variation? If not, what type of problem does it indicate?

9. What would be indicated by a 2+ shower of fibrillation potentials in muscles innervated by the ulnar nerve distal to the elbow?

10. What EMG findings might be found in muscles innervated by the fifth lumbar nerve root that was severely compressed by a herniated lumbar disk 18 days earlier?

REFERENCES

1. Brown MC, Ironton R. Suppression of motor nerve terminal sprouting in partially denervated mouse muscles. *J Physiol.* 1977; 272:70.
2. Weddell G, Feinstein B, Pattle RE. The electrical activity of voluntary muscle in man under normal and pathological conditions. *Brain.* 1944; 67:178.
3. Buchthal F, et al. Motor unit territory in different human muscles. *Acta Physiol Scand.* 1959; 45:82.
4. Henneman E, Somjen G, Carpenter DO. Functional significance of cell size in spinal motorneurons. *J Neurophysiol.* 1965; 28:560–580.
5. DeLuca CJ, Lefever RS, McCue MP. Behavior of human motor units in different muscles during linearly varying contractions. *J Physiol.* 1982; 329:113–128.
6. Magladery JW, MacDougla DB Jr. Electrophysiological studies of nerve and reflex activity in normal man: identification of certain reflexes in electromyogram and conduction velocity of peripheral nerve fibers. *Bull Johns Hopkins Hosp.* 1950; 86:265.
7. Hoffmann P. Uber die Beziehungen der Sehnenreflexe zur willkurlichen bewegung and zum tonus. *Z Biol.* 1918; 68:351.
8. Crone C, Hultborn, H, Illert, M. Reciprocal Ia inhibition ankle flexors and extensors in man. *J Physiol.* 1987; 389:163–185.
9. Leonard CT, Moritani T. H reflex testing to determine the neural basis of movement disorders of neurologically impaired individuals. *Electro Clin Neurophysiol.* 1992; 32:341–349.
10. Johnson EW, ed. *Practical Electromyography.* Baltimore, MD: Williams & Wilkins; 1988.

11. Crone C, Nielsen J. Methodological implications of the post activation depression of the soleus H-reflex in man. *Exp Brain Res.* 1989; 78(1):28.

12. Braddom RL, Johnson EW. Standardization of H reflex and diagnostic use in S1 radiculopathy. *Arch Phys Med Rehabil.* 1974; 55:161.

13. Schuchmann JA. H reflex latency in radiculopathy. *Arch Phys Med Rehabil.* 1978; 59:185.

14. Kugelberg E. Facial reflexes. *Brain.* 1952; 75:385.

15. Kimura J, Powers JM, Van Allen MW. Reflex response of orbicularis occuli muscle to supraorbital nerve stimulation. *Arch Neurol.* 1969; 21:193.

16. Lyon LW, VanAllen MW. Alterations of the orbicularis occuli reflex by acoustic neuroma. *Arch Otolaryngol.* 1972; 95:100.

17. Desmedt J ed. *New Developments in Electromyography and Clinical Neurophysiology.* Basel, Switzerland: Karger; 1973.

18. Brooke M. *A Clinician's View of Neuromuscular Diseases.* Baltimore, MD: Williams & Wilkins; 1977.

19. Sumner AJ. Axonal polyneuropathies. In: Sumner AJ, ed. *The Physiology of Peripheral Nerve Diseases.* Philadelphia, PA: WB Saunders; 1980:340–57.

20. Lambert EH, Eaton LM, Rooke ED. Defect of neuromuscular conduction associated with malignant neoplasm. *Am J Physiol.* 1956; 187:617.

21. Nelson RM, Currier DP. *Clinical Electrotherapy.* 2nd ed. Norwalk, CT: Appleton & Lange; 1991.

22. Goodgold J, Eberstein A. *Electrodiagnosis of Neuromuscular Disease.* 3rd ed. Baltimore, MD: Williams & Wilkins; 1983.

23. Elmqvist D, Lambert EH. Detailed analysis of neuromuscular transmission in a patient with the myasthenic syndrome sometimes associated with bronchogenic carcinoma. *Mayo Clin Proc.* 1968; 443:689.

24. Kugelberg E, Taverner D. Comparison between voluntary and electrical activation of motor units in anterior horn cell diseases on central synchronization of motor units. *Electroenceph Clin Neurophysiol.* 1950; 2:125.

25. Halliday AM. *Evoked Potentials in Clinical Testing.* Edinburgh, UK: Churchill Livingstone; 1982.

26. Davis HL. Is electrostimulation beneficial to denervated muscle? a review of results from basic research. *Physiother Can.* 1983; 35:306.

27. Pachter BR, Eberstein A, Goodgold J. Electrical stimulation effect on denervated skeletal myofibers in rats: a light and electron microscopic study. *Arch Phys Med Rehabil.* 1982; 63:427.

28. Kosman AJ, Osborne SL, Ivy AC. The effect of electrical stimulation on denervated muscle in rat. *Am J Physiol.* 1946; 145:447.

SECTION 5

ADDITIONAL

PHYSICAL AGENTS

This section contains five commonly used physical agents which the authors felt should be included in this text but which could not accurately be placed in any of the three previous sections. The modalities discussed previously were categorized according to the major physical components influencing their use as patient treatments. They included modalities using heat and cold, water or other fluids, and electrical currents passing through the patients for the purpose of benefiting their conditions.

EMG BIOFEEDBACK was not placed in the Electrotherapy Section for, although the *feedback* is obtained through electronic circuitry, the stimuli is the electrical firing from the patients' muscles; it is not activated by an electrical stimulator. Although the LASER which is used in physical therapy, and the ULTRAVIOLET modalities are radiation therapies, they were not placed in the Thermal Section because they do not utilize wave lengths in the *thermal* range of the Electromagnetic Spectrum. The TRACTION and INTERMITTENT PNEUMATIC COMPRESSION modalities involve the application of physical forces, distraction, compression and pressure, as the primary beneficial components. For these reasons these five modalities were placed in this section OTHER PHYSICAL MODALITIES.

24

Electromyographic Biofeedback for Motor Control

Lynn Geisel, PT, BS and
Dina Fine Rhodes, PT, MA

The EMG Signal

Equipment

Placement of Electrodes

Application to Treatment

  Examples Using One Channel of IEMG Information

Examples Using Two Channels of IEMG Information

Treatment Considerations

Conclusion

Key Terms

*B*iofeedback is the nearly instantaneous return of information to a person about physiological functions of which he or she might otherwise be unaware. This information provides the potential for more active self-control over the function that is being monitored.

Different kinds of biofeedback devices are available to monitor different biological functions. The more common ones are (1) thermal feedback for skin temperature, (2) galvanic skin response (GSR) feedback for electrical conductance of the skin, and (3) electromyographic (EMG) feedback for muscle activity. These kinds of biofeedback have been used by different health professionals for a variety of different treatment purposes.[1] One way all three kinds of biofeedback have been used is in training for generalized relaxation for the treatment of stress-related disorders such as hypertension, headaches, and chronic pain. *EMG feedback* in the hands of a rehabilitation professional such as a physical or occupational therapist also can be used to help train patients with physical disabilities to improve their motor control. This topic will be the focus of this chapter.

Fig. 24–1 indicates the various information loops that are ongoing during a physical therapy session using EMG feedback. After the therapist has placed surface electrodes over the desired muscle or muscles, the electrical signal generated by the muscle is detected by the electrodes and conveyed by cables to the EMG feedback machine. The machine processes the signal and displays the information (that is, "feeds it back") to the patient by visual or auditory means, or both. In this way, knowledge of the results helps the patient learn how to control the muscle consistently. It also helps the therapist provide suggestions or therapeutic interventions that will help the patient improve and ultimately achieve the desired movement.

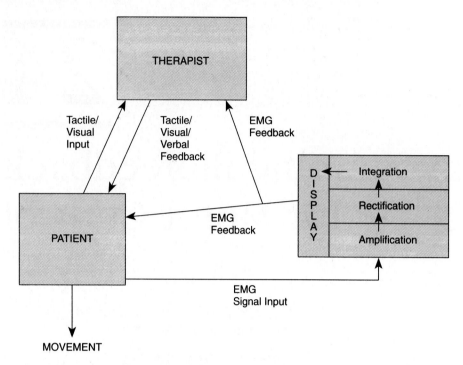

Figure 24–1. Schematic representation of the various information loops during a P.T. session using EMG biofeedback.

THE EMG SIGNAL

An EMG signal gives a measure of motor unit activation of a muscle. Because this signal can be hard to quantify, it is altered to be more meaningful to the patient and therapist. The raw EMG signal, which contains positive and negative phases, is rectified and then integrated (see Fig. 24–2). Through *rectification,* the positive and negative aspects of the summated action potentials are made unidirectional. The resultant signal then undergoes *integration:* that is, the area under the curve of the signal is computed. This gives a representation of both the amplitude and duration of the signal. The integration occurs at periodic time intervals and displays a measurement of muscle activity in units of "microvolt-seconds." These values are what is displayed as the EMG feedback signal.

EQUIPMENT

Commercially available EMG feedback equipment varies in complexity. Basic units have only one channel of integrated electromyographic (IEMG) information (see Fig. 24–3). The more sophisticated units have two channels so that two muscles can be monitored simultaneously. All units give a visual or auditory presentation, or both, of the IEMG signal. The means of visual display may be a fluctuating needle meter read-out, flashing numbers, or a series of progressively lit lights. On more sophisticated and detailed displays, the signal is traced on an oscilloscope or computer screen. The advent of software programs that present EMG signals processed by computer offers an even wider range of visual displays.

Auditory feedback is usually of either the "threshold" or "proportional" type. The threshold mode functions by turning a tone on or off when the IEMG amplitude reaches a level predetermined by the therapist. The proportional mode produces a sound that modulates proportionally to the IEMG amplitude. For example, the sound may be a changing rate of clicks or a changing amplitude of tone. Most EMG feedback units will employ some sort of sensitivity or "gain" adjustment that

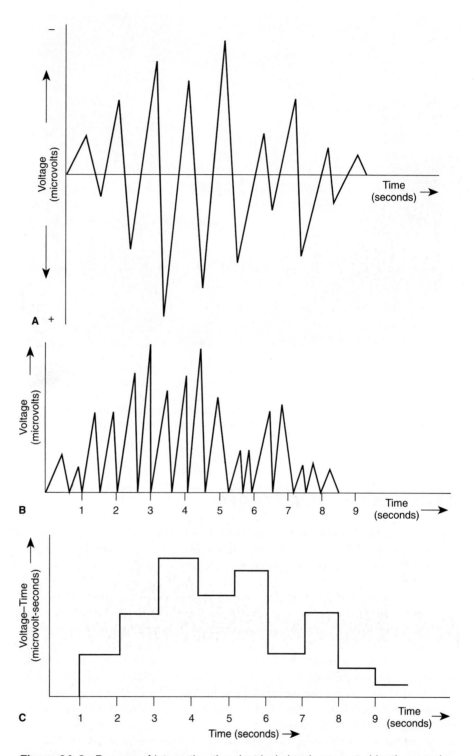

Figure 24–2. Process of integrating the electrical signals generated by the muscle. **(A)** Representation of the raw EMG signal. **(B)** The EMG signal is rectified. **(C)** The rectified signal is then integrated.

magnifies or compresses the IEMG signal to fit within the scale of the feedback display.

The surface electrodes used are made of a conductive metal and are usually cupped to hold a conducting gel that enhances skin-electrode contact. A single muscle hookup for one channel of IEMG information consists of three electrodes: two active and one reference or ground. Each set of three electrodes can be either permanently attached to the input cable or detachable.

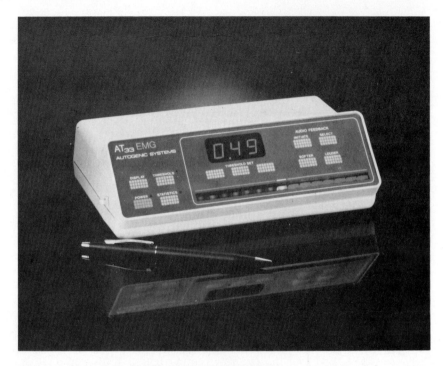

Figure 24–3. A single-channel portable EMG biofeedback unit with (1) controls for collection and analysis of EMG activity occurring during treatment (left), (2) visual feedback (digital readout in the center and light bar across the bottom of the panel), and (3) audio feedback controls (right). Leads connect the unit to surface electrodes placed on the skin over the muscles. The electrodes are not shown. (*Reproduced with permission from GE Miller Inc., Yonkers, NY.*)

PLACEMENT OF ELECTRODES

A general rule for placing the electrodes is to place the two active electrodes over the motor point or belly of the muscle to be monitored. Because surface rather than needle electrodes are used, the problem of multiple muscle activation being detected may arise. Placement of electrodes over small or narrow muscles increases the probability of this occurring. For a more isolated detection of IEMG activity in these cases, better results may be obtained by placing the electrodes in an area where only the desired muscle is located, even though this may not be over its motor point. Monitoring for activity in the long flexor muscle of the fingers is an example. Because the muscle bellies of the finger and wrist flexors are both in the proximal portion of the anterior forearm, detection of isolated finger flexor activity may be difficult. Placing the electrodes on the lower half of the forearm may still pick up activity of the finger flexor fibers present in that area, but it avoids adding wrist muscle activity to the signal.

An additional problem in using surface electrodes is that only superficial muscles can be monitored reliably. Deeper muscles can be detected, but the resultant IEMG signal will be a composite of the deeper muscle and any superficial muscle that is activated at the same time.

The distance between the active electrodes will affect the amplitude and specificity of the signal. Electrodes placed close together will sample a smaller area of muscle and therefore give a smaller signal; however, the signal will be more precise. Electrodes placed further apart will yield a larger signal but may reflect activation of more than one muscle. Thus, the size of the muscle to be monitored and the proximity of other muscles will contribute to the decision regarding placement of the electrodes. Generally, spacing the electrodes 1–5 cm apart yields an effective reading.

Before attaching the electrodes, the skin must be cleaned with alcohol to remove surface dirt and oils. Skin hair over the muscles may have to be shaved to reduce electrical impedance. Occasionally, light abrasion with fine sandpaper may be needed in the presence of extremely thick skin for the same reason.

APPLICATION TO TREATMENT

The physical therapist can use EMG biofeedback to treat a multitude of physical disorders, including a variety of neurological, orthopedic, and respiratory problems. An in-depth description of all the possible uses of EMG feedback for improving motor control is beyond the scope of this chapter. There is also no "cookbook" method of steps to follow when using EMG feedback as part of a treatment regimen. Therapists must use their skills of observation and knowledge of normal and abnormal kinesiology to decide when and how to use the EMG information. Thus, the following examples serve as illustrative guidelines.

Before using EMG biofeedback as an aid to treatment, therapists should be familiar with what normal motor unit activation looks or sounds like on the particular EMG feedback device they are using. Therefore, it is important for therapists to spend some time monitoring their own muscles with the device during various movements and exercises: How much of a muscle contraction or movement is required to cause a change in the IEMG signal at different gain (sensitivity) settings? They also should experience the response time of the unit: How quickly does the IEMG signal respond to a change in muscle activation? These are important factors to be aware of when instructing patients and subsequently interpreting their IEMG tracings.

Examples Using One Channel of IEMG Information

A simple scenario that demonstrates the utilization of single-channel EMG feedback in a physical therapy setting is when the IEMG information is used to monitor appropriate activation or relaxation of a muscle that is neurologically intact. A first example would be instructing a patient with a knee problem to contract the quadriceps muscle isometrically (known in the profession as performing a "quad set").

The therapist explains the purpose of the feedback device to the patient, with instructions that the visual or auditory signal will increase proportionally with the appropriate increase in muscle contraction and decrease with decreased contraction (that is, increased relaxation) of that muscle. The patient should understand that the machine will not help to cause the muscle contraction but will simply monitor the muscle's activity. If the patient is fearful about having the electrodes applied to a postoperative or painful site, another muscle group can be used to demonstrate how the EMG feedback unit works. Possible sites are the same muscle in the contralateral limb, the biceps brachii muscle for elbow flexion, or the thenar eminence muscle group for thumb abduction or opposition.

Once the electrodes are applied to the quadriceps muscle, the therapist gives the usual instructions to teach the patient to contract the muscle. In this scenario, the EMG feedback signal serves as a powerful positive reinforcer to the patient. It also helps the patient and therapist by quantifying the amount of muscle activation achieved. Once a good contraction is obtained, the "threshold mode" (see "Equipment") can then be used to help the patient repeatedly deliver the same high level of muscle contraction for muscle strengthening. In this way, the use of EMG feedback can enhance the patient's motivation and compliance for optimal improvement. Research has shown that monitoring the quadriceps muscle with EMG feedback both before and after a meniscectomy surgery aids in patient recovery.[2]

A second relatively simple example of using EMG feedback, this time to reduce muscle activity, involves a patient with tension or spasm of the upper trapezius muscle that contributes to cervical pain. Monitoring the trapezius muscle for reduction of IEMG activity can aid in lessening the pain and "stiffness." First, the patient is instructed in how the EMG feedback machine functions in the scenario above. The therapist then instructs the patient regarding what motions of the shoulder and neck activate the trapezius muscle. The patient is guided into relaxing the trapezius muscle by verbal and possibly tactile cueing: for example, "let the shoulders gently drop down, away from the ears." Progression to slow gentle stretching of the muscle or small-range head motions could follow, as the EMG signal continues to give information regarding the continued relaxation of the muscle. This sequence may take place within the same session or over a few sessions, depending on the patient's skill in learning to control the muscle.

A third way to use EMG feedback in a physical therapy session is to aid in the reduction of antagonistic muscle contractions during attempts to passively stretch a painful joint. For instance, a patient with restricted passive range of motion in a shoulder joint may be unaware of tensing the pectoralis major muscle when the therapist attempts to stretch the joint into abduction. Monitoring the muscle for activation with EMG feedback can help teach the patient to eliminate this undesirable muscle contraction.

When working with the neurologically involved patient, a common treatment goal is to increase the shifting of weight onto a lower extremity when standing and walking. This can be augmented with EMG feedback by monitoring the quadriceps muscle for increased activation as the patient shifts more weight onto the limb with the knee in slight flexion (not hyperextended). The therapist determines the desired level of IEMG activation of the quadriceps muscle by helping the patient shift an acceptable amount of weight onto the affected side and observing how much of a signal is produced. The threshold level for the auditory signal can then be set to that level. Next, the patient is asked to make the EMG feedback device consistently produce an auditory tone each time he or she attempts to shift his or her weight. This can be expanded to other activities, such as increasing weight-bearing while changing from a sitting to a standing position and the reverse. In this way, the patient takes more responsibility for producing the desired motion, rather than relying on the therapist's manual guidance to achieve the appropriate degree of weight shift.

Examples Using Two Channels of IEMG Information

More sophisticated treatments can be performed by using two channels of IEMG information. Returning to the arena of orthopedic knee problems, good results have been reported using EMG feedback to train patients for improved tracking of the patella in the patellofemoral joint.[3] Increasing the activation of the vastus medialis oblique head of the quadriceps muscle, which will pull the patella medially, is the goal. However, this task must be accomplished selectively so that the pull of the vastus lateralis is not increased to an equal degree. Therefore, monitoring only one muscle for increased activity is insufficient. Two channels of EMG information are required, one for each of the two heads of the quadriceps muscle that are of interest. This presents a greater challenge to both patient and therapist to achieve the desired motor control.

The example just cited introduces the concept of using EMG biofeedback to train for *motor control* or coordination rather than for simple muscle strengthening or relaxation alone. This concept becomes especially important when treating patients with complex motor control problems such as those seen after damage to the central nervous system. Many aspects of the IEMG signal can contribute to improved motor control. These include appropriate rises or falls in signal amplitude, peak activation and relaxation times, time of maintained activation or relaxation, and the relationship between the contractions of the two muscle groups being monitored. In other words, how high or low can the signals be made to go, how quickly do they get there, how long can they be kept there, and which muscles are contracting and in what order? This type of information helps to train the neuromuscular complex to a point that more closely approximates optimal muscle functioning. The term "neuromuscular reeducation" is a familiar one to physical therapists, and EMG biofeedback is an ideal adjunct to a treatment program that helps patients to achieve this.

Describing to therapists how to employ two-channel EMG feedback to treat neurologically impaired patients can be difficult. This is because there is no one right way to train a patient. The approaches vary, depending on which overall treatment approach the therapist favors and on the patient's particular "package" of motor control problems. EMG feedback cannot cause muscles to work if the patient is neurologically incapable of accessing them, whether the cause is brain damage, spinal cord injury, or peripheral nerve injury. What the EMG feedback does offer, however, is the increased ability to maximize whatever degree of muscle functioning or motor control the patient is capable of.

EMG Feedback to Treat Hemiplegia

The first example of the use of two channels of EMG feedback with neurological patients is to train those with hemiplegia to improve the control of their upper extremity. This has been the subject of investigation by a number of researchers.[4–7] Much of the early use of EMG feedback focused on monitoring antagonistic muscles around a single joint for appropriate responses. For example, the biceps and triceps brachii muscles might be monitored during elbow extension to increase activation of the triceps and reduce biceps spasticity. Similarly, muscles that flex and extend the wrist may be monitored for increased extension with decreased flexor spasticity. Whereas this has proved to be useful for some patients, most notably those with relatively high levels of motor control, disappointing results are often the case for others.

Broader approaches that dovetail more closely with current principles of treating hemiplegia within the physical therapy profession can benefit a larger population of patients. The biceps muscle can be monitored for decreased hyperactivity while the patient is taught to assume a more symmetrical trunk posture, or the upper trapezius can be monitored concurrently for decrease of involuntary contraction. Monitoring the triceps for elbow extension during upper extremity weight bearing can help the therapist determine whether the desired activation is actually occurring; concurrent monitoring of the biceps on a second IEMG channel can provide additional useful information. Asking a patient with a relatively high level of motor control to increase the EMG signal of finger extensors can be done while the triceps is monitored for unwanted synergistic activity, thus making the finger motion more functional. In all of these examples, patients are asked to produce a movement or at least to be aware of what is occurring in other areas of their bodies in addition to the joint that is the main concern.

EMG Feedback to Treat Other Conditions

EMG feedback has been used successfully for a variety of other neurological conditions, including cerebral palsy, spinal cord injury,[8] and facial paralysis.[9] For example, it can be used to monitor weakened muscles in a patient with Guillain-Barré syndrome or a brachial plexus injury to strengthen without substitution by unwanted muscle groups. It can assist a patient with multiple sclerosis to drink from a cup with reduced tremor in the upper extremity. It can aid patients in learning muscle control that would otherwise be beyond the reach of more traditional physical therapy treatments—these include patients with focal dystonias or dyskinesias such as spasmodic torticollis or dystonic writer's cramp.[10,11]

Thus, EMG feedback can serve multiple roles in working with neurologically involved patients. It may help clarify a particular patient's abnormal motor pattern, provide guidance regarding which physiotherapeutic approaches actually enhance the desired outcome in that patient, and, finally, heighten the patient's awareness regarding proper versus improper movements and how to better attain them. In addition, it is important for the therapist to remember to use the IEMG information not only to train for appropriate muscle response but also to apply the improved movement to functional tasks. Automatic carryover does not occur magically. If the tibialis anterior muscle is being trained for ankle dorsiflexion to improve ambulation, the movement must progress from supine to sitting to actual gait. If the biceps brachii is trained to improve elbow flexion, the patient should eventually practice the movement while trying to hold a package. Furthermore, the patient must be weaned from relying on the EMG feedback unit when practicing or using the newly acquired motor skills.

TREATMENT CONSIDERATIONS

Three factors warrant consideration when deciding to use EMG biofeedback as part of a physical therapy session: treatment setting, duration of the session, and patient selection.

The setting in which EMG biofeedback can be used can vary from a private, quiet room to a busy gym area. The more the patient is expected to interact with the EMG biofeedback and the more difficult the requested motor task is, the more a quiet setting is needed. This is especially true when working with two channels of IEMG information, which require greater concentration and greater motor skill.

Sessions of 30–45 minutes have proved to be optimal. This gives the therapist time to connect the patient to the equipment and allows for sufficient practice of the motor task. Longer sessions can be overly tiring, both mentally and physically, for the patient.

A final consideration of primary importance is the patient's cognitive or communication capability to interact meaningfully with the EMG feedback information. A patient can be screened by monitoring an unaffected muscle or pair of muscles with the EMG feedback unit, and then asking him or her to manipulate the signals appropriately. The therapist can discern whether the patient understands the relationship between the EMG signal and the muscular control over it. This is especially relevant when two channels of information are used.

CONCLUSION

EMG biofeedback is an invaluable tool for the physical therapist in clarifying and accelerating improvement in many patients. Its value has proven to be significant according to both clinical reports by therapists and empirical research findings. The authors' years of experience in its use support this view. Hopefully, the information presented here will encourage other physical therapists to take advantage of EMG biofeedback in the treatment of their own patients.

■ KEY TERMS

biofeedback	integration
EMG biofeedback	motor control
rectification	

■ REVIEW QUESTIONS

1. How is the raw EMG signal adapted for use in biofeedback?
2. EMG biofeedback is being used to reeducate the muscles in the leg of a patient with foot-drop. What are some possibilities for electrode placement?

3. What are some ways in which EMG biofeedback can be incorporated into a physical therapy treatment program for a patient with hemiplegia?

REFERENCES

1. Basmajian JV, ed. *Biofeedback: Principles and Practice for Clinicians.* 3rd ed. Baltimore, MD: Williams & Wilkins; 1989.
2. Krebs D. Clinical electromyographic feedback following meniscectomy: a multiple regression experimental analysis. *Phys Ther.* 1981; 61:1017–1021.
3. Wise H, Fiebert I, Kates J. EMG Biofeedback as Treatment for Patellofemoral Pain Syndrome. *J Orthop Sports Phys Ther.* 1984; 6:95–103.
4. LeCraw DE. Biofeedback in stroke rehabilitation. In: Basmajian JV, ed. *Biofeedback: Principles and Practice for Clinicians.* 3rd ed. Baltimore, MD: Williams & Wilkins; 1989:105–117.
5. Brudny J, Korein J, et al. Helping hemiparetics to help themselves. *JAMA.* 1979; 242:814–818.
6. Honer J, Mohr T, Roth R. Electromyographic biofeedback to dissociate an upper extremity synergy pattern: a case report. *Phys Ther.* 1982; 62:299–303.
7. Wolf LS, Baker MP, Kelly JL. EMG biofeedback in stroke: a one year follow-up on the effect of patient characteristics. *Arch Phys Med Rehabil.* 1980; 61:351–355.
8. Nacht MB, Wolf SL, Cooglerr CE. Use of electromyographic biofeedback during the acute phase of spinal cord injury: a case report. *Phys Ther.* 1982; 62:290–294.
9. Brown DM, Nahai F, Wolf S, et al. Electromyographic feedback in the re-education of facial palsy. *Am J Phys Med.* 1978; 57:183–190.
10. Brudny J, Korein J, et al. EMG feedback therapy: review of treatment of 114 patients. *Arch Phys Med Rehabil.* 1976; 57:55–61.
11. Korein J, Brudny J. Integrated EMG feedback in the management of spasmodic torticollis and focal dystonia: a prospective study of 80 patients. In: Yahr M, ed. *The Basal Ganglia.* New York: Raven Press; 1976:385–424.

25

Ultraviolet Irradiation

Joseph Weisberg, PT, PhD

T he use of sunlight for healing purposes is ancient. References to sun gods are found in the writings of ancient Egypt and Greece. In 525 BC, Herodotus concluded that the energy of the sun affected bone growth. Throughout the centuries that followed, sun bathing was prescribed for conditions such as arthritis, sciatica, weight loss, ulcers, scurvy, rickets, and general weakness. In 1877, Downes and Blunt proved that sun rays could kill bacteria.[1]

Artificial ultraviolet light was developed during the 19th century. In 1859 the relationship between artificial ultraviolet irradiation and erythema was discovered. In 1893 Niels Finsen introduced the use of artificial ultraviolet light from a carbon arc to treat skin disorders such as lupus vulgaris, for which he received the Nobel Prize. The mercury vapor lamp was developed early in the 20th century.[2] Today, ultraviolet light is readily available to the general public, mostly for tanning purposes, and to the medical profession for specific therapeutic purposes, primarily tissue repair, exfoliation, and wound healing. However, the reasons for administering UV therapy are decreasing because more efficient methods of achieving the same treatment goals have been developed.

PHYSICAL PRINCIPLES

The term ultraviolet (ultra = beyond) was first used by J. Ritter (1801). This term is misleading because the wavelengths referred to are actually below the wavelength of visible light (less than 400 nm); thus, a more accurate term would be infraviolet. Angström (1868) was the first to map out the wavelengths of this part of the spectrum. The unit of measurement used to describe the wavelength was the angstrom unit (Å) (1 Å = 10 nm). At present, a nanometer is the unit of measure used (1 nm = 0.1 Å).

The range of radiant energy designated as *ultraviolet* (UV) extends from approximately 180 nm to approximately 400 nm. The frequencies range from approximately 1.65×10^{15} cycles per second (CPS) to approximately 7.5×10^{14} CPS[3] (CPS has now been replaced by Hz) The ultraviolet rays are in the range immediately below violet of the visible spectrum (Fig. 25–1). Within the ultraviolet range, the longer wavelengths are referred to as *near ultraviolet* rays because they are nearer to the visible light and are considered to be beneficial to life in general (between 290 nm–400 nm). For example, UV at this range helps with the production of vitamin D and photosynthesis in general. The shorter wavelengths are referred to as the *far ultraviolet* rays because they are farther away from the visible light (between 180 nm–290 nm) and are generally considered to be harmful to life. For example, UV light at this range is used to sterilize instruments. Some authors separate the ultraviolet radiation into three bands: UV-A (320–400), UV-B (290–320), and UV–C (200–290).[4,5]

Ultraviolet light is produced when the electrons in stable atoms are activated to move to higher orbits, thus creating an unstable state. As these electrons move back to their original orbit, energy is given up as electromagnetic radiation. This energy has the property of both discrete particles (photons) and continuous waves. The emission and transmission of this energy has been explained by the quantum and electromagnetic wave theories (see Chapter 5).

The sun is the natural source of UV light. 5–10% of the sun's energy is in the UV range (180 nm–400 nm).[6] The ozone layer of the earth's atmosphere filters most of the harmful UV rays. Most, but not all of the sun's UV rays that reach the earth's surface after filtration range from 290 nm to 400 nm. UV-A (320 nm–400 nm) accounts for 6.3% of the sunlight during the summer, whereas UV-B (290 nm–320 nm) accounts for only 0.5%. Both can be involved in sunburn and skin diseases.[7] The actual UV rays from the sun reaching the earth will depend on (1) variation in the amount of energy radiated from the sun, (2) variation in the earth's distance from the sun (season of the year), (3) the time of day, (4) the condition of the atmosphere (the ozone layer, dust, moisture), (5) the latitude, and (6) the altitude. For example, the larger the ozone layer or the more acute the angle of the rays reaching the earth's surface, the less the sun's UV rays will affect life on earth.

PHYSIOLOGIC AND PSYCHOLOGICAL EFFECTS

In biologic tissue, UV rays are absorbed within 0.22 mm of the surface. Therefore, when normal skin is exposed to UV radiation, 80–90% reaches the dermis. In addition, it is important to realize that skin reflects the shorter wavelength rays more

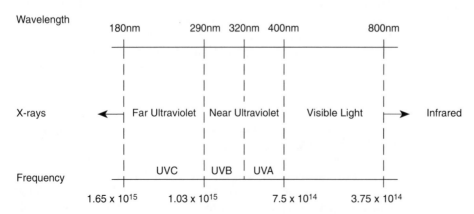

Figure 25–1. Portion of the electromagnetic spectrum containing ultraviolet and visible light.

than it reflects the longer wavelength rays. Therefore, the amount of UV rays with shorter wavelengths affecting the skin is proportionally less.[8] The UV rays absorbed by the tissue are capable of breaking chemical bonds, which leads to the formation of new chemical bonds, thus producing photochemical effects. This process is caused by a chain of reactions; therefore, the net effect of UV treatment is delayed, appearing over a period of time after the treatment is given. The specific photochemical effect produced by UV rays differs at various wavelengths. For example, rays of 254 nm or 299 nm are the most effective wavelengths for producing tanning (Fig. 25–2). Rays of 254 nm or 297 nm are the most effective in producing erythema (Fig. 25–3). Rays of wavelength between 250–270 nm have a predominantly bactericidal effect. Some bands obviously have a multiple effect (Fig. 25–4).[9]

The specific effect of UV light depends on the wavelength. For example, a relatively long wavelength (297 nm) will produce erythema that will develop slowly (within 24 hours) and will disappear slowly (in more than 10 days). A shorter wavelength (254 nm) will produce peak erythema in 6 hours, which will disappear within 4 days.[9,10]

The beneficial effects of ultraviolet can be summarized as follows:

Erythema. Erythema is defined as redness of the skin produced by congestion of the capillaries. Erythema promotes wound healing by increasing the blood supply to the treated area. If the dosage is sufficiently high, the UV rays will initiate an inflammatory response.[11] It is believed that the vasodilation is caused by the liberation of histaminelike substances and other vasodilators.[12] This, in turn, stimulates the formulation of granular tissue, leading to tissue repair. Note that erythema occurs as a result of enlargement and engorgement of minute blood vessels in the corium (the superficial layer of the dermis), not as a thermal reaction. Erythema is best achieved with wavelengths of 254 nm and 297 nm (see Fig. 25–3).

Pigmentation. Pigmentation is the production of melanin in the deeper strata of the epidermis. The melanin ascends into the more superficial zones, causing a darkening of the skin (tanning) and thickening of the corneum. In turn, this par-

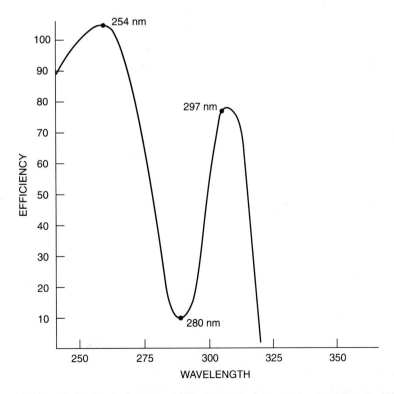

Figure 25–2. Production of pigmentation in relationship to the wavelength. Wavelengths of 254 nm or 299 nm are the most effective tanning rays. (*Adapted from S Licht.*[3])

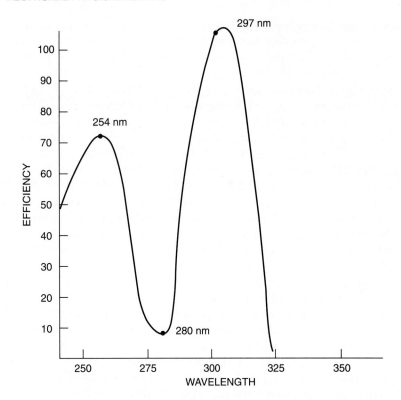

Figure 25–3. Production of erythema in relationship to the wavelength. Wavelengths of 254 nm and 297 nm are the most effective in producing erythema. (*Adapted from S Licht.*[3])

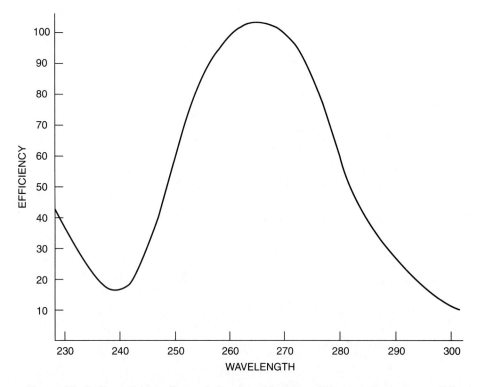

Figure 25–4. Bactericidal effects of ultraviolet irradiation. Wavelengths between 250 nm and 270 nm are most effective.

tially blocks penetration of UV light, thus providing protection from sunburn. Tanning is best achieved with wavelengths of 254 nm and 299 nm (see Fig. 25–2).

Destruction of bacteria. The destructive effect of UV rays on bacteria was demonstrated as early as 1877 by Downes and Blunt. The bactericidal effect is best achieved with wavelengths ranging from 250 nm to 270 nm (Fig. 25–4). These rays exterminate bacteria by suppressing their synthesis of DNA and RNA.[9] Ultraviolet rays in these ranges can be used to sterilize air and water. Clinically, UV light is used to destroy bacteria in ulcers and other types of wounds. Furthermore, it increases the resistance to airborne infection by stimulating reticuloendothelial cells, which increases the production of circulatory antibodies.[13] In addition, the destruction of bacteria enhances the tissue repair process.

Wound healing. Nutini suggested that UV rays in the range of 260–280 nm are helpful in the healing process and that they promote tissue growth.[14] **Note:** ultraviolet rays in the range of 260–270 nm are bactericidal, which by itself might contribute to the healing effect.

Thickening of the epidermis. Ultraviolet light causes thickening of the epidermis in all layers, with the exception of the basal layer.[15] This may have a protective function, but its usefulness is questionable.

Exfoliation of epidermal cells. Ultraviolet light causes the exfoliation or sloughing off of dead epithelial cells at the stratum corneum, the most superficial layer of the epidermis. Thus, it is used to treat acne vulgaris.[8]

Formation of vitamin D. Historically, UV light was useful in treating patients with a deficiency of vitamin D. Currently, however, this vitamin is readily available in the diet and supplements.

Increased production of red cells. Even though this effect has been demonstrated, ultraviolet is not currently used for this purpose.[9]

Stimulation of steroid metabolism. Ultraviolet radiation promotes vasomotor responses causing an antirachitic effect.[16]

Psychological effects. Sunshine in general promotes the feeling of well-being. Many people equate tanning with health; thus, we can say that UV light promotes the feeling of well-being.[8]

The photochemical effect of excessive doses of UV irradiation can lead to shock.[11] This condition reduces the pulse rate, respiration, and blood pressure and can be a life-threatening condition. The early, clinically observable sign is that the patient suddenly becomes pale. Even doses within the clinical range can, at times, cause an extreme reaction in patients who have preexisting conditions that make them photosensitive. The student is reminded of the inverse square law and the cosine law, both of which apply to UV radiation. The distance of the application from the surface of the body and the angulation of the rays will affect the dose the body receives.

In the event that the patient is overexposed, some authors suggest that the patient should be treated within 1 hour by luminous infrared lamp or fluorescent light for at least 10 minutes. This has been claimed to cause photoreactivation, which will thus diminish the effect of UV irradiation.[17]

CONTRAINDICATIONS AND PRECAUTIONS

Because the cornea absorbs UV wavelengths over 295 nm, the eyes of the patient and operator must be well protected with goggles at all times. Ultraviolet irradiation is contraindicated for only a few conditions:

- Photosensitivity (photosensitive patient, such as one with albinism, might not tolerate even a minimum dosage).
- Porphyrias (a rare metabolic disorder).

- Pellagra (dermatitis due to severe niacin deficiency).
- Discoidlupus erythematosus (inflammatory dermatitis due to lupus).
- Sarcoidosis or xeroderma pigmentosum (chronic progressive granulomatous reticulosis involving organs including the skin).
- Fever, active pulmonary tuberculosis, severe cardiac involvement, acute diabetes, and acute skin pathologies.

PRECAUTIONS

Caution should be taken with patients who have any of the preexisting conditions listed below because each condition increases their sensitivity to UV rays. When it is necessary to treat such patients with UV rays, the overall dosage should be lowered.

- Patients with little pigmentation, often seen in blonds and redheads. (A patient with albinism may not tolerate even a minimum dosage.)
- Patients with conditions such as syphilis or alcoholism because of photochemical hypersensitivity; cardiac or renal diseases because their tolerance is lower; initial acute onset of psoriasis; acute eczema, herpes simplex, systemic lupus erythematosus; active pulmonary tuberculosis because UV may exacerbate it; hyperthyroidism and diabetes because UV causes itching; cancer because UV may increase anemia; and infants, the elderly, or patients receiving chemotherapy because of low tolerance.
- Patients who have ingested certain foods such as strawberries, eggs, or shellfish before the treatment.
- Patients who are taking any of the following medications: birth control pills (because of hormonal changes, UV can produce undesirable blotching), sulfonamides, sulfonylurea, griseofulvin, tetracycline, quinine, endocrines, gold or other heavy metals, diuretics, insulin, phenothiazines, psoralens, or using tar. Exposure to UV light while taking these medications heightens the effect of the medication. (When in doubt, consult the physician, pharmacologist, or the *Physicians' Desk Reference*.)
- Patients who received superficial heat treatment (hot pack infrared) before the UV treatment.[18]

EQUIPMENT

Most UV generators that are used clinically are made of a quartz tube filled with argon gas and some liquid mercury. The quality of the quartz tube is such that it permits the UV rays to go through to affect the target tissue. When the lamp is turned on, the argon gas is heated by the passing current. The heat produced vaporizes the mercury, causing the emission of the UV and visible violet rays.

Two common UV generators are in clinical use; they are referred to as "hot quartz" and "cold quartz" generators. The hot quartz generator (see Fig. 25–5) is an air-cooled, high-pressure mercury vapor lamp. This type of generator uses low voltages (30–110 V) and high currents (5 A). The UV rays emitted under these conditions are in both the near and the far bands.

The other common type of generator, the cold quartz generator, operates in a manner similar to the hot quartz generator but at a lower temperature. It uses a high voltage (as high as 3000 V), low current (15 mA), low temperature, and low pressure. More than 90% of its emission after filtration is 253.7 nm, which is bactericidal.[17] These generators are smaller than hot quartz generators, they are portable, and they can be used in close proximity to the body (see Fig. 25–6).

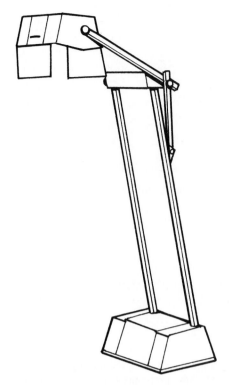

Figure 25–5. A hot quartz generator. (*Reproduced with permission from GE Miller, Inc.*)

DOSAGE

Method of Determining the Minimal Erythemal Dose

To determine the therapeutic dosage for each patient, the following procedure should be performed:

1. Prepare an *erythrometer*, which can be made from a piece of paper, cardboard, exposed x-ray film, or fabric measuring 4 inches by 8 inches. Cut small holes approximately ¾ of an inch wide in six different shapes about ¾ of an inch apart (see Fig. 25–7).
2. Clean and dry the surface to be tested. Make certain that the skin of the area selected for the test has not been previously exposed to UV radiation. Tape the erythrometer to the flexor aspect of the forearm or to the lower abdomen. Use the lower abdomen if the forearm is too small or if it is unavailable for another reason. These are the areas of choice because they are flat and are rarely exposed to the sun and are more photosensitive.
3. Cover all the holes in the erythrometer.
4. Drape the patient completely.
5. Put on goggles and give a pair to the patient.

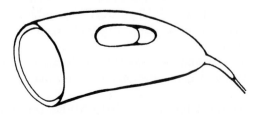

Figure 25–6. A cold quartz generator. (*Reproduced with permission from GE Miller, Inc.*)

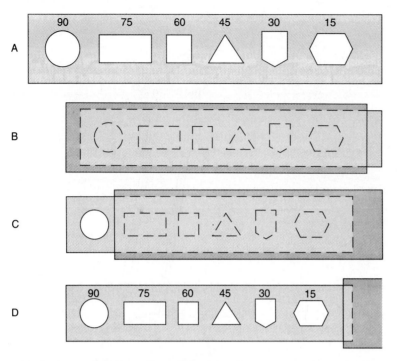

Figure 25–7. An erythrometer. (**A**) The cardboard with the cut holes. (**B**) The cardboard with the cover. (**C**) The cardboard with one hole exposed. (**D**) The cardboard with all holes exposed and the time exposures labeled in seconds.

6. Position the UV lamp directly over the area (so it is perpendicular) and 30 inches (76 cm) away.
7. Turn on the generator to preheat for 5 minutes.
8. Open the shutters and expose the first hole, keeping the remaining holes covered. After 15 seconds, uncover the second hole. Continue uncovering each subsequent hole at 15-second intervals until all the holes are uncovered.
9. When 90 seconds have elapsed since the first hole was uncovered, cover the patient and close the shutters. In this way, the first hole will have received 90 seconds of exposure, the last hole only 15 seconds.
10. Instruct the patient to check the area every 2 hours while awake and to record which symbols appeared, which ones faded, and the times that each one appeared and faded. This information is used to determine the patient's *minimal erythemal dose (MED)*, or the amount of infrared exposure required to show erythema lasting up to 48 hours.

Ultraviolet Doses

The parameters for the various doses are listed below:

- Suberythemal dose (SED), no evidence of erythema.
- Minimal erythemal doses (MED), evidence of erythema lasting 24 hours.
- First-degree erythemal dose (E1) (2.5 × MED), evidence of erythema lasting as long as 48 hours.
- Second-degree erythemal doses (E2) (5 × MED), evidence of intense erythema with edema, peeling, and pigmentation that will last as long as 72 hours.
- Third-degree erythemal doses (E3) (10 × MED), produces erythema with severe blistering and exudation and should be limited to an area no larger than 25 sq cm. **Note:** Change in pigmentation may occur simultaneously.

Generalized Exposure

When treatment is sought for conditions such as generalized dermatitis or localized psoriasis, the following procedures must be adhered to:

1. Position the patient in the supine position with the face turned to one side and with the palms up. Cover the patient, providing an extra protective covering over the nipples, umbilicus, genitalia, hair, and eyes.
2. Center the lamp over the superior half of the patient's body 30 inches (76 cm) away from the sternum.
3. Expose the upper part of the body for the dosage indicated, using the anterior superior iliac spine as the borderline between the upper and the lower part of the body.
4. Close the shutters and cover the patient.
5. Position the generator over the lower part of the patient's body.
6. Expose the lower area for treatment.
7. Close the shutters and cover the patient.
8. Do the same for the back, using the posterior superior iliac spine as the dividing landmark, and expose the upper and lower parts in the same manner as before while the patient is prone. Make certain that the arm is now positioned with the palm down and the other side of the face is now exposed. (To avoid double exposure, record the original position.) Be extra careful with obese patients because landmarks are not clearly visible. Furthermore, fat rolls and the umbilicus area should be exposed with care.
9. Subsequent treatments should be conducted in the same manner, but the duration per area usually can be increased by 5 seconds each time. The increment by which the dosage is increased will depend on the patient's sensitivity to UV radiation. When the total exposure for each area reaches 3 minutes, the distance can then be reduced to avoid increasing the exposure time further.

PROCEDURES

General Instructions

1. The treatment room should be well ventilated to eliminate the accumulation of poisonous ozone gas[3] from the warm-up. (Short UV wavelengths, 184.9 nm, are readily absorbed by the oxygen in the air to form ozone and nitrogen oxides.
2. Wipe off the envelop (bulb) and the reflectors at least once a day (if in use), preferably with 95% ethyl alcohol. Use nap- or lint-free toweling to avoid leaving any fibers behind. Any dust, oil, or water film on the envelope or the reflector will diminish the amount of UV energy reaching the patient.
3. Position the lamp perpendicular to the area to be treated. Measure the distance from the lamp to the highest surface of the area (A distance of 30 inches, 76 cm, is commonly used at the start.)
4. Clean the skin to be treated.
5. Completely cover all skin area (including hair) until treatment time, when the involved area will be exposed for a timed dose.
6. Protect the patient's and your own eyes with special goggles designed for this purpose. Other glasses and sunglasses do not protect from reflection from the side. Eyes need this protection because of poor circulation in the superficial structure of the eye. Thus, the energy absorbed from the UV rays concentrates in a small volume of tissue and damages that tissue.
7. The hot quartz generators should be warmed up 5 to 10 minutes (or as indicated by the manufacturer's manual) before the treatment, with the shutters closed to protect the patient and yourself.

8. Begin timing as soon as the shutters are open and treatment time is on.
9. Carefully monitor the exposure time. The dose is determined according to the MED. (Remember that the dose can be intensified by increasing the exposure time or shortening the distance between the lamp and the patient.)
10. Immediately cover the exposed area after the treatment and close the shutter.
11. Record the exposure time and lamp distance. If the office has more than one lamp, specify the lamp used.

While treating the patient, the therapist should avoid exposing part of his or her body. In addition, the therapist must remember that hot quartz lamps must cool sufficiently to reestablish the original gaseous state before they are turned on again. The lamps should be restandardized by the company representative after every 100 treatment hours.

Local Treatment With Hot Quartz

The procedures for treating local conditions are the same as for generalized exposure, but the UV rays are applied to a local area. Closer distances can be used for this type of treatment, and the exposure time should be recalculated according to the formula

$$T2 = T1 \left(\frac{(d2)^2}{(d1)^2} \right)$$

Where T2 = new exposure time, T1 = initial exposure time, d1 = initial distance, and d2 = new distance.

Never use a hot quartz generator closer than 15 inches (about 38 cm) to the patient because the intensity of the UV will be extremely high, and regulating the dosage will be difficult. No dose should be repeated until the erythemal effect of the previous dose has disappeared.

The therapist is responsible for positioning the patient carefully for treatment to avoid over- or underexposure. Duplication of exposure can easily occur if one is not careful, especially if whole-body irradiation is used. One-half of the face, either the anterior or the posterior surfaces of the upper extremities, and the lateral aspect of the lower extremity are especially vulnerable.

When treating local areas, it is important to keep a precise record of the area treated to avoid overexposure in subsequent treatments. Charting the area by means of bony landmarks is helpful.

Underexposure can occur if the lamp or body part is not clean or is not optimally positioned. For example, in treating the ventral surface of the arm, the neutral position of the arm (that is, with the lateral aspect perpendicular to the lamp) is not optimal. The UV rays will be parallel to the volar surface of the arm, leading to underexposure.

Local Treatment with Cold Quartz

Cold quartz is used most commonly to treat decubitus ulcers for the bactericidal healing effects. Because the UV is applied to an open wound, the skin is not a mediating factor. There is no need to determine the MED for this treatment. Exposure time for the different doses is predetermined.

The MED for cold quartz from a distance of 1 inch (2.5 cm) is 12–15 seconds, E1 = 36–45 seconds, E2 = 72–90 seconds, and E3 = 135–180 seconds. When this generator is used in direct contact with the body, 55% of the dosage should be used. This may be appropriate when deeper penetration is desired.

When operating the cold quartz generator, the therapist should carry out the following steps:

1. Wash the area with soap and water and clean the wound of any debris.
2. Dry the area thoroughly.
3. Cover the area with a sterile drape when treating open wounds.
4. Put on the goggles and give the patient a pair.
5. Drape the bulb end of the unit.
6. Turn on the unit for 1–3 minutes to warm it up.
7. Position the lamp perpendicular to the skin surface at a distance of 1 inch (2.5 cm). You can insure the correct distance either by placing the lamp on doughnut gauze that is 1 inch thick or by taping tongue depressors that protrude 1 inch (2.5 cm) (see Fig. 25–8).
8. Expose the wound for the required time.
9. Turn off the lamp.

The dose with the cold quartz method depends on the condition. Healing wounds can be treated with a MED of E3. Exposure of the intact skin to UV radiation may require more exposure to get the same effect. Generally, mucosal surfaces can tolerate a dose that is twice as high as the epidermal surfaces can tolerate. However, because there is no epidermal covering that might thicken, the dosage remains the same.

The effectiveness of the UV treatment also depends on the output of the lamps. Their output diminishes as they age. The effectiveness of the lamp is reduced long before the bulb is completely burned out. That is why the lamp must be checked after every 100 hours of use or at least once a year.

Many large facilities have their own meters to calibrate UV lamps.[19] Commercial calibration facilities serve those users without in house facilities.

COMMON INDICATIONS

Psoriasis (not in the acute stage of the first manifestation).[20] One common use of UV radiation is in the treatment of psoriasis. Ultraviolet radiation can be used alone to achieve exfoliation or in conjunction with medication, tar paste, or ointment.[21–24] The two types of UV treatments for psoriasis that are considered to be safest and most effective are the TUVAB and the PUVA. TUVAB is an acronym for tar and ultraviolet A and B, three antipsoriatic agents also known as the Goeckerman regimen. The treatment involves the application of tar ointment, followed by exposure to ultraviolet light. With this type of treatment, it is theorized that the light damages the DNA, thus inhibiting the cells from proliferating as rapidly. PUVA is an acronym for psoralen and UV-A. The patient ingests psoralen and is then exposed to UV-A. It is theorized that the psoralen binds to the DNA and damages it when it is irradiated with UV light. Patients must be warned that for 24 hours after ingesting psoralen, they must wear UV-opaque goggles to protect the lens of the eyes.[25] It is important to note that PUVA has recently been associated with an increased incidence of skin cancer, liver disease, and some tumors. However, it is still an acceptable treatment, but only for selected severe cases.[26]

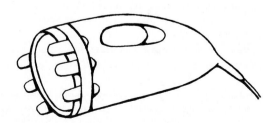

Figure 25–8. A cold quartz generator with taped tongue depressors used as spacers. The tongue depressors all protrude 1 inch from the generator to provide the desirable distance of 1 inch.

Acne vulgaris. Ultraviolet light is used to achieve exfoliation.[11] The treatment for this condition involves local or general body irradiation three times a week, beginning with a MED and progressively increasing the dosage with subsequent treatment (up to 16–20 MED). It has been suggested that patients who show spontaneous remission of the acne during the summer are better candidates for this treatment. Obviously, the treatments are given during the winter.

Ulcers. Ultraviolet light is used to treat ulcers, especially decubitis ulcers, because of its bactericidal effect and its positive effect on healing. The treatment for this condition depends on the condition of the ulcer. If granulations are present, a suberythemal dose is required daily or every other day. If the ulcer is still spreading, a first-degree erythemal dose or even a second-degree erythemal dose once or twice a week may be required to initiate granulation. Then a smaller, suberythemal daily dose is used to promote healing.

Uremic Pruritus. Ultraviolet irradiation has proved to be helpful to patients who have uremic pruritis.[27] The treatment for this type of itching involves general body irradiation with a suberythemal dose every 3 or 4 days.

Jaundice. Ultraviolet irradiation also is used to help prevent jaundice in newborns.

■ KEY TERMS

ultraviolet
  near ultraviolet
  far ultraviolet

erythrometer
minimal erythemal dose (MED)

REFERENCES

1. Licht S. History of ultraviolet therapy. In: Licht S, ed *Therapeutic Electricity and Ultraviolet Radiation.* 2nd ed. New Haven, CT: Elizabeth Licht; 1967:200.
2. Harber LC, Bickers DR. Introduction to photobiology. In: *Photosensitivity Diseases: Principles of Diagnosis and Treatment.* Philadelphia, PA: WB Saunders; 1981:3–9.
3. Anderson WT. Instrumentations for ultraviolet therapy. In: Licht S, ed. *Therapeutic Electricity and Ultraviolet Radiation.* 2nd ed. New Haven, CT: Elizabeth Licht; 1967:214–215.
4. Anderson TG, Wadinger TP, Voorhees JJ. UV-B phototherapy: an overview. *Arch Dermatol.* 1948; 120:1502–1507.
5. Schafer V. Artificial production of ultraviolet radiation, introduction and historical review. In: Urback F, ed. *The Biological Effects of Ultraviolet Radiation, with Emphasis on the Skin.* New York, NY: Pergamon Press; 1969:93.
6. Brown I, Meng MJ. *Fundamentals of Electrotherapy: Course Guide.* Madison, WI: American Printing & Publishing; 1972:10.
7. *Monthly Skin News.* June 1988; 1(4).
8. Scott BO. Clinical uses of ultraviolet radiation. In: Stillwell KG, ed. *Therapeutic Electricity and Ultraviolet Radiation.* 3rd ed. Baltimore, MD: Williams & Wilkins, 1983:234.
9. Fischer E, Solomon S. *Physiological Effects of Ultraviolet Radiation.* 2nd ed. New Haven, CT: Elizabeth Licht; 1967:258–273.
10. Hausser KW, Vahle W. Sunburn and suntanning. In: Urback F, ed. *The Biologic Effects of Ultraviolet Radiation, with Emphasis on the Skin.* New York, NY: Pergamon Press; 1969:7.
11. Scriber WJ. *A Manual of Electrotherapy.* Philadelphia, PA: Lea & Febiger; 1975:49.
12. Holti G. Measurements of the vascular responses in skin at various time intervals after damage with histamine and ultraviolet radiations. *Chem Sci.* 1955; 14:143–155.
13. Kahn J. Physical agents: electrical, sonic and radiant modalities. In: Scully RM, Barnes MR, eds. *Physical Therapy.* Philadelphia, PA: JB Lippincott; 1989:894–897.
14. Nutini LG: Tissue repair. In: Glasser O, ed. *Medical Physics II.* Chicago, IL: Yearbook Publisher; 1950:1124.

15. Daniels F Jr, Brophy D, Lobitz WC. Histochemical responses of human skin following ultraviolet irradiation. *J Invest Dermatol.* 1961; 37:351.

16. Wadsworth H, Channugam A. *Electrophysical Agents in Physiotherapy.* New South Wales, Australia: Science Press; 1980.

17. Griffin JE, Karselis TC. *Physical Agents for Physical Therapists.* 3rd ed. Springfield, IL: Charles C Thomas; 1982:269.

18. Montgomery PC. The compounding effects of infrared and ultraviolet irradiation upon normal human skin. *Phys Ther.* 1973; 53:489–496.

19. *Safety Bulletin.* New York: Columbia University, Department of Environmental Health and Safety. June 1985. Health Sciences Revision #6.

20. Bryant BG. Treatment of psoriasis. *Am J Hosp Pharm.* 1980; 37:814–820.

21. Solomon WM, Netherton EW, Nelson PA, *et al.* Treatment of psoriasis with the Goeckerman technique. *Arch Phys Med Rehabil.* 1955; 36:74–77.

22. Fusco RU, Jordan PA, Kelly A, *et al.* PUVA treatment for psoriasis. *Physiotherapy.* 1980; 66(2):39–40.

23. Klaber MR. Ultraviolet light for psoriasis. *Physiotherapy.* 1980; 66(2):36–38.

24. Shurr DG, Zuehlke RI. Photochemotherapy treatment of psoriasis. *Phy Ther.* 1981; 62(1):33–36.

25. Psoriasis update. *J Coll Phys Surg Columbia Univ.* 1986; 6(1).

26. Psoriasis therapy linked to cancer. *PT Bull.* October 5, 1988.

27. Gilchrest BA, Rowe JW, Brown RS. Relief of the uremic pruritis with ultraviolet phototherapy. *N Engl J Med.* 1977; 297(3):136–138.

26

Lasers

Joseph Weisberg, PT, PhD

Physical Principles	**Indications, Contraindications, and Precautions**
Physiological Effects	**Key Terms**
Types Used in Physical Therapy	
Procedures	

L aser technology is rapidly advancing, and its usage in medicine is constantly growing. Recently, a low-power laser was introduced in the United States with the claim that the device could help reduce pain, spasm, and inflammation and could promote healing. Although a low-power laser with an output of less than 1 mW has been used in Europe for more than a decade, its effectiveness has not been established.[1,2] Most of the therapeutic claims attributed to this modality are based on empirical observation. At present, the Food and Drug Administration (FDA) has classified the low-power laser as a Class III medical device. Therefore, practitioners who want to use this type of a device must obtain an investigational device exemption, as stated in FDA regulation 812.2(b).

PHYSICAL PRINCIPLES

The word *laser* is an acronym for "light amplification by stimulated emission radiation." The low-power laser is a form of electromagnetic energy with a wavelength that may fall within the visible or the infrared section of the electromagnetic spectrum. However, lasers have three unique qualities that distinguish them from ordinary light: coherence, monochromaticity, and a collimated beam.

Coherence. Coherent light, unlike ordinary light, consists of parallel waves that propagate with a high degree of order approximating the same phase (temporal) and the same direction (spatial) (Fig. 26–1). These properties, referred to as *temporal and spatial coherence,* minimize divergence and focus the energy so that it is concentrated in one area. Figs. 26–1 and 26–2 show the difference between laser light and ordinary light.

Monochromaticity. Each laser device emits energy of one wavelength. For example, the Helium-Neon (HeNe) device produces a red laser beam with a wavelength of 632.8 nm, and the Gallium-Arsenide (GaAs) device produces an infrared laser beam with a wavelength of 910 nm. Ordinary light is a mixture of many wavelengths. The significance of the *monochromaticity* of light is found in reports suggesting that certain wavelengths have certain characteristics that affect biological tissue in a particular way. For example, Wolbarsht[3] suggested that a wave-

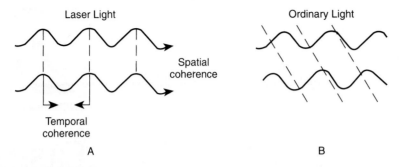

Figure 26–1. (**A**) Phase characteristics of laser light. The wavelengths have temporal coherence—all the waves emitted by individual gas molecules have the same wavelength. The wavelengths also have spatial coherence: that is, all the waves travel in the same direction. (**B**) Phase characteristics of ordinary light.

length of 632.8 nm is "in tune with the resonance of the biological tissue," thus affecting it in a positive way, enhancing its healing.[4]

Collimated beam. Collimation refers to the minimal divergence or moving apart of the photons in a laser beam. Laser beams can be produced by applying electrical, mechanical, or chemical energy to various forms of matter. The stimulus (energy) can bring about a change in the position of an electron within the atom of a substance, forcing the electron to move momentarily to an outer orbit, which is at a higher energy level. At this point, the atom is said to be in an "excited" (unstable) state. When the electron returns to its original orbit, photons are released. The released photons may then collide with other atoms, causing the release of more photons. This stimulation leads to a chain reaction that cumulatively causes the emission of radiant energy (see Fig. 26–3).

Laser beams, like any other form of radiant energy, can be absorbed, reflected, or transmitted. To achieve temporal and spatial coherence, the photons are aligned in a reflecting chamber. The photons are then reflected back and forth between mirrors to achieve amplification before being ejected through a fiberoptic cable or a diode to reach the area to be treated.

PHYSIOLOGICAL EFFECTS

The effects of laser beams on biologic tissue are directly related to the wavelength of the beam, the depth to which it penetrates, the dosage (ie, the intensity and the duration of the treatment), and the total number of treatments. In addition, the condition of the tissue plays an important part in the outcome of the treatment; for example, a poor blood supply to the treated area reduces the amount of energy absorbed by that tissue.

Lasers are available in high or low power. Lasers with a power of more than 60 mW are considered to be high-power lasers (CO^2, Argon, and YAG lasers) and can cause thermal responses and can damage tissues (burning, dehydration, evaporation, or coagulation of proteins). These lasers are not used by physical thera-

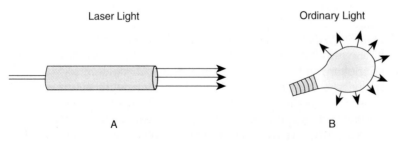

Figure 26–2. Wave direction of (**A**) laser light and (**B**) ordinary light.

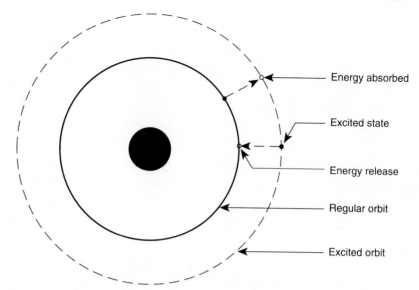

Figure 26–3. Excited state of electrons and the release of energy.

pists; they are used in surgery. Low-power (HeNe and GaAs) lasers (cold lasers) use less than 60 mW and cause minimal or no thermal responses.

Low-power lasers are used in physical therapy at 1 mW or less. At peak intensity, they continue to stimulate at 1 mW while the output of the pulsed mode is about 0.5 mW. The human skin absorbs as much as 99% of the radiation; dark skin absorbs more than light skin.[5]

Recently, the case for the use of low-power lasers for therapeutic purposes has been strengthened by theories and scientific investigations. The physiological effects attributed to low-power laser treatments include pain reduction, accelerated tissue healing related to an increased rate of collagen synthesis and vascularization, and a decrease in microorganisms. However, the research is in its early stages, and more well-controlled studies are needed. Kleinkort and Foley[6] suggested that low-power laser treatments have a local effect on cells within the treatment area and a systemic effect on the body in general. This effect is probably the result of the acceleration of photobiologic or photochemical processes or both. This theory has gained some support from more recent, controlled studies: Snyder-Mackler and Bork[7] demonstrated that low-power laser treatments cause an increase in the sensory nerve latency response. Vizi *et al.*[8] demonstrated that low-power laser radiation on nerve plexus caused an increase in the release of acetylcholine. Walker[9] demonstrated that low-power laser stimulation increased the release of serotonin and endogenous opiates, thus affecting pain. Snyder-Mackler and Bork[10] also demonstrated a decrease in skin impedance after low-power laser stimulation. Seitz and Kleinkort[11] have shown that low-power laser can lower the temperature of tissue at a distal site. In addition, the treatment also affects urine secretion both qualitatively and quantitatively. King et al[12] have demonstrated that low-power auriculotherapy reduces the pain threshold. Goldman[13] found that low-power laser therapy reduces most of the symptoms secondary to rheumatoid arthritis.

TYPES USED IN PHYSICAL THERAPY

The most common low-power laser available today for physical therapy treatments is the HeNe laser (see Fig. 26–4). The red laser light in this device is produced in a tube filled with helium and neon gases (atoms). Electrical stimulation of these gases causes the emission of radiation at a wavelength of 632.8 nm, which is in the red range of visible light. The light beam produced is amplified as it passes through multiple silver resonator mirrors. From there, the light is directed through

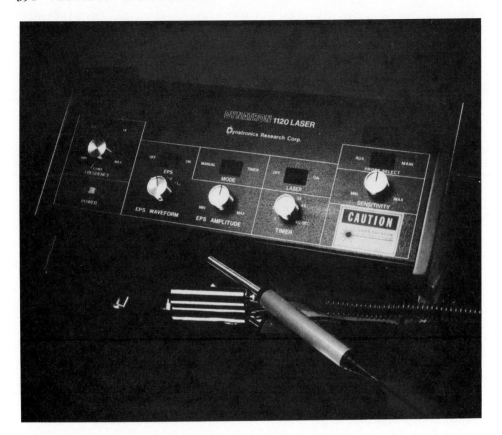

Figure 26–4. Helium-Neon (HeNe) laser. (*Reproduced with permission from Dynatron Research Co.*)

a flexible monofilament fiberoptic system to the tip of a hand-held wand that directs the laser beam toward the tissue to be stimulated. This laser penetrates directly into the tissue to a depth of about 0.8 mm, but some claim that it affects tissues to a depth of 15 mm.[11,14] Note that although the GaAs laser produces a beam in the infrared band, it is not a thermal modality. The low power used and the fact that the beam is pulsed negate any heating effect.

The literature suggests that low-power lasers may have many applications. Some reports indicate successful use of the HeNe laser to treat musculoskeletal pain.[15] Other reports suggest that the cold laser may be an effective treatment for local and systemic inflammation,[11,13] burns,[16] migraine headaches,[11] ulcers, and other wounds.[17,18]

PROCEDURES

Operating the unit. The operation of the laser unit is simple. For example, the procedures for operating the Dynatron 1120 HeNe laser unit are described below:

1. Expose and clean the skin and explain the procedure to the patient.
2. Turn the power switch on.
3. Set the timer to the selected duration (for pain, 16–20 seconds; for wounds, 20–30 seconds per area).[18]
4. Select the frequency (5–20 pulses per second, pps, for tissue healing and 20–80 pps for pain).
5. Find the low-impedance spots on the skin when the treatment requires it.
6. Activate the laser by pressing the button on the wand (point finder). A light will stay on for the duration selected.
7. Turn off the power and place the wand back in its holder.

Measuring skin impedance. The Dynatron 1120 has within it an electronic circuit that can measure skin impedance. To find the low impedance spots, the therapist must have the patient hold an inactive electrode in one hand while the therapist completes the circuit by holding the wand used to find the spot. As the therapist moves the tip of the point finder along the skin in the suspected area, the low impedance values of the trigger points and acupuncture points are significant relative to the impedance values of the surrounding tissue.

Determining the dosage. The dosage (joules/sq cm) is determined by the condition, the surface of the area to be irradiated, the total treatment time, and the mode and the type of laser. For tissue healing, the periphery of the wound can be stimulated with a HeNe laser for 30 seconds every half inch every other day. Some therapists may choose to grid the wound with 30-second continuous strokes; both techniques are recommended by the manufacturers. Treatment continues until healing is complete.

For pain, the trigger and acupuncture points related to the pain can be stimulated with a HeNe laser for 30 seconds for each point with a continuous mode. Treatment continues until the pain subsides. If no improvement occurs after four to six treatments, however, treatment should be discontinued.

INDICATIONS, CONTRAINDICATIONS, AND PRECAUTIONS

Many claims have been made regarding the effectiveness of the low-power laser in promoting tissue healing and many different techniques have been proposed.[17-19] For example, some claim that the device is useful for managing pain associated with muscle spasm, headaches, local inflammation, and systemic inflammation;[7,11,13,15,16] others claim that it effectively reduces musculoskeletal inflammation.[11,13]

The fact that the FDA has classified low-powered lasers as Class III devices means that they pose an insignificant risk to humans exposed to them unless the beam is directed toward the cornea of the eye. However, because little is known about the long-term effects, the physical therapist should avoid using lasers on pregnant women, the fontanelles of babies, and cancerous tissue.

The use of the low-power laser as a therapeutic modality in physical therapy is an exciting new development. However, more research is obviously necessary to substantiate the claims about its usefulness. Because of the FDA regulations, data from investigative clinicians has been accumulating and will soon be analyzed. In addition, many research studies are currently in progress. If the data from these sources support earlier claims, the use of lasers by physical therapists will become unrestricted.

■ KEY TERMS

laser
coherent light
temporal and spacial coherence

monochromaticity
collimation

REFERENCES

1. FDA Office of Training and Assistance, Center for Devices and Radiological Health: Fact Sheet: *Laser Biostimulation.* August 1985.
2. Krikorian DJ, Hartshorne MF, Stratton SA, et al. Use of He-Ne laser for treatment of

soft tissue trauma: evaluation by Gallium-67 citrate scanning. *Orthop Sports Phys Ther.* 1986; 8:93–96.

3. Wolbarsht ML, ed. *Laser Application in Medicine and Biology.* Vol 33. New York: Plenum Press; 1977.

4. Il'Asora S. Effect of He-Ne laser beam in post radiation repair in skeletal muscle tissue. *Bul Exp Biol Med* (It) 1980; 89:212–222.

5. Goldman L, Rockwell JR. *Lasers in Medicine.* New York: Gordon & Breach; 1971.

6. Kleinkort JA, Foley RA. Laser acupuncture: its use in physical therapy. *Am J Acupuncture.* 1984; 12:51–56.

7. Snyder-Mackler L, Bork CE. Effect of helium-neon laser irradiation on peripheral sensory nerve latency. *Phys Ther.* 1988; 68:223–225.

8. Vizi ES, Mester E, Tisza S, et al. Acetylcholine releasing effect of laser irradiation on Auerbach's plexus in guinea pig ileum. *J Neural Trans.* 1983; 40:339–344.

9. Walker JB. Relief from chronic pain by low power laser irradiation. *Neuroscience.* 1983; 43:339–344.

10. Snyder-Mackler L, Bork CE, Bourbon B, et al. Effect of helium-neon laser on musculoskeletal trigger points. *Phys Ther.* 1986; 66:1087–1090.

11. Seitz LM, Kleinkort JA. Low-power laser: its application in physical therapy. In: Michlovitz SL, ed. *Thermal Agents in Rehabilitation.* Philadelphia, PA: FA Davis; 1990:232.

12. King CE, Clelland JA, Knowles CJ, et al. Effect of helium-neon laser auriculotherapy on experimental pain threshold. *Phys Ther.* 1990; 20:24–30.

13. Goldman JA, Chiapella J, Casey H, et al. Laser therapy of rheumatoid arthritis. *Lasers Surg Med.* 1980; 1:93–101.

14. Demers LM. Overview of laser biostimulation and its application in physical therapy. In: Michlovitz SL, ed. *Thermal Agents in Rehabilitation.* 2nd ed. Philadelphia, PA: FA Davis; 1990.

15. Kroetlinger M. On the Use of Laser in Acupuncture. *Acupuncture and Electrotherapeutic Res Int J.* 1980; 5:297–311.

16. Kleinkort JA. Clinical use of laser in chronic pain and tissue healing. *Stimulus,* 1982; 7:2.

17. Mester E. Effect of laser rays on wound healing. *Am J Surg.* 1971; 122.

18. Shaw CJ. The effects of low-power lasers on wound healing: a review of the literature. Student paper, *New York University Physical Therapy Program,* December 1982.

19. Saperia D, Glassberg E, Lyons RF, et al. Demonstration of elevated type I and type III procollagen MRNA levels in cutaneous wounds treated with helium-neon laser. *Biochem Biophys Res Common.* 1986; 138:1123–1128.

27

Spinal Traction (Distraction)

Joseph Weisberg, PT, PhD

Types of Traction

Results of Treatment

Application

Indications and Contraindications

Lumbar Traction

Cervical Traction

Traction is the application of a force or a system of forces to the spine in a way that separates or attempts to separate the vertebrae and elongates the surrounding soft tissue. A more appropriate term would be distraction.[1]

Traction is an ancient therapeutic tool that was described at the time of Hippocrates. Until 1990, however, traction was used mainly to treat fractures, dislocations, and deformities of the spine. At the beginning of the 20th century, traction was used before casting and for stretching of the soft tissue surrounding the spine of scoliosis patients. Since then, traction has been refined and has become a treatment designed to manage specific disorders. In the 1950s, Cyriax[2] popularized the use of traction for lumbar disc lesions. However, follow-up studies on the use of spinal traction to treat chronic and acute musculoskeletal disorders of the spine failed to establish its effectiveness.[3–12] Over the past 25 years, the interest in traction has grown, and new methods have been developed.[13–19]

The use of gravity as the tractional force has been refined,[20] and techniques for spinal traction such as positional traction, inversion traction, Goodly polyaxial traction, Goodly-Shement lumbar lift, the Cottrell 90/90 Backtrac, and autotraction have been developed. These new methods apply precise and more gentle forces that are based on sound neurophysiological and biomechanical principles. With these techniques, the patient is positioned in a way that promotes maximal separation between the vertebrae, and some of the units permit the patient to exercise while in traction.

The new traction techniques, combined with the clinician's improved abilities to evaluate and tailor precise treatment to specific disorders enables today's physical therapist to treat patients with traction more effectively. This chapter covers the lumbar and cervical traction techniques that are used for many musculoskeletal and neurogenic disorders, excluding fractures and dislocations.

The literature supports the fact that spinal traction can elongate the spine.[21–23] To elongate the spine, the muscles and the ligaments must be elongated and the space between the vertebral bodies, the articulating facets, and the intervertebral foramen must be increased. These changes are claimed to promote relaxation in the paraspinal muscles, reduce the bulging in a herniated disc,[24, 25] and reduce the pressure on nerve roots in the area of the intervertebral foramen.[26]

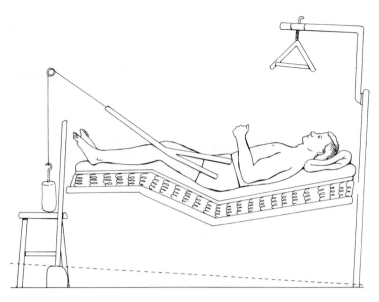

Figure 27–1. Continuous lumbar traction. This type of traction is applied continuously with a constant force for several hours each day, usually for 10–14 days. (*Adapted with permission from* Low Back Pain Syndrome *R Caillet. 1978, FA Davis.*)

TYPES OF TRACTION

Many different types of traction are available. The following are the different types of spinal traction:

Continuous traction is applied with a constant force (weight) for several hours each day, usually for 10–14 days. Because of the long duration, only a small amount of force can be applied. The purpose of this type of traction is to reduce the pressure exerted on the spine by muscles and other soft tissues while the patient is kept in complete bed rest. (Figs. 27–1 and 27–2).

Sustained traction also is applied continuously, but usually for no longer than 45 minutes. Because of this relatively short duration, greater forces can be applied.

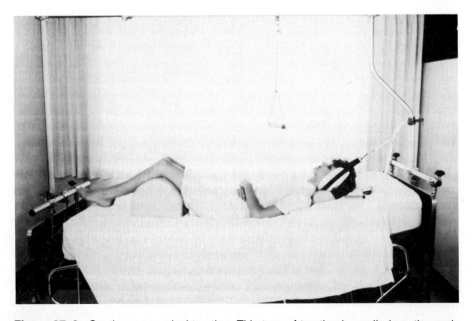

Figure 27–2. Continuous cervical traction. This type of traction is applied continuously with a constant force for several hours each day, usually for 10–14 days. (*Neck Track Hospital Set courtesy of Lossing Orthopedic Co.*)

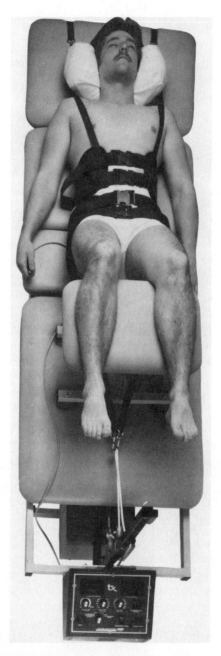

Figure 27–3. Intermittent lumbar traction. (*Reproduced with permission from Chattanooga Co.*)

With this type of traction, relaxation of muscles can be achieved, soft tissue can be stretched, and separation of bony surfaces is possible.

Intermittent mechanical traction involves a mechanical device that alternately applies and releases the traction for brief intervals, usually from 15–60 seconds. This form of traction also uses relatively high forces. Its purpose is to separate bony surfaces, mobilize the joint, stretch soft tissues, and relax the muscles around the joints. The duration of treatment is usually 10–30 minutes (Figs. 27–3 and 27–4).

Manual traction is applied by the therapist, usually for 15–60 seconds or as a sudden thrust. The forces are also relatively high. This type of traction also can be used to determine whether mechanical traction is indicated. As a trial, it should be given in various positions to find the most comfortable one (Figs. 27–5, 27–6, and 27–7).

Positional traction is applied by positioning the patient in a way that will affect the relationship of the bony surfaces in the area treated. The purpose is to alleviate pressure on an entrapped nerve and relax the muscle in spasm. This can be done

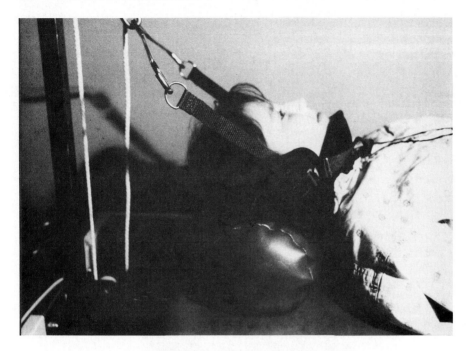

Figure 27–4. Intermittent cervical traction.

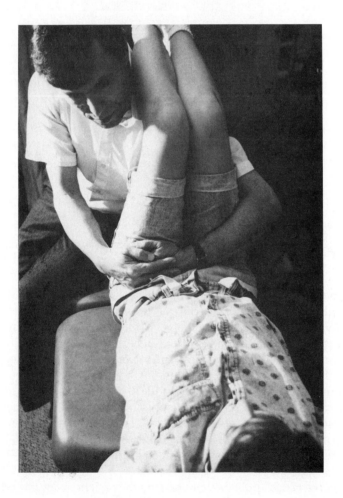

Figure 27–5. Manual lumbar traction.

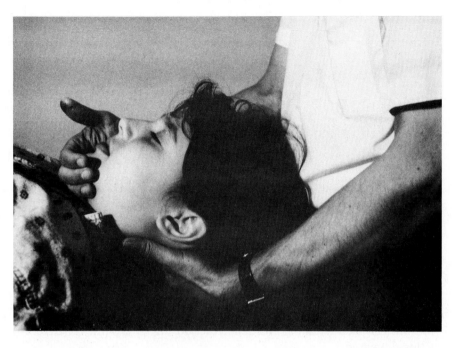

Figure 27–6. Manual cervical traction while the patient is in the supine position.

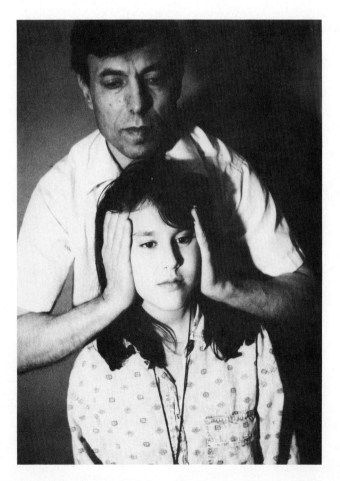

Figure 27–7. Manual cervical traction while the patient is in the sitting position.

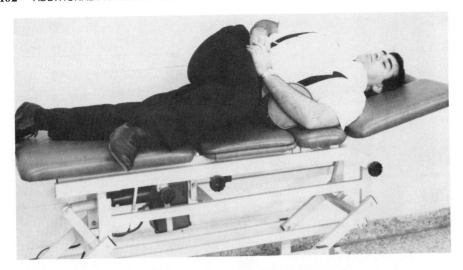

Figure 27–8. Unilateral positional lumbar traction.

unilaterally or bilaterally. The duration of treatment is usually 5–30 minutes. Fig. 27–8 shows unilateral lumbar positional traction, Fig. 27–9 shows bilateral cervical positional traction.

Gravity-assisted traction is among the newest techniques and can be applied in most situations. With this type of traction, the patient is placed in a position that favors distraction. Treatment duration is usually 10–30 minutes. In addition, the traction device is applied in a way that permits gravity to help the overall distraction of the targeted tissue. Some of these units permit the patient to regulate the amount of pull, thus preventing the possibility of exceeding the tolerance of the tissue. Fig. 27–10 shows gravity-assisted cervical traction, and Fig. 27–11 shows gravity-assisted lumbar traction.

Traction by inversion requires the patient to be held in an inverted position by the ankles and another part of the lower extremities. The traction force is gravity. During the treatment, the patient can exercise the trunk muscles while in the inverted position. The duration of treatment is usually 5 to 15 minutes. This type of traction may stress the cardiovascular system and cause a temporary rise in blood pressure. Fig. 27–12 shows lumbar traction by inversion.

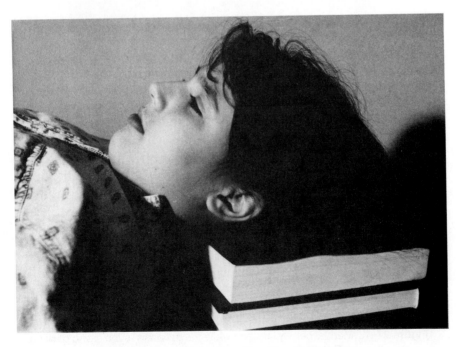

Figure 27–9. Bilateral positional cervical traction.

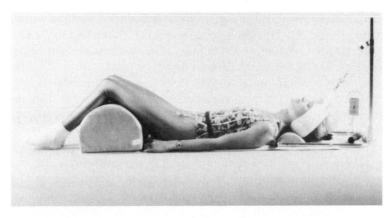

Figure 27–10. Gravity-assisted cervical traction. (*Reproduced with permission from Lossing Orthopedic Co.*)

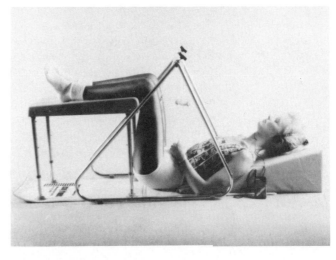

Figure 27–11. Gravity-assisted lumbar traction. (*Reproduced with permission from Lossing Orthopedic Co.*)

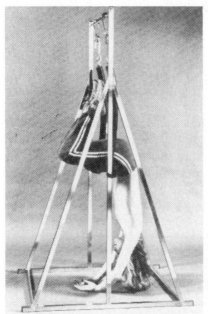
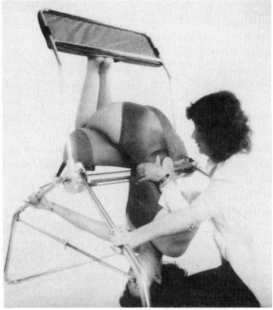

A   B

Figure 27–12. Examples of traction by inversion. (A) without exercise (B) with exercise. (*Reproduced with permission from Lossing Orthopedic Co.*)

Traction in water requires the patient to be suspended vertically in the water with a floating ring around the chest while weights are attached to the ankles. The duration of treatment is usually 6–30 minutes. The warm water can help relax the muscle (see Figs. 27–13, lumbar traction in water).

Autotraction is a multiplane automatic traction with a force determined by the patient.[3] The autotraction table has two sections that can be set at different angles in different planes. In addition, the table can be manipulated from the horizontal to the vertical position, and the patient can lie on it in a prone, supine, or side-lying position. These characteristics of the autotraction table permit the therapist to position the patient passively in a position that is most comfortable and utilizes the principles of positional traction and gravity-assisted traction. The duration of treatment is usually 20–60 minutes. This type of traction also permits the use of exercise techniques to rehabilitate the patient. Fig. 27–14 shows the autotraction table.

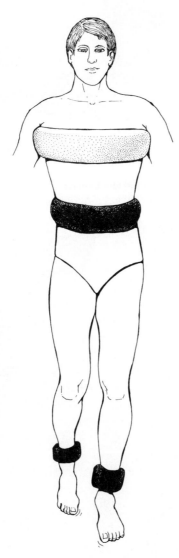

Figure 27–13. Lumbar traction in water. Weight can be placed on either the waist or the ankles.

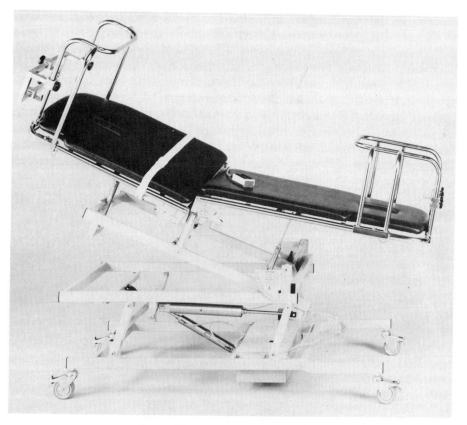

Figure 27–14. Table for autotraction.

RESULTS OF TREATMENT

The result of traction depends on the strength and direction of the applied force, the length of time the force is applied, the inertial state of the body (at rest or in motion), the contour and texture of the body surfaces, and the surface on which the patient rests.

The amount, duration, and direction of the applied force for any given treatment depends on the following:

- The pathology (eg, disk herniation, osteoarthritis, muscle spasm).
- The spinal level at which pathology is present.
- The weight and the position of the part being treated.
- The nature of the surface on which the body part is resting. (The force of friction that opposes the movement differs from surface to surface; it is equal to the product of the body weight and the coefficient of friction of the surfaces—skin, cloth, and the material on the surface of the treatment table.)
- The size of the area that is in contact with the treatment table.
- The type of traction (continuous, intermittent).
- The patient's condition (general health, age, sex).
- The patient's tolerance.

APPLICATION

In general, when applying traction, one should aim for maximum results with the minimum amount of force. This will reduce some of the complications, such as skin lacerations, pressure on blood vessels, and pain, arising from the use of high forces, thus permitting more patients to benefit from this type of treatment. To accomplish this goal, it is necessary to do the following:

- Minimize the amount and duration of force needed to overcome friction and to achieve separation. The magnitude of the force will be directly proportional to the frictional resistance of the surfaces and to the resistance of the soft tissue. Surface resistance to traction depends on the weight of the body segment undergoing traction and on the frictional coefficient of the surfaces. Usually half the body weight is required to overcome friction.[27]
- Ensure that the direction of the applied force is in line with the desired direction of distraction.
- Ensure that the joint is placed in a neutral position so that the ligaments of the joint will be relaxed.

The application of these principles is explained in the section on techniques.

The choice of a traction technique depends on the desired result. The following choices are also summarized in Table 27–1.

1. Distraction and separation of bony surfaces: Continuous, sustained, intermittent, and manual traction and positional autotraction will accomplish this result.
2. Stretching of soft tissue: Continuous, sustained, manual, and positional traction and intermittent autotraction can be used.
3. Relaxation of skeletal muscles: Sustained, intermittent, manual, positional, and continuous traction and autotraction can be used (results might not be immediate).
4. Mobilization of joints: Intermittent and manual traction can be used.
5. Immobilization and rest: Continuous traction is the only technique that accomplishes this result.
6. Temporary relief of compression in the intervertebral foramen caused by edema, herniation, inflammation or spasm: Intermittent, sustained, manual, and positional traction and autotraction techniques can be used.

INDICATIONS AND CONTRAINDICATIONS

Indications. Traction has been well documented as a successful technique for many indications. The following are examples:

- Nerve root impingement (herniated disc, narrowing of the intervertebral foramen, osteophyte encroachment, ligament encroachment, spondylolisthesis) because the separation of vertebrae eliminates the stress from the impinging tissues.
- Subacute joint pain because gentle mobilization of the joints cause a positive neurophysical effect.
- Degenerative joint disease (subacute stage) because traction improves the range of motion.
- Discogenic pain because separation of the vertabrae reduces the pain.
- Compression fracture (chronic state) because elongation of the spine reduces the compressive forces.

TABLE 27–1. The Effects of Using Different Traction Techniques

Effects	Technique							
	Continuous Sustained	Sustained	Intermittent	Manual	Positional	Gravity Assisted	Inversion	Traction in Water
Distraction		X	X	X	X	X	X	X
Stretching soft tissue	X	X	X	X	X	X	X	X
Relaxing muscles	X	X	X	X	X	X	X	X
Mobilizing joints			X	X				
Immobilization	X							
Temporary relief of compression		X	X	X	X	X	X	X

- Joint hypomobility because the intermittent pull improves the mobility of the joint.
- Paraspinal muscle spasm because traction force also stretches the spinal musculature.

Contraindications. Like any other treatment modality, traction should not be used indiscriminately and is contraindicated in some disease processes and some conditions for which movement may be harmful. For example, traction is contraindicated for the following:

- Patients with local and systemic diseases affecting joints, ligaments, bones and muscles such as tumors, infections, rheumatoid arthritis, and osteoporosis because the structure may not be strong enough to sustain the forces of the traction.
- Patients with acute sprains or strains because treatment may interfere with the healing process.
- Patients with acute inflammation. Treatment might irritate the joint, increasing the inflammatory process.
- Patients with hypermobility because the treatment may aggravate the condition.
- Patients with vascular conditions because the pressure of the halter or harness may compromise the circulation even further.
- Patients whose symptoms increase during traction.
- Patients with postsleeve fibrosis in the lumbar area that would receive cervical traction.
- Patients for whom the pressure of a lumbar and thoracic harness are hazards: for example, pregnant women and patients with hiatus hernia or cardiac or pulmonary disorders.
- All forms of traction except for continuous traction are contraindicated in conditions where movement is not allowed.
- Treatment should not be given unless the patient can tolerate it comfortably.
- Patients with temporomandibular joint dysfunction.

Patients with temporomandibular joint dysfunction must be provided with vertical support between their molars before conventional cervical traction can be administered. The support will transmit the forces from the chin part of the halter to the skull through the maxilla, bypassing the temporomandibular joint. However, some units transmit all the forces directly to the skull without a chin halter, thus avoiding the application of pressure on the temporomandibular joint (See Fig. 27–15).

The remainder of this chapter discusses mechanical traction to the lumbar and cervical areas. The discussion includes the rationale for the treatment and specific instructions concerning its application.

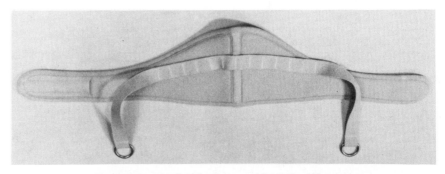

Figure 27–15. Cervical strap without the chin strap.

LUMBAR TRACTION

To apply traction effectively, the technique must be tailored to the disorder. The type of traction, continuous or intermittent, must be considered. We have found that disk pathology responds better to brief continuous traction (10 minutes), whereas a facet dysfunction responds better to intermittent traction (15–20 minutes).

Distraction in the lumbar area also can be achieved by positional traction,[28] inversion,[29] or other gravitational traction systems such as the Cottrell 90/90 traction or lumbar lift. A full discussion of these systems is beyond the scope of this book.

Position

Lumbar traction can be administered in the supine or prone position with equal effectiveness. The patient's comfort will determine the choice of position. Traction can be applied unilaterally or bilaterally. With unilateral dysfunctions such as hypomobility of a facet joint or muscle spasm, unilateral traction is more effective.[29] The position of the patient's spine (flexion, extension, or neutral) depends on the dysfunction. When positioning the patient for treatment, the therapist must consider two principles: (1) the patient's position should provide optimum separation between the articulation surfaces and (2) the joint position should be as close to midrange or neutral as possible because the more relaxed the joint capsule and the ligaments, the less force required to achieve the desired amount of distraction.

There are no standard treatment approaches to traction; each treatment must be tailored to the individual patient and to the specific pathology involved. For example, the degree of disk herniation can vary from patient to patient, and it can occur in different directions. The position of the patient will depend on his or her tolerance. Ideally, the prone position should be used because the spine can be extended and the forces are directed on the disk anteriorly (see Fig. 27–16). However, this will be the position of choice only if the patient can tolerate the position well

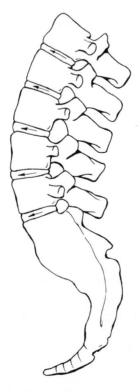

Figure 27–16. Lateral view of the lumbar spine in extension.

and benefit from it. Only then can the therapist assume that the herniation may be reduced by the treatment. For patients who cannot tolerate the extended position, the neutral position should be attempted. The neutral position is a midrange position between flexion and extension and can be assumed while in either the prone or supine position. If the patient cannot tolerate the neutral position, the flexed position should be attempted with caution. The reader should recall that most herniations are in a posterolateral direction, which is why a force on the disk that is applied anteromedially may help to reduce the herniation. During extension of the spine, the forces on the disk are directed anteriorly. Adding lateral bending toward the affected side by applying unilateral positional traction might further direct the herniation medially (ie, toward the center of the disk) and thus be more effective. A patient may not tolerate a particular position because the forces applied are not moving the nucleus pulposus in the intended direction, but instead are exerting even more pressure and thus producing more pain. In such a situation, the therapist should explore another position.

An optimal position for treating patients with encroachment on the intervertebral foramen with traction is one that will permit maximal opening of this foramen. For bilateral conditions such as a paraspinal muscle spasm, the spine at the level of the encroachment should be in a neutral position. In a unilateral dysfunction, side bending toward the unaffected side and rotation of the upper part toward the affected side will increase the amount of opening of the foramen at the affected side (see Fig. 27–8). We have found clinically that dysfunction of the joint facet is best treated in flexion. The amount of flexion is determined by the level of the facet being treated. This is done by positioning the patient on the table and flexing the hip slowly with one hand while the other hand is on the spine at the appropriate segmental level. As the hip is flexed, the spine will begin to flex at some point. The movement will begin from below L_5–S_1 and move upward. Once the movement reaches the involved segmental levels, it can be felt by the palpating hand. The segment then will continue to move to the extent that the structure permits. At the midpoint between the beginning and end of the range of movement is the neutral position of this segmental level—the point at which the ligaments around the joints are lax. It has been observed clinically that the L_5–S_1 segmental level requires about 45°–60° of hip flexion to achieve laxity in the joints involved. To achieve laxity at the L_4–L_5 segmental level, 60°–75° of hip flexion is required. To achieve laxity at the L_3–L_4 segmental level, 75°–90° of hip flexion is required. With the respective degree of hip flexion, one can assume that each respective facet is in the mid (neutral) position. In this position, the ligaments of the facets and the joint capsule are lax, thus permitting separation of joint surfaces.

Equipment

The following apparatus is available to provide lumbar traction:

- A pelvic corset that fits snugly over the iliac crests.
- A thoracic harness that fits around the lower thoracic ribs below the xiphoid process.
- A spreader bar with a rope attached at each end.
- A machine that continuously or intermittently applies the pulling force.
- A traction table.

Both the pelvic and the thoracic harnesses should be placed next to the patient's skin to eliminate slippage. These harnesses should be strapped in such a way as to overlap slightly (see Fig. 27–17).

The most effective traction table is one that splits in the middle, thus minimizing the resistance of the friction force to the traction (Fig. 27–18). Because the coefficient of friction between a human body and a mattress is approximately 0.5, traction on a similar surface will require a force of one-half the patient's body weight to move that part of the body horizontally. During lumbar traction, only about half

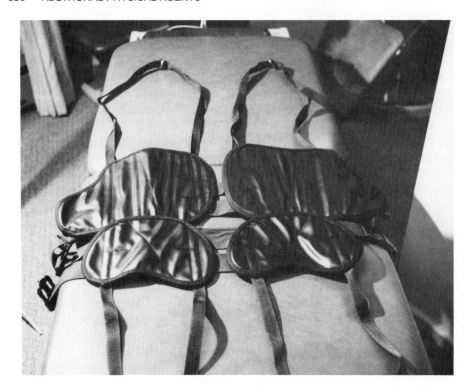

Figure 27–17. Overlapping harnesses.

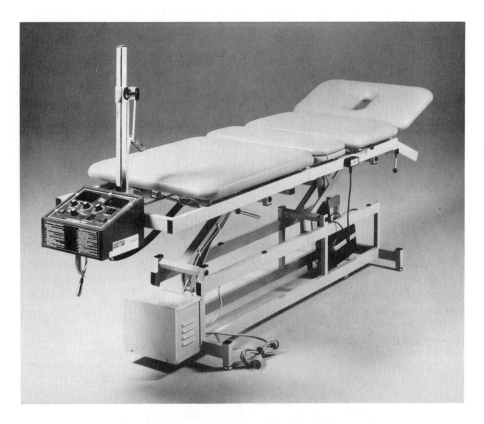

Figure 27–18. A split traction table.

of the body weight is pulled; in other words, a traction force of about one- fourth of the total body weight is required just to overcome the frictional force.[30] Applying lumbar traction on a table that is split virtually eliminates this force; thus, the traction force applied is used almost totally to distract the tissue.

At the beginning of the treatment, the table should be closed. This is done to ensure that the slack from the harnesses has been removed during the first few pulls. Once the table is opened by releasing the catch, the treatment begins.

Force and Frequency

A large amount of force is required to affect structural changes in the lumbar spine. For some disorders, such as severe nerve root involvement, 25 to 60 pounds is sufficient to achieve beneficial effects. Most authors agree that to separate segmental levels effectively, the force must be greater than 65 pounds; some authors indicate that a force as high as 200 pounds may be required.[31, 32] However, low force should be used during the first treatment so that the patient's reaction can be observed. Once the therapist has established that the patient is tolerating the low forces (25–50 pounds) well, higher forces can be administered to achieve a therapeutic effect. The setting of the on-and-off cycle is determined by the patient's condition and tolerance. Disk involvement requires longer on-times (60 seconds) and shorter off-times (20 seconds). Joint involvement requires a shorter on-time (15 seconds) and the same amount of off-time (15 seconds). The frequency of treatment can range from twice daily to once a week.

Procedure for Conventional Systems

Before initiating the treatment, the therapist should carry out the following steps:

1. Arrange the pelvic corset and the thoracic harness on the table in the position that they will be placed on the patient.
2. Place the patient on the table in the desired position (flexion, neutral, or extension) and put a pillow under the patient's head.
3. Attach the lumbar corset first, then apply the thoracic harness and let it overlap slightly to allow for the minor slippage that will occur. Both appliances must fit snugly, however.
4. Attach the rope to the corset with the hook or the spreader bar.
5. Select the amount of force, the on-off cycle, and the duration of the treatment. The parameters chosen must be within the patient's tolerance and comfort.
6. Turn on the machine and let it pull for a few seconds to remove the slack from the straps.
7. Release the catch of the table to allow the lower part to move.

When the treatment is completed, **slowly** reduce the tension on the rope. When the rope is slack, undo the corset and the harness and encourage the patient to rest for a few minutes before getting up.

CERVICAL TRACTION

Documentation

Cervical traction is used to treat facet disk and soft-tissue dysfunctions and is guided by the same basic principles discussed in the section on lumbar traction. In addition, however, it is advisable to perform the vertebral artery test (Fig. 27–19), which determines whether the vertebral artery might be compromised in certain head positions.

A comparison of the patient's pain before and after treatment can be one criterion in measuring the patient's response to cervical traction. However, changes in

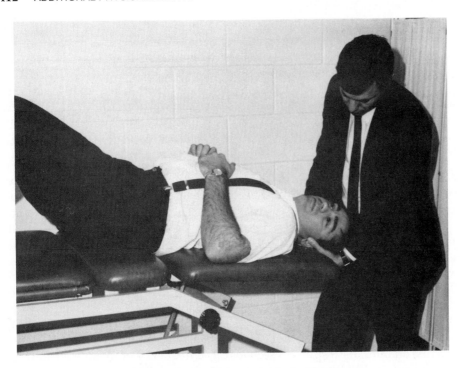

Figure 27–19. The vertebral artery test.

range of motion or in functional abilities are more objective. Measurements should be taken before and after traction and should be recorded. Usually, the response to treatment is immediate, but it does not always last; only repetitive treatments now bring lasting relief.

Although the effects of cervical traction have been studied for many years, more research is needed to determine its effects on specific dysfunctions. Studies that are currently underway not only may increase our understanding about the effects of traction but help us to be more precise in its application as well.

Position

When the treatment is administered, the patient is positioned both for comfort and security. This will promote relaxation. If the patient's paraspinal muscles are not relaxed, other modalities (eg, hot pack, cold pack, ultrasound) can be used before the traction to help achieve relaxation. Relaxing the muscles before traction is preferable because it permits better distraction from the onset of the treatment.

Cervical traction can be administered to patients in the sitting or the supine position; however, the supine position is clearly preferred.[33, 34] In the sitting position, the weight of the head (approximately 12–14 pounds) must be overcome before any distractive forces of the traction can affect the tissues. In the supine position, the head rests on the traction table and more of the traction force is directed toward distraction of the tissues. At times, however, the patient may prefer the sitting position.

When treating facet dysfunction, the cervical spine should be in a flexed position. As with the lumbar traction, the purpose of the flexion position is to put the involved facet joint capsule in the most lax position. As the neck is flexed forward, the facets of C_1 and C_2 begin to move; further flexion brings movement at the segmental level C_2 and C_3, then level C_3 and C_4 and C_5, and so on. Obviously, the higher the level involved, the less flexion necessary to position the joints in the midrange.

The therapist must determine the specific amount of flexion for each patient. This is done by slowly flexing the patient's neck with one hand while placing the other hand between the spinous processes at the involved segmental level. The

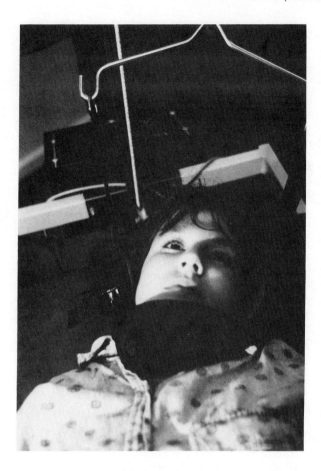

Figure 27–20. The unilateral cervical position.

therapist should feel when movement relative to the two spinous processes begins, when it ends, and when it approximates the midrange. The following are estimated ranges of degrees per segmental levels: Occiput (C_1–C_2) is 0°–5°, midcervical (C_2–C_5) is 10°–20°, and low cervical (C_5–C_7) is 25°–30°. In these positions, the ligaments and the joint capsules of the respective facets are in a relatively lax position, thus permitting better distraction of the joint surfaces.

Intervertebral foramen encroachment can be treated best when the patient is in a position that promotes maximal opening of the intervertebral foramen; namely, flexion, lateral bending toward the unaffected side, and rotation toward the affected side (Fig. 27–20).

Disk dysfunction is treated best when the cervical spine is in a neutral (postural) position. In this position, the ligaments of the spinal column are lax, thus permitting better distraction of the vertebrae.

Equipment

The apparatus available to provide mechanical cervical traction consists of the halter that fits the patient's head and a machine that intermittently or continuously applies the pulling force to the halter by means of a rope and a spreader bar (Fig. 27–21).

To apply traction correctly, a proper head halter must be used. The most appropriate halter seems to be one that positions the head in some flexion, enabling the traction pull to be exerted from the occiput, **not** the chin. This type of halter concentrates the traction force posteriorly, where it is most beneficial. In addition, the rope should be arranged at the predetermined angle for optimal results (Fig. 27–22).

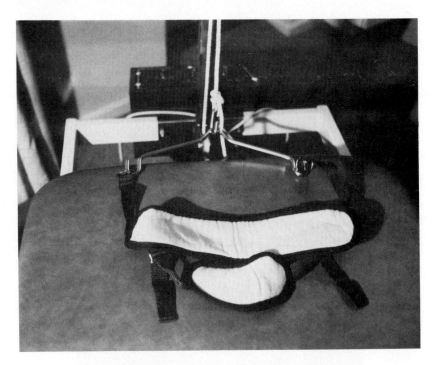

Figure 27–21. Mechanical cervical traction apparatus.

Force and Frequency

The amount of force necessary to demonstrate a change in the upper cervical area is 10–15 pounds. In the middle and low cervical region, it is 25–50 pounds.

The treatment time is relatively brief, usually 5–10 minutes for disk dysfunction and 10–15 minutes for other conditions. The patient's comfort is the determining factor when establishing the duration of the treatment.

Unilateral traction can be incorporated in the treatment of unilateral dysfunctions. With this technique, the therapist is able to direct a stronger force to one side of the cervical spine. With this technique, a stabilizing strap must be used over the patient's chest so that he will not align himself with the angle of the rope (see Fig. 27–20).

Some traction units such as Goodly Polyaxial Traction and Necktrac use gravity as the force and thus are more gentle and precise (Fig. 27–23). The patient can control the amount of force applied and have it operate intermittently (Fig. 27–24). These treatments are usually tolerated well.

The two units just mentioned and the Chattanooga Cervical Traction, Model 7080, can be applied to the skull without a chin strap (see Fig. 27–23). These traction devices enhance the patient's comfort. Moreover, because none of their traction forces are directed at the temporomandibular joint, they should be used with patients who suffer from temporomandibular joint dysfunction. When traction with a chin strap is the only available unit, the therapist should separate the upper

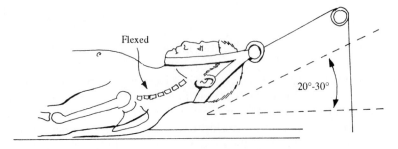

Figure 27–22. Using the angle of pull to achieve cervical flexion.

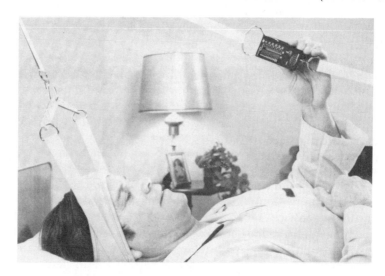

Figure 27–23. Gravity-assisted cervical traction.

and lower molars with a material such as gauze or cotton, which will maintain the separation but will not damage the teeth. This will reduce the forces passing through the chin strap toward the temporomandibular joint. Further discussion of these traction units is beyond the scope of this book.

Procedures for Traction in the Supine Position

Before initiating the treatment, the therapist must carry out the following steps:

1. Prepare the table, adjusting the angulation of the rope for the specific dysfunction. Place a pillow under the patient's head when flexion is desired. Another pillow under the knees can be used to promote relaxation.
2. Remove the patient's dentures and use a mouth piece or several layers of gauze to absorb the pressure that might be exerted on the temporomandibular joint, especially if the patient is sensitive in that area.

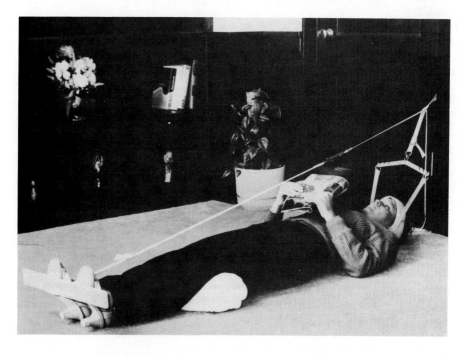

Figure 27–24. The patient applies intermittent traction.

3. Position the patient and adjust the halter under the occiput and the mandible.

4. Attach the halter to the spreader bar. The rope must be slack to attach the spreader bar, but the slack should be removed before the treatment.

5. Select the force, the duration on the on-off cycle, and the duration of the treatment. The suggested amount of force to use initially is 10–15 pounds. Then increase the force to achieve the desired amount of pull the patient can tolerate.

6. Turn on the machine and make certain that the pull the patient experiences comes from the occiput.

Rotation exercises can be done during the traction phase, but the patient must maintain the original cervical angle. At the conclusion of the treatment, release the rope gradually, then remove the bar and halter from the patient, and instruct the patient to rest for a few minutes before getting up. The frequency of treatment will depend on the patient's response. The traction can be administered from twice daily to once a week.

Administering traction while the patient is in a sitting position must be done with the proper angulation of the rope. The instructions for cervical traction in a sitting position are the same as those for the supine position except for the amount of flexion, which is determined by the position of the chair in relation to the line of pull. Care must be taken to ensure that the patient follows instructions, especially those regarding the specific head position. If the patient's neck is not aligned, the effectiveness of the treatment will be reduced.

The therapist should instruct the patient to report all symptoms, not just pain. Nausea, visual changes, and dizziness can be triggered by traction. If these symptoms or any other neurological symptoms occur, the traction should be stopped.

REFERENCES

1. Saunders MD. Lumbar traction. *J Orthop Sports Phys Ther* 1979; 1(1):36.
2. Cyriax J. The treatment of lumbar disc lesions. *Br Med J.* 1950; 2:1434.
3. Christy B. Discussion on treatment of backache by traction. *Proc R Soc Med.* 1955; 48:811.
4. Larsson V, Sholer U, Lindstrom A, et al. Auto traction for treatment of lumbago-sciatica. *Acta Orthop Scand.* 1980; 51:791.
5. Lindstrom A, Zachrisson M. Physical therapy on low back pain and sciatica: an attempt at evaluation. *Scand J Rehabil Med.* 1970; 2:37.
6. Mathews J, Heckling H. Lumbar traction: a double-blind control study for sciatica. *Rheumatol Rehabil.* 1975; 14:222.
7. Weber H. Traction therapy in sciatica due to disc prolapse. *J Oslo City Hosp.* 1973; 23(10):167.
8. Ljunggren AE, Walker L, Weber H, et al. Manual traction versus isometric exercises in patients with herniated intervertebral lumbar discs. *Physiother Theroy Pract.* 1992; 8:207.
9. Pal B, Magnion P, Hossian MA, et al. A controlled trial of continuous lumbar traction in the treatment of back pain and sciatica. *Br J Rheumatol.* 1986; 25:181.
10. Crisp EJ. discussion of the treatment of backache by traction. *Proc R Soc Med.* 1955; 43:805.
11. Andersson BJG, Schulz AB, Machemson A. Intervertabrae disc pressures during traction. *J Rehabil Med.* 1988; 9(suppl):88.
12. Goldie I, Landquist A. Evaluation of the effect of different forms of physiotherapy in cervical pain. *Scand J Rehabil Med.* 1970; 2–3:117.
13. Lind G. *Auto-Traction Treatment of Low Back Bain and Sciatica.* University of Linkoping; Linkoping, Sweden; 1974. Thesis.
14. Larsson U, Choler U, Lindstrom A. Auto-traction for treatment of lumbago-sciatica. *Acta Orthop Scand.* 1980; 51:791.
15. Nossi L. Inverted spinal traction. *Arch Phys Med Rehabil.* 1978; 59:367.

16. Kaltenborn F. In: Kent B, ed. *Proceedings of the International Federation of Orthopedic Manipulative Therapists.* Vail, Colorado; 1977.
17. Saunders H. Evaluation, treatment and prevention of musculoskeletal disorders. In: *Educational Opportunities.* Minnesota; 1985.
18. Saunders H. Unilateral lumbar traction. *Phys Ther.* 1981; 61:221.
19. Oudenhoven RC. Gravitational lumbar traction. *Arch Phys Med Rehabil.* 1978; 59:510.
20. Alice MK, Wong M, Chaupeng I. The traction angle and cervical intervertebral separation. *Spine.* 1992; 17(2):136.
21. Basmagian JV. *Manipulation, Traction and Massage.* 3rd ed. Baltimore, MD: Williams & Wilkins;1985:174.
22. Colachis SC Jr, Strohan BR. Cervical traction relationship of time to varied tractive force with constant angle of pull. *Arch Phys Med Rehabil.* 1965; 46:815.
23. Colachis SC Jr, Strohan BR. Effects of intermittent traction on separation of lumbar vertebrae. *Arch Phys Med Rehabil.* 1969; 50:251.
24. Judovich B. Herniated cervical disc: a new form of traction therapy. *Am J Surg.* 1952; 84:646.
25. Mathews JA. The effects of spinal traction. *Physiotherapy.* 1972; 58:64.
26. Christie BGB. Discussion on the treatment of backache by traction. *Proc R Soc Med. (Physical Med).* 1972; 58:64.
27. Judovich BD. Lumbar traction therapy and dissipated force factor. *Lancet.* 1954; 74:411.
28. Paris S. Spinal dysfunction: etiology and treatment of dysfunction including joint manipulation. *Manual of Course Notes.* Atlanta 1979.
29. Saunders H. Unilateral lumbar traction. *Phys Ther.* 1981; 61:221.
30. Judovitch BD. Lumbar traction therapy: Elimination of physical factors that prevent lumbar stretch. *JAMA.* 1955; 159,459.
31. Lehmann JF, Brenner GD. A device for the application of heavy lumbar traction: its mechanical effects. *Arch Phys Med Rehabil.* 1958; 39:696.
32. Cyriax JH. Discussion on the treatment of backache by traction. *Proc R Soc Med* (Phys Rehabil). 1955; 45:808.
33. Deets D, Hands K, Hopp S. Cervical traction: a comparison of sitting and supine positions. *Phys Ther.* 1977; 57:255.
34. Colachis S, Strokes M. Cervical traction. *Arch Phys Med.* 1965; 46:815.

28

Intermittent Pneumatic Compression

Diana Fond, and Bernadette Hecox

Equipment

Technique of Application

Pretreatment

Posttreatment

Dosage

Indications and Contraindications

Indications

Contraindications

Modified Units

Documentation

P hysical therapists have been using the concept of compression for years. Elastic bandages have been used to shape amputated limbs to prepare them for prosthetic fitting. After long periods of bed rest, patients who are placed in an upright position for the first few times, either on a tilt table or in the parallel bars, may have their lower extremities wrapped in ace bandages to prevent orthostatic hypotension. When a patient sustains a traumatic injury such as ligamentous tear in the ankle rest, ice, compression, and elevation are used to prevent swelling and the resulting pain which would follow.

In Chapter 3 the pathophysiologic basis for the formation of edema was discussed and various agents for controlling swelling were mentioned. One of these agents, the intermittent pneumatic compression pump (IPC) is discussed in this chapter. The use of IPCs has increased since the early 1970s. In addition to being used to control or reduce edema, these pumps are used to treat many other peripheral problems, including traumatic edema (subacute and chronic), venous insufficiency, lymphedema, leg ulcers, amputated limbs, wound healing, arterial insufficiency, contractures and possibly to prevent thrombophlebitis. These pumps also are used for dialysis patients.

EQUIPMENT

Intermittent pneumatic compression (IPC) units, as the name implies, are basically air pumps. They intermittently force air into inflatable sleeves or boots into which an upper or lower extremity has been inserted. Thus, the air pressure surrounding the extremity increases. In turn, this applied pressure increases the pressure of the fluids in the interstitial spaces to a level higher than that of the lymph and blood vessels. The resulting pressure gradient encourages the fluids in the interstitial spaces to return to the venous and lymphatic vessels. Because the air pressure is applied intermittently, it acts somewhat like a pump, moving fluids back toward the heart.

The following items are required for IPC:

- An IPC unit containing (1) an on-off switch, (2) a dial to control pressure, (3) a dial to control inflation-time (time on), (4) a dial to control deflation time (time off), and (5) a pressure or air outlet to which rubber hosing is attached (Figs. 28–1, 28–2, 28–3, and 28–4).
- Inflatable sleeves and boots.
- A sphygmomanometer and stethoscope to measure the patient's blood pressure before treatment.
- Marking pencils for marking the skin, and a tape measure for measuring the part being treated before and after treatment.
- Standardized charts or paper for recording the measurements (see Fig. 28–5).
- A stockinette to be placed on the part being treated for absorption of perspiration and for hygiene.
- Pillows, an incline board, or another device for elevating the part being treated.

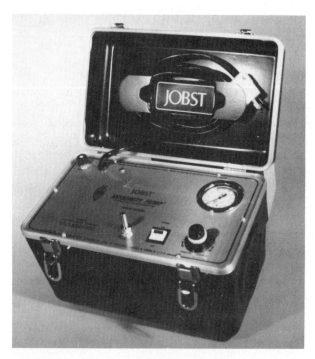

Figure 28–1. Portable intermittent compression extremity unit. (*Reproduced with permission from the Jobst Institute, Inc., Toledo, OH.*)

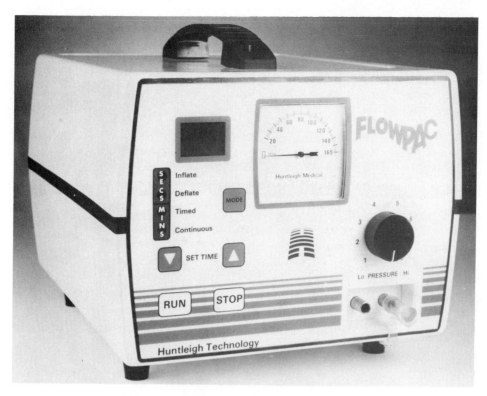

Figure 28–2. Intermittent compression extremity pump for clinical use. (*Reproduced with permission from Huntleigh Technology Inc., Manalapan, NJ.*)

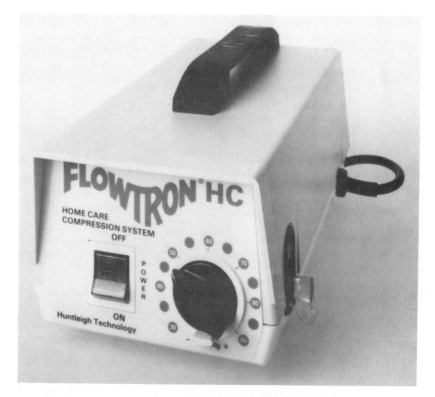

Figure 28–3. Intermittent compression extremity pump for home use. (*Reproduced with permission from Huntleigh Technology Inc., Manalapan, NJ.*)

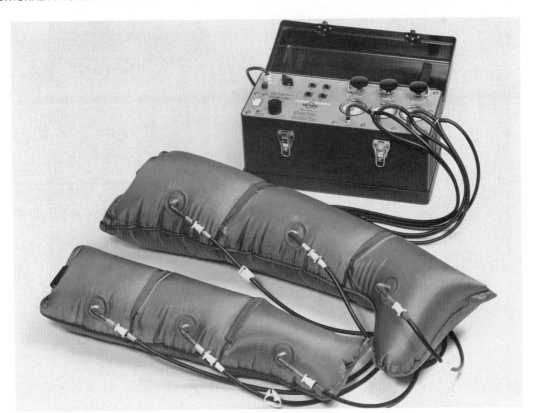

Figure 28–4. Intermittent compression pump with sequential air filling. Note that the compression garment has divided sections (cells). The pressure varies in each cell; it is highest in the distal cell and is lower in each more proximal cell. (*Reproduced with permission from Wright Linear Pump, Imperial, PA.*)

CHART INFORMATION

Patient Name _____ Diagnosis _____

ID# _____

(other pertinent information) _____

Extremity being treated: Right Lower Extremity _____

		Treatment Dates	9/12/93		9/13/93		9/15/93		9/18/93		9/22/93	
			Pre-tx	Post-tx	Pre-tx	Post-tx	Pre-tx	Post-tx	Pre-tx	Post-tx	Pre-tx	Post-tx
Locations to be marked for measuring on lateral aspects of the extremity	Example	9″ prox to LE	35″	34½″	35″	34Æ	35″	34″	34″	33½″	33½″	32½″
		6″ prox to LE										
		3″ prox to LE										
		At LE										
		9″ prox to LM										
		6″ prox to LM										
		3″ prox to LM										
		1″ prox to LM										
		4″ prox to MH										
		2″ prox to MH										
		At MH										

Figure 28–5. A sample chart for recording pre- and posttreatment measurements of the girth of a lower extremity. The patient information at the top of the chart may vary, depending on the clinic. The points to be measured will vary according to the patient's size. LE = lateral epicondyle, LM = lateral malleolus, MH = head of the fifth metatarsal, PRE TX = pretreatment, POST TX = post treatment, PROX = proximal.

TECHNIQUE OF APPLICATION

Pretreatment

Before initiating the treatment, the therapist should carry out the following steps:

1. Explain to the patient the procedure and the sensations of pressure likely to be experienced and advise the patient about the duration of treatment. Some therapists suggest that patients move their fingers or toes occasionally during the "inflation off" periods.
2. Place the patient in a comfortable position, because the treatment may last a relatively long time.
3. Take the patient's pulse and blood pressure. It is recommended that the pressure from the unit not exceed the diastolic pressure because it could occlude return of blood. However, the Jobst Corporation, which produces one of the compression units that will be discussed, claims that the diastolic pressure can be exceeded because the pressure is on for a relatively short time when in the intermittent compression mode.
4. Remove jewelry and inspect the skin. Any open wounds should be covered with sterile gauze.
5. Test the limb for pressure sensation. If the limb is extremely pressure sensitive, the patient will have to be monitored closely. If a **deep thrombus** is suspected, do not treat without consulting a physician.
6. Use bony prominences for reference points and mark the skin approximately every 2 or 3 inches. Measure and record the girth at each marking. (Fig. 28–5).
7. Connect the unit to the wall outlet.
8. Place the stockinette on the part being treated and smooth out all wrinkles. When an amputated limb is treated, the stockinette is often placed over the elastic bandage used to shape the stump.
9. Apply the boot or sleeve. Some slide on, whereas others have zippers.
10. Elevate the treated limb to a horizontal position or higher to allow gravity to help drain the fluids.
11. Attach the rubber hose to the garment and to the air outlet on the IPC unit.
12. Set the on-off dials to the desired inflation-deflation times. (Home units may have the inflation and deflation times preset in a ratio of 3:1—90 seconds on, 30 seconds off.)
13. Turn the power on.
14. Turn the pressure dial to the desired pressure. It will register **only** when the machine is in the inflation cycle.
15. Stay with the patient for the first few inflations and deflations to make certain that the patient is not uncomfortable or experiencing tingling or pain and that the pressure output is stabilized at the desired level.

Posttreatment

All of the following procedures should be completed while the limb is still elevated: in other words, before the patient assumes a dependent position that might allow fluids to flow distally again.

1. At the end of treatment, turn the pressure off when the machine is in the deflation cycle.
2. Turn the power off.
3. Disconnect the tubing from the machine.
4. Remove the garment and stockinette.
5. Check the skin for pressure areas or creases from the stockinette.
6. Remeasure and record the girth of the limb at distances previously marked to determine if the treatment made progress in decreasing swelling.

7. Apply a compression garment or ace bandage. (Before applying compression garments, many therapists have patients perform range of motion or resistive exercises or both with the treated part in the elevated position.

The usual treatment time for massive edema is at least 2 to 4 hours; however, the treatment time will depend on the problem addressed. Continue the treatments, always comparing the before- and-after measurements to determine progress and the point at which a plateau is reached in the circumference of the limb. At that point, the patient should be ready to be fitted with a custom-made compression garment.

DOSAGE

Pressure on the upper extremity usually should not exceed 40–60 mm Hg; pressure on the lower extremity usually should not exceed 40–70 mm Hg. The dosages shown on tables 28–1 and 28–2 are based on those suggested by The Jobst Institute- and Huntleigh Inc. All companies that produce IPC units provide their own guidelines for each model, and they will provide more detailed treatment guides on request. Therapists should follow the guidelines for the specific model being used.

TABLE 28–1. Treatment Guidelines Recommended by the Jobst Institute, Inc.*

Indications	Pressure (mm Hg)	Recommended Treatment Periods	Inflation Time (on)	Deflation Time (off)
Postmastectomy lymphedema	30–50	Two treatment periods a day for 3 hrs	80–100 s	25–35 s
Edema of lower extremities	30–60	Two treatment periods a day for 3 hrs	80–100 s	25–35 s
Peripheral edema and venous stasis ulceration	85	One treatment period for 2½ hrs three times a week	80–100 s	30 s
Stump reduction	30–60	Three treatment periods a day for 4 hrs	40–60 s	10–15 s
Hand edema	30–50	Two treatment periods a day of 30 min to 1 hr each	Extension position: 5–10 minutes	Flexion position: 5–10 min

TABLE 28–2. Treatment Guidelines Recommended by Huntleigh Technology Inc.*

Indications	Pressure (mmHg)	Treatment Minimum/Day	Treatment Total
Venous ulcers	50	Two 2 hr periods	As necessary (not less than 6 wks)
Edema (venous)	40–80	Two 2 hr periods	4–8 wks
Lymphatic edema	70–90	2 hrs	As necessary (not less than 6–8 wks)
Traumatic edema	50	2 hrs	As necessary
Stump forming	20–50	1 hr	4–6 wks

*These lists should be used only as a guide. Pressure and treatment periods can be varied to suit the individual requirements. The system should be used intensively initially, then reduced as improvements are obtained. The use of elasticized stockings to maintain control between treatments is recommended for certain conditions. In traumatic edema the use of ice packs may greatly aid in the reduction of pain and swelling.

Note: In general, pressures for the upper extremity should not exceed 40–60 mm Hg, and pressures for the lower extremity should not exceed 40–70 mm Hg. Pressures lower than 30 mm Hg are usually not recommended.

INDICATIONS AND CONTRAINDICATIONS

Indications

Traumatic edema. Following soft tissue injury, mechanical compression may be applied to help reduce swelling that leads to pain and immobility; however, compression should not be used in the acute phase, when pressure may cause resumption of bleeding.

Chronic edema. Lack of movement can cause chronic edema, such as seen in patients with severe neurological diseases who cannot move their limbs.

Lymphedema. Flow of lymph may be impeded because lymph nodes have been removed or lymph vessels have been blocked, as after a radical mastectomy or an inguinal lymphadectomy. Massive swelling can cause pain, immobility, and decreased function of the involved extremity. Infection also can occur as a secondary result. Therefore, external pressure is helpful in decreasing swelling and lessening the possibility of infection from a break in the skin of the affected extremity.[1, 2]

Stasis ulcers. Leg ulcers can develop when there is prolonged presence of fluid in the interstitial spaces. Outside pressure from a pump can aid in circulation, resulting in increased nutrients to tissues and removal of waste materials, both of which lead to healing.

Amputated limbs. The stumps of amputated limbs tend to swell when in the dependent position. In conjunction with elastic wraps, compression pumps can be used to hasten the shaping and reduce the edema in the stump in preparation for prosthetic fitting.[3]

Prevention of thrombophlebitis. Postoperatively, compression pumps are used to reduce the possibility that a patient will develop deep vein thrombosis because of inactive muscles in the leg and coagulation of blood.[4, 5]

Wound healing. Patients who have undergone orthopedic or vascular surgical procedures may have reduced swelling and pain and therefore faster wound healing at the suture. In such cases, a lower pressure should be used to avoid recurrent bleeding.[6]

Arterial insufficiency. It has been suggested that the arterial-venous pressure gradient is maintained by providing external pumping for increasing venous return, thus enhancing arterial flow in patients such as those with intermittent claudications. Patients who tend to have pain during walking also are helped.[7] Note that the compression time should be brief so that a vessel is not occluded.

Contractures and edema of the hand. Physical therapists often treat contractures and edema of the hand caused by trauma, stroke, or surgery with passive range of motion and stretching procedures. These conditions are now treated with compression pumps, especially in Europe. The interphalangeal joints are mobilized, and the edema that is often the result of lack of use is decreased. A similar technique can be used to increase the range of motion of other joints such as the elbow or the knee.

Renal Insufficiency. Because patients on dialysis tend to develop hypotension and extremely edematous extremities, compression applied to the lower extremities may help overcome these problems.

Contraindications

The following are contraindications to the use of intermittent compression:

Acute pulmonary edema. Because IPC brings more fluid to the already overburdened area, it could increase stress on the heart and lungs.

Congestive heart failure. IPC could increase stress on the heart and lungs.

Recent or acute deep vein thrombosis. IPC could dislodge the clot and cause the embolus to travel to and lodge in the heart, lungs, or brain.

Acute fracture. IPC could cause movement of the fracture site and interfere with healing.

Acute local dermatological infections. IPC could spread the infection because of increased perspiration in the stockinette and garment.

Edema immediately after a traumatic injury. IPC might increase the pressure at the injury site to a degree that is sufficient to augment the inflammatory process.

MODIFIED UNITS

In addition to the standard models of IPC, some units have extra features: for example, the Wright linear pump, the Huntleigh sequential system, and the Jobst Cryo/Temp unit (Fig. 28–6). The Wright linear pump (see Fig. 28–4) may increase the elimination of edema because it offers compression through different "cells" in the garment that give more pressure distally than proximally: eg, 90 mm Hg at the ankle, 70 mm Hg at the knee, and 50 mm Hg at the proximal thigh. The most distal cell has the highest pressure, which is the mean of the systolic and diastolic blood pressures.[8] Theoretically, this gradient pressure promotes the flow of fluid (edema) from the distal to the proximal part of a limb. This type of unit can be useful in the treatment of lymphedema because it prevents the backflow or reverse flow "to the areas of relatively decreased resistance."[9] Dr. Milton Klein and his colleagues[9] reported that the Wright Linear Pump was effective in treating lower extremity lymphedema in adults.

The Huntleigh Sequential System has three chambers; each is filled sequentially, starting with the distal and moving to the proximal chamber. Theoretically, this should enhance the movement of fluid in a limb in a proximal direction.

The Jobst Cryo/Temp therapy system combines two components of the RICE treatment described in Chapter 14: cooling of a limb with either intermittent or continuous controlled compression (Fig. 28–6).[10] Two types of Cryo/Temp units are available. The large "professional" or hospital unit stands 32" high; has its own refrigeration mechanism, which does not require ice or water; and comes with different-sized sleeves that remain completely dry and fit on different limbs. The temperature is adjustable and thermostatically controlled and ranges from 32° F (0° C) to room temperature. A compression on-off-time cycle allows compression to be on for as long as 180 seconds and off for as long as 60 seconds. Gauges indicate the temperature and pressure. Two separate controls allow two different limbs to be treated simultaneously.

A smaller portable or home Cryo/Temp unit also is available for foot, ankle, knee, hand, wrist, and elbow injury treatment. With this unit, only one injured part can be treated at a time. Like the hospital unit, the temperature and pressure of this unit are adjustable. However, it offers only intermittent compression at a preset time of 90 seconds on and 30 seconds off. The unit also has a gauge to indicate pressure. The temperature is determined by the injury. If a deep muscle or joint is involved, a low temperature should be used.

If continuous pressure is used, the pressure dial should be lowered to zero once the treatment is completed so that the sleeve or garment can be removed easily. The temperature dial should be turned down.

The combination of cold and compression may help to reduce the bleeding and edema and, in turn, reduce the pain caused by the pressure of the edema on structures in and around the injured area. The home unit can be useful for patients who cannot come to the clinic often.

The combination does have a few disadvantages. Some patients cannot tolerate cold, however, as was mentioned previously, the temperature can be controlled. The amount of pressure must be low and carefully selected if there is any danger that bleeding can be exacerbated. If treatment is applied over a fracture site, one must be assured that the fracture is well aligned. Physical therapists usually do not treat such cases.

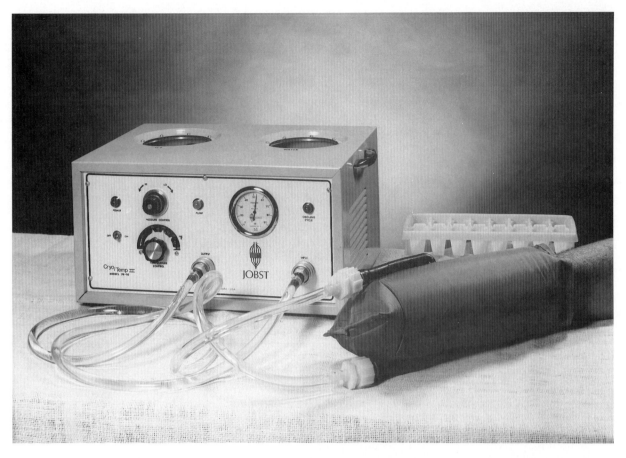

Figure 28–6. The Cryo/Temp therapy system, which combines intermittent pressure with cooling. (*Reproduced with permission from the Jobst Institute, Inc., Toledo, OH.*)

DOCUMENTATION

As in other areas of physical therapy, ample clinical documentation demonstrates positive results with using IPC. The manufacturers have supported research to substantiate these benefits. In 1990 an independent study comparing the effects of IPC and electrical stimulation on posttraumatic hand edema showed significant reduction of edema with IPC.[11] This study supports the findings of previous studies and clinical observations; however, further investigations must still be conducted. At present, the comparison of girth measurements before and after treatment and from treatment to treatment is a good clinical indication of the effectiveness of IPC.

In physical rehabilitation, IPC is an accepted treatment whenever the danger of excessive or prolonged swelling warrants its use: for example, after a mastectomy or surgery on a shoulder or ankle. As was mentioned in Chapter 4, tissues stretch accordingly when edema is prolonged, thus encouraging more edema. Aggressive physical therapy, including IPC treatments, active exercise, proper positioning, and compressive garments can do much to prevent the development of chronic swelling.

■ REVIEW QUESTIONS

1. Why is intermittent pneumatic compression (IPC) contraindicated for patients with a congestive heart problem?
2. Why is IPC contraindicated for patients with thrombosis?
3. When using IPC on a patient who has arterial insufficiency, what precautions must be taken?
4. When using IPC to treat a patient who has stasis ulcers in the leg, what pressure and treatment periods are recommended? For how long should treatment continue?
5. A 40-year-old woman is being treated with IPC after a radical mastectomy. How can IPC help reduce the postoperative lymphedema? How much pressure should be applied, and for how long?
6. Why is a stockinette placed on the part to be treated with IPC?
7. For what cases would the combination of cold and compression, as with the Cryo/Temp, be useful?
8. Before treating chronic edema in a 45-year-old man's leg, his blood pressure proves to be 140/120. What effect, if any, would these pressures have on the amount of pressure selected for the IPC treatment?

REFERENCES

1. Sanderson R, Fletcher W. Conservative management of primary lymphedema. *Northwest Med.* 1965; 64:584–588.
2. McNair TJ, Martin IJ, Orr JD. Intermittent compression for lymphedema of arm. *Clin Oncol* 1976; 2:339–342.
3. Redford JB. Experiences in use of a pneumatic stump shrinker. *Inter-clin Inform Bull Prosth Orthot.* July 1973; 12(1).
4. Allenby E, Pflug J, Boardman G, et al. Effects of external pneumatic intermittent compression on fibrinolysis in man. *Lancet.* December 22, 1973; 2:1412–1414.
5. Clark WB, et al. Pneumatic compression of the calf and post-operative deep vein thrombosis. *Lancet.* July 6, 1974; 2:5.
6. Pflug J. Intermittent compression: a new principle in the treatment of wounds? *Lancet.* August 10, 1974.
7. Henry JP, Windos T. Compensation of arterial insufficiency by augmenting the circulation with intermittent compression of the limbs. *Am Heart J.* 1965; 70(1); 77–88.
8. Klein M, Alexander M, Wright J, et al. Treatment of lower extremity lymphedema with the Wright linear pump: statistical analysis of a chronic trial. *Arch Phys Med Rehabil.* 1988; 69:203–206.
9. Alexander M, Wright E, Wright J, et al. Lymphedema treated with linear pump: pediatric case report. *Arch Phys Med Rehabil.* 1983; 64:132–133.
10. Cryo/Temp Therapy Systems. *Product News.* Toledo, OH: Jobst Institute.
11. Griffin J, Newsome L, Stralka S, et al. Reduction of post-traumatic hand edema: a comparison of high voltage pulsed current, intermittent pneumatic compression and placebo treatments. *Phys Ther.* 1990; 70:279–286.

SECTION 6

CLINICAL PROBLEMS FOR REVIEW AND LABORATORY EXPERIMENTS

The practicing physical therapist must be able to evaluate a patient, understand well the pathology being treated, and decide on the best mode of treatment. This section has been written in an effort to identify the role of physical agents within a total treatment. The physical therapist must learn the proper rationale for and use of modalities. To help the reader develop the skills to integrate physical agents in treatment decision making, we developed the clinical problems presented in Chapter 29. As the need to verify the benefits of various physical agents becomes increasingly obvious, an effort must be made to focus on experimental research. With this in mind, Chapter 30 presents several laboratory experiments that have been set up using a basic research design. These experiments are designed to introduce students to clinical experimental procedures and can be performed easily and realistically. The treatments and experiments presented in this section should only be done with the approval and supervision of the course instructor and should follow the safety criteria and procedures for the academic or clinical facility in which they are used.

The aim of research in physical agents is to know that what we do is or is not beneficial. We must be able to validate why we, as practitioners, choose one method of treatment over another. Many therapists rely on the fact that a modality has been used in a certain way "for years" and that "it works." We do not want to minimize clinical evidence; however, we do wish to emphasize that experimental proof of the actual results of our techniques will validate our work to our colleagues and to the rest of the medical community as well. On the other hand, it may force us to let go of "cherished" beliefs. As Eugene Michaels said:

> Expert opinion, private opinions, and opinion based upon physiological rationale are not enough to justify what we do. We must evaluate our treatment methods, and to do this we should establish standards for judging the value, importance, and usefulness of what we do. Among these standards should be one that calls for research evidence of the effectiveness of physical therapy methods. (Evaluation and research in physical therapy. JAPTA. 1982; 62(6):828)

29

Clinical Problems

Bernadette Hecox, PT, MA, Tsega Andemicael Mehreteab, PT, MS and
Joseph Weisberg, PT, PhD

T his chapter provides the student and the therapist with clinical problems that will require choices of modalities, keeping in mind the pathology, the effects of each physical agent, and the precautions that must be addressed. We are aware that some states require prescriptions for physical therapy, others require referrals, and still others permit direct access to patients. Therefore, the ability to make appropriate choices is extremely important.

The following case studies are presented in a progressive order designed to increase students' ability to plan treatment procedures. The cases involving superficial heat, diathermy and ultraviolet radiation are the most structured ones because they are presented as prescriptions, whereas the cases involving ultrasound are presented as referrals that give the student more latitude in decision making. The remaining cases require progressively more independent treatment planning. To encourage thoughtful approaches to treatment, many clinical problems are followed by directive questions.

Having read this text, students are aware that many methods of treating any problem are available and controversy exists in many instances. The answers given here demonstrate this situation. They are presented both as a guide for selecting modalities and as a stimulant for discussions that may enhance students' ability to integrate information and decide on the course of treatment.

The cases that lack answers are meant to encourage discussion and decision making by instructors and student readers without influencing them with our selections. To maximize the benefits of discussing these case studies, readers are advised to consult the related chapters.

CASE STUDIES 1–9. PHYSICAL THERAPY REFERRALS WITH PRESCRIBED MODALITIES

Case Studies 1–9 are presented as physical therapy referral slips. The information is given exactly as it was copied from referrals received in a physical therapy department. Because abbreviations are commonly used on referral slips, they are retained. The meanings of the abbreviations are given in Table 29–1. (Proposed answers to Case Studies 1–9 are found after Case Study 9.)

TABLE 29–1. THE MEANING OF ABBREVIATIONS OFTEN USED ON REFERRAL SLIPS

c/o	complains of	MM	muscle
$\bar{c}$	with	OA	osteoarthritis
$\bar{s}$	without	RA	rheumatoid arthritis
Hx	history	LBP	low-back pain
Dx	diagnosis	$\bar{p}$	post
Rx	prescription	s/p fx	status post fracture
Tx	treatment	p/o	post operation
♂	male	x 6 mo	for 6 months or 6 months' duration
♀	female	AA	active assistive
y.o. or y/o	year-old	ROM	range of motion
EXER.	exercise	MMT	manual muscle test
L-S	lumbosacral	Bil	bilateral
pt.	patient	RLE	right lower extremity
ER	emergency room	LUE	left upper extremity
NN	nerve		

CASE STUDY 1

Referral Slip

Hx: 25 y/o obese ♂, employed as a furniture mover, c/o diffuse LBP × 2 wks. Pain is nonradiating and increases $\bar{c}$ strenuous lifting.
Dx: Lumbosacral muscle spasms.
Rx: Hot packs to L-S area.
   Massage.
   EXER. program.
   Instruct proper body mechanics.

PT Procedures

A. Evaluate skin condition, sensory status, especially tactile and thermal, low back eval. Any other?
B. Tx as per referral.

Questions

1. How would you position the patient for a hot pack application?
2. What benefits could be derived from the hot pack?

CASE STUDY 2

Referral Slip

Hx. 45 y/o R-handed ♀, employed as a computer operator, injury to R hand $\bar{p}$ 3 mo, c/o progressive loss of function of R hand.
Dx: Post traumatic R hand laceration, diminished strength & range.
Rx: Paraffin.
   AA ROM exercises.

PT Procedures

A. Evaluate ROM, MMT, skin conditions, tactile and thermal sensation, hand function.
B. Tx as per referral.

Questions

1. Why was heat prescribed for this case?
2. Why was paraffin chosen rather than a hot pack?
3. Compare the use of paraffin, Fluidotherapy, and a hot pack for this case.

CASE STUDY 3

Referral Slip

Hx: 82 y/o ♂ broke hip 1 year ago—good recovery—no therapy given at that time. c/o weakness & pain in area and ambulation difficulty.
Dx: s/p fx. R femoral neck.
Rx: Hot packs.
  AA exercise.

PT Procedures

A. Evaluate ROM and functional ability, tactile and thermal sensation, skin condition, and patient's ability to report.
B. Tx as per referral.

Questions

1. Why was a hot pack presribed for this patient?
2. How would you position this patient for the hot pack?
3. What other heat modalities might be used?

CASE STUDY 4

Referral Slip

Hx: 30 y/o ♀ c/o LBP, 3-month duration.
Dx: Paraspinal muscle spasms c̄ sciatica.
Rx: Shortwave diathermy
  Appropriate exercises.

PT Procedures

A. Evaluate (bear in mind SWD).
B. Tx as per referral.

Questions

1. What evaluation procedures must be performed?
2. Which method of shortwave diathermy and which placement of electrodes would you select?

CASE STUDY 5

Referral Slip

Hx: 35 y/o ♂ shoe factory shipping clerk.
Dx: (L) middle and lower trapezius fibromyalgia.
Rx: SWD to area—use inductance method.
 Active Exercise.
 Postural and body mechanics instructions.

PT Procedures

A. Evaluate tactile and thermal sensation, check skin condition for scarring that might imply embedded metal, palpate, ROM.
B. Tx as per referral.

Questions

1. Do you think induction is an appropriate diathermy treatment method?
2. How would you position the patient?

CASE STUDY 6

Referral Slip

Hx: 23 y/o ♀ high-fashion model, c/o pain in R shoulder, and shoulder ROM limited due to pain.
Dx: Chronic subdeltoid bursitis.
Rx: Microwave to area.
 ROM.

PT Procedures

A. Evaluate.
B. Treat as per referral.

Questions

1. What is the rationale for selecting microwave diathermy?
2. What director shape would you select? Why?

CASE STUDY 7

Referral Slip

Hx: 45 y/o Vietnam veteran employed as interior decorator; c/o red, itching rash over forearms and hands. Present exacerbation × 6 mo. This condition interferes c̄ patient's occupation in addition to being painful.
Dx: Chronic psoriasis.
Rx: Ultraviolet radiation.

PT Procedures

    A. Evaluate skin condition, sensation, ROM.
    B. Tx as per referral.

Questions

    1. What important evaluation pertaining to this modality must be done before tx?
    2. What dosage of UV radiation would you give for this condition?

CASE STUDY 8

Referral Slip

Hx: 16 y/o ♂ high school student. Has had "bad complexion" for 3 years.
Dx: Acne vulgaris on forehead, chin, and both cheeks.
Rx: UV radiation.
    Instructions in daily hygiene.

PT Procedures

    A. Evaluate skin condition and sensation.
    B. Tx as per referral.

Questions

    1. How would you determine the UV dosage? What do you have to consider and why?
    2. How would you position the patient?
    3. What would you advise the patient with regard to (A) eating, (B) medication, and (C) hygiene?

CASE STUDY 9

Referral Slip

Hx: 62 y/o woman with RA; admitted to hospital 10 days ago c̄ a large decubitus ulcer over the sacral area. She has been receiving hydrotherapy tank treatments for cleansing and debridement before application of fresh dressings.
Rx: Non healing sacral decubitus ulcer.
Tx: Replace hydro with daily UV treatment for bactericidal effects.

PT Procedures

    A. Evaluate.
    B. Tx as per referral.

Questions

    1. In treating this open wound, which type of unit would you use? Why?
    2. How do you determine the initial dosage, and how do you treat consequently?
    3. What other physical agents might be used for this case?

ANSWERS TO QUESTIONS IN CASE STUDIES 1–9

The reader is again reminded that the following are not the only solutions or answers.

CASE STUDY 1

1. The position depends on the cause of pain or spasms. The prone position, with a pillow under the stomach, or side lying in the fetal position will put the lumbar area in a relaxed midrange, or flexed position. If one wishes to encourage passive extension, the prone position without pillows under the abdomen may be preferred. The supine position with the knees bent is **not** advised because extra precautions must be taken if a hot pack is placed under the back.
2. Increased cutaneous circulation and analgesic and sedative effects that promote relaxation. Significant temperature changes will not occur in deep back muscles.

CASE STUDY 2

1. The probable goal of heat in this case was to increase ROM and the extensibility of collagen tissues.
2. Paraffin is a fluid. If the palm and the fingers have flexion contractures, the fluid would reach all flexor surfaces; therefore, paraffin is better than a hot pack.
3. Although studies have shown differences in the depth of heating of paraffin, Fluidotherapy, and hot packs (see Chapter 11), no clinical studies have yet determined which one may be most effective in increasing joint ROM or hand function. Either paraffin or fluidotherapy could get heat into the palm better than a hot pack. Fluidotherapy would allow the patient to move the hand while still experiencing the heat; with paraffin or a hot pack, movement must wait until after heat is removed. Convenience and the patient's preference also must be considered. If evaluation indicates thermal sensory involvement, all three modalities should be used cautiously. The benefit of mild heating is questionable.

CASE STUDY 3

1. To relax the patient and relieve pain so that the patient could more easily do therapeutic exercises.
2. In a semiprone or semisupine position on the left side, which would be comfortable and would place the right hip in a convenient position to place and secure a hot pack around the hip area.
3. Possibly diathermy for deeper heating if no surgical or other metal implants are present. IR might be risky because there may be bony prominences in the area and circulation may be diminished. Ultrasound is not recommended. Why?

CASE STUDY 4

1. In addition to evaluating for skin condition, tactile and thermal sensations, and back evaluation procedures, the therapist must check for menstrual period, pregnancy, and metal implants, including an IUD.

2. Either the condenser field or the induction field method could be used. If the condenser field method is selected, place one plate superior and one inferior to the area of pain or spasm (parallel position). If the induction field method is used, either the monode or the diplode could be positioned over the back in the same area. Some authorities believe that the induction method might reach deeper muscle; however, this has not been determined conclusively.

CASE STUDY 5

1. Yes. Induction would probably heat the trapezious effectively.
2. In either the prone or sitting position. In either position, the arms and head should be placed in a supported position to relax cervical and posterior shoulder girdle muscles as much as possible.

CASE STUDY 6

1. If this fashion model is thin, she will have a minimal thickness of subcutaneous fat. Microwave diathermy may heat the superficial muscles at the shoulder. The chronic condition may be relieved by elevating the tissue temperature in this area. The sensation of warmth directed to the area also may be beneficial.
2. A circular director will focus most of the energy to the muscles around the bursa (deltoid), and only approximately 50% of the energy is directed toward the bursa itself if the center of the director is positioned over the bursa area. This is desirable because elevating the temperature in the bursa might aggravate the inflammatory condition, augmenting the symptoms, and the patient might not be able to tolerate the treatment.

CASE STUDY 7

1. A MED test. This test **must** be given.
2. E_1 (first erythema dosage). This is sometimes administered in conjunction with psoralen (the PUVA procedure).

CASE STUDY 8

1. A MED test will determine the dosage because patient sensitivity varies. It is important to consider the patient's medical history and skin pigmentation, the food the patient ate before coming for treatment, medications, and sensitivity to light.
2. If the patient is positioned with the head turned to one side, the facial surfaces will be exposed more evenly. The treatment is given to one side of the face, then to the other side. If the patient is positioned with the entire face **up,** the nose must be protected and the cheeks near the temples will not be radiated effectively because the rays will be parallel to the cheeks. Remember, in any position, the patient must wear goggles, and the rest of the body must be completely covered.
3. (A) Do not eat foods such as strawberries, eggs, or shellfish for 24 hours before treatment. (B) Be sure to notify the therapist of any change in the intake of medication, especially any of the following: sulfa, quinine, tetracyclines, endocrine medications, gold, or other heavy metals. (C) Be sure to wash your face before treatment; otherwise, some of the rays might be reflected by the oil on your skin.

CASE STUDY 9

1. Cold quartz, because it emits more rays in the bactericidal range.
2. The minimal effective dose (MED) is determined in relation to the distance from the wound. At a distance of 1 inch, the MED is 12–15 seconds: E_1, 36–45 seconds; E_2, 72–90 seconds; E_3, 135–180 seconds. To treat this condition, E_1 or, at a maximum, E_2 should be used. Treatment on contact should be 55% of these dosages.
3. High-voltage or low-intensity direct-current (LIDC) electrical stimulation should be used instead of, or in addition to, UV, using the recommended dosage and techniques for wound healing. Other agents could include an extremely mild dosage of infrared at a greater distance and for a longer time (40 inches × 40 minutes) or a cold laser (the therapist must follow the FDA's guidelines for the use of experimental equipment).

CASE STUDIES 10–13. LESS STRUCTURED REFERRALS: ULTRASOUND

For Case Studies 10–13, the referrals are less structured and each treatment includes the use of ultrasound. In some of these cases, the prescribed treatment may conflict with your judgment. Such controversial prescriptions are presented here to give you practice in making critical judgments when selecting modalities. In a clinical setting, should you have opposing opinions concerning the prescribed modality or dosage, consult with the referring physician and be prepared to give a sound rationale that is backed up by scientific evidence.

For each of these case studies, you should be able to answer the following questions.

1. What evaluations should be performed for each patient?
2. Why is ultrasound indicated for this patient?
3. Would the direct or the indirect (immersion) method be better?
4. What dosage and frequency of treatment is appropriate?
5. Can you suggest a better or alternative modality? Why?

(Case Study 10 is used to illustrate how one might answer these questions.)

CASE STUDY 10

Referral Slip

Hx: 34 y/o ♀ beautician. No longer able to work.
Dx: Scleroderma c̄ development of flexion contractures of fingers and palm of R hand.
Rx: US (indirect) to R hand.
ROM exercises.

ANSWERS TO QUESTIONS IN CASE STUDY 10

1. In addition to sensory testing, range of motion and hand function should be evaluated.
2. Ultrasound is indicated. The mechanical effects may prevent or retard the binding down of subcutaneous tissues; the heat may enhance extensibility of these tissues.
3. Indirect ultrasound could more easily direct the energy into the flexor side

of the fingers and palm. It would be difficult to get the sound head directly on flexor tissues with the direct method.

4. For this patient, daily treatment should be given with an aggressive dosage: ie, an intensity as high as the patient can tolerate and a duration at the maximal end of the range (5 minutes rather than 3 minutes), to obtain maximum TTR and increase tissue extensibility.

5. This would be the treatment of choice, especially because it is given under water. Thus, the ultrasound could be followed by movement and stretching procedures in the water.

CASE STUDY 11

Referral Slip

Hx: 49 y/o ♀ s/p radical mastectomy (R). c/o R shoulder pain especially with shoulder elevation activities.

Dx: Adhesive capsulitis (R) shoulder.

Rx: U.S. continuous or pulsed to (R) shoulder.
    AA ROM.

CASE STUDY 12

Referral Slip

Hx: 42 y/o ♂, hospital administrator.

Dx: p/o repair for traumatic laceration of (L) quadricep at the area of common tendon in the suprapatellar region.

Rx: US to scar area 1.5 watts/cm^2/5 min. 5x/wk.
    ROM, passive & active.

CASE STUDY 13

Referral Slip

Hx: 25 y/o marathon runner, c/o pain in area of (L) Achilles tendon.

Dx: Bursitis of Achilles tendon.

Rx: US in whirlpool
    Exercise to (L) ankle.

CASE STUDIES 14–17. CLINICAL JUDGMENTS

The following cases are presented for discussion and practice in problem solving and making clinical judgments. Treatments for Case Studies 14 and 15 involve traction, those for Case Study 16 involves the laser, and those for Case Study 17 involves TENS. (Answers to the questions are given after Case 17.)

CASE STUDY 14

A 36-year-old male shipping-room clerk is referred to your office with a diagnosis of L$_5$–S$_1$ disc herniation with irritation of the right sciatic nerve. After evaluating the patient, you decide that the most appropriate treatment is traction.

1. Which traction technique would you use? Why?
2. What position would you prefer for the patient? Why?
3. What should the initial poundage be? and What other factors should be considered?

CASE STUDY 15

A 45-year-old female is referred to your office for cervical traction to reduce severe spasms in her neck. After examining the patient, you realize that she also exhibits signs and symptoms of temporomandibular joint (TMJ) synovitis bilaterally.

1. Will you administer cervical traction? How and why?
2. What will your initial poundage be? Which factors will you have to consider to determine this poundage?

CASE STUDY 16

A 60-year-old woman is referred to your office after spraining her back. The patient suffers severe pain and paraspinal muscle spasms. After evaluating the patient, you decide that the laser is the modality of choice.

1. How would you use the modality?
2. What other ways of using the laser are possible if the patient doesn't respond to this treatment?

CASE STUDY 17

A 72-year-old man is referred to your office for pain management. He was diagnosed as having osteoarthritis in both knees. You evaluate the patient and conclude that TENS is the modality of choice.

1. Which technique will you use initially? Why?
2. What will be your instructions to the patient? Why?

ANSWERS TO QUESTIONS IN CASE STUDIES 14–17

CASE STUDY 14

1. Four different traction techniques can be applied in this case: intermittent, sustained, manual, and positional. To determine which technique will be most effective, actual trials will be necessary. The most common technique used is intermittent traction because of the high forces, as much as 200 pounds, that can be applied. The use of unilateral traction might make this treatment even more effective.
2. The position of choice will ultimately be determined by the patient's comfort. If the patient can hyperextend his lumbar spine, the prone position should be considered first. In this position, the vertebrae apply forces on the disc that are directed anteriorly; thus, there is a tendency to reduce the herniation.
3. The poundage will be determined by the patient's weight and medical condition, the amount of friction that must be overcome, and the patient's toler-

ance. On the first visit, begin with less poundage, observe the patient's reaction; then you might decide to go to the optimal level. For example, if the patient weights 150 pounds, begin with approximately 25–30 pounds of force, then increase to 40–50 pounds with progressive treatments.

CASE STUDY 15

1. Yes. However, make sure that the traction forces bypass the TMJ. This can be done two ways: by using a traction system that does not place force on the mandible or by providing support for the molars so that the forces from the mandible will go to the cranium via the maxillary molars and bypass the T.M.J.
2. In a sitting position, 10–14 pounds (weight of the head). In the supine position, 5–10 pounds (to reduce weight of the head).

CASE STUDY 16

1. Using the point finder or palpation, find the trigger points in the area of pain. Once the exact points are found, 15 seconds of laser stimulation at 80 pulses per second (pps) is given to each point.
2. The same technique can be used with acupuncture points.

CASE STUDY 17

1. Begin with conventional TENs because it may be effective and is easily tolerated by the patient.
2. Explain the procedure to allay all the patient's anxieties about the treatment. When patient is capable of using TENs at home between clinical visits, instruct the patient concerning dosage (or preset the dosage parameters) and when to discontinue treatments. To avoid skin irritation, instruct the patient to keep the skin and electrodes clean and to avoid placing the electrodes too close together. Should the patient develop skin irritation, suggest alternative electrode placement, another coupling media, or both to stop the irritation.

CASE STUDIES 18–20: SELECTION OF TREATMENT PROGRAMS

For Case Studies 18 through 20, the student must select the **entire treatment program** to be given as well as the modality or modalities to be used. Questions included in these cases studies emphasize the selection of modalities and their incorporation into total treatment planning. (Answers to the questions in each case study follow Case Study 20.)

CASE STUDY 18

A 75-year-old woman with painful arthritic changes in both hands comes to you for treatment. You would like to use a physical agent before initiating therapeutic exercise. Which modality would you choose? Why?

CASE STUDY 19

You are working at the annual runners marathon. A runner has just sprained the lateral collateral ligaments of his right ankle. What is the treatment of choice? Why?

CASE STUDY 20

A hemiplegic patient with severe spasticity in the left biceps comes to your department for treatment. You are planning to have the patient work on weight bearing on the upper extremities. What might you do before beginning the therapeutic exercise regime?

ANSWERS TO QUESTIONS IN CASE STUDIES 18-20

CASE STUDY 18

Either the whirlpool or Fluidotherapy. Heat could decrease the joint stiffness, and the patient can do ROM activities while still being heated rather than afterward. If the whirlpool is used, the buoyancy may enhance the movements. Paraffin gloves are commonly used for arthritic hands and may be best if the patient has dry skin. However, no hand exercises can be done while the gloves are on, and after they are removed, the hands may have cooled down considerably.

CASE STUDY 19

The total treatment is RICE (rest, ice, compression, and elevation). The physical agent is an ice pack or chemical cold pack to reduce pain, bleeding, and edema.

CASE STUDY 20

Position the patient in a way that will neurologically inhibit flexor spasticity and apply a cold pack to the biceps to inhibit the spasticity further.

CASE STUDIES 21-31. RATIONALES FOR TREATMENT

For Case Studies 21–31, a variety of treatment programs have been selected. Discuss the rationale for each treatment and for possible combinations of two or more treatments.

CASE STUDY 21

A 29-year-old woman was bending to lift a heavy clothes basket when she sustained an acute onset of low back pain and could not straighten up. She presented to the E.R. and was immediately referred to your department for relief of pain. She is 3 months pregnant. What is the rationale for using each of the following: (1) an ice or cold pack because of the acuteness of injury, followed by gentle massage or

(2) a hot pack or infrared radiation if the patient cannot tolerate cold, followed by gentle massage?

Note: With either treatment, consider positioning: the patient may be unable to tolerate the prone position although she is only 3 months pregnant.

CASE STUDY 22

A 42 y.o. male presents to your department after sustaining a trimalleolar fracture of the ankle 6 mos s/p. The hardware used to immobilize the ankle was removed 4 weeks ago, and the fx is well healed. The scars across both malleoli have closed well but are "stuck" to the underlying tissue. Ankle range of motion is extremely limited. What is the rationale for using each of the following: whirlpool for heat and hydro exercise, (2) deep friction massage, (3) mobilization, or (4) Fluidotherapy?

CASE STUDY 23

A 33-year-old man sprained his lower back while playing tennis. He has had no relief from pain using a heating pad at home and has been admitted to the hospital for bed rest and conservative management of low-back pain. He is currently in the subacute stage. He has no other medical problems. The patient's history indicates that superficial heat is ineffective. What is the rationale for using each of the following: (1) ultrasound or shortwave diathermy, (2) electrical stimulation (HVS or LVAC) to paraspinal muscles, followed by a cold pack, or (3) massage to the low-back region and TENS?

CASE STUDY 24

A 55 y.o. male caught (L) hand in a machine at work. He has had numerous operations and skin grafts to repair the traumatized hand and forearm. He now presents with an extremely stiff hand with fibrotic intrinsic muscles and limited movement; several tendons are contracted. Although the grafts and incisions are well healed, he is hypersensitive to extreme temperatures. What is the rationale for using each of the following: (1) a whirlpool at a moderate temperature (96–98° F), (2) underwater ultrasound, or (3) deep friction massage?

NOTE Do not use paraffin because the temperature is too high for new skin.

CASE STUDY 25

A 69-year-old woman presents to your department with an exacerbation of her cervical osteoarthritis, causing pain, particularly in the neck, right upper trapezius, and arm. The patient has high blood pressure and a pacemaker. What is the rationale for each of the following: (1) a hot pack, (2) massage, or (3) gentle range of motion in the cervical area and postural exercises? Which modalities are contraindicated for patients with pacemakers? Why?

CASE STUDY 26

A 58-year-old woman is admitted to the hospital for treatment of depression and anxiety neurosis. She complained to her physician of pain in her neck that radiated up the back of her head and into her forehead and temples. The order is to evaluate and treat (1) massage and (2) mild superficial heat: via infrared radiation to the face and hot packs to the neck. What is the rationale for each of the following?

CASE STUDY 27

The patient is a 45-year-old man who plays tennis on weekends. He presents with lateral epicondylitis. What is the rationale for each of the following treatments: (1) whirlpool and underwater ultrasound, (2) ice massage followed by friction massage, and (3) phonophoresis and therapeutic exercise.

CASE STUDY 28

A 25-y.o. woman involved in a car accident sustained a whiplash injury 2 weeks ago. Her x-rays are negative. She has pain in her neck and trapezius area, and reduced range in all neck motions. She has headaches and pain when she attempts to move her neck and holds her head stiffly while walking. What is the rationale for each of the following treatments: (1) a hot pack to the cervical area and massage of the upper back, neck, and facial muscles, (2) a hot pack plus ultrasound to the levator scapulae trapezius and rhomboid areas, and (3) electrical stimulation: LVAC, HVS, &/or TENS.

CASE STUDY 29

The patient is a 28-year-old man who jogs daily and plays football on weekends. He has a history of pain in the back of his left knee when climbing stairs and walking quickly. Upon examination, you find ecchymosis over the lateral hamstring area, pain to palpation, and minimal weakness in the knee flexors (the weakness appears to be the result of pain). What is the rationale for each of the following treatments: (1) ultrasound to the tendon and massage of the hamstring tendons, and calf and (2) electrical stimulation and active exercise for hamstrings.

CASE STUDY 30

The patient is a 50 y.o. female who underwent a radical mastectomy of her right breast 3 wks ago. Pt has swelling of entire RUE—pain in shoulder and at surgical site (sutures still intact), and reduced active ROM. What is the rationale for each of the following treatments: (1) UE massage, active UE exercises, dangling precautions and (2) TENS, intermittent compression, and exercise with arm in an elevated position.

CASE STUDY 31

The patient is a 20-year-old waiter who complains of heel pain with weight bearing, especially while walking, with residual pain at rest. His gait is antalgic, and x-rays reveal calcaneal spurs. What is the rationale for each of the following treatments: (1) ultrasound to the calcaneal spur area and hot whirlpool with active exercise, (2) shoe modification or orthotic inserts, (3) iontophoresis (acetic acid), and (4) phonophoresis (hydrocortisone).

CASE STUDIES 32–34. ELECTRICAL EVALUATIONS AND TREATMENTS

For Case Studies 32 through 34, describe an initial treatment program. For each case, include either one evaluative or treatment procedure in the program. (Suggestions follow Case 34.)

CASE STUDY 32

The patient is a 30-year-old woman with notable dropping of the right side of her mouth and an inability to close her right eyelid. The diagnosis is Bell's palsy.

CASE STUDY 33

A 32 y.o. doorman involved in an accident suffering traumatic injury to (L) elbow with ulnar nerve involvement.

CASE STUDY 34

A 65-year-old man with history of diabetes presents with a nonhealing, but non-infected, wound of the dorsum of (R) foot that has persisted for 3 weeks.

SUGGESTED PROCEDURES FOR CASE STUDIES 32–34

CASE STUDY 32

Evaluations
Sensory and motor testing, both manual and electrical. (Chronaximetry, strength-duration test, or nerve conduction velocity test or all of these.)
Treatment
1. Carefully monitored infrared radiation.
2. Electrical stimulation to the facial nerve.
3. Facial massage.
4. Muscle reeducation (active assistive exercise while looking in a mirror.

CASE STUDY 33

Evaluations
1. Nerve conduction velocity test of the ulnar nerve.
2. Chronaximetry to record the patient's recovery progress.
3. Strength-duration test.
Treatment
1. Whirlpool and active assistive exercise.
2. Neuromuscular Electrical Stimulation (NMES) (alternating current, interrupted direct current, or High Voltage Stimulation)

CASE STUDY 34

Evaluations
1. Sensory and motor evaluations.
2. Nerve conduction velocity test.
3. Measurement of the size of the wound or photographs to record progress.

Treatment
1. Low-intensity direct current or high-voltage pulsed electrical stimulation.
2. Whirlpool and exercise (avoid very warm or hot water).

CASE STUDIES 35–37. HEAT MODALITIES FOR HOME TREATMENT PROGRAMS.

Heat treatments can be given at home. Five modalities readily available in homes are (1) immersion in tubs or buckets, (2) hot water bottles, (3) heating pads, (4) hot packs, and (5) lamps radiating infrared rays. Case studies 35–37 concern patients with knee problems. Each problem and each patient is different. Using your knowledge of the effectiveness of heat, which modalities that are available at home would you advise for each patient? (The treatments are discussed following Case Study 37.)

CASE STUDY 35

George X is a college football player who tore some fibers of his rectus femoris muscle approximatley 2 inches proximal to the patella. He is otherwise in good physical condition. The vascular supply to his thigh is excellent. In an effort to hasten healing of his injury, heat is to be applied. Which home modality would you select for George?

CASE STUDY 36

Mrs. Y is an obese 52-year-old bank clerk who stands or sits at a desk all day and has arthritis in her right knee. Her circulation is good. You want to apply enough heat to increase the joint motion in her knee. Select a home modality for Mrs. Y.

CASE STUDY 37

Mr. B is a thin 68-year-old retired waiter who complains of leg cramps and has knee pain. The pain is caused by chondromalacia. Select a home modality for him.

DISCUSSIONS FOR CASE STUDIES 35–37

CASE STUDY 35

Because the rectus femoris is a superficial muscle, under certain situations heat might conduct to that depth, thus increasing the local metabolic rate and circulation, which may hasten healing. However, George has good circulation, so heat may be convected away so quickly that there will be little increase in the metabolic rate. A hot water bottle does not contain much heat. If heat did penetrate to the muscle, it would do so only for a brief period; thus, there would be little increase in tissue temperature. With a heating pad, there is only a slight temperature gradient between the thigh and the pad; thus, there would be a slow rate of conduction and the heat will easily be convected away. A heat lamp may reflect and diverge energy toward the patella. Because the patella is a bony prominence, it may become overheated unless covered. However, it could be covered with a reflective material such as a white smooth fabric. Immersion in hot water would most likely heat the muscle best. If George can position his leg in a tub so that he is comfortable for a period of time, this treatment would be suggested. However, positioning oneself to immerse one leg may be difficult. A tub soak would heat more of the body and produce systemic effects, and a bucket is not tall enough to cover the knee. A hot pack, if properly applied, is a possibility. Because the rectus femoris is a superficial muscle, if George has a minimal layer of fat, the muscle might be heated sufficiently to cause some increase in metabolic rate, but certainly not enough to produce significant increase in blood flow. Deep heat modalities, which would be more effective, are not available for home use.

CASE STUDY 36

Because Mrs. Y is likely to have a thick subcutaneous fat layer, perhaps the periarticular structures could be heated by immersion without overheating superficial tissues. Fluidotherapy might be useful, but it is not available for home treatments, and positioning of the local area would be difficult with either tub or Fluidotherapy. However, Mrs. Y may obtain sensory relief, and her joint stiffness can be reduced with any superficial modality.

CASE STUDY 37

Because Mr. B's leg cramps may be a symptom of diminished circulation, only mild local heat, if any, should be used. A vigorous dose of heat will **not be safe.** Furthermore, with the possible exception of immersion, no superficial heat modality could reach the underside of the patella. Ultrasound could be helpful, but it obviously is not available for home use.

In all three cases, the application of any mild heat modality can be used to relax the patient and thus decrease the pain and muscle spasms. Even if deeper problem areas are not heated, the ability to move and exercise will in turn increase the metabolic rate and blood flow in the muscle, thus hastening healing and increasing range of motion and circulation of the joint.

30

Laboratory Experiments

Bernadette Hecox, PT, MA, Tsega Andemicael Mehreteab, PT, MS and
Joseph Weisberg, PT, PhD

I. Effect of Electrical Stimulation on Skin Temperature

Equipment and Materials

Procedures

II. Effect of Electrical Stimulation on Hyperemia

Equipment and Materials

Procedures

III. Tolerance to Electrical Stimulation

Equipment and Materials

Procedures

IV. Effect of Heat Modalities on Respiratory Rate, Pulse Rate, and Skin Temperature

A. Hot Packs

Equipment and Materials

Procedures

B. Infrared Treatment

Equipment and Materials

Procedures

C. Paraffin Treatment

Equipment and Materials

Procedures

V. Effects of Dry Versus Moist Towel Spacing on the Thermal Conductivity of Hot Packs

Equipment and Materials

Procedures

VI. Effect of Duration of Soaking of Hot Packs on Skin Temperature

Equipment and Materials

Procedures

VII. Effect of Hot Pack Application on Local and Distal Skin Temperatures

Equipment and Materials

Procedures

VIII. Effect of Applying Cold Packs Adjacent to a Hot Pack on Local and Distal Skin Temperatures

Equipment and Materials

Procedures

IX. Effect of Different Water Temperatures on the Vital Signs of a Patient Immersed in a Hubbard Tank

Equipment and Materials

Procedures

X. Effect of Ice Massage on Respiratory Rate, Pulse Rate, and Skin Temperature

Equipment and Materials

Procedures

XI. Effect of Cervical or Lumbar Traction on Range of Motion

Equipment and Materials

Procedures

XII. Effect of Cold Laser Treatment on Pain

Equipment and Materials

Procedures

XIII. Effect of Transcutaneous Electrical Nerve Stimulation (TENS) on Range of Motion Limited by Musculoskeletal Pain

Equipment and Materials

Procedures

This final chapter presents suggestions for experimentation with various aspects of physical agents. The suggestions are proposed as student laboratory experiments as a means of introducing students to clinical experimental methods and providing topics for in-depth research. These projects may enhance the students' problem-solving abilities as well as their basic knowledge. Furthermore, they may help students understand the rationale for the use of the various physical agents and techniques of application. Basically, the experiments are arranged in the following order: electrical stimulation, application of heat, application of cold, and the effects of modalities (traction, laser, and TENS) on pain. Because clinical experiments take readers beyond the mere gathering of information, we regard this chapter as an essential part of the text.

The purpose of these experiments is to establish the effects of the modalities or to compare the effectiveness of different techniques of application. To enhance the accuracy of the data:

1. Note the room temperature because the ambient temperature can affect experimental results. Try to maintain the room at about the same temperature for all stages of the experiments.
2. Have the same student measure the same variable (eg, skin temperature, respiratory rate, pulse rate, range of motion, manual muscle test) whenever possible before, during, and after application. Use a skin thermometer when measuring the temperature of the part being treated.
3. Record all measurements immediately after taking them.
4. Repeat the treatment and measurements on several students using similar equipment for all subjects in each experiment. (See the instructions regarding "group selections" in Experiments III, VI, XI, XII, and XIII.
5. Compile the data.
6. Compare the data: note individual and group differences and determine the average for each individual and for each group. Realize that the results indicate effects only for the subjects or groups tested. The greater the number of subjects, the more the results apply to a larger population of young healthy subjects.

For **safety,** all the experiments should be performed under the conditions described in earlier chapters. All indications, contraindications, and precautions should be carefully noted.

I. EFFECT OF ELECTRICAL STIMULATION ON SKIN TEMPERATURE

Equipment and Materials

1. Electric stimulator with biphasic and electric stimulator with monophasic waveform stimulus output.

   2. Four electrodes (3″ × 3″) and leads.
   3. Surface (skin) thermometer.
   4. Timer.
   5. Pencil and paper for recording data.

Procedures

A. 1. Record room temperature.
     2. Position the subject supine and place a roll of toweling under each knee.
     3. Measure the skin temperature over the quadriceps in the area to be stimulated.
     4. Stimulate the right quadriceps, using the bipolar technique, with monophasic pulses at 30 pps and surged at 20/min. Increase the amplitude gradually to the minimal visible contraction (MVC).
     5. Stimulate for 5 minutes.
     6. Remove the electrodes and immediately measure and record the skin temperature under each electrode.
     7. Note any other changes in the stimulated areas.
B. Using the same setup as in A, stimulate the left quadriceps with biphasic 30 pps and surged at 20/min. Increase the amplitude to MVC. Stimulate for 5 minutes. Measure and record the results as in A.
C. Compare the results with the results in A. Discuss the results of the experiment.

Similar experiments can be done to compare the effects of other electrical stimulators.

II. EFFECTS OF ELECTRICAL STIMULATION ON HYPEREMIA

Equipment and Materials

Same equipment as in Experiment I.

Procedures

A. 1. Conduct the experiment in a well-lit room.
     2. Position the subject comfortably with the right arm supported.
     3. Observe the skin color and condition in bicep area of arm before stimulating. Record these subjective observations.
     4. Using bipolar technique, stimulate the right biceps with monophasic pulses at 30 pps and surged at 20/min.
     5. Increase the amplitude until the MVC is observed.
     6. Stimulate for 5 minutes.
     7. Remove the electrodes and observe the reaction to the stimulation.
     8. Rate the extent of skin hyperemia using a scale of 0–3, where 0 represents no change in skin color, 1 is minimal hypermia, 2 is moderate hyperemia, and 3 is marked hypermia.
     9. Record the results.
    10. Compare the results with the contralateral nonstimulated area.
B. Using the same procedure as in A, stimulate the left biceps with biphasic pulses at 30 pps and surged at 20/min.
C. Compare the results with those in A and discuss the rationale for this reaction.

III. TOLERANCE TO ELECTRICAL STIMULATION

The objective of this experiment is to compare the tolerance of a subject to various types of electric stimulation.

Equipment and Materials

1. Electric stimulator with biphasic and electric-stimulator with monophasic waveform stimulus output.
2. Four small (2" × 2") electrodes.
3. Timer.
4. Pencil and paper for recording data.

Procedures

A. Apply the electrical stimulation to two groups of subjects. Subjects should be randomly selected to each group.

Group 1. Apply monophasic pulses at 30 pps first, followed by biphasic pulses, at 30 pps, as described below.

Group 2. Reverse the order of stimulators used: Apply the biphasic pulses first, followed by the monophasic pulses.

B. 1. Explain to the subject the scale of comfort or tolerance to be used. Use a scale of 1 to 4, where 1 is least comfortable and 4 is most comfortable.
2. Position the subject comfortably in a supine position.
3. Prepare the area to be stimulated.
4. Locate the motor point of the right anterior tibialis muscle, using the bipolar technique, with the monophasic pulses and stimulate.
5. Increase the intensity until maximum muscle contraction and full dorsiflexion of the ankle occurs.
6. Repeat the stimulation 10 times.
7. Ask the subject to rate the comfort of this stimulation on the scale of 1–4.
8. Record the subject's response.
9. Remove the electrodes and observe any change in the tissues stimulated.

Repeat the same procedures but stimulate *left* anterior tibialis with biphasic pulses at 30 pps. Increase the intensity until maximum contraction and full dorsiflexion occur. Have the subject rate the comfort of this stimulation, as described above. Again remove the electrodes and observe any change in the stimulated tissue.

C. Compare the tolerance levels for each form of electrical stimulation.

Similar experiments can be done to compare tolerance to stimulation of other electrical stimulators such as the high volt pulse current and interferential current. These experiments can be done without letting the subject know which stimulator is being used.

IV. A. EFFECT OF HOT PACK TREATMENT ON RESPIRATORY RATE, PULSE RATE AND SKIN TEMPERATURES.

Equipment and Materials

1. Stop watch.
2. Skin thermometer.
3. Hot water tank thermostatically controlled.
4. Hot packs that have been soaked in Hydrocollator for 30 minutes.
5. New hot pack covers (envelopes).
6. Towels.
7. Pencil and paper for recording data.

Procedures

1. Record the room temperature and the temperature of the water in hot water tank.

2. Position and drape the subject for treatment to the low back area.
3. Instruct the subject to report any pain or discomfort, in which case the treatment will be discontinued.
4. Measure and record the respiration rate, pulse rate, and skin temperature in the area of the application of the pack.
5. Measure the temperature of the hot pack.
6. Apply the hot pack with eight layers of toweling (or an envelope cover and extra toweling) between the pack and the subject's skin.
7. Measure and record the respiration rate, pulse rate, and skin temperature again 10 minutes into the treatment. (Momentarily remove the pack to remeasure the temperature at the treatment site.)
8. Remove the pack after 20 minutes and repeat the measurement procedures for respiration rate, pulse rate, and skin temperature.
9. Remeasure the temperature of the hot pack.
10. Record all final measurements
11. Compile and compare the data for individual subjects and determine the average.

IV B. EFFECT OF INFRARED TREATMENT ON RESPIRATORY RATE, PULSE RATE, AND SKIN TEMPERATURE

Equipment and Materials

1. Luminous infrared unit.
2. Stop watch.
3. Skin thermometer.
4. Tape measure.
5. Towels.
6. Pen and pencil for recording.

Procedures

1. Follow procedures 1–4 as in Part A.
2. Position the lamp so the beam is directed perpendicular to the treatment area.
3. Select a distance between 30–36 inches and measure and record the exact distance between the lamp and the treatment area on the subject.
4. Turn the lamp on and immediately begin timing a 30-minute treatment.
5. Monitor the skin every 5 minutes and, using a towel, wipe away any perspiration.
6. Repeat the measurements of the subject 10 and 20 minutes into the treatment as in Part A, Procedure 4, and record them.
7. After 30 minutes, terminate the treatment and repeat the measurements.
8. Record all measurements.
9. Compile and compare data as in Part A, Procedure 11.

IV. C. EFFECTS OF PARAFFIN TREATMENT ON SKIN TEMPERATURE, RESPIRATORY RATE, AND PULSE RATE

Equipment and materials

1. Paraffin unit with thermometer.
2. Paraffin solution at 127° F (52.8° C).
3. Plastic bags.
4. Towels.
5. Pencil and paper for recording.

Procedures

1. Follow procedures 1–4, as in Part A but position and drape for treatment to hand-forearm area.
2. Follow the procedures given in Chapter 11 for the paraffin glove method. (Treatment time = 30 minutes.)
3. Measure and record the respiration and pulse rates 10 and 20 minutes into treatment.
4. Remove the paraffin after 30 minutes and immediately measure and record the skin temperatures, respiration, and pulse rates.
5. Compile and compare the data.

Similar experiments can be done to compare the effects of deep heat modalities (shortwave diathermy, microwave diathermy, ultrasound) on vital signs. The results can be compared with the results of the superficial heat modalities experiments.

V. EFFECTS OF DRY VERSUS MOIST TOWEL SPACING ON THE THERMAL CONDUCTIVITY OF HOT PACKS

Equipment and Materials

1. Hot water tank thermostatically controlled and hot packs.
2. Towels.
3. Skin thermometer.
4. Timer.
5. Pencil and paper for recording.

Procedures

A. 1. Record the room temperature.
    2. Follow procedures 2–5 in Experiment IV, Part A (Omit measuring the respiration and pulse rates.)
    3. Apply a specific sized hot pack that has been heated for at least 1 hour and immediately wrapped in eight layers of fresh *dry* towels.
    4. Remove the pack momentarily to measure and record the skin temperature every 2 minutes for the duration of a 20-minute treatment period.
B. At least 24 hours later, repeat the identical procedures under the same environmental conditions with identical equipment and temperatures, but use *moist towels* instead of dry ones. Towels can be moistened by wrapping them around another hot pack for 15 minutes before application.
C. Compare the changes in skin temperature and time for procedures A and B.

The experiment can be varied by comparing temperature changes using a different number of towel layers or by comparing changes using terrycloth spacing and the commercially made hot pack covers.

VI. EFFECT OF DURATION OF SOAKING OF HOT PACKS ON SKIN TEMPERATURE

Equipment and materials:

Same as for Experiment V.

Procedures

A. 1. Randomly divide the subjects into three groups.
   2. Apply hot packs to all subjects in the three groups as follows: Group 1, a hot pack soaked in hot water overnight; Group 2, a hot pack soaked in hot water for 30 minutes; Group 3, a hot pack soaked in hot water for 10 minutes.
B. 1. Follow procedures 1–6 in Experiment IV Part A, omitting measurements of pulse, respiration, and the temperature of distal skin area.
   2. Measure the temperature of the skin in the area treated after the pack is on for 10 minutes, then for 20 minutes (momentarily removing pack), and again immediately after terminating a 30-minute treatment.
   3. Compare the changes in the skin temperature of the different groups.

The same experiment can be performed measuring respiratory rate, pulse rate, or both.

VII. EFFECT OF HOT PACK APPLICATION ON LOCAL AND DISTAL SKIN TEMPERATURES

Equipment and Materials:

Same as for Experiment V.

Procedures

A. 1. Record the room temperature.
   2. Measure and record the skin temperature of the area to be treated and at a specifically designated distal location.
   3. Apply the hot pack to the area to be treated.
   4. Remove it after 20 minutes.
   5. Immediately measure the skin temperatures again at both the treated area and the distal site.
   6. Record these temperatures.
B. Compare the pre- and posttreatment temperatures at both the treated and the distal sites.
C. This experiment can be varied by using infrared or a deep heat modality in place of the hot packs.

Similar experiments can be done to compare the effects of a deep heat (shortwave diathermy, microwave diathermy, ultrasound) versus a superficial heat (hot pack, infrared) on local and distal skin temperatures.

VIII. EFFECTS OF APPLYING COLD PACKS ADJACENT TO A HOT PACK ON LOCAL AND DISTAL SKIN TEMPERATURES

Equipment and materials

   1. Hot water tank thermostatically controlled unit and hot packs.
   2. Cold pack unit ($-5°$ C) and cold packs.
   3. Towels.
   4. Skin thermometer.
   5. Timer.
   6. Pencil and paper for recording.

Procedures

A. Repeat the procedures described in Experiment VII, Part A.

B. Repeat the procedures described in Experiment VII, Part B.

C. Twenty-four hours later, repeat the same procedures, but, in addition, place a cold pack in the areas both proximal and distal to the area being heated.

D. Compare the results of the hot pack alone with those of the hot pack applied simultaneously with cold packs on the skin temperature of the heated and the designated distal areas.

IX. EFFECT OF DIFFERENT WATER TEMPERATURES ON THE VITAL SIGNS OF A SUBJECT WHO IS IMMERSED IN A HUBBARD TANK

Equipment and Materials

1. Hubbard tank with water level sufficient for full immersion.
2. Towels.
3. Oral thermometer.
4. Stop watch.
5. Blood pressure measuring equipment.

Procedures

A. 1. Divide the subjects into three groups. Designate each group for immersion in one of the following water temperatures: Group 1, 93° F (33.9° C); Group 2, 99° F (37.2° C); Group 3, 104° F (40° C).
2. Take the subjects' vital signs before immersion: oral temperature, blood pressure, and pulse and respiration rates.
3. Have the subjects sit quietly in the tank, neck high in water, for 20 minutes.
4. Have the subjects get out of the water after 20 minutes and wrap themselves in dry towels.
5. Take vital signs again immediately.

B. 1. Compare changes in vital signs between individuals in the same group.
2. Calculate the mean of each vital sign for each group.
3. Compare the means for each vital sign between groups.

The same experiment can be varied by comparing changes in vital signs while doing various grades of activities rather than while at rest in the water. Similar experiments can be done while sitting in whirlpool tanks instead of Hubbard tanks, with the water at various temperatures, at various water levels, or both: for example, waist level water.

Note: Because changing the water temperature in a Hubbard tank is time consuming, it may be necessary to extend this experiment over three or more laboratory sessions, using a different water temperature each day.

X. EFFECT OF ICE MASSAGE ON RESPIRATORY RATE, PULSE RATE, AND SKIN TEMPERATURE.

Equipment and Materials

1. Ice cubes.
2. Towels.
3. Skin thermometer.
4. Pencil and paper for recording.

Procedures

1. Record the room temperature.
2. Position and drape the subject for treatment to the low-back area.
3. Measure and record the respiration rate, pulse rate, and skin temperature in the area to receive the massage.
4. Perform ice massage to the lumbosacral area following the procedures described in Chapter 14.
5. Measure and record the skin temperature after 5 minutes of treatment.
6. Discontinue the ice massage after 10 minutes and repeat the measurements, as in Procedure 3.
7. Compile and compare the data from individuals and determine the average.

Similar experiments can be done to study the effects of chemical cold packs, vapocoolant sprays, or both and to compare the results of the various modalities.

XI. EFFECT OF CERVICAL OR LUMBAR TRACTION ON RANGE OF MOTION

Equipment and Materials:

1. Motorized traction unit.
2. Traction table.
3. Stool.
4. Head halter with TMJ protectors and lumbar traction harness.
5. Pillow.
6. Goniometer.
7. Pencil and paper for recording.

Procedures

A. 1. Use a goniometer to measure and record the active range of motion of the cervical spine of all subjects and select those who demonstrate a limited range.
2. Divide the subjects randomly into two groups (experimental and controlled)
3. Subject the experimental group to 15 minutes of cervical traction (line of pull, 30° flexion) in the supine position.
4. Subject the control group to 15 minutes of rest in the supine position.
5. Remeasure and record the active range of motion in all subjects.
B. Compare the pre- and posttreatment results in both groups and statistically analyze these results.
C. Using the same methods and procedures, determine the effects of lumbar traction.

Similar experiments can be done to compare different techniques of traction (eg, sitting vs lying, prone vs supine position).

XII. EFFECT OF COLD LASER TREATMENT ON PAIN

Equipment and Materials

1. Pain scale questionnaire.
2. Cold laser unit.
3. Treatment table.
4. Pillow.

5. Curtain.
6. Pencil and paper for recording.

Procedures

A. 1. Select students who have experienced musculoskeletal pain for more than 24 hours.
  2. Divide the subjects randomly into two groups (controlled and experimental).
  3. Ask subjects to fill out the pain questionnaire.
  4. Position each subject behind a curtain so that he or she cannot see the modality or benefit from any body language that the operator might inadvertently use.
  5. Expose only the part of the body to be treated.
  6. Treat all subjects with a cold laser in the way suggested in Chapter 26 (the cold laser device will be "off" for the control group).
  7. Ask all subjects to fill out the questionnaire again immediately after the treatment.
B. 1. Compare the pre- and posttreatment data.
  2. Analyze the results statistically.

Similar experiments can be done to compare different treatment approaches (eg treating acupuncture points vs. pain areas).

XIII. EFFECT OF TRANSCUTANEOUS ELECTRICAL NERVE STIMULATION (TENS) ON RANGE OF MOTION LIMITED BY MUSCULOSKELETAL PAIN

Equipment and Materials

1. Two-channel TENS units.
2. Four electrodes and leads.
3. Treatment table.
4. Towels.
5. Pillows.
6. Goniometer.
7. Timer.
8. Pencil and paper for recording.

Procedures

A. 1. Select students who have limited range of motion because of musculoskeletal pain.
  2. Use a goniometer to measure and record the range of motion of the part affected by the pain.
  3. Divide the subjects into two groups (experimental and controlled).
  4. Apply the TENS in accordance with one of the techniques discussed in Chapter 21.
  5. Turn on the unit for the experimental subjects for 30 minutes (with unit turned off the control subjects lie down in a similar position for 30 minutes).
  6. Remeasure and record the range of motion of the part treated for all subjects immediately after the treatment.
  7. Remove the electrodes and observe the area stimulated for any skin irritation.

B. Compare the pre- and posttreatment data of both groups and statistically analyze the results.

Similar experiments can be done with different treatment approaches (see Chapter 21).

It is the hope of the authors that their efforts in developing this text will enhance the students' and clinicians' understanding of the theories underlining physical agents, their clinical application and to also further research interest in this area. The authors hope that physical agents continue to hold a major interest in physical therapy and that this text book contributes to that end.

Index